# Soft Tissue Sarcomas

# Soft Tissue Sarcomas

## A Pattern-Based Approach to Diagnosis

**Angelo Paolo Dei Tos**
University of Padua School of Medicine, Italy

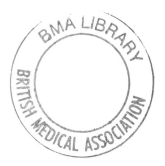

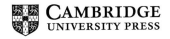
CAMBRIDGE
UNIVERSITY PRESS

# CAMBRIDGE
## UNIVERSITY PRESS

University Printing House, Cambridge CB2 8BS, United Kingdom

One Liberty Plaza, 20th Floor, New York, NY 10006, USA

477 Williamstown Road, Port Melbourne, VIC 3207, Australia

314–321, 3rd Floor, Plot 3, Splendor Forum, Jasola District Centre, New Delhi – 110025, India

79 Anson Road, #06–04/06, Singapore 079906

Cambridge University Press is part of the University of Cambridge.

It furthers the University's mission by disseminating knowledge in the pursuit of education, learning, and research at the highest international levels of excellence.

www.cambridge.org
Information on this title: www.cambridge.org/9781107040809
DOI: 10.1017/9781316535097

First published 2019

Printed and bound in Great Britain by Clays, St Ives plc, Elcograf S.p.A.

*A catalogue record for this publication is available from the British Library.*

*Library of Congress Cataloging-in-Publication Data*
Names: Dei Tos, Angelo Paolo, author.
Title: Soft tissue sarcomas : a pattern-based approach to diagnosis / Angelo Paolo Dei Tos.
Description: Cambridge, United Kingdom ; New York, NY : Cambridge University Press, 2019. | Includes bibliographical references and index.
Identifiers: LCCN 2018019497| ISBN 9781107040809 (alk. paper) | ISBN 9781107040809 (mixed media) | ISBN 9781316535097 (Cambridge Core)
Subjects: | MESH: Sarcoma – diagnosis
Classification: LCC RC270 | NLM QZ 345 | DDC 616.99/4075–dc23
LC record available at https://lccn.loc.gov/2018019497

ISBN 978-1-107-04080-9 Print Online Bundle
ISBN 978-1-316-53509-7 Cambridge Core

This book is dedicated to my beloved family:

To my wife, Antonella; to my daughters, Virginia and Irene; and to Kimi

# Contents

# Contributors

**Valérie Bousson MD, PhD**
Service de Radiologie Ostéo-Articulaire
Hôpital Lariboisière
Paris, FRANCE

**Paolo G. Casali MD**
University of Milan Department of Oncology and Hemato-Oncology & Fondazione IRCCS Istituto Nazionale dei Tumori
Milan, ITALY

**Marco Gambarotti MD**
Department of Pathology,
IRCCS Istituto Ortopedico Rizzoli
Bologna, ITALY

**Alessandro Gronchi MD**
Department of Surgery
Fondazione IRCCS Istituto Nazionale dei Tumori
Milan, ITALY

**Jean-Denis Laredo MD**
Service de Radiologie Ostéo-Articulaire
Hôpital Lariboisière
Paris, FRANCE

**Alberto Righi MD**
Department of Pathology,
IRCCS Istituto Ortopedico Rizzoli
Bologna, ITALY

**Marta Sbaraglia MD**
Department of Pathology
Azienda ULSS 2 Marca Trevigiana
Treviso, ITALY

**Daniel Vanel MD**
Institute Gustave Roussy
Paris, FRANCE

# Preface

Soft tissue tumors represent one of the most challenging fields of oncologic diagnostic pathology. Pathologic diagnosis is the result of a complex combination of morphologic observation, immunohistochemistry, and molecular genetics. A major factor hampering diagnostic accuracy is represented by rarity. As overall sarcoma incidence is fewer than 6 cases/100,000/year, to achieve sufficient diagnostic expertise is unavoidably difficult. Mesenchymal neoplasms are also affected by intrinsic challenges. For example, they often tend to deviate from the classic criteria of malignancy that are applicable to epithelial tumors. Mitotic activity, hypercellularity, and even nuclear pleomorphism do not necessarily equate to malignancy when dealing with a soft tissue tumor. As a consequence, whatever the latitude, published data indicate a rate of diagnostic inaccuracy approaching 30%. Proper therapeutic planning in oncology is based on precise pathologic classification; any effort should therefore be made to reduce diagnostic uncertainty.

The aim of this book is to focus on malignant as well as intermediate malignant soft tissue neoplasms underlying the most relevant diagnostic pitfalls. Benign tumors are discussed whenever they pose significant challenges in terms of differential diagnoses. The reader won't find herein a systematic approach based on "histogenetic" classification. By offering a practical format, I organized the content according to the approach I use in my daily diagnostics. This means considering the shape of the cells, how they organize, and in which background they are set. Of course, diagnostic pathology cannot be framed by rigid rules, and exceptions tend to be numerous. However, a pattern-based approach allows one to narrow significantly the differential diagnoses and to guide rationally the choice of immunostains as well as of molecular tests. Whereas both immunomorphology and molecular genetics are discussed in detail, I sincerely hope that the reader will be able to appreciate the great diagnostic power of microscopic observation. In the era of the explosion of molecular testing, a competent use of this "not at all obsolete" technique still represents an invaluable tool for providing sarcoma patients with the best possible therapeutic option.

# Acknowledgments

Writing a book certainly represents a significant effort; however, it also represents a unique chance to share ideas, opinions, and experiences with many colleagues.

First of all, I wish to thank all the friends who contributed to the content. A special thank you goes to Marta Sbaraglia for her invaluable help in the creation of the iconography as well as for her remarkable support in the development of several chapters. I also wish to express my gratitude to Paolo Casali and Alessandro Gronchi, two outstanding sarcoma clinicians who have significantly broadened my understanding of soft tissue sarcomas as a disease. Thanks go to Professor Fabio Facchetti of the Department of Pathology, University of Brescia School of Medicine for providing Figures 9–47; 9–51, 9–52;9–58; 9; 9–60; 9–61; 9–63; and 9–64.

I would never have started my long journey through sarcoma pathology without having met Christopher Fletcher. His unique teaching skills, coupled with an unsurpassed generosity in sharing his formidable expertise, still represent major drivers of my passion for this unique field of oncologic pathology.

I also wish to thank the many friends and colleagues who during the past 25 years have shared with me their most challenging cases. Without them, I would have never been able to build on and strengthen my own diagnostic skills.

# Introduction

Angelo Paolo Dei Tos MD

Soft tissue sarcomas represent a heterogeneous group of rare malignancies with an overall incidence of about 5/100,000/year. Incidence tends to vary according to age, ranging from approximately 2/100,000/year in the first two decades to 15–20/100,000/year in the elderly population. Soft tissue sarcomas can occur at any anatomic location; however, approximately half of all sarcomas occur in the limbs (wherein the thigh is by far the most common site), 30% occur intra-abdominally (including the retroperitoneum), and 15% arise in the trunk and in the head and neck region. As will be discussed in more detail, both incidence and site of occurrence are strongly influenced by the specific histotype. For example, alveolar rhabdomyosarcoma occurs most often in children, myxoid liposarcoma occurs most often in the thigh of adults in their third decade, dedifferentiated liposarcoma tends to occur in the retroperitoneum with a peak incidence in the fourth and fifth decades, and myxofibrosarcoma tends to occur in the superficial soft tissues of elderly patients.

Soft tissue sarcomas are aggressive neoplasms capable of local destructive growth, recurrence, and distant metastases, most often to lungs, liver, bone, soft tissue, and brain. Lymph node metastases are comparatively more rare, and tend to be associated with a relatively limited number of distinctive histologies, such as epithelioid sarcoma, clear cell sarcoma, alveolar rhabdomyosarcoma, and succinate dehydrogenase-deficient gastrointestinal stromal tumors (SDH-deficient GISTs). In approximately 20–30% of cases there is local recurrence, whereas about 30–50% of cases metastasize. Five-year overall survival varies between 55 and 65%, regardless of stage and histology.

Mesenchymal tumors have always been regarded as diagnostically challenging, rarity and morphologic heterogeneity representing the main factors affecting diagnostic accuracy. As a consequence, sufficient expertise can be achieved only through access to a large number of cases. To avoid major mistakes, careful evaluation of clinical presentation and integration of immunohistochemistry and molecular genetics whenever relevant are mandatory. As accurate classification increasingly correlates with the choice of specific treatments, every effort should be made to achieve diagnostic accuracy.

Soft tissue sarcomas are currently classified on the basis of the 2013 World Health Organization's (WHO) classification of soft tissue tumors, which has further expanded and refined the concepts that were pioneered in the 2002 WHO classification, and which has collected and distilled all the major advances generated in the past 15 years. WHO classifies the different entities on the basis of histomorphology and includes all available immunophenotypic and genetic data. This perfectly matches a diagnostic approach that integrates sequentially the microscopic features of the lesion with its immunophenotype and its genetic profile. The changes that have occurred since publication of the latest WHO classification will be specifically addressed in the context of the discussion of the single tumor entities; however, it is useful at this stage to summarize the major changes introduced thus far. Soft tissue sarcomas and soft tissue tumors of intermediate malignancy currently recognized by the WHO 2013 classification are listed in Table 1.1.

**Table 1.1** Intermediate (locally aggressive and/or rarely metastasizing) and malignant soft tissue tumors recognized by the 2013 WHO Classification of Soft Tissue Tumors

### Intermediate Adipocytic Tumors
Atypical lipomatous tumor/well-differentiated liposarcoma

### Malignant Adipocytic Tumors
Dedifferentiated liposarcoma
Myxoid liposarcoma
Pleomorphic liposarcoma

### Intermediate Fibroblastic/Myofibroblastic Tumors
Superficial fibromatosis
Desmoid-type fibromatosis
Lipofibromatosis
Giant cell fibroblastoma
Dermatofibrosarcoma protuberans and variants
Solitary fibrous tumor
Inflammatory myofibroblastic tumor
Low-grade myofibroblastic sarcoma
Myxoinflammatory myofibroblastic tumor
Infantile fibrosarcoma

### Malignant Fibroblastic/Myofibroblastic Tumors
Adult fibrosarcoma
Myxofibrosarcoma
Low-grade fibromyxoid sarcoma
Sclerosing epithelioid fibrosarcoma

### Intermediate So-Called Fibrohistiocytic Tumors
Plexiform fibrohistiocytic tumor
Giant cell tumor of soft tissues

### Malignant Smooth Muscle Tumors
Leiomyosarcoma

Table 1.1 (cont.)

**Malignant Skeletal Muscle Tumors**

Embryonal rhabdomyosarcoma
Alveolar rhabdomyosarcoma
Pleomorphic rhabdomyosarcoma
Spindle cell/sclerosing rhabdomyosarcoma

**Intermediate Vascular Tumors**

Kaposiform hemangioendothelioma
Retiform hemangioendothelioma
Papillary intralymphatic angioendothelioma
Composite hemangioendothelioma
Pseudomyogenic (epithelioid sarcoma-like)
hemangioendothelioma
Kaposi sarcoma

**Malignant Vascular Tumors**

Epithelioid hemangioendothelioma
Angiosarcoma of soft tissue

**Malignant Chondro-Osseous Tumors**

Extraskeletal mesenchymal chondrosarcoma

**Gastrointestinal Stromal Tumors**
**Malignant Nerve Sheath Tumors**

Malignant peripheral nerve sheath tumor
Epithelioid malignant peripheral nerve sheath tumor
Malignant triton tumor
Malignant granular cell tumor
Ectomesenchymoma

**Intermediate Tumors of Uncertain Differentiation**

Hemosiderotic fibrolipomatous tumor
Atypical fibroxanthoma
Angiomatoid fibrous histiocytoma
Ossifying fibromyxoid tumor
Mixed tumor
Myoepithelioma
Myoepithelial carcinoma
Phosphaturic mesenchymal tumor

**Malignant Tumors of Uncertain Differentiation**

Synovial sarcoma
Epithelioid sarcoma
Alveolar soft parts sarcoma
Clear cell sarcoma of soft tissues
Extraskeletal myxoid chondrosarcoma
Ewing sarcoma
Desmoplastic small round cell tumor
Extrarenal rhabdoid tumor
PEComa
Intimal sarcoma

**Undifferentiated/Unclassified Sarcomas**

Undifferentiated spindle cell sarcoma
Undifferentiated pleomorphic sarcoma
Undifferentiated round cell sarcoma
Undifferentiated epithelioid sarcoma

## Adipocytic Tumors

One of the major conceptual shifts introduced after 2002 is the use of a stricter terminological definition of "well-differentiated liposarcoma," which represents the most common liposarcoma subtypes. It has been clarified that the terms **atypical lipomatous tumor** and **well-differentiated liposarcoma** are synonyms, and that the latter term should be used only for lesions that occur in the retroperitoneum/mediastinum or in other anatomic sites where complete resectability is unachievable. The use of the term "atypical lipomatous tumors" for resectable lesions is justified by the fact they never recur and are most often cured by complete (even marginal) surgical excision. In 2002, it was recognized that in **dedifferentiated liposarcoma** (defined as morphologic progression from well-differentiated liposarcoma to high-grade non-lipogenic sarcoma), a low-grade dedifferentiation can also be observed. In 2013, the concept of homologous dedifferentiation (represented by the occurrence of lipogenic, high-grade morphology somewhat mimicking pleomorphic liposarcoma) was fully acknowledged. A major change also involved **myxoid liposarcoma**, which, until 2002, was kept separated from **round cell liposarcoma**. To reflect the fact that both lesions actually represent the ends of a morphologic spectrum of a genetically distinct histology, in 2002 myxoid and round cell liposarcoma merged into a single entity. In 2013 the term "round cell liposarcoma" was eliminated and replaced by **high-grade myxoid liposarcoma** to underscore the fact that clinical outcome depends on the amount of hypercellularity and not on the shape of neoplastic cells, which can be either rounded or spindled.

## Fibroblastic/Myofibroblastic Tumors

An important conceptual change in 2002 was represented by the inclusion of **hemangiopericytoma** (HPC) within the WHO's chapter on solitary fibrous tumors, because the borders between those lesions had become increasingly blurred. It was felt that the very concept of HPC was at risk of extinction, because it represented a collection of unrelated, benign as well as malignant, simple lesions sharing an HPC-like vascular network. Most cases (at any location) would currently be reclassified as **solitary fibrous tumors**, and the entity labeled as **lipomatous HPC** is considered a variant of solitary fibrous tumor. As a logical consequence of this conceptual evolution, in 2013 the label "hemangiopericytoma" (HPC) was completely abolished. Currently, the original (still valid) idea generated by Arthur Purdy Stout of the existence of lesions composed mainly of contractile cells organized in a perivascular pattern of growth survives within the label **myopericytoma**.

**Fibrosarcoma** also experienced a significant remodeling. Whereas it is currently recognized that most superficially located fibrosarcomas actually represent examples of **fibrosarcomatous dermatofibrosarcoma protuberans** (FS-DFSP), **infantile fibrosarcoma** is confirmed as a clinically, pathologically, and genetically distinct entity. However, new distinctive sarcoma subtypes featuring fibroblastic/myofibroblastic differentiation have been introduced. These are **low-grade fibromyxoid sarcoma, myxoinflammatory fibroblastic sarcoma, sclerosing epithelioid fibrosarcoma**, and **low-grade myofibroblastic sarcoma**.

## So-Called Fibrohistiocytic Tumors

After reappraisal of malignant fibrous histiocytoma (MFH) and its variants, the label malignant fibrous histiocytoma was abolished in 2013. As discussed in depth in Chapter 7, **pleomorphic MFH**, once the most commonly diagnosed sarcoma, is now synonymous with high-grade undifferentiated pleomorphic sarcoma and it should not exceed approximately 5% of newly diagnosed sarcomas. **Myxoid MFH** is now included within the morphologic spectrum of myxofibrosarcoma. In addition, the so-called **giant cell variant of MFH** appears to be a heterogeneous collection of clinically as well as morphologically distinctive lesions – namely, giant cell tumor of soft tissue, extraskeletal osteosarcoma, and spindle cell sarcoma (most often leiomyosarcoma) featuring osteoclast-like giant cells. The **inflammatory variant of MFH** most often represents examples of inflammatory dedifferentiated liposarcoma. **Angiomatoid MFH**, the latest addition to the MFH family, is no longer considered a malignancy and has therefore been downgraded to the intermediate category. As its line of differentiation remains unknown, it has also been moved to the category of mesenchymal tumors of uncertain differentiation.

The existence of a broader category of **undifferentiated sarcomas** (pleomorphic, epithelioid, round cell, and spindle cell) is now fully acknowledged. Those round cell sarcomas harboring the *CIC-DUX4* or the *BCOR-CCNB3* translocation are temporarily classified under the heading "undifferentiated round cell sarcomas." In consideration of the new data accumulated, these sarcomas are covered in Chapter 6 as separate entities.

## Vascular Tumors

In the past two decades, several new entities have been characterized, particularly in the intermediate malignancy category, including **kaposiform, retiform**, and **composite hemangioendotheliomas**. Since the 2002 WHO classification, **epithelioid hemangioendothelioma** (EHE) has been reclassified as malignant because of its considerable metastatic rate that ranges between 15 and 30%. **Endovascular papillary angioendothelioma** (so-called Dabska tumor) has been renamed **papillary intralymphatic angioendothelioma**. **Pseudomyogenic hemangioendothelioma**, a novel, genetically distinct entity characterized by multifocality as well as relatively indolent clinical behavior, has been added to the group of vascular neoplasms of intermediate malignancy.

## Tumors of Uncertain Differentiation

Tumors of uncertain differentiation is a category that contains tumors without a clear line of differentiation or without a normal cellular counterpart. Obviously, several new entities have been described since 1994, including **myoepithelioma of soft tissue** and **PEComa**. Because we now know more about divergent differentiation in various sarcoma subtypes, the category of **malignant mesenchymoma** is also losing ground, as it is currently acknowledged that heterologous differentiation may occur in the context of specific entities such as malignant peripheral nerve sheath tumors (MPNSTs) and dedifferentiated

liposarcoma. The morphologically rather elusive category of **intimal sarcoma** was introduced as a new entity in this group.

## Principles of Sarcomagenesis

The pathogenesis of the vast majority of soft tissue sarcomas is still unknown and most of them seem to arise de novo without an apparent causative factor. In rare cases, genetic and environmental factors such as radiation, lymphedema (secondary angiosarcoma of the breast), viral infections (human herpesvirus 8 infection is associated with Kaposi sarcoma), exposure to chemicals (vinyl chloride is linked to hepatic angiosarcoma), and immunodeficiency (Epstein-Barr virus infection in immunodeficient subjects is associated with the development of smooth muscle tumors) have been identified as risk factors. It is broadly accepted that trauma does not represent a predisposing factor and that, at best, it can simply draw attention to the presence of a pre-existing mass.

Genetic susceptibility plays a role in a minority of soft tissue sarcomas. Neurofibromatosis type 1 (NF1) and Li-Fraumeni syndromes represent two good examples. In NF1, up to 10% of patients will develop MPNSTs as well as multiple GISTs. The autosomal dominant Li-Fraumeni syndrome (wherein germline mutations of the *TP53* gene occur) has been shown to predispose the development of malignant tumors, one-third of which are represented by bone and soft tissue sarcomas. Recent data have shown that approximately half of patients with sarcoma have putatively pathogenic monogenic and polygenic variation in known and novel cancer genes, among which are *TP53, ATM, ATR, BRCA2*, and *ERCC2*.

In the past two decades, molecular genetics has greatly contributed to the elucidation of some of the molecular mechanisms associated with the development of soft tissue sarcomas. Significant subsets of mesenchymal malignancies are associated with **chromosome translocations**, the presence of which is currently being exploited for diagnostic confirmation (Table 1.2). A smaller group of lesions is characterized by the presence of **simple karyotypes associated with mutations**. Good examples are represented by **desmoid fibromatosis** (the vast majority of which are associated with mutations of either the *CTNNB1* or *APC* gene) and **gastrointestinal stromal tumors** (most often associated with mutations of the *KIT* and *PDGFRA* genes and far less often of the *BRAF, SDH*, and *NF1* genes). A third (large) group of sarcomas exhibits **variably complex karyotypes**. In this context, particularly relevant is the occurrence of gene copy number alterations as observed in well-differentiated/dedifferentiated liposarcoma, wherein the amplification of the *MDM2, CDK4*, and *HMGA2* genes represents the key driver genetic event.

## Principles of Pathologic Diagnosis

Sarcomas are currently classified on the basis of their morphology, their immunophenotype, and their molecular status. The integration of conventional morphology with immunohistochemistry and molecular genetics represents the major contribution of the WHO classification since 2002 and this approach has been further confirmed in 2013. For practical reasons, the

**Table 1.2** Gene fusions in soft tissue neoplasms

| Tumor | Gene fusion | Cytogenetics |
|---|---|---|
| Lipoma | EBF1-LOC204010 | t(5;12)(q33;q14) |
| | HMGA2-CXCR7 | t(2;12)(q37;q14) |
| | HMGA2-EBF1 | t(5;12)(q33;q14) |
| | HMGA2-LHPF | t(12;13)(q14;q13) |
| | HMGA2-LPP | t(3;12)(q28;q14) |
| | HMGA2-NFIB | t(9;12)(p22;q14) |
| | HMGA2-PPAP2B | t(1;12)(p32;q14) |
| | HMGA2-LPP | t(3;6)(q27;p21) |
| | LPP-C12orf9 | t(3;12)(q28;14) |
| Lipoblastoma | COL1A2-PLAG1 | t(7;8)(q21;q12) |
| | HAS2-PLAG1 | Del(8)(q12;q24) |
| | PLAG1-RAD51L1 | t(8;14)(q12;q24) |
| | COL3A1-PLAG1 | t(2;8)(q31;q12.1) |
| Chondroid lipoma | C11orf95-MKL2 | t(11;16)(q13;p13) |
| Myxoid/round liposarcoma | FUS-DDIT3 | t(12;16)(q13;p11) |
| | EWSR1-DDIT3 | t(12;22)(q13;q12) |
| Soft tissue angiofibroma | AHRR-NCOA2 | t(5;8)(p15;q13) |
| | GTF2I-NCOA2 | t(7;8;14)(q11;q13;q31) |
| Dermatofibrosarcoma protuberans | COL1A1-PDGFB | t(17;22)(q21;q13) |
| Low-grade fibromyxoid sarcoma | FUS-CREB3L2 | t(7;16)(q34;p11) |
| | FUS-CREB3L1 | t(7;16)(p11;p11) |
| | EWSR1-CREB3L1 | t(11;22)(p11;p12) |
| Solitary fibrous tumor | NAB2-STAT6 | inv(12)(q13;q13) |
| Infantile fibrosarcoma | ETV6-NTRK3 | t(12;15)(p13;q25) |
| Sclerosing epithelioid fibrosarcoma | FUS-CREB3L2 | t(7;16)(q34;p11) |
| | FUS-CREB3L1 | t(11;16)(p13;p11) |
| | EWSR1-CREB3L1 | t(11;22)(p11;p12) |
| Myxoinflammatory fibroblastic sarcoma/ Hemosiderotic fibrolipomatous tumor | MGEA5-TGFBR3 | der(10)t(1;10)(p22;q24) |
| Inflammatory myofibroblastic tumor | CARS-ALK | t(2;11)(p23;p15) |
| | SEC31A-ALK | t(2;4)(p23;q21) |
| | ATIC-ALK | inv(2)(p23;q35) |
| | RANBP2-ALK | t(2;2)(p23;q13) |
| | CLTC-ALK | t(2;17)(p23;q23) |
| | TPM3-ALK | t(1;2)(q21;p23) |
| | TPM4-ALK | t(2;19)(p23;p13) |
| | PPFIBP1-ALK | t(2;12)(p23;p11) |
| | RREB1-TFE3 | t(X;6)(p11;p24) |

**Table 1.2** (cont.)

| Tumor | Gene fusion | Cytogenetics |
|---|---|---|
| Myxofibrosarcoma | KIAA2026-NUDT11 | t(9;X)(p24;p11) |
| | CCBL1-ARL1 | t(9;12)(q34;q23) |
| | AFF3-PHF1 | t(2;6)(q12;p21) |
| Tenosynovial giant cell tumor | COL6A3-CSF1 | t(1;2)(p13;q37) |
| Pericytoma with t(7;12)t(7;12) | ACTB-GLI1 | t(7;12)(p22;q13) |
| Alveolar rhabdomyosarcoma | PAX3-FOXO1 | t(2;13)(q35;q14) |
| | PAX7-FOXO1 | t(1;13)(p36;q14) |
| | PAX3-FOXO4 | t(X;2)(q13;q36) |
| | PAX3-NCOA1 | t(2;2)(p23;q36) |
| | PAX3-NCOA2 | t(2;8)(q36;q13) |
| | FOXO1-FGFR1 | t(8;13;9)(p11;q14;q32) |
| Spindle cell rhabdomyosarcoma | SRF-NCOA2 | t(6;8)(p21;q13) |
| | TEAD1-NCOA2 | t(8;11)(q13;p15) |
| Angiomatoid fibrous histiocytoma | EWSR1-CREB1 | t(2;22)(q33;q12) |
| | FUS-ATF1 | t(12;16)(q13;p11) |
| | EWSR1-ATF1 | t(12;22)(q13;q12) |
| Ossifying fibromyxoid tumor | EP400-PHF1 | t(6;12)(p21;q24) |
| | MEAF6-PHF1 | t(1;6)(p34;p21) |
| | ZC3H7B-BCOR | t(X;22)(p11;q13) |
| Myoepithelioma/ mixed tumor | EWSR1-ATF1 | t(12;22)(q13;q12) |
| | EWSR1-PBX1 | t(1;22)(q23;q12) |
| | EWSR1-POU5F1 | t(6;22)(p21;q12) |
| | EWSR1-ZNF444 | t(19;22)(q13;;q12) |
| | EWSR1-KLF17 | t(1;22)(p34.1;q12) |
| | EWSR1-PBX3 | t(9;22)(q12.2;q33.3) |
| | FUS-KLF17 | t(1;16)(p34.1;p11) |
| | LIFR-PLAG1 | t(5;8)(p13;q12) |
| | SRF-E2F1 | t(20;6)(q11;p21) |
| Clear cell sarcoma | EWSR1-ATF1 | t(12;22)(q13;q12) |
| | EWSR1-CREB1 | t(2;22)(q33;q12) |
| | IRX2-TERT | del(5)(p15.33) |
| Synovial sarcoma | SS18-SSX1 | t(X;18)(p11;q11) |
| | SS18-SSX2 | t(X;18)(p11;q11) |
| | SS18-SSX4 | t(X;18)(p11;q11) |
| | SS18L1-SSX1 | t(X;20)(p11;q13) |
| Biphenotypic sinonasal sarcoma | PAX3-MAML3 | t(2;4)(q35;q31.1) |
| | PAX3-NCOA1 | t(2;2)(q35;p.23) |
| | PAX3-FOXO1 | t(2;13)(q35;q14) |
| Alveolar soft part sarcoma | ASPSCR1-TFE3 | t(X;17)(p11;q25) |
| Extraskeletal myxoid chondrosarcoma | EWSR1-NR4A3 | t(9;22)(q31;q12) |
| | TAF15-NR4A3 | t(9;17)(q31;q12) |
| | TFG-NR4A3 | t(9;3)(q31;q12) |
| | TCF12-NR4A3 | t(9;15)(q31;q21) |
| | HSPA8-NR4A3 | t(9;11)(q31;q24) |

**Table 1.2** (cont.)

| Tumor | Gene fusion | Cytogenetics |
|---|---|---|
| Desmoplastic small round cell tumor | EWSR1-WT1 | t(11;22)(p13;q12) |
| Ewing sarcoma and Ewing-like sarcomas | EWSR1-FLI1 | t(11;22)(q24;q12) |
| | EWSR1-ERG | t(21;22)(q22;q12) |
| | FUS-ERG | der(21)t(16;21) |
| | EWSR1-ETV1 | t(7;22)(p21;q12) |
| | EWSR1-ETV4 | t(17;22)(q21;q12) |
| | EWSR1-FEV | t(2;22)(q35;q12) |
| | EWSR1-NFATC2 | t(20;22)(q13;q12) |
| | EWSR1-PATZ1 | inv(22) (q12q12) |
| | EWSR1-SMARCA5 | t(4;22) (q31;q12) |
| | EWSR1-POU5F1 | t(6;22) (p21;q12) |
| | EWSR1-SP3 | t(2;22)(q31;q12) |
| | FUS-FEV | t(2;16)(q35;p11) |
| | CIC-DUX4 | t(4;19)(q35;q13) |
| | CIC-FOXO4 | t(X;19)(q13;q13) |
| | BCOR-CCNB3 | inv(X) (p11.4p11.22) |
| | FUS-NCATc2 | t(16;20) (p11;q13) |
| Gastrointestinal stromal tumor | ETV6-NTRK3 | t(12;15)(p13;q25) |
| Perivascular epithelioid cell tumor | SFPQ-TFE3 | t(X;1)(p11;p34) |
| Soft tissue chondroma | HMGA2-LPP | t(3;12)(q28;214) |
| Mesenchymal chondrosarcoma | HEY1-NCOA2 | del(8)(q13;q21) |
| | IRFBP2-CDX1 | t(1;5)(q42;q32) |
| Epithelioid hemangioma | ZFP36-FOSB | t(19;19)(q13.32; q13.2) |
| Epithelioid hemangioendo-thelioma | WWTR1-CAMTA1 | t(1;3)(p36;q25) |
| | YAP1-TFE3 | t(x;11)(p11;q22) |
| Pseudomyogenic hemangioendo-thelioma | SERPINE1-FOSB | t(7;19)(q22;q13) |
| Angiosarcoma | CIC-LEUTX | t(19;19)(q13.11; q13.2) |

classification scheme follows a histogenetic approach, even though currently it is no longer believed that a given mesenchymal neoplasm actually originates from a mature normal counterpart. Interestingly, the list of lesions of unknown histogenesis (i.e., unknown line of differentiation) has increased in size, reflecting the uncertainties surrounding the mechanisms of sarcomagenesis.

Microscopic observation of hematoxylin- and eosin-stained slides obtained from formalin-fixed, paraffin-embedded material still represents the mainstay of sarcoma classification. The amount of information provided by this technically simple step is invaluable. Any other ancillary technique (immunohistochemistry and/or molecular pathology/genetics), even the most sophisticated, certainly represents an important complement to, but under no circumstances a replacement for, classic morphologic observation. It should be also noted that macroscopic observation also plays a fundamental role – first in providing accurate reporting of the status of surgical margins, and second in guiding proper sampling, and therefore acting as the milestone for correct classification. It is very important that any area showing a distinct gross appearance is sampled so that no relevant information is missed. It is also possible that in the near future, similar to what already occurs for osteosarcoma and Ewing sarcoma, the morphologic evaluation of tumor response to systemic treatment will gain significant clinical relevance.

## Microscopic Examination of Soft Tissue Sarcomas

The diagnosis of mesenchymal malignancies represents a true challenge. This is largely owing to their rarity, a fact that hampers the chance to develop expert skills outside high-volume referral centers. Moreover, sarcomas relatively often exhibit a tendency to violate some of the common rules of malignancy that we routinely apply to non-mesenchymal cancers. Just imagine a lesion occurring in the forearm of a young adult that is clinically characterized by rapid growth, and that microscopically is composed of a spindle cell proliferation featuring both hypercellularity and high mitotic activity (Fig. 1-1). Understandably, in the absence of specific expertise, these morphologic (and clinical) features would all lead to a diagnosis of malignancy. However, those characteristics actually fit perfectly with the clinicopathologic presentation of nodular fasciitis, an entirely benign myofibroblastic proliferation that, in fact, is frequently mislabeled as a sarcoma. Several other examples of benign tumors mimicking malignant lesions are discussed in this book whenever appropriate (Table 1.3). At the opposite end, try to imagine a deep-seated mass featuring a hypocellular spindle cell proliferation with minimal atypia and irrelevant mitotic activity. The presence of cellular variation as well as of fibromyxoid background is of great help to the expert pathologist to suspect a low-grade fibromyxoid sarcoma (also known as Evans tumor). In less experienced hands, however, most of these cases are unrecognized and so diagnosed as benign (Fig. 1-2). Locally aggressive or malignant soft tissue lesions mimicking benign processes are listed in Table 1.4.

Despite the intrinsic challenge of sarcoma diagnosis, it is still possible to achieve a correct classification in most instances, provided that cases are approached following a rigorous methodology. The diagnosis of sarcoma relies upon the evaluation as well as the integration of four main features:

1. Predominant shape of the neoplastic cells
2. Pattern of growth
3. Quality of the background
4. Architecture of the vascular network

**Table 1.3** Clinically benign soft tissue lesions mimicking malignancy

Nodular fasciitis

Proliferative fasciitis

Proliferative myositis

Ischemic fasciitis

Myositis ossificans

Pleomorphic angiectatic hyalinizing tumor

Pseudosarcomatous proliferation of urinary bladder

Cellular schwannoma

Atypical fibroxanthoma

PEComa

Pleomorphic lipoma

**Table 1.4** Intermediate and malignant soft tissue lesions mimicking benign tumors

Desmoid fibromatosis

Low-grade fibromyxoid sarcoma

Low-grade myxofibrosarcoma

Low-grade myxoid liposarcoma

Epithelioid hemangioendothelioma

Epithelioid sarcoma, classical type

Low-grade malignant peripheral nerve sheath tumor

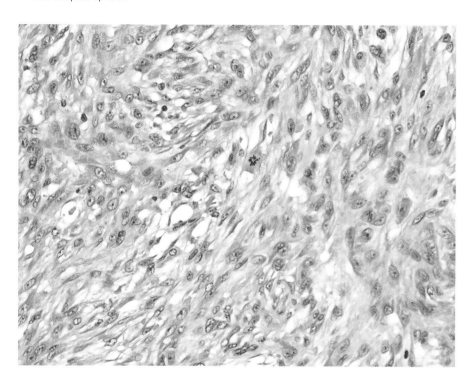

**Fig. 1-1.** Nodular fasciitis. Hypercellularity and mitotic activity certainly represent worrisome morphologic features. However, they are the morphologic hallmark of this entirely benign mesenchymal neoplasm.

This approach possesses the great merit of reducing dramatically the number of diagnostic options, also allowing a rational choice of ancillary immunohistochemical and molecular tests.

Of course, this approach needs some degree of flexibility because numerous entities may at times exhibit a combination of different major morphologic features.

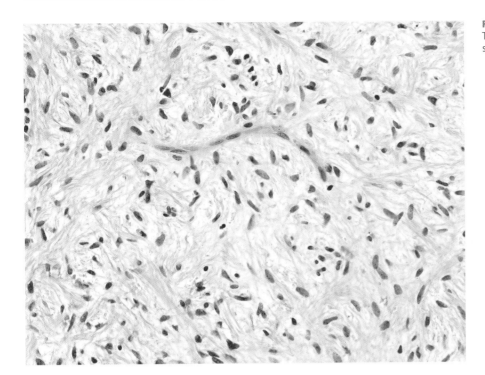

**Fig. 1-2.** Low-grade fibromyxoid sarcoma. The absence of nuclear atypia contrasts with the significant aggressiveness of this tumor entity.

## The Shape of Neoplastic Cells

Neoplastic cells can be classified on the basis of their shape into four main categories: spindle, epithelioid, round, and pleomorphic.

1. **Spindle cells** are defined by the presence of an elongated cytoplasm, harboring oval nuclei that can be *blunt ended* (as typically seen in smooth muscle tumors) (Fig. 1-3), *tapering* (as seen in myofibroblastic tumors) (Fig. 1-4), or *pointed* (as seen most often in neural neoplasms) (Fig. 1-5). Soft tissue malignancies featuring a predominantly spindle cell morphology are listed in Table 1.5 and described in Chapter 4.

2. **Epithelioid cells** are defined by the presence of polygonal, abundant cytoplasm, most often harboring a round-shaped nucleus (Fig. 1-6). Soft tissue malignancies featuring predominantly epithelioid cell morphology are listed in Table 1.6 and described in Chapter 5.

3. **Round cells** are defined by the presence of circular, scanty cytoplasm, harboring centrally located, round nuclei (Fig. 1-7). Soft tissue malignancies featuring predominantly round cell morphology are listed in Table 1.7 and described in Chapter 6.

4. **Pleomorphic cells** are defined on the basis of marked nuclear atypia represented by extreme variation of nuclear size with or without macronucleolation and nuclear hyperchromasia (Fig. 1-8). Soft tissue malignancies featuring a predominantly pleomorphic morphology are listed in Table 1.8 and described in Chapter 7.

**Table 1.5** Intermediate and malignant soft tissue neoplasms featuring spindle cell morphology

Dermatofibrosarcoma protuberans (DFSP)

Fibrosarcomatous dermatofibrosarcoma protuberans (FS-DFSP)

Giant cell fibroblastoma

Angiomatoid "malignant" fibrous histiocytoma

Low-grade myofibroblastic sarcoma

Desmoid fibromatosis

Phosphaturic mesenchymal tumor

Gastrointestinal stromal tumor (GIST)

Leiomyosarcoma

Solitary fibrous tumor

Synovial sarcoma

Infantile fibrosarcoma

Malignant peripheral nerve sheath tumor (MPNST)

Spindle cell liposarcoma

Spindle cell/sclerosing rhabdomyosarcoma

Intimal sarcoma

Undifferentiated spindle cell sarcoma

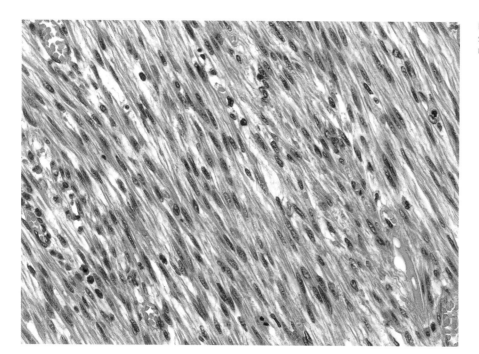

**Fig. 1-3.** Leiomyosarcoma. In spindle cell sarcomas, spindle cells are elongated. In smooth muscle lesions, nuclei tend to be blunt ended.

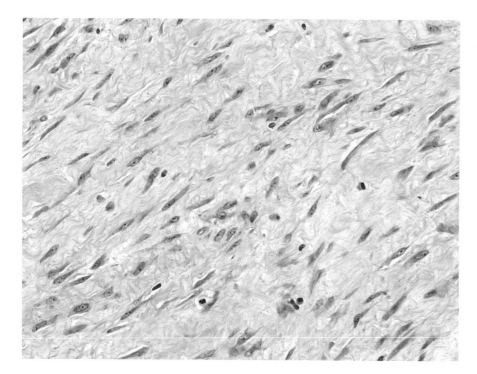

**Fig. 1-4.** Desmoid fibromatosis. Spindle cells in myofibroblastic proliferation most often exhibit tapering nuclei.

**Table 1.6** Intermediate and malignant soft tissue neoplasms featuring epithelioid cell morphology

Epithelioid sarcoma, classical type

Epithelioid sarcoma, proximal type

Malignant rhabdoid tumor

Malignant myoepithelioma (myoepithelial carcinoma)

Pseudomyogenic hemangioendothelioma (can be spindled)

Epithelioid hemangioendothelioma

Epithelioid angiosarcoma

Epithelioid malignant peripheral nerve sheath tumor

Clear cell sarcoma of soft parts

Clear cell sarcoma of gastrointestinal tract (malignant gastrointestinal neuroectodermal tumor)

Sclerosing epithelioid fibrosarcoma

Alveolar soft part sarcoma

PEComa

Epithelioid pleomorphic liposarcoma

Epithelioid GIST

Epithelioid myxofibrosarcoma

Epithelioid leiomyosarcoma

Epithelioid rhabdomyosarcoma

Epithelioid inflammatory myofibroblastic sarcoma

Undifferentiated epithelioid sarcoma

**Table 1.7** Malignant soft tissue neoplasms featuring round cell morphology

Ewing sarcoma

CIC-DUX4-associated round cell sarcoma

BCOR-CCNB3-associated round cell sarcoma

Extraskeletal mesenchymal chondrosarcoma

Desmoplastic small round cell tumor

Alveolar rhabdomyosarcoma

Poorly differentiated round cell synovial sarcoma

High-grade myxoid (formerly, round cell) liposarcoma

**Table 1.8** Malignant soft tissue neoplasms featuring pleomorphic morphology

Pleomorphic rhabdomyosarcoma

Pleomorphic liposarcoma

Dedifferentiated liposarcoma

Extraskeletal osteosarcoma

Pleomorphic high-grade myxofibrosarcoma

Pleomorphic leiomyosarcoma

Pleomorphic malignant peripheral nerve sheath tumor

Undifferentiated pleomorphic sarcoma

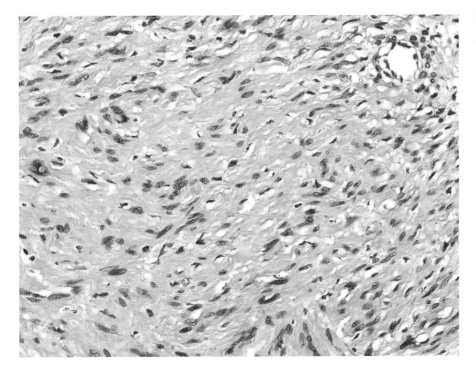

**Fig. 1-5.** Schwannoma. In neural neoplasms, nuclei tend to be irregularly shaped and often feature a pointed end.

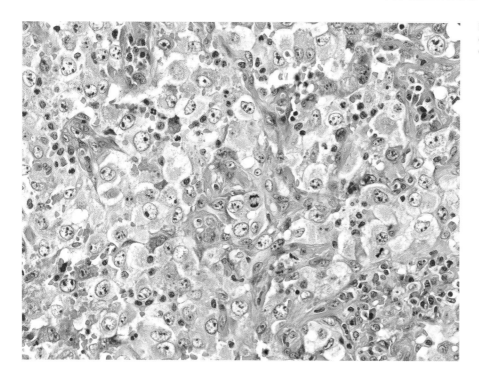

**Fig. 1-6.** Epithelioid angiosarcoma. Epithelioid cells exhibit abundant polygonal cytoplasm, most often harboring rounded nuclei.

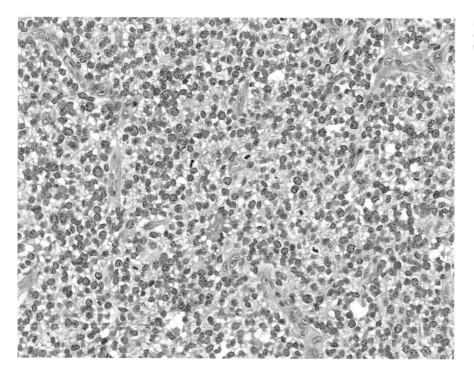

**Fig. 1-7.** Ewing sarcoma. Round cell sarcomas are characterized by the presence of round nuclei. Cytoplasm tends to be scanty.

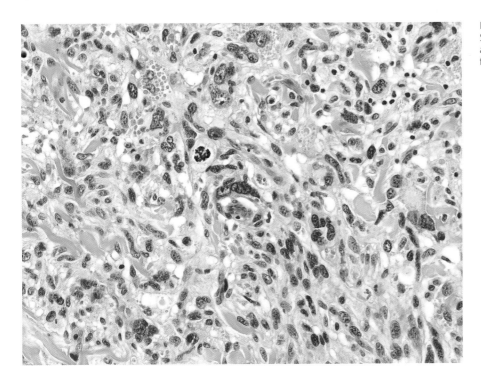

**Fig. 1-8.** Undifferentiated pleomorphic sarcoma. Significant nuclear pleomorphism is often associated with the presence of atypical mitotic figures.

## The Patterns of Growth

The patterns of growth of the neoplastic cell population are extremely important, as they help to further refine the possible diagnostic options. Main growth patterns are as follows:

1. **Fascicular**: neoplastic cells are arranged in parallel to form fascicles of variable length. This pattern is typically observed in leiomyosarcoma and malignant peripheral nerve sheath tumors (Fig. 1-9).

2. **Herringbone**: neoplastic cells are arranged in long, intersecting fascicles. This pattern of growth is typically observed in the fibrosarcomatous variant of dermatofibrosarcoma protuberans (FS-DFSP) (Fig. 1-10).

3. **Storiform**: neoplastic cells are arranged in intersecting fascicles of variable length. This pattern is typically observed in DFSP but is also seen in undifferentiated pleomorphic sarcoma (Fig. 1-11).

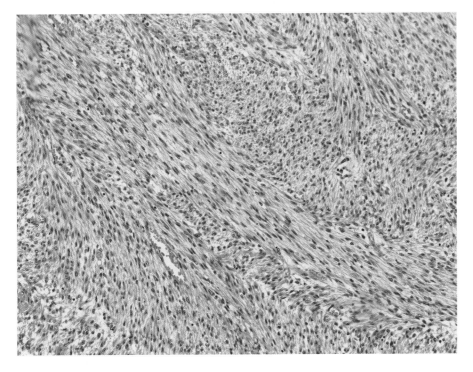

**Fig. 1-9.** Leiomyosarcoma. A fascicular pattern of growth occurs when neoplastic cells (most often spindled) form long fascicles arranged in parallel.

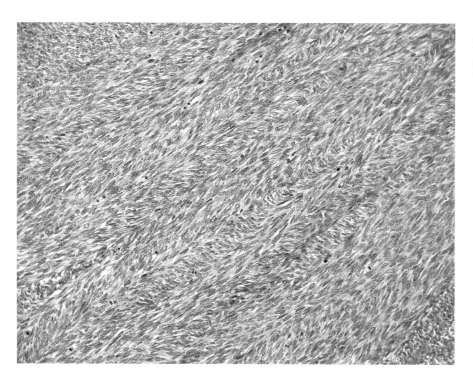

**Fig. 1-10.** Fibrosarcomatous dermatofibrosarcoma protuberans (FS-DFSP). The formation of intersecting long fascicles of spindle cells generating a herringbone apperance is the morphologic hallmark of FS-DFSP.

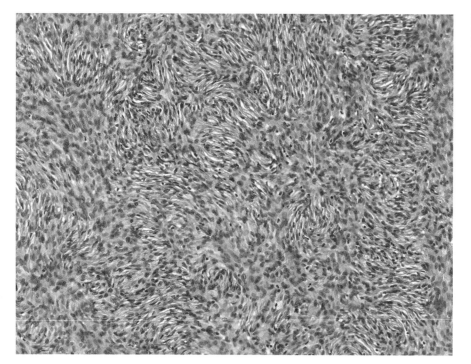

**Fig. 1-11.** Dermatofibrosarcoma protuberans. When neoplastic cells grow in short intersecting fascicles, they may generate the so-called storiform pattern.

4. **Alveolar**: neoplastic cells form roundish aggregates often surrounded by vascularized stroma. Loss of cohesion at the center of the neoplastic aggregate may occur, somewhat reminiscent of a lung alveolus. This pattern of growth is typically observed in alveolar soft part sarcoma and alveolar rhabdomyosarcoma (Fig. 1-12).
5. **Solid**: neoplastic cells are arranged in solid sheets of variable dimension (Fig. 1-13).
6. **Biphasic**: neoplastic cells are organized in two (rarely more) patterns. The prototype is represented by biphasic synovial sarcoma wherein a spindle cell component is organized in fascicles, whereas an epithelioid cell component forms glands or gland-like structures (Fig. 1-14). A biphasic pattern is typically observed in mesenchymal chondrosarcoma (cartilage plus high-grade round/spindle cell proliferation) but it can also be observed in dedifferentiated liposarcoma and in malignant peripheral nerve sheath tumors, wherein several types of heterologous differentiation may occur.

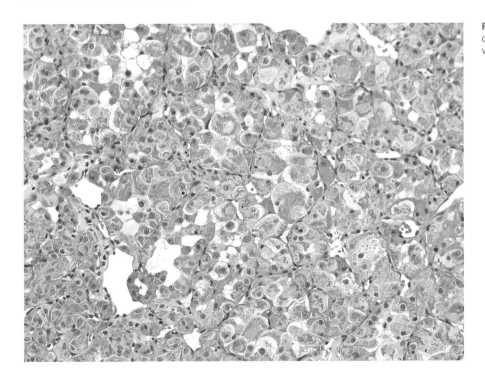

**Fig. 1-12.** Alveolar soft part sarcoma. Neoplastic cells organize in clusters, surrounded by thin, vascularized, fibrous septa.

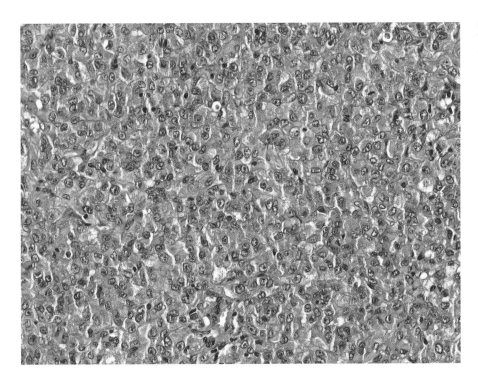

**Fig. 1-13.** Epithelioid sarcoma, proximal type. The cell population at times may assume a carcinoma-like, solid pattern of growth.

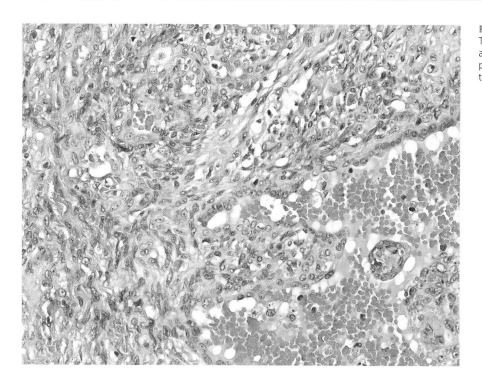

**Fig. 1-14.** Biphasic synovial sarcoma. The presence of a spindle cell proliferation associated with glandular structures is one of the possible biphasic presentations of soft tissue tumors.

## The Quality of the Background

The quality of the background refers to the characteristics of the extracellular stroma in which the neoplastic cell population is embedded.

1. **Fibrous**: neoplastic cells are set in a variably collagenized stroma. Collagen fibers can be of variable thickness, from thin and fibrillary to coarse. A fibrillary background is typically observed in the sclerosing subtype of well-differentiated liposarcoma (Fig. 1-15). Collagen fibers are typically coarser in solitary fibrous tumor (Fig. 1-16). The distribution of the collagen is also of great help in recognizing specific entities. The presence of pericellular collagen is, for example, associated with synovial sarcoma (Fig. 1-17), whereas the presence of perivascular collagen is most often observed in solitary fibrous tumor (Fig. 1-18) and in benign schwannoma (Fig. 1-19).

2. **Sclerotic**: neoplastic cells are set in a heavily collagenized stroma that acquires a solid, somewhat glassy appearance of an osteogenic-mimicking matrix. A sclerotic background is typically observed in sclerosing epithelioid fibrosarcoma (Fig. 1-20), and sclerosing rhabdomyosarcoma (Fig. 1-21).

3. **Myxoid**: neoplastic cells are set in a stroma rich in mucin. Myxoid degeneration of the stroma is rarely observed in virtually all soft tissue tumors. However, as the presence of a myxoid background characterizes distinctive subtypes of soft tissue malignancies such as myxoid liposarcoma, myxofibrosarcoma, and extraskeletal myxoid chondrosarcoma (Fig. 1-22; Table 1.9), they are discussed separately in Chapter 8.

4. **Myxochondroid**: neoplastic cells are set in a stroma rich in mucin. In addition, the stroma assume a more condensed texture, somewhat similar to the chondrogenic matrix. This type of stroma can be observed in epithelioid hemangioendothelioma (Fig. 1-23).

5. **Osteogenic**: neoplastic cells are surrounded by a dense eosinophilic matrix most often organized in a lace-like configuration. The presence of an osteogenic matrix represents a prerequisite to the diagnosis of extraskeletal osteosarcoma (Fig. 1-24).

**Table 1.9** Malignant soft tissue neoplasms featuring a myxoid background

Myxofibrosarcoma

Myxoinflammatory fibroblastic sarcoma

Low-grade fibromyxoid sarcoma

Myxoid liposarcoma

Extraskeletal myxoid chondrosarcoma

Ossifying fibromyxoid tumor

Embryonal rhabdomyosarcoma

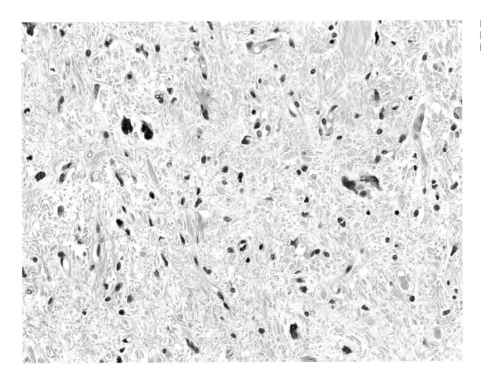

**Fig. 1-15.** Well-differentiated sclerosing liposarcoma. Neoplastic cells are set in a dense background featuring a distinctive fibrillarity.

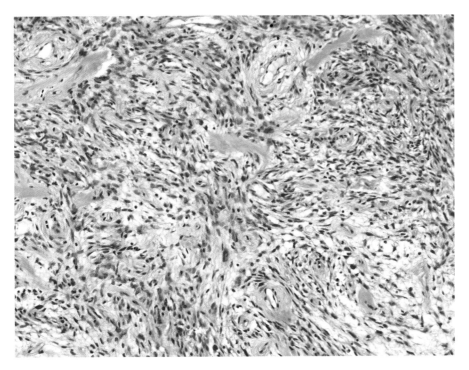

**Fig. 1-16.** Solitary fibrous tumor. Neoplastic cells are set in dense, fibrous stroma. Collagen forms coarse bundles.

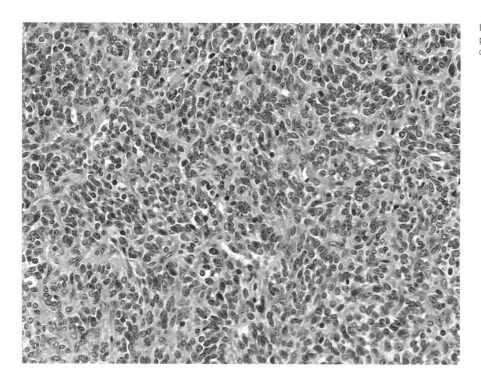

**Fig. 1-17.** Synovial sarcoma. The presence of pericellular collagen represents one of the distinctive features of synovial sarcoma.

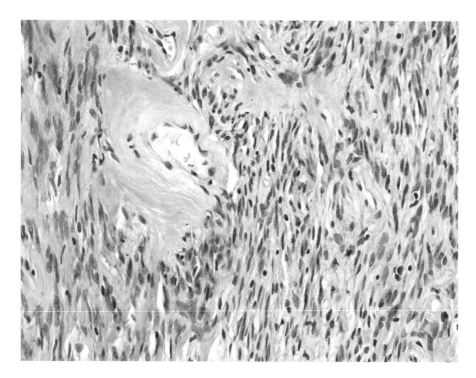

**Fig. 1-18.** Solitary fibrous tumor. Perivascular hyalinization represents a relatively common morphologic feature.

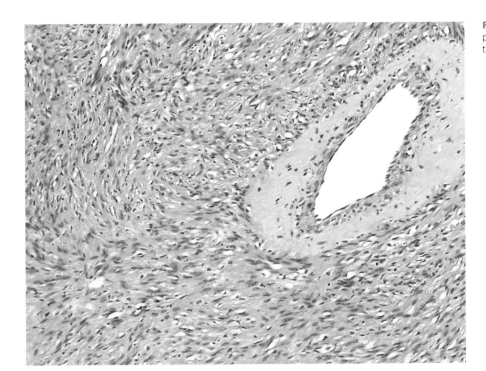

**Fig. 1-19.** Schwannoma. The presence of perivascular hyalinization is a distinctive feature of the vast majority of benign schwannian neoplasms.

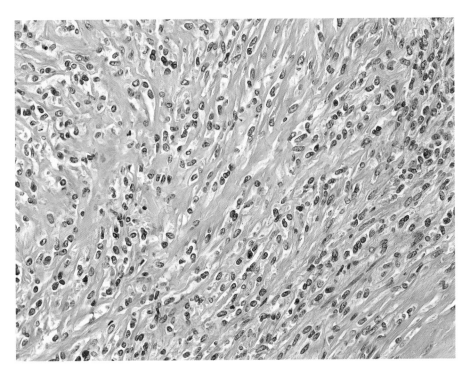

**Fig. 1-20.** Sclerosing epithelioid fibrosarcoma. Neoplastic cells are embedded in an abundant, dense sclerotic background.

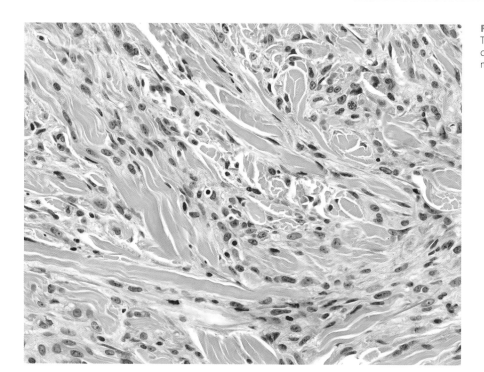

**Fig. 1-21.** Sclerosing rhabdomyosarcoma. The presence of a variable amount of coarse collagen bundles contributes to the distinctive morphology of this variant of rhabdomyosarcoma.

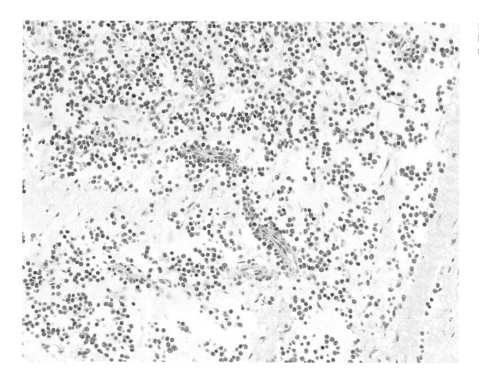

**Fig. 1-22.** Extraskelatal myxoid chondrosarcoma. Neoplastic cells appear to float in an abundant, mucin-rich myxoid matrix.

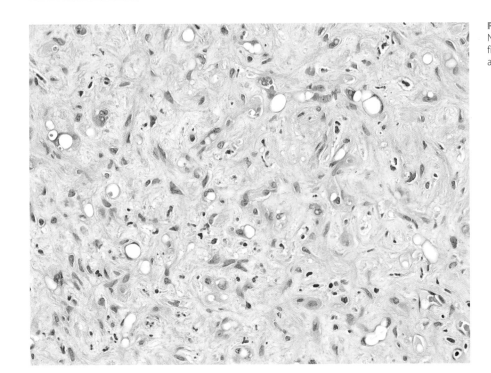

**Fig. 1-23.** Epithelioid hemangioendothelioma. Neoplastic cells are set in a stroma that exhibits both fibrous and myxoid features, somewhat mimicking a chondrogenic matrix.

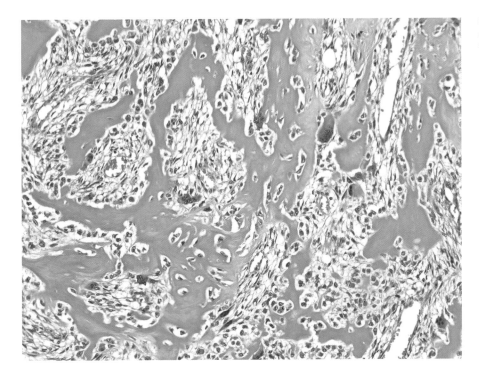

**Fig. 1-24.** Extraskeletal osteosarcoma. Neoplastic cells are set in a background featuring osteogenic differentiation.

# The Architecture of the Vascular Network

Blood vessels can variably organize to form a plexiform, archiform, or HPC-like architecture. These features can be extremely helpful in recognizing specific tumor entities, at least to address the differential diagnosis within a limited number of options.

1. **Plexiform architecture:** blood vessels are capillary sized and organized to form a richly anastomosed network. This pattern has been variably labeled as "chicken wire" or "crow's feet," depending on the imagination of the pathologist. This architecture is typically observed in myxoid liposarcoma (Figs. 1-25 and 1-26).

2. **Archiform architecture:** blood vessels are capillary sized and exhibit an archiform shape. This architecture is typically observed in myxofibrosarcoma (Figs. 1-27 and 1-28).

3. **Hemangiopericytoma-like architecture:** blood vessels are branching, dilated, and thin walled, generating

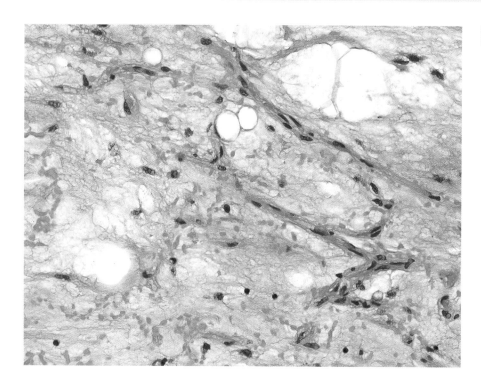

**Fig. 1-25.** Myxoid liposarcoma. Capillary-sized blood vessels form a rich plexiform network.

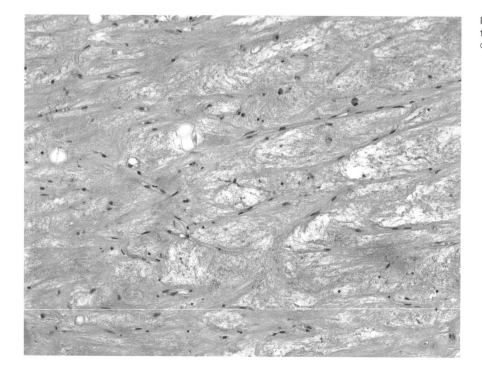

**Fig. 1-26.** Myxoid liposarcoma. Anastomosing, thin-walled blood vessels may form the so-called chicken-wire pattern.

a "staghorn" configuration. This architecture is observed in several (from benign to malignant) tumor entities but most often in solitary fibrous tumor and synovial sarcoma (Fig. 1-29). The lesions associated with an HPC-like vascular network are listed in Table 1.10.

The integration of the aforementioned morphologic features reduces significantly the number of diagnostic options to the extent that, in some instances, ancillary technique may play a rather limited role. As an example, a hypocellular spindle cell proliferation set in a myxoid background and associated with a plexiform vascular

**Table 1.10** Soft tissue neoplasms featuring an HPC-like vascular network

**Benign soft tissue neoplasms featuring an HPC-like vascular network**
Myofibroma/myofibromatosis
Myopericytoma
Deep-seated benign fibrous histiocytoma

**Malignant soft tissue neoplasms featuring an HPC-like vascular network**
Solitary fibrous tumor
Phosphaturic mesenchymal tumor
Synovial sarcoma
Extraskeletal mesenchymal chondrosarcoma
Malignant peripheral nerve sheath tumor
Infantile fibrosarcoma

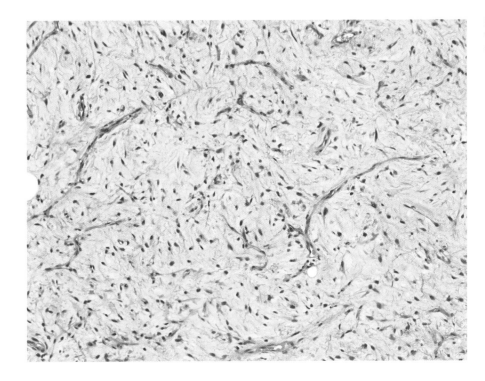

**Fig. 1-27.** Myxofibrosarcoma. Thin-walled blood vessels assume a distinctively archiform architecture.

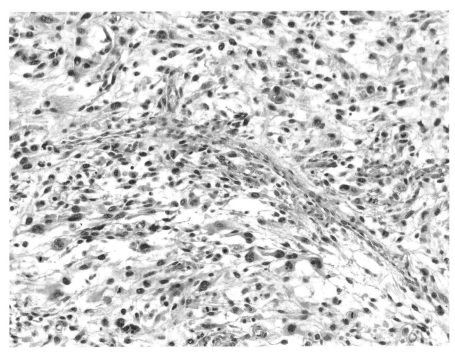

**Fig. 1-28.** High-grade myxofibrosarcoma. The presence of archiform, capillary-sized blood vessels is also retained in high-grade forms of myxofibrosarcoma.

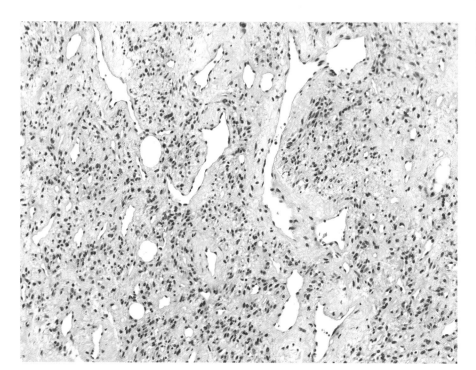

**Fig. 1-29.** Solitary fibrous tumor. The presence of a vascular network featuring dilated, branching blood vessels defines the hemangiopericytoma-like pattern.

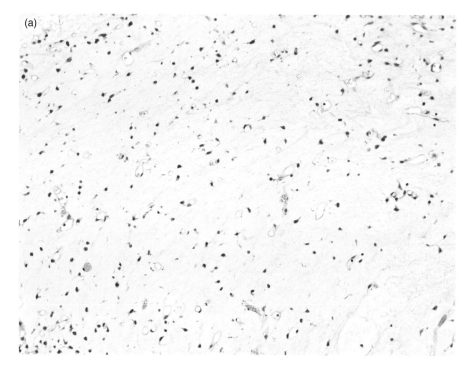

(a)

**Fig. 1-30A.** Myxoid liposarcoma. A hypocellular spindle cell proliferation is seen at low power.

network has the greatest chance to represent an example of myxoid liposarcoma (Fig. 1-30A–B). Following the same approach, a spindle cell proliferation set in a fibrous background, exhibiting variation in cellularity, and featuring an HPC-like vascularization most often represents an example of solitary fibrous tumors (Fig. 1-31A–B). However, in most situations an accurate diagnosis may require a second step represented by the application of a variable (ideally relatively limited) number of immunohistochemical stains.

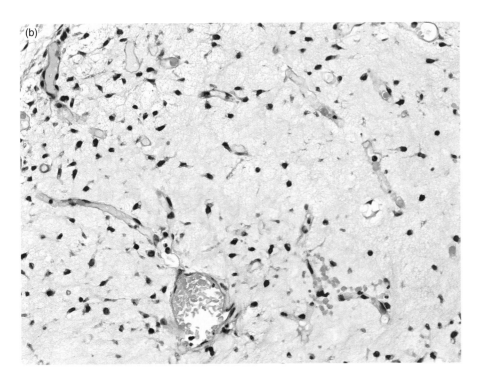

**Fig. 1-30B.** Myxoid liposarcoma. At high power, the distinctive plexiform vascular network is appreciated. This combination of morphologic features identifies almost unequivocally a myxoid liposarcoma.

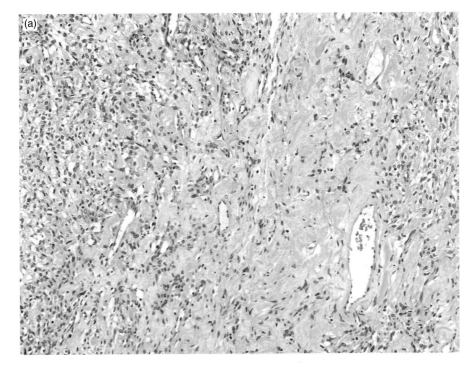

**Fig. 1-31A.** Solitary fibrous tumor. At low power, a spindle cell proliferation set in a fibrous background and featuring variation of cellularity is seen.

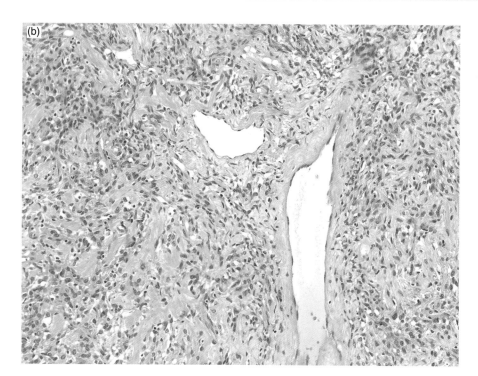

**Fig. 1-31B.** Solitary fibrous tumor. The association of the morphologic features described in Fig. 1-31A with the presence of a hemangiopericytoma-like vascular network almost certainly identifies a solitary fibrous tumor.

## Immunohistochemical Characterization of Soft Tissue Tumors

Immunohistochemical characterization plays a key role in the diagnostic workup of soft tissue sarcomas. However, a blind application of a broad range of immunophenotypic markers unsupervised by morphology most often leads to diagnostic errors. The determination of the line of differentiation is crucial in order not only to ensure proper classification but also to provide prognostic and/or predictive information. The number of potential diagnostic markers has grown exponentially through the years; in consideration of the natural evolution of the field, however, some markers have lost their role, while others have gained diagnostic relevance. It has to be underlined that, with some exceptions that will be discussed, the majority of classic differentiation markers tends to show good sensitivity, although associated with rather limited specificity. This may not represent a problem if interpretation is strictly handled in context with morphology.

We will herein focus on those differentiation markers showing major diagnostic as well as clinical relevance. Of course, more details will be given while discussing the specific tumor entities. The use of a panel of immunostains driven by morphology is felt to represent the most efficient approach. We will briefly describe the application of time-honored (however, still valid) differentiation markers as well as of newly reported ones, focusing on those having a consolidated diagnostic utility.

## Myogenic Differentiation Markers

Demonstration of myogenic (both smooth muscle and striated) differentiation is clinically relevant in the following situations:

1. To differentiate between rhabdomyosarcoma and non-rhabdomyosarcoma pediatric soft tissue tumors (those two broad groups definitely undergo distinct systemic treatments).
2. To recognize adult myogenic sarcomas in general. As is discussed in depth in Chapter 7, the separation of both pleomorphic leiomyosarcoma and rhabdomyosarcoma from the undifferentiated pleomorphic sarcoma category is also relevant, as they represent prognostically unfavorable histologic subtypes.
3. To identify rhabdomyoblastic differentiation in malignant peripheral nerve sheath tumors, as it is associated with worse prognosis.
4. To identify myogenic differentiation in dedifferentiated liposarcoma, wherein it also seems to associate with poorer outcome.

Classic myogenic markers are basically represented by **smooth muscle actin, muscle specific actin, desmin**, and **h-caldesmon**.

**Smooth muscle actin** immunopositivity is observed in most smooth muscle tumors and in myofibroblastic, myoepithelial, and pericytic neoplasms. **Muscle specific actin** (HHF-35) also stains smooth muscle lesions; however, it also represents a very sensitive marker of striated muscle differentiation, staining up to 90% of rhabdomyosarcomas of all subtypes (embryonal, alveolar, and pleomorphic). **Desmin** belongs to the category of intermediate filaments and represents a valid marker for both smooth muscle and striated muscle lineage. A subset of myofibroblastic neoplasms may also express desmin. Expression of desmin is also observed in non-myogenic lesions such as desmoplastic small round cell tumor and angiomatoid fibrous histiocytoma,

**Box 1.1 Pitfalls in the detection of myogenic differentiation**

1. Focal smooth muscle actin positivity can be observed in a broad variety of spindle cell mesenchymal and even non-mesenchymal neoplasms (i.e., sarcomatoid carcinoma and sarcomatoid melanoma).
2. Desmin is consistently expressed in non-myogenic neoplasms such as desmoplastic small round cell tumor and angiomatoid fibrous histiocytoma.
3. Myogenin expression in pleomorphic rhabdomyosarcoma can be limited to a few cells and therefore can be easily overlooked.
4. Myogenin expression is retained by infiltrated and degenerated normal striated muscle fibers, and therefore it can be misinterpreted as evidence of rhabdomyoblastic differentiation.
5. Rhabdomyoblastic differentiation does not equate to rhabdomyosarcoma as it can be seen as a heterologous component in MPNSTs (so-called malignant triton tumor), Wilms' tumor, dedifferentiated liposarcoma, mullerian adenosarcoma, malignant mullerian mixed tumor of the genital tract (so-called carcinosarcoma), biphenotypic sinonasal sarcoma, and, in malignant phyllodes, tumor of the breast.

**Table 1.11** Neoplasms featuring S100 immunopositivity

**Benign neoplasms featuring S100 immunopositivity**

Melanocytic nevi
Benign neural neoplasms
Benign adipocytic neoplasms
Granular cell tumor
Langerhans cell histiocytosis
Rosai-Dorfman disease

**Malignant neoplasms featuring S100 immunopositivity**

Malignant melanomas
Clear cell sarcomas (both soft tissue and GI tract)
Alveolar rhabdomyosarcoma
Epithelioid malignant peripheral nerve sheath tumor (100%)
Synovial sarcoma (30%)
Ossifying fibromyxoid tumor
Myoepithelial carcinoma
Extraskeletal myxoid chondrosarcoma (20%)
Malignant peripheral nerve sheath tumors (30%)
Biphenotypic sinonasal sarcoma
Myxoid liposarcoma
Langerhans cell sarcoma
Interdigitating reticulum cell sarcoma

wherein it represents a great diagnostic help. **h-Caldesmon** immunoreactivity is observed in most smooth muscle neoplasms. In contrast to other smooth muscle markers, it tends to be negative in myofibroblastic lesions as well as in rhabdomyoblastic neoplasms. h-Caldesmon positivity is consistently observed in GIST and glomus tumors.

The most specific and sensitive markers to demonstrate rhabdomyoblastic differentiation remains **myogenin (MYF4)**, a lineage-restricted nuclear transcription factor involved in striated muscle differentiation. Recently, it was shown that **MyoD1 (MYF3)**, an alternative nuclear transcription factor involved in the development of striated muscle, represents the most sensitive marker for the spindle cell variant of rhabdomyosarcoma, wherein *MyoD1* gene homozygous mutations have been shown to occur.

## Neural Differentiation Markers

Paradoxically, the best use of the prototypic schwannian differentiation markers, namely, **S100 protein** (named after its 100% solubility in ammonium sulphate), is achieved out of context of recognition of malignant peripheral nerve sheath tumors (MPNSTs). In fact, approximately only 30% of MPNSTs exhibit S100 positivity, which is usually limited to less than 30% of neoplastic cells. Epithelioid MPNST represents an important exception, as S100 usually decorates most neoplastic cells. It has to be stressed that S100 exhibits a distinctive multispecificity (Table 1.11) to the extent that its evaluation needs to be strictly performed in context with morphology.

The best use of S100 immunostains is as follows:

**Box 1.2 Pitfalls in the detection of neural differentiation**

1. Approximately 30% of monophasic synovial sarcomas may also exhibit S100 immunopositivity, causing significant immunophenotypic overlap with MPNSTs.
2. S100 immunopositivity in a cutaneous spindle cell "sarcomatous" tumor supports metastatic sarcomatoid melanoma rather than MPNST that virtually never occurs as a primary cutaneous neoplasm.
3. S100 immunopositivity is associated with expression of melanocytic markers HMB45 and Melan-A in clear cell sarcoma (CCS) of soft tissue; however, the same association seems to be absent in most (but not all) examples of CCSs of the gastrointestinal tract.
4. SOX10 immunoreactivity is also observed in melanocytic as well as myoepithelial neoplasms.

1. Recognition of benign neural neoplasms.
2. Support in the diagnosis of cellular schwannoma (that in contrast to MPNSTs expresses S100 diffusely).
3. Recognition of metastatic sarcomatoid melanoma (wherein commonly used melanocytic differentiation markers such as HMB45 and Melan-A can be lost).
4. Support (in association with expression of epithelial differentiation markers) in the recognition of myoepithelial differentiation.
5. Identification (in association with the expression of melanocytic markers) of clear cell sarcoma of soft tissue, with the important caveat that clear cell sarcoma of the GI tract most often lacks expression of melanocytic markers.
6. Recognition (along with loss of nuclear expression of INI1) of epithelioid MPNST.

7. Support in the recognition of interdigitating dendritic cell sarcoma.
8. Recognition of cartilaginous differentiation (particularly useful in identifying the focal heterologous component in MPNST and dedifferentiated liposarcoma).

Another member of the group of the intermediate filaments, **glial fibrillary acidic protein** (GFAP) is also detectable in Schwann cells. When dealing with soft tissue neoplasms, it may stain a minority of MPNSTs; however, its sensitivity does not exceed that of S100. GFAP immunopositivity can also be observed in myoepithelial neoplasm.

**SOX10** and **H3K27me3** (histone 3K27 trimethylation) represent more recently introduced markers that can be used in the diagnosis of neural soft tissue neoplasm. SOX10 represents a transcription factor belonging to the SRY-related HMG-box family. SOX10 is involved in melanogenesis and schwannian differentiation, and has been proposed as a valid immunohistochemical marker for both melanocytic and neural neoplasms. SOX10 tends to immunostain the vast majority of benign neural mesenchymal lesions, whereas when dealing with MPNSTs its sensitivity is much lower, with approximately 20% of cases showing positivity in a minority of neoplastic cells. Importantly, SOX10 immunopositivity is also observed in myoepithelial neoplasms, astrocytic tumors, and metaplastic and basal-like breast carcinomas. H3K27me3 expression tends to be lost in approximately half of MPNSTs as a consequence of homozygous inactivation of the polycomb repressive complex 2 (PRC2). H3K27me3 seems to show relatively good specificity but it does not offer greater sensitivity than other neural markers.

## Epithelial Differentiation Markers

Any soft tissue neoplasm featuring true epithelial differentiation or epithelioid morphology is characterized by variable expression of epithelial differentiation markers, namely, **cytokeratin** and **epithelial membrane antigen** (EMA). Cytokeratin expression is observed in up to 80% of classic synovial sarcomas and in about half of those that are poorly differentiated. Cytokeratins actually represent a family of

---

**Box 1.3** Pitfalls in the detection of epithelial differentiation

1. Focal expression of cytokeratin can be observed in a variety of unrelated neoplasms featuring sarcomatoid morphology such as melanoma and carcinoma.
2. Expression of epithelial differentiation markers in sarcomatoid carcinoma can be limited to a few neoplastic cells and therefore easily overlooked.
3. Poorly differentiated synovial sarcoma is often keratin negative, whereas EMA expression is retained in the vast majority of cases.
4. EMA positivity within plasma cells can be misinterpreted as expression in neoplastic cells.

---

molecules classically catalogued by Moll into 20 types. The most widely used is the multispecific cytokeratin cocktail AE1/AE3 that recognizes keratins 9–17 (AE1) and keratins 1–8 (AE3). Importantly, AE1/AE3 does not recognize keratin 18. Cytokeratin AE1/AE3 decorates virtually all examples of epithelioid sarcomas, desmoplastic small round cell tumors, and pseudomyogenic hemangioendotheliomas. It is also observed in half of epithelioid angiosarcomas and, less frequently, in epithelioid hemangioendotheliomas (EHEs). Importantly, expression of cytokeratin is relatively commonly observed in histotypes wherein it is somewhat unexpected, such as leiomyosarcoma, retroperitoneal schwannomas, inflammatory myofibroblastic sarcoma, alveolar rhabdomyosarcoma, and Ewing sarcoma. Epithelial membrane antigen also stains most epithelioid sarcomas, and 90% of synovial sarcomas (including those that are poorly differentiated), therefore representing the most sensitive marker of epithelial differentiation in this context. By contrast, in sarcomatoid carcinoma cytokeratin expression can be very limited and therefore easily overlooked. EMA is also expressed consistently in meningothelial cells, perineurial cells, and subsets of plasma cells.

## Endothelial Differentiation Markers

Demonstration of endothelial differentiation appears crucial when dealing with poorly differentiated vascular neoplasms, in particular epithelioid angiosarcoma that may often lack overt vasoformative morphology. **CD34, CD31,** and **FlI1** represent time-honored but still valid markers. The use of **factor VIII-RA**, despite its high specificity, is strongly limited by a relatively low sensitivity. CD34 is a sialomucin expressed in the precursors of hematopoiesis, endothelial cells, and various subsets of fibroblasts. When dealing with vascular neoplasms, CD34 is very sensitive, but it has to be stressed that it is also expressed in half of epithelioid sarcomas in addition to an endless list of non-vascular, spindle cell neoplasms (Table 1.12). Much more specific and extremely sensitive is the transmembrane glycoprotein CD31 (also known as platelet-endothelial cell adhesion molecule-1 [PECAM-1]); however, it is consistently expressed by histiocytes, megakaryocytes, and subsets of myeloblasts. **FLI1** represents an ETS-related transcription factor that shows high sensitivity in detecting normal as well as neoplastic endothelium. Importantly, FLI1 immunopositivity is observed in most Ewing sarcomas, lymphoblastic lymphomas, and, more rarely, in melanomas and carcinomas. **ERG** (another member of the ETS-related family of nuclear transcription factors) represents a recently developed, sensitive endothelial marker. ERG specificity is also reasonably good, with a major caveat represented by the fact that ERG also stains prostatic adenocarcinomas, a small subset of Ewing sarcomas carrying the *EWSR1-ERG* translocation, and approximately 40% of epithelioid sarcomas.

Important diagnostic adjuncts in the context of the diagnosis of vascular lesions are represented by nuclear detection of **human herpesvirus 8** (HHV-8) in Kaposi sarcoma that appears to be very specific and of **c-MYC** in post-radiation cutaneous angiosarcoma.

**Table 1.12** Non-vascular soft tissue neoplasms exhibiting CD34 immunopositivity

| Tumor entity | Potential pitfalls |
| --- | --- |
| Dermatofibrosarcoma protuberans | FS-DFSP may show reduced expression. A small minority of cellular fibrous histiocytoma may feature CD34 immunoreactivity. |
| Solitary fibrous tumor (SFT) | Malignant SFT may show reduced expression. |
| Spindle cell/ pleomorphic lipoma | In myxoid variants, expression may be weaker. |
| Neurofibroma | CD34-positive component may be abundant. Diffuse form may be confused with DFSP or with spindle cell liposarcoma. |
| Epithelioid sarcoma | There is partial overlap with epithelioid angiosarcoma. |
| Myxofibrosarcoma | There is a differential diagnosis with myxoid DFSP. |

In recent years, as a byproduct of new insights in the molecular pathogenesis of vascular neoplasms, a number of new diagnostic immunohistochemical markers have been made available. The recognition of EHE is currently greatly helped by the detection of the nuclear expression of **CAMTA1** that is observed in those cases harboring a *WWTR1-CAMTA1* gene fusion. **TFE3** nuclear expression is observed in a subset of EHEs carrying the *YAP1-TFE3* gene fusion. **FOSB** expression is consistently observed in pseudomyogenic hemangioendothelioma (associated with a *FOSB-SERPIN1* gene fusion) as well as in a subset of epithelioid hemangioma (associated with a *ZFP36-FOSB* gene fusion).

**Box 1.4 Pitfalls in the detection of endothelial differentiation**

1. CD34 is expressed in dermal fibroblasts and in a broad variety of spindle cell neoplasms. By contrast, it can be negative in a variety of vascular neoplasms, particularly in epithelioid angiosarcomas.
2. CD34 expression is observed in approximately 50% of epithelioid sarcomas, leading to potential diagnostic confusion with epithelioid angiosarcomas.
3. CD31 is consistently expressed in intra-tumoral histiocytes, potentially leading to overdiagnosis of vascular malignancies.
4. CD31 is expressed in platelets where the antigen can be absorbed on the outer surface of neoplastic cells.
5. ERG is consistently expressed in prostatic adenocarcinomas as well as in up to 40% of epithelioid sarcomas.

**Box 1.5 Pitfalls in the detection of melanocytic differentiation**

1. Most melanocytic differentiation markers such as Melan-A and HMB45 tend to be negative in sarcomatoid melanoma.
2. Melanocytic markers are strongly expressed in clear cell sarcoma of soft tissue but much less in those lesions arising in the GI tract.

## Melanocytic Differentiation Markers

Despite total lack of specificity, S100 remains the most sensitive marker of melanocytic differentiation. HMB45, Melan-A (MART1), and MITF1 all represent sensitive melanocytic differentiation; however, their sensitivity drops significantly when dealing with sarcomatoid variants of malignant melanomas, wherein S100 is most often the only expressed diagnostic marker. Negativity of S100 in "bona fide" examples of metastatic melanomas may occur, but it represents a much more rare event. They not only play an obvious role in the differential diagnosis of malignant melanoma, but they have also proved extremely helpful in recognizing the members of the clinically and morphologically heterogeneous family of PEComas, as well as being helpful in the proper classification of clear cell sarcomas.

## Other Useful Immunohistochemical Markers

There exists an increasing number of immunohistochemical markers that despite variable specificity play a major role in the differential diagnosis of soft tissue sarcomas.

### ALK (Anaplastic Lymphoma Kinase)

Cytoplasmic expression of the tyrosine kinase ALK plays a key role in supporting the diagnosis of inflammatory myofibroblastic tumors (IMTs), including the aggressive epithelioid subtypes. The pattern of staining (cytoplasmic, perinuclear, membrane) may predict the underlying genetic aberration. Its presence is also potentially relevant from a therapeutic standpoint to justify its use in the metastatic setting of ALK inhibitors. Unfortunately, approximately half of IMTs lack ALK expression. In addition to anaplastic large cell lymphomas and to a small subset of lung adenocarcinomas, ALK expression is also observed in alveolar rhabdomyosarcoma and in epithelioid benign fibrous histiocytoma.

### Beta-catenin

Nuclear expression of beta-catenin (a 92 KDa protein that normally localizes in the cytoplasm wherein it acts both as an intracellular signal transducer in the Wnt signaling pathway and in cadherin-mediated cell adhesion) represents an extremely valuable confirmatory finding in the diagnosis of desmoid fibromatosis. Nuclear accumulation is due to mutation of the *CTNNB1* gene (found in up to 90% of sporadic desmoid fibromatosis) or, alternatively, of the *APC* gene (in the context of Gardner syndrome). A major pitfall is represented by the fact that beta-catenin expression can be observed in approximately one-third of solitary fibrous tumors, in synovial sarcoma, and in low-grade myofibroblastic sarcoma. Interestingly, nuclear expression of beta-catenin (associated with *CTNNB1* gene mutations) occurs in sinonasal hemangiopericytoma.

## Brachyury (T)

Brachyury is a protein acting as a transcriptional activator of notochordal development. Nuclear expression of brachyury represents a key diagnostic feature in the recognition of chordoma and is very helpful in the differential diagnosis with chondrosarcoma, metastatic carcinoma, and myoepithelial neoplasms.

## CD63

The most relevant diagnostic application of CD63 is in the recognition of cellular neurothekeoma. CD63 is not specific because it is also commonly seen in melanocytic lesions.

## CD68

CD68 (a 110 kDa glycoprotein) represents a lysosome-specific marker and therefore is generally used as a histiocytic differentiation marker. However, CD68 tends to be positive in several lysosome-rich lesions such as granular cell tumor and neural and melanocytic neoplasms.

## CD163

CD163 represents a specific as well as sensitive histiocytic marker that at variance with CD68 exhibits very limited expression in non-histiocytic lesions.

## CD99

When dealing with the differential diagnosis of small round cell sarcomas, CD99 (a cell surface glycoprotein normally expressed on thymic T cells) represents a powerful diagnostic marker. In fact, virtually all Ewing sarcomas exhibit strong CD99 immunopositivity, to the extent that such a diagnosis should be regarded as doubtful in case of CD99 negativity. However, it has to be underlined that CD99 is expressed rather broadly, and among potential mimics of Ewing sarcoma, CD99 is also detectable in 90% of synovial sarcomas (including the poorly differentiated round cell variant), in 40% of Merkel cell carcinomas, in lymphoblastic lymphomas, and in mesenchymal chondrosarcoma. Importantly, immunopositivity in all these lesions tends to be more diffuse, rarely matching the thick membrane staining typically observed in Ewing sarcoma.

## Cyclin-B3

Expression of the cell cycle regulator cyclin-B3 seems to be useful in the recognition of a small subset of poorly differentiated round cell sarcomas associated with a *BCOR-CCNB3* gene fusion.

## DOG1

DOG1 (discovered on GIST 1, also known as anoctamin 1 [ANO1] and TMEM16A) represents a useful and sensitive marker for diagnosis of GIST. DOG1 is a calcium-activated chloride channel and is expressed in the interstitial cells of Cajal. DOG1 is extremely helpful in rescuing at least half of KIT-negative GIST cases. Importantly, DOG1 immunopositivity can be observed in smooth muscle tumors of the retroperitoneum as well as in synovial sarcoma.

## INI1 (SMARCB1)

INI1 (integrase interactor 1, also known as SMARCB1) is a member of the BAF molecular complex that contributes to the process of chromatin remodeling and plays a key role in regulating transcription of DNA. Loss of INI1 nuclear expression is consistently observed in malignant rhabdoid tumors (including atypical teratoid rhabdoid tumors of the central nervous system) as a consequence of INI1 biallelic inactivation. Loss of INI1 is also observed in up to 95% of both classical and proximal variants of epithelioid sarcoma wherein it tends to be associated with homozygous deletion of the INI1 locus. INI1 negativity has been described in up to 70% of epithelioid MPNSTs, in 10 to 35% of myoepithelial carcinomas, and in almost all renal medullary carcinomas.

## KIT (CD117)

KIT represents a tyrosine kinase receptor that is involved in the development of mast cells, melanocytes, and interstitial cells of Cajal. KIT has become one of the most clinically relevant phenotypic markers. In fact, its expression in GIST permits the accurate recognition of this once orphan tumor, offering proper selection of patients for treatment with tyrosine kinase inhibitors. KIT expression does not predict response to tyrosine kinase inhibitors and can be observed in unrelated neoplasms such as seminoma, thymic carcinoma, melanocytic neoplasm, and mast cell disorders.

## MDM2

MDM2 (murine double minutes) is the product of the MDM2 proto-oncogene, the main function of which is to promote cell proliferation via inhibition of *TP53*. Both well-differentiated liposarcoma and dedifferentiated liposarcoma are characterized by strong nuclear overexpression of MDM2 as a consequence of *MDM2* gene amplification. MDM2 immunopositivity is most often associated with CDK4 overexpression. A possible pitfall is represented by the fact that MDM2 multifocal immunopositivity (unrelated to gene amplification) can be observed in MPNST, rhabdomyosarcoma, and myxofibrosarcoma. Among mesenchymal malignancies, MDM2 overexpression associated with gene amplification is also observed in intimal sarcoma and in low-grade central osteosarcoma of bone.

## MUC4

MUC4 (mucin 4) is a high molecular weight transmembrane glycoprotein normally expressed in epithelial cells. The major diagnostic role of MUC4 is represented by diagnostic confirmation of both low-grade fibromyxoid sarcoma and sclerosing epithelioid fibrosarcoma, wherein gene expression profiling has identified its upregulation. MUC4 expression is not observed in spindle cell lesions that enter the differential diagnosis with LGFMS (Low Grade Fibromyxoid Sarcoma), perineurioma, low-grade myxofibrosarcoma, and desmoid fibromatosis; nor in other tumors associated with prominent sclerotic background such as sclerosing epithelioid rhabdomyosarcoma. Expression of MUC4 is, however, observed in the epithelial component of biphasic synovial sarcoma. MUC4 immunostaining (along with SATB2) is also helpful in the differential diagnosis with extraskeletal osteosarcoma, a lesion in which distinguishing osteogenic matrix from sclerotic collagen is not always an easy task.

## RB

RB (retinoblastoma gene product) is the product of the *RB* tumor suppressor gene that acts as a potent negative regulator of the cell cycle. From a diagnostic standpoint, loss of nuclear expression of RB is observed in spindle cell and pleomorphic lipomas. The same phenomenon is also observed in atypical spindle cell lipomatous tumor.

## SATB2

Nuclear expression of SATB2 (special AT-rich sequence-binding protein 2) is observed in neoplasm featuring osteogenic differentiation. Normal function of SATB2 is to enable osteoblast lineage commitment. Importantly, SATB2 expression is shared by both normal and neoplastic osteoblasts and therefore plays no role in the differential diagnosis between benign and malignant osteogenic neoplasms. SATB2 is best used whenever hematoxylin and eosin (H&E) stain does not discriminate unequivocally between osteoid and sclerotic collagen, or when osteoid is either minimally represented or not represented in the sample.

## STAT6

Nuclear expression of STAT6 (signal transducer and activator of transcription-6) is consistently expressed in all variants of solitary fibrous tumors. Nuclear relocation of STAT6 nuclear expression is determined by the occurrence of the *NAB2-STAT6* gene fusion.

## TFE3

TFE3 (transcription factor E3) decorates the neoplastic cell population of alveolar soft part sarcoma (as a consequence of the presence of the *ASPSCR1-TFE3* gene fusion that leads to the overexpression of the TFE3 protein) but it is not an entirely specific marker. In fact, it is also expressed in Xp11 translocated renal cell carcinomas, in a small subset (approximately 5%) of perivascular epithelioid cell tumors (PEComa), and, as already discussed, in a subset of epithelioid hemangioendothelioma.

## TLE1

TLE1 (transducing-like enhancer of split 1) is a transcriptional co-repressor that inhibits Wnt signaling. Gene profiling studies have demonstrated high levels of TLE1 in synovial sarcoma that can be detected immunohistochemically. An important potential pitfall is represented by the fact that TLE1 has limited as well as weak immunopositivity may also be observed in unrelated sarcomas such as MPNSTs or solitary fibrous tumors.

## WT1

Nuclear expression of the c-terminus WT1 (Wilms' tumor 1) can be used as a confirmatory tool in the diagnosis of desmoplastic small round cell tumor.

## Molecular Characterization of Soft Tissue Tumors

The marriage of molecular genetics and soft tissue tumor pathology certainly represents one of the most fruitful events of the past decade. The close relationship between morphology (including immunohistochemistry) and molecular genetics was certified by the 2002 WHO classifications of bone and soft tissue tumors and further expanded in the 2013 update.

This integration has had an impact on several aspects of pathology:

1. Created a more accurate definition of disease entities and validation of classification schemes.
2. Improved diagnostic accuracy.
3. Identified molecular predictive and prognostic markers.
4. Discovered and validated therapeutic molecular targets.

## Definition of Disease Entities and Validation of Classification Scheme

Molecular genetics has contributed greatly to a more robust definition of histologic subtypes. This is particularly true whenever new entities are described and also applies to the revision of classification schemes. As an example, the fact that the morphologic description of pseudomyogenic hemangioendothelioma has been followed by the identification of a "disease-specific" *FOSB-Serpine1* gene fusion has greatly contributed to the credibility of this newly identified entity. In addition, molecular genetics has contributed greatly to refining and modifying histologic classification. The merging of myxoid liposarcoma and round cell liposarcoma into a single entity (first generated by morphologic observations) has been greatly supported by the detection in both lesions of the same rearrangement involving the *CHOP* gene. Similarly, identification of *MDM2* gene amplification in so-called inflammatory MFH has represented a key finding, allowing reclassification of those malignancies as an inflammatory variant of dedifferentiated liposarcoma.

## Improvement of Diagnostic Accuracy

From a diagnostic standpoint, during the past two decades it has become clear that molecular testing may add diagnostic accuracy in important subsets of challenging soft tissue tumors. In fact, many of these lesions are known to harbor a variety of relatively specific point mutations, gene amplifications, and chromosome translocations. Gene fusion seems to be particularly frequent in soft tissue neoplasms, the most common of which are listed in Table 1.2. Their occurrence can be routinely assessed for diagnostic purposes via fluorescence in situ hybridization (FISH) and/or polymerase chain reaction (PCR) techniques. It can be foreseen that next-generation sequencing (NGS) technology will greatly contribute to a comprehensive genetic evolution of mesenchymal malignances.

The diagnostic utility of molecular genetics can be best exemplified in the following situations:

1. Distinguishing specific subtypes of sarcomas.
2. Supporting diagnosis in non-canonical clinical presentations.
3. Distinguishing sarcomas from benign mimickers.

## Distinguishing Specific Subtypes of Sarcomas

The distinction of specific sarcoma subtypes is becoming increasingly important as more specific local as well as systemic treatments are being developed. Molecular genetics/pathology has proved diagnostically useful in all morphologic groups of mesenchymal malignancies. Round cell sarcomas represent the perfect example to underscore how clinically relevant molecular diagnostics has become. Round cell sarcomas include Ewing sarcoma, desmoplastic small round cell tumor (DSRCT), alveolar rhabdomyosarcoma, poorly differentiated round cell synovial sarcoma (PDSS), *CIC*-rearranged and *BCOR*-rearranged undifferentiated round cell sarcomas, and a minority of cases of high-grade liposarcomas featuring a round cell morphology. They all represent aggressive neoplasms, and their distinction is crucial because therapeutic approaches may differ significantly. As morphologic overlap may be at times extreme, to the extent that even immunohistochemical characterization cannot help in achieving a definitive classification (i.e., keratin positive Ewing sarcoma vs. poorly differentiated round cell synovial sarcoma), molecular genetics may play a key diagnostic role. As shown in Table 1.2, all these entities harbor relatively specific genetic aberrations that can be routinely assessed, contributing to increased diagnostic accuracy. The demonstration by FISH of *EWSR1*, *SS18*, and *FOXO1* rearrangements in Ewing sarcoma, rhabdomyosarcoma, and PDSS, respectively, or, alternatively, of specific chimeric transcripts by PCR-based techniques or via an NGS-based approach, is of great help in achieving a correct diagnosis. As far as FISH analysis of the *EWSR1* gene is concerned, a major caveat is represented by the fact that its rearrangement can occur in a variety of unrelated lesions

(Table 1.2). As a consequence, any result needs to be mandatorily interpreted in context with morphology and immunohistochemical findings.

The detection of translocations is not the only diagnostically relevant genetic event. The identification of **gene copy number variations** has also proved extremely helpful. The perfect example is represented by dedifferentiated liposarcoma (DDLPS), a pleomorphic, usually (but not exclusively) retroperitoneal adipocytic malignancy that, in contrast to other sarcomas such as leiomyosarcoma, exhibits the tendency to recur locally with a comparatively lower rate of metastatic spread. As a consequence, the surgical treatment of retroperitoneal dedifferentiated liposarcoma is currently based on multivisceral resection aimed at prolonging the time period until a local destructive recurrence. The recognition of dedifferentiated liposarcoma is generally based on the identification of a well-differentiated (WD) lipogenic component associated with a high-grade, most often non-lipogenic, sarcoma. In consideration of the increasing tendency to use core biopsies for diagnostic purposes, the well-differentiated lipogenic component is often not made available. In this context, the detection of *MDM2* amplification by FISH or quantitative RT-PCR certainly represents a useful diagnostic adjunct. *MDM2* testing is also potentially useful in distinguishing between myxoid liposarcoma (consistently *MDM2* negative and most often instead characterized by a *DDIT3/CHOP* gene rearrangement) and WD/DDPLS with myxoid change, as well as to separate homologous dedifferentiated liposarcoma from pleomorphic liposarcoma. In most of these situations, it must be stressed that MDM2 immunohistochemistry (under corrrect laboratory conditions) matches both in terms of sensitivity and specificity of molecular techniques.

## Supporting Diagnosis in Non-canonical Clinical Presentations

As a result of the widespread use of molecular pathology as a confirmatory diagnostic tool, the range of clinical presentations of many entities has broadened. In fact, the combination of morphologic criteria and genetics validates the recognition of rare diseases even when arising at non-canonical anatomic locations. This is particularly true for referral centers wherein challenging cases tend to concentrate. Molecular genetics has undoubtedly greatly contributed, for instance, to the identification of primary Ewing sarcoma of the skin, kidney, and meninges, as well as of synovial sarcomas occurring at visceral sites such as the lungs and the gastrointestinal tract.

## Distinguishing True Sarcomas from Benign Mimics

As mentioned, the morphologic appearance of mesenchymal lesions does not always reflects the clinical behavior. The distinction of sarcomas from benign mimics most often relies on morphologic criteria; however, in a minority of cases molecular genetics may also prove diagnostically helpful. This is particularly true when dealing with low-grade fibromyxoid sarcoma (LGFMS), a deceptively bland-looking spindle cell mesenchymal malignancy characterized by an aggressive clinical behavior on a long-term basis. The differential diagnosis of LGFMS includes benign lesions such as perineurioma, neurofibroma, cellular myxoma, and nodular fasciitis, as well as locally aggressive neoplasms such as desmoid fibromatosis. Even if MUC4 expression is currently regarded as a key diagnostic feature, the identification of *FUS* rearrangement via interphase FISH or the identification of either FUS-CREB3L2 or FUS-CREB3L2 transcripts represents an extremely useful diagnostic tool. As mentioned, desmoid fibromatosis enters the differential diagnosis, and it should be therefore noted that in addition to immunohistochemical detection of nuclear accumulation of β-catenin, mutational analysis of the *CTNNB1* gene may also represent a valuable diagnostic tool.

## Identification of Molecular Predictive and Prognostic Markers

During the past decade, several attempts have been made to determine the prognostic value of molecular genetic findings. Most analyses have focused on Ewing sarcoma, alveolar rhabdomyosarcoma, and synovial sarcoma. Following initial enthusiasm, we have to admit that subsequent results have been contradictory and at this point no meaningful molecular prognostic stratification can be foreseen. The attempt to correlate molecular status and clinical behavior in desmoid fibromatosis has proved controversial. A potential exception is represented by a recently published molecular signature, complexity index in sarcomas (CINSARC), which reportedly allows better separation of grade 2 sarcomas. Nonetheless, this attempt was based on the use of a relatively complex technique (comparative genomic hybridization [CGH]-array) and requires availability of fresh material. Both factors may unfortunately hamper a large-scale clinical application of CINSARC.

An extremely important, clinically relevant exception is represented by gastrointestinal stromal tumors (GISTs), wherein the types of mutations involving both the *KIT* and *PDGFRA* genes are associated with distinctive outcomes. As examples, it is now well known that deletions occurring at exon 11 of the *KIT* gene are associated with more aggressive disease, whereas mutations of exon 18 of the *PDGFRA* gene generally identify a more indolent clinical course. Again, GIST represents the best example of successful prediction of response to treatment in sarcomas. Distinct mutation types reflect different objective response rates (greater for the *KIT* exon 11 mutation and much lower for so-called wild-type GIST) as well as different progression-free survival and overall survival. The presence of specific mutations of exon 18 of the *PDGFRA* gene (D842V) predicts primary resistance to tyrosine kinase inhibitors. Considering that imatinib is currently administered as an adjuvant treatment, the molecular assessment of GIST assumes a central role in clinical decision making. Mutational analysis in GIST also has an impact on dose selection; in fact, the progression-free survival of GIST patients with *KIT* exon 9 mutations is known to be significantly better in patients treated with 800 mg as compared with 400 mg per day.

More recent examples are represented by the use of crizotinib in inflammatory myofibroblastic tumors wherein assessment of

**Table 1.13** FNCLCC grading system

### Tumor differentiation

| | |
|---|---|
| Score 1 | Sarcoma closely resembling normal adult mesenchymal tissue |
| Score 2 | Sarcoma for which histologic typing is certain |
| Score 3 | In myxoid variants, expression may be weaker |

### Mitotic count

| | |
|---|---|
| Score 1 | 0–9 mitoses/10HPF |
| Score 2 | 10–19 mitoses/10HPF |
| Score 3 | ≥ 20 mitoses/10HPF |

### Tumor necrosis

| | |
|---|---|
| Score 0 | No necrosis |
| Score 1 | < 50% tumor necrosis |
| Score 2 | > 50% tumor necrosis |

### Histologic Grade

| | |
|---|---|
| Grade 1 | Total score: 2 to 3 |
| Grade 2 | Total score: 4 to 5 |
| Grade 3 | Total score: 6 to 8 |

*ALK* gene status may represent an important diagnostic confirmatory finding as well as a key biomarker of prediction.

It must be stressed how molecular pathology/genetics represents the most valuable tool used to identify and validate new therapeutic targets. Good examples are represented by MDM2 and CDK4 in dedifferentiated liposarcoma, the mTOR pathway in malignant PEComa and lymphangioleiomyomatosis, PDGFB in DFSP, KDR in angiosarcoma, NTRK3 in GIST, and CSF1 in giant cell tumor of tendon sheath.

## The Grading of Soft Tissue Sarcomas

Soft tissue sarcomas tend to behave aggressively and metastasize in a large percentage of cases. Tumor size, location, depth, and histologic type are all prognostic factors in terms of metastatic risk and overall survival.

With many exceptions, histologic typing does not provide sufficient information for predicting the clinical course of the disease and, therefore, grading systems based on histologic parameters were introduced to provide a more accurate estimation of the degree of malignancy of tumors.

Several different grading systems have been developed. The most successful have been the National Cancer Institute (NCI) and the Fédération Nationale des Centres de Lutte Contre le Cancer (FNCLCC) (French Federation of Cancer Centers Sarcoma Group) systems. Both are three-tiered systems. The FNCLCC system, created in 1984 and updated in 1997, was chosen for use in European Organisation for Research and Treatment of Cancer (EORTC) trials and advocated in both the 2002 and 2013 versions of the WHO classification. It offers slightly better discrimination between low- and high-grade sarcomas, the intermediate group being smaller. The FNCLCC grading system is based on the evaluation of three main parameters: (1) Differentiation; (2) Mitotic count per high-power fields (HPF); (3) Presence of necrosis. As summarized in Table 1.13, each parameter generates a score, the sum of which determines a final score that assigns the tumor to one of the three groups.

The main limitations of the FNCLCC system (actually, of any grading system) are as follows:

1. Many sarcoma subtypes are ungradable. A typical example is alveolar soft part sarcoma, an aggressive lesion that by applying the FNCLCC system would be rated as G1.

2. The concept of differentiation is rather subjective and therefore hampered by poor reproducibility.

3. The FNCLCC system has been devised for surgical specimens from untreated patients. In real life, pathologic diagnosis is increasingly based on core biopsy, wherein no grading system has yet been validated. The same concept applies to surgical specimens from patients treated with neoadjuvant systemic therapy, wherein the presence of necrosis may actually reflect the effect of chemotherapy instead of an intrinsic quality of the tumor itself.

4. The FNCLCC system is not applicable to metastasis. The rationale is rather simple and based on the assumption that a metastatic tumor has already shown its potential for aggressiveness. Relatively often, however, metastases exhibit a morphology that does not match with that of the primary lesion and actually clearly indicates morphologic progression. Interestingly, clinicians tend to show increased interest in the morphologic features of metastatic lesions as a parameter for modulating systemic treatments.

Prognostic monograms that recently have incorporated the revised WHO classification of soft tissue tumors represent an additional, valuable clinical tool. From one of these monograms, there is now a freely downloadable application for portable devices called Sarculator.

## Chapter 1 Selected Key References

- Ballinger ML, Goode DL, Ray-Coquard I, et al. International Sarcoma Kindred Study. Monogenic and polygenic determinants of sarcoma risk: an international genetic study. *Lancet Oncol.* 2016;**17**:1261–71.

- Barretina J, Taylor BS, Banerji S, et al. Subtype-specific genomic alterations define new targets for soft-tissue sarcoma therapy. *Nat Genet.* 2010;**42**(8):715–21.

- Brenca M, Maestro R. Massive parallel sequencing in sarcoma pathobiology: state of the art and perspectives. *Expert Rev Anticancer Ther.* 2015;**15**:1473–88.

- Callegaro D, Miceli R, Bonvalot S, et al. Development and external validation of two nomograms to predict overall survival and occurrence of distant metastases in adults after surgical resection of localised soft-tissue sarcomas of the extremities: a retrospective analysis. *Lancet Oncol.* 2016;**1**:671–80.

- Cancer Genome Atlas Research Network. Comprehensive and integrated genomic characterization of adult soft tissue sarcomas. *Cell.* 2017;**171**:950–65.e28.

- Casali PG, Dei Tos AP, Gronchi A. Gastrointestinal stromal tumor. In DeVita VT Jr, Lawrence TS, Rosenberg SA, editors. *DeVita, Hellman, and Rosenberg's Cancer: Principles & Practice of Oncology.* 10th ed. New York: Wolters Kluwer; 2015. pp. 745–56.

- Chibon F, Lagarde P, Salas S, et al. Validated prediction of clinical outcome in sarcomas and multiple types of cancer on the basis of a gene expression signature related to genome complexity. *Nat Med.* 2010;**16**:781–7.

- Coindre JM, Terrier P, Guillou L, et al. Predictive value of grade for metastasis development in the main histologic types of adult soft tissue sarcomas: a study of 1240 patients from the French Federation of Cancer Centers Sarcoma Group. *Cancer.* 2001;**91**:1914–26.

- Dei Tos AP. Classification of pleomorphic sarcomas: where are we now? *Histopathology.* 2006;**48**:51–62.

- Dei Tos AP. A current perspective on the role for molecular studies in soft tissue tumor pathology. *Semin Diagn Pathol.* 2013;**30**:375–81.

- Dei Tos AP. Liposarcomas: diagnostic pitfalls and new insights. *Histopathology.* 2014;**64**:38–52.

- Fletcher CD. The evolving classification of soft tissue tumours an update based on the new 2013 WHO classification. *Histopathology.* 2014;**64**:2–11.

- Fletcher CDM, Bridge JA, Hogendoorn PCW, Mertens F, editors. *Pathology and Genetics of Tumours of Soft Tissue and Bone. WHO Classification of Tumours of Soft Tissue and Bone.* 4th ed. Lyon: IARC Press; 2013.

- Fletcher CDM, Unni KK, Mertens F, editors. *Pathology and Genetics of Tumors of Soft Tissue and Bone. WHO Classification of Tumours.* Lyon: IARC Press; 2002.

- Gatta G, van der Zwan JM, Casali PG, et al; the RARECARE working group. Rare cancers are not so rare: the rare cancer burden in Europe. *Eur J Cancer.* 2011;**47**:2493–511.

- Guillou L, Coindre JM, Bonichon F, et al. Comparative study of the National Cancer Institute and French Federation of Cancer Centers Sarcoma Group grading systems in a population of 410 adult patients with soft tissue sarcoma. *J Clin Oncol.* 1997;**15**:350–62.

- Hornick JL. Novel uses of immunohistochemistry in the diagnosis and classification of soft tissue tumors. *Mod Pathol.* 2014;**27**:S47–S63.

- Miettinen M. Immunohistochemistry of soft tissue tumors – review with emphasis on 10 markers. *Histopathology.* 2014;**64**:101–18.

- Neuville A, Ranchère-Vince D, Dei Tos AP, et al. Impact of molecular analysis on the final sarcoma diagnosis: a study on 763 cases collected during a European epidemiological study. *Am J Surg Pathol.* 2013;**37**:1259–68.

- Ray-Coquard I, Montesco MC, Coindre JM, et al. Sarcoma: concordance between initial diagnosis and centralized expert review in a population-based study within three European regions. *Ann Oncol.* 2012;**23**:2442–9.

- Singer S, Nielsen, TO, Antonescu CR. Molecular biology of sarcomas. In DeVita VT Jr, Lawrence TS, Rosenberg SA, editors. *DeVita, Hellman, and Rosenberg's Cancer: Principles & Practice of Oncology.* 10th ed. New York: Wolters Kluwer; 2015. pp. 1241–52.

# Imaging of Tumors and Pseudotumors of Soft Tissues

Valérie Bousson MD, PhD, Jean-Denis Laredo MD, and Daniel Vanel MD

Soft tissue tumors and pseudotumors represent a relatively common finding. From a radiologic point of view, this broad topic can be addressed by asking three main questions:

1. How do I investigate a soft tissue mass?
2. Is it a benign or a malignant lesion?
3. What are the main diagnostic pitfalls?

## 1. How do I investigate a soft tissue mass?

The first step is clinical, encompassing the questioning and physical examination of the patient. It aims at collecting key information such as age, past history, background of occurrence, evolutionary pattern, unicity or multiplicity of lesions, location, and size of the lesion.

The second step consists of imaging the lesion to specify exact location and size and to analyze both tissue organization and composition. In practice, radiographs and ultrasound examination will be obtained first and completed, if needed, with a magnetic resonance (MR) imaging.

## A. Clinical Information and Physical Examination

All the available clinical information should be carefully collected, as all such information contributes to the characterization of the lesion – namely, age, sex, history of previously excised lesion, clinical presentation, and physical examination. Generally, the proportion of malignant tumors tends to increase with age. Some histologic subtypes tend to predominate in a particular age-group. For instance, tumors and malformations of blood vessels are most often found in children and young adults, whereas elastofibroma and liposarcoma (with the notable exception of the myxoid subtype) are observed more frequently in middle-aged and elderly patients.

Be aware of the patient's past history that may prove decisive in the diagnostic approach: for instance, history of previous malignancy (subcutaneous or intramuscular metastases); previous radiation therapy (radiation-induced sarcoma) (Fig. 2-1); primary or secondary chronic lymphedema (Stewart-Treves syndrome); history of multiple myeloma; personal or familial syndrome such as type 1 neurofibromatosis (benign or malignant peripheral nerve sheath tumors), hypercholesterolemia (xanthomas), and Gardner syndrome (association of familial intestinal polyposis and abdominal desmoid tumors); Mazabraud syndrome (fibrous dysplasia and soft tissue myxoma) (Fig. 2-2); Ollier disease (multiple enchondromas) (Fig. 2-3); Maffucci disease (enchondromas

and hemangiomas); or a systemic disease such as gout (tophi) or sarcoidosis (nodular sarcoid myositis).

Clinical presentation requires special attention, for instance, a history of anticoagulant treatment (hematoma), a recent trauma (hematoma or myositis ossificans), an infectious disease (abscess), or skin wound (abscess, foreign body reaction). Soft tissue sarcomas often develop slowly over several years before being recognized. This is especially true for synovial sarcoma. A lesion demonstrating a rapid growth is most often inflammatory in nature. Reduction in size suggests a benign process that is being resolved. Fluctuations in size evoke a ganglion cyst or a vascular malformation. If the mass is painful, an inflammatory process must first be considered. By contrast, soft tissue sarcomas often present as a painless mass.

The anatomic location of the disease can also support some specific diagnosis. For example, a mass at the tip of the scapula would suggest an elastofibroma; a lesion located at the intercapitometatarsal space would suggest a Morton neuroma, whereas a mass in the subungueal bed most often represents a glomus tumor.

Physical examination may also provide important clues. A superficially located mass is most often benign or even nonneoplastic, whereas a deep-seated lesion tends to be more suspicious for malignancy. Of course, as with any clinical feature, this is not an absolute rule and several exceptions may occur. Lesions that can be superficial at presentation include the following: ordinary lipoma (Fig. 2-4), slow-flow vascular malformations (Fig. 2-5), benign peripheral nerve sheath tumors (Fig. 2-6), inflammatory conditions such as erythema nodosum and granuloma annulare, benign fibrous histiocytoma, nodular fasciitis (Fig. 2-7), calcifying epithelioma of Malherbe, non-Hodgkin lymphoma, dermatofibrosarcoma protuberans (Fig. 2-8), myxofibrosarcoma, and metastases (most often from breast, cutaneous malignant melanoma, lungs). The etiologies of deep lesions are specified with imaging.

The presence of multiple lesions is rather in favor of a benign process but again this is not an absolute rule. Actually, the differential diagnosis of multiple masses is somewhat limited and includes vascular malformations (particularly venous malformations), vascular tumors (including the low-grade malignant pseudomyogenic hemangioendothelioma), superficial or deep fibromatosis, benign tumors of peripheral nerve sheath (Fig. 2-9), lipomas (Fig. 2-10), rheumatoid nodules (in friction zones) (Fig. 2-11), sarcoids, xanthomas, gout tophi, amyloid deposits, myxomas (see Fig. 2-2), glomus tumors, and elastofibromas (most often

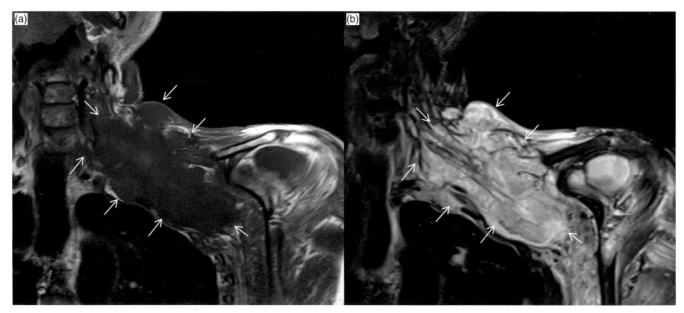

**Fig. 2-1.** Malignant peripheral nerve sheath tumor occurring 20 years after radiation therapy for lymphoma. (a) Coronal T1-weighted and (b) coronal fat-suppressed T2-weighted MR images showing a solid mass of the left brachial plexus (*arrows*).

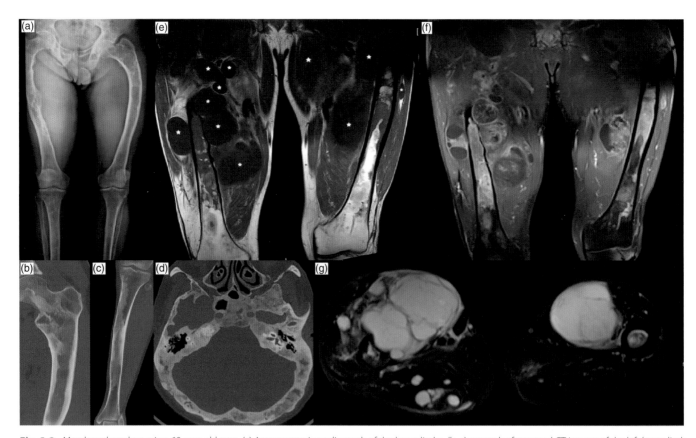

**Fig. 2-2.** Mazabraud syndrome in a 69-year-old man. (a) Anteroposterior radiograph of the lower limbs, (b, c) coronal reformatted CT images of the left lower limb, and (d) axial reformatted CT image of the cranial base showing fibrous dysplasia lesions with bone deformities and typical ground glass appearance. (e) Coronal T1-weighted, (f) fat-suppressed post-contrast T1-weighted, and (g) axial fat-suppressed T2-weighted MR images showing multiple intramuscular masses (*stars*) that are "cyst-like" on T1- and T2-weighted sequences. Note the scalloping of the medial cortex of the right femur. These soft tissue masses are myxomas; the patterns of enhancement vary across myxomas. The medullary cavity of both femurs is occupied by dysplastic fibrous tissue.

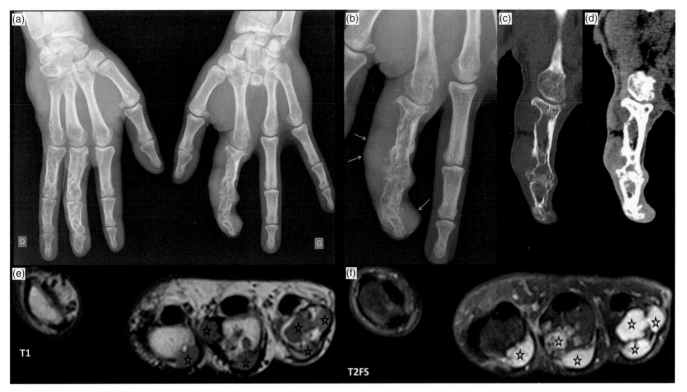

**Fig. 2-3.** Ollier disease in a 29-year-old man. (a) Conventional radiograph of the hands and (b) radiograph of the second and third left fingers, showing multiple chondromas of the bone and soft tissues. Small foci of calcifications are visible within the lesions (*arrows*). Two fingers were amputed for treatment of chondrosarcomas. (c, d) Coronal reformatted CT images of the second left finger, and (e) axial T1-weighted, and (f) axial fat-suppressed T2-weighted MR images showing multiple chondromas (*stars*) of the bone and soft tissues.

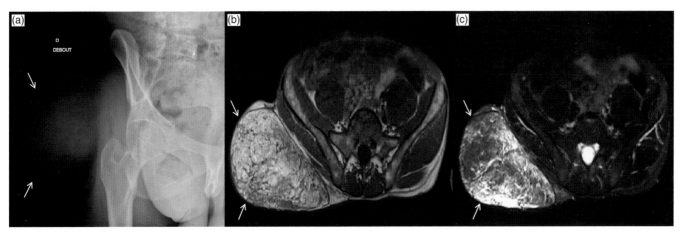

**Fig. 2-4.** Large superficial lipoma in a 45-year-old man. (a) Conventional radiograph, (b) axial T1-weighted, and (c) axial fat-suppressed T2-weighted MR images showing a large superficial mass containing fat (*arrows*). Percutaneous biopsy diagnosed a lipoma.

located in the interscapular region). Kaposi sarcoma, dermatofibrosarcoma protuberans, and mixofibrosarcoma may also present as multiple superficial masses.

## B. Imaging

Useful information obtainable from imaging studies, especially at MR, includes the following: (1) origin of the mass; (2) shape of the lesion; (3) margins; (4) presence of liquid-liquid levels; (5) presence of ossification or calcification; (6) presence of peripheral edema; and (7) signal intensity.

The variety of "intramuscular" masses is rather broad and includes lesions such as hematoma, benign lipoma (see Fig. 2-10), slow-flow vascular malformation, intramuscular myxoma (see Fig. 2-2), sarcoids, metastasis, and soft tissue sarcomas. Deep "intermuscular" masses are most often represented by ganglia cysts, benign and malignant peripheral nerve sheath tumors, and soft tissue sarcomas (myxoid liposarcoma is the most common). A deep "juxta-articular" mass suggests a ganglion cyst, a juxta-articular myxoma, crystalline apatite/pyrophosphate deposits, gout tophi, tumor calcinosis, and, among sarcomas, synovial sarcoma.

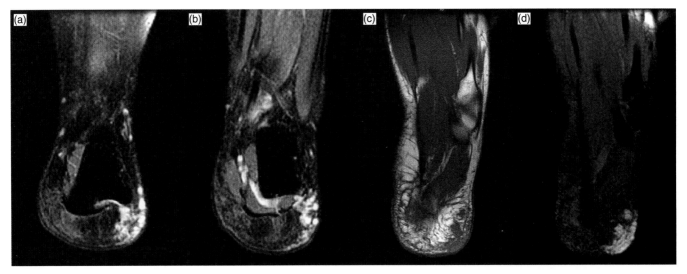

**Fig. 2-5.** Slow-flow vascular malformation of the left foot in a 27-year-old woman. (a, b) Coronal fat-suppressed T2-weighted, and (c) axial T1-weighted, and (d) axial fat-suppressed T2-weighted MR images showing a superficial and deep soft tissue mass with vascular spaces related to plantar veins. No phlebolith was present on radiograph.

The exact location of the mass deserves particular attention. Indeed, identification of a specific origin limits the differential diagnoses. When the mass is centered on the superficial fascia, there are three main diagnoses: nodular fasciitis (see Fig. 2-7), superficial fibromatosis (Fig. 2-12), and Morel-Lavallée effusion. Myxofibrosarcomas, especially those with a superficial origin, produce a tail-like pattern on gadolinium MRI. The tail sign represents a thick fascial enhancement extending from the margin of a myxofibrosarcoma and is related to the infiltrative growth pattern of the tumor. When the mass is centered on a peripheral nerve with the nerve entering and exiting the mass, a peripheral nerve sheath tumor is the diagnosis of choice (see Fig. 2-6). Other possible diagnoses are a fibrolipomatous hamartoma of the nerve (Fig. 2-13) or a lymphoma (Fig. 2-14). When the mass is centered on a tendon sheath, especially in the hand and foot, the primary diagnosis is giant cell tumor of tendon sheath (Fig. 2-15). Other possible diagnoses are a fibroma of tendon sheath or a chondromatosis.

The shape of the lesion may be of interest. For instance, a fusiform, dumbbell-shaped, or moniliform mass suggests a peripheral nerve sheath tumor; a piriform mass, a Morton neuroma; a serpiginous mass, a slow-flow vascular malformation (see Fig. 2-5); a mass with soap bubbles, a lipoma arborescens; and a digitiform mass, a plexiform neurofibroma or a deep fibromatosis (Fig. 2-16). The presence of irregular margins also suggests a deep fibromatosis (Fig. 2-16).

The presence of liquid-liquid levels within the mass is related to the occurrence of cystic or hemorrhagic components. They can be observed inside a broad variety of lesions that include hematoma, myositis ossificans, tumoral calcinosis (Fig. 2-17), slow-flow vascular malformation, aneurysmal cyst of soft tissue, myxoma, benign fibrous histiocytoma, and benign peripheral nerve sheath tumors. They can also be observed in malignant tumors, especially synovial sarcoma and angiosarcoma, as well as in myxofibrosarcomas,

undifferentiated high-grade sarcomas, and malignant peripheral nerve sheath tumors.

Ossifications reproduce the normal structure of bone and include both trabecular and compact bone. This should not be confused with calcifications that simply correspond to amorphous deposits of calcium. Unfortunately, it is not always easy to distinguish ossification from calcification, particularly when the lesion is small. Ossifications and calcifications are visible on CT scans or X-rays, but usually go unnoticed with MRI because of their low signal intensity. Ossifications can be observed in hematoma, lipoma (ossifying lipoma), metastases (particularly from stomach and bladder cancers), and sarcomas, most often synovial sarcoma, liposarcoma, malignant peripheral nerve sheath tumors, and extraskeletal osteosarcoma. The pattern of mineralization is also very important: peripheral mature ossification occurring 6 to 8 weeks after onset of symptoms strongly supports the diagnosis of myositis ossificans (Fig. 2-18). Calcifications are common in slow-flow vascular malformation (phlebolites), tumoral calcinosis (usually associated with liquid levels) (see Fig. 2-17), chondroma (Fig. 2-19), synovial chondromatosis, chondrosarcoma (cartilage matrix), and synovial sarcoma (Fig. 2-20). The resorption of apatite calcification at MRI provides a broad and intense edema of the soft tissue and adjacent bone, edema in which the calcification is barely visible.

Important information can also be gathered by a careful analysis of the surroundings of the mass. For instance, a peripheral rim of fat indicates that the origin of the mass is in the neurovascular bundle or in the intermuscular space. A cap of fat and a ring of edema are characteristic of myxomas. Muscular atrophy can be observed at the periphery of a myxoma or in muscle innervated by a nerve affected by a tumor.

Finally, the signal intensity represents an extremely important feature by which to orientate the diagnosis. The radiologist should be able to identify a relatively high T1-weighted signal

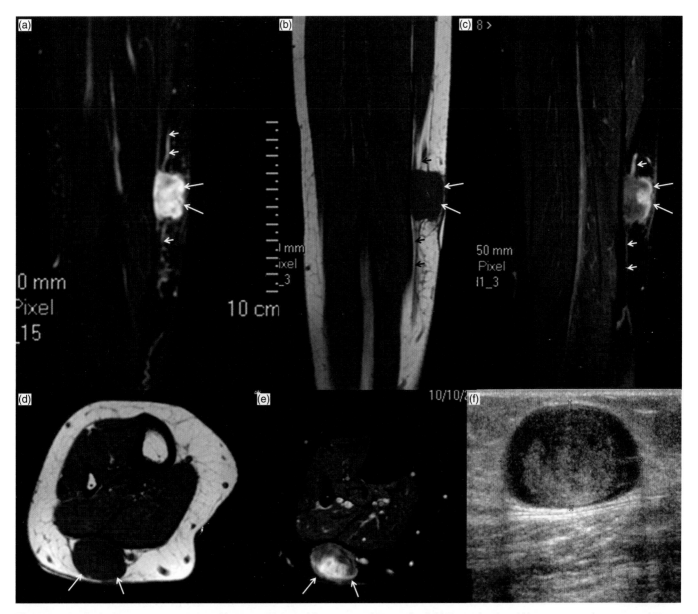

**Fig. 2-6.** Superficial schwannoma in a 56-year-old woman. (a) Sagittal fat-suppressed T2-weighted, (b) T1-weighted, and (c) post-contrast fat-suppressed T1-weighted MR images, (d) axial T1-weighted, and (e) post-contrast fat-suppressed T1-weighted MR images showing a mass in the subcutaneous fat. The mass is related to a small neurovascular bundle. The signal intensity is slightly higher than that of muscles on (b) T1-weighted images. (f) Ultrasonography shows a well-defined, partly hypoechoic solid mass.

intensity (relative to muscles), or a low T2-weighted signal intensity, or a high T2-weighted signal intensity (signal intensity of liquids). Four categories of lesions can feature a high signal on T1-weighted images: (1) those *containing fat*: lipoma and variants (see Figs. 2-4, 2-10; Fig. 2-21), liposarcoma, peripheral nerve sheath tumor, and phosphaturic mesenchymal tumor; (2) those *containing proteinaceous fluid*: ganglion cysts (Fig. 2-22), synovial cysts, abscesses, and neural tumors (Fig. 2-23); (3) those *containing methemoglobin or slow blood flow*: hematomas, slow-flow vascular malformations (Fig. 2-24), and tumors or pseudotumors with hemorrhage (Figs. 2-25, 2-26); and (4) those *containing melanin pigment*: melanoma, clear cell sarcoma, and melanotic schwannoma. Lesions with foci of low signal intensity on all pulse sequences are lesions containing either *calcifications and/or ossifications* (gout tophi, dystrophic calcifications [see Fig. 2-17],

chondroma [see Fig. 2-19], synovial sarcoma [see Fig. 2-20]), or *fibrosis* (superficial and deep fibromatosis [see Figs. 2-12, 2-16], elastofibroma, amyloidosis, rheumatoid pannus, lymphoma) or *hemosiderin* (villonodular synovitis [Fig. 2-27], giant cell tumor of tendon sheaths [see Fig. 2-15], hematoma or hemorrhagic tumors [Fig. 2-25], synovial sarcoma [see Fig. 2-20]). Among lesions that are totally or partially hyperintense on T2-weighted images, there are true cystic lesions such as ganglion cyst, epidermal cyst, seroma, or abscesses, and there are pseudocystic lesions. Pseudocystic lesions may contain *myxoid matrix* [myxoma (see Fig. 2-2), nodular fasciitis, peripheral nerve sheath tumor (Fig. 2-28), myoepithelioma (Fig. 2-29), myxoid liposarcoma (Fig. 2-30), myxofibrosarcoma, extraskeletal myxoid chondrosarcoma (Fig. 2-26), low-grade fibromyxoid sarcoma, myxoid leiomyosarcoma] or *necrosis* (Fig. 2-31).

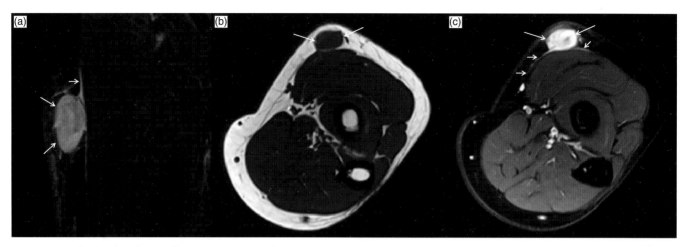

**Fig. 2-7.** Superficial nodular fasciitis of the elbow. (a) Coronal fat-suppressed T2-weighted, (b) axial T1-weighted, and (c) axial post-contrast fat-suppressed T1-weighted MR images showing a superficial mass (*arrows*) with signal intensity that is identical to that of skeletal muscles on T1-weighted images, higher than that of skeletal muscles on T2-weighted images, and markedly enhanced after contrast administration. Note the thickening and contrast enhancement of the superficial fascia (*short arrows*).

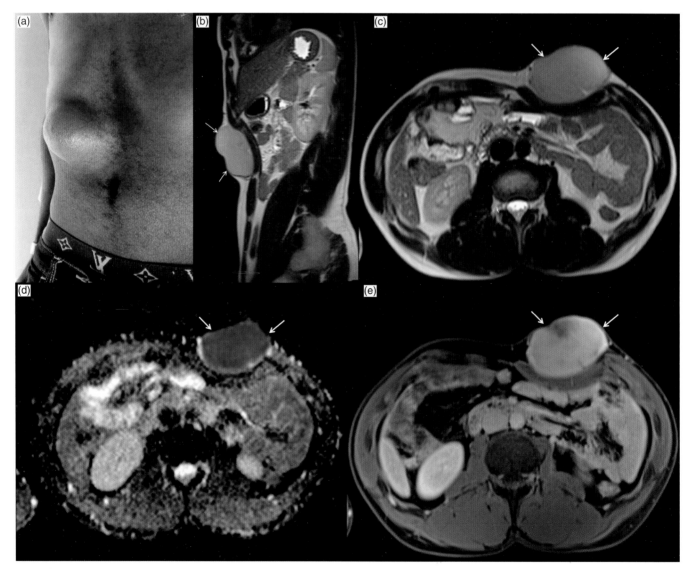

**Fig. 2-8.** Dermatofibrosarcoma protuberans in a 29-year-old man. (a) Photograph of the mass. (b, c) Sagittal and axial T2-weighted MR images showing a nodular mass (*arrows*) involving the skin and subcutaneous tissues of the abdominal wall. Apparent diffusion coefficient (d) is low, in favor of a highly cellular tumor. (e) Axial post-contrast fat-suppressed T1-weighted MR image demonstrating marked enhancement of the mass.

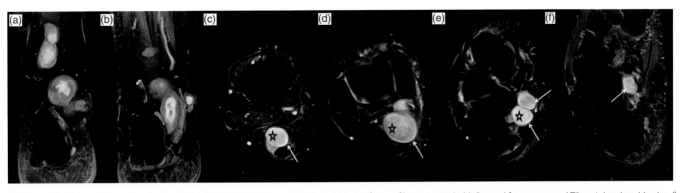

**Fig. 2-9.** Multiple schwannomas in the ankle of a 55-year-old woman with no history of neurofibromatosis. (a, b) Coronal fat-suppressed T2-weighted and (c, d, e, f) axial fat-suppressed T2-weighted MR images showing multiple soft tissue masses related to the right posterior tibial nerve. The masses demonstrate a thin peripheral rim of high signal intensity (*arrows*), and a fascicular sign on axial images (*stars*).

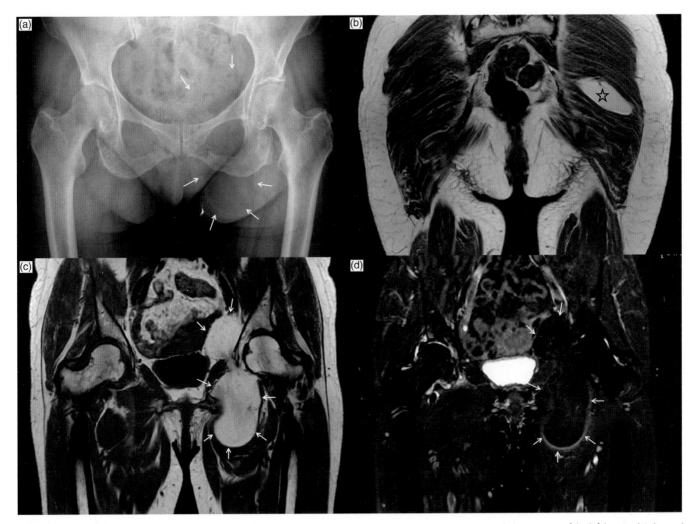

**Fig. 2-10.** Two deep lipomas in a 65-year-old woman. (a) Anteroposterior radiograph of the pelvis showing a large radiolucent mass of the left hemi pelvis (*arrows*). (b, c) Coronal T1-weighted images showing a lipoma located in the left gluteus maximus muscle (*star*), and a second one, located in the proximal left thigh, extending into the pelvis (*arrows*) and infitrating the hip. The masses demonstrate a signal intensity similar to that of subcutaneous fat on T1-weighted images. (d) On the coronal fat-suppressed T2-weighted MR image, the hyperintense area is suppressed.

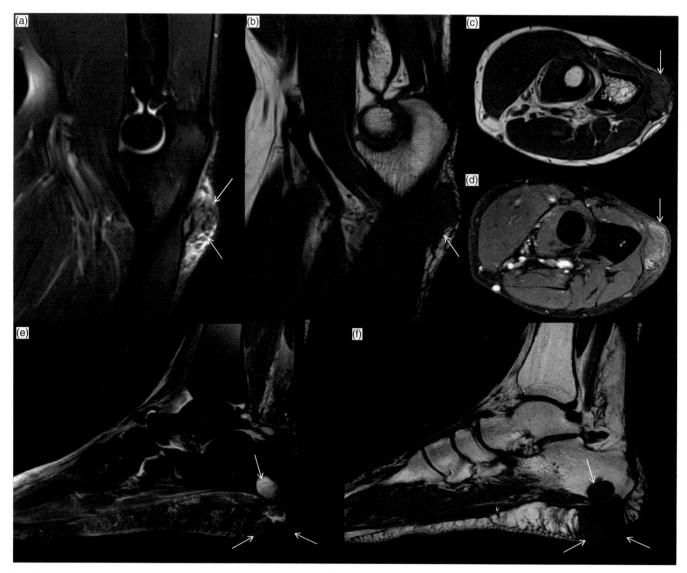

**Fig. 2-11.** Two rheumatoid nodules in a 68-year-old woman with rheumatoid arthritis. (a) Sagittal fat-suppressed T2-weighted and (b) T1-weighted MR images, (c) axial T1-weighted and (d) axial post-contrast fat-suppressed T1-weighted MR images of the elbow. (e) Sagittal fat-suppressed T2-weighted and (f) T1-weighted MR images of the angle. The images show two non-specific heterogeneous masses (*arrows*) in friction areas. Medical history provides the diagnosis of rheumatoid nodules.

## 2. Is it a benign or a malignant lesion?

Clinical data and imaging findings together may allow an accurate diagnosis in a reasonable number of soft tissue lesions. But when findings are not typical for a specific diagnosis, the radiologist should be extremely cautious and should ask whether it is a benign or a malignant lesion, a question that is often difficult to answer. Although no criterion is sufficient by itself, there are numerous radiologic features that deserve attention. The most relevant criteria are the following:

1. Superficial masses are usually benign; deep masses are suspected to be malignant. Exceptions: lymphoma, myxofibrosarcoma, and dermatofibrosarcoma protuberans (see Fig. 2-8) may be superficially located. By contrast, benign lipoma can extend more deeply.

2. The involvement of more than one anatomic compartment by crossing of fascia is usually a feature of malignancy.

However, slow-flow vascular malformations are able to occupy several different spaces.

3. Large size suggests malignancy (Fig. 2-32). Indeed, only 5% of benign tumors are larger than 5 cm. But benign lipomas again represent the exception, as they can often attain a large size (see Fig. 2-4). The opposite condition (small size) tends to be meaningless, as malignant tumors are small before becoming large.

4. Unlike bone malignancies, in soft tissue lesions the presence of infiltrative margins represents a poor criterion. In fact, sarcomas often have sharp boundaries because of the presence of a pseudocapsule that results from the compression of the adjacent connective tissue with or without associated inflammation (see Figs. 2-20 and 2-31). Some locally aggressive, non-metastasizing tumors, such as desmoid tumors, actually have irregular boundaries (see Fig. 2-16).

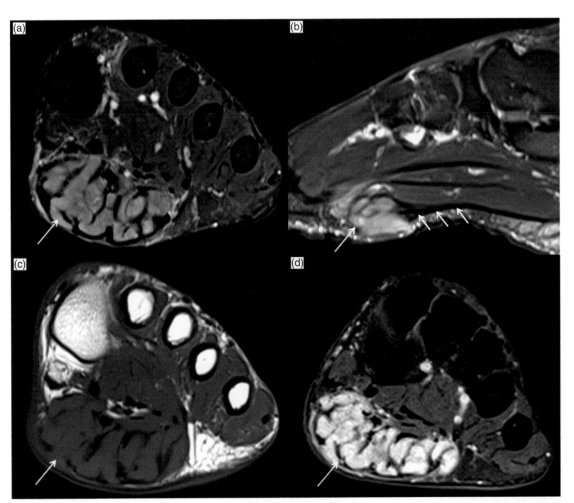

**Fig. 2-12.** Plantar fibromatosis. (a, b) Coronal and sagittal fat-suppressed T2-weighted, (c) coronal T1-weighted, and (d) post-contrast fat-suppressed T1-weighted MR images showing a soft tissue mass (*arrows*) located in the plantar fascia (*short arrows*), suggesting the diagnosis of plantar fibromatosis. The mass contains areas of very low signal intensity on all pulse sequences. Marked enhancement after contrast administration is seen.

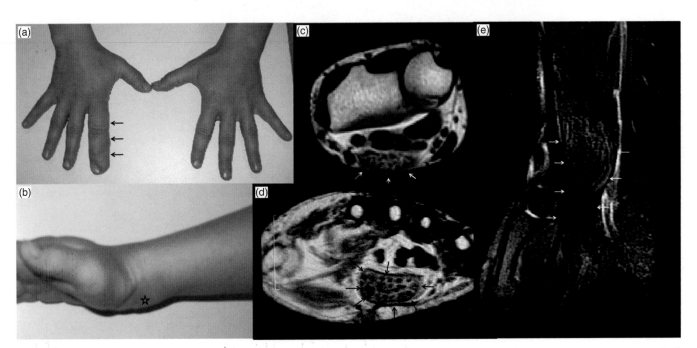

**Fig. 2-13.** Macrodystrophia lipomatosa and neural fibrolipoma of the median nerve. (a, b) Photographs of the hands and right wrist showing an overgrowth of the second right finger (*black arrows*), and a soft tissue mass (*star*) of the wrist. (c, d) Axial T1-weighted and (e) coronal fat-suppressed T2-weighted MR images showing dramatic enlargement of the median nerve (*arrows*) with fatty and fibrous tissue overgrowth dissecting nerve fascicles.

5. The heterogeneity of signal intensity on T1- and/or T2-weighted images suggests malignancy (see Figs. 2-1, 2-20, 2-30, 2-31, 2-32; Fig. 2-33). Septa of low T2-signal intensity has also been described as suggestive of malignancy.

6. Measuring the apparent diffusion coefficient (ADC) represents a powerful tool to guide the diagnosis. A low ADC means a high cellularity and therefore it evokes malignancy (see Fig. 2-8). A high ADC means that the distribution of water is free and consequently it evokes a benign process. However, the correct interpretation of ADC values requires comparison of T1-weighted, T2-weighted, and post-contrast T1-weighted MR images. Indeed, the diagnostic performance of the ADC is high for non-myxoid tumors, with a truly significant difference of the ADC values between benign and malignant tumors. However, some benign processes such as an abscess, a recent hematoma, or a giant cell tumor may indeed demonstrate a relatively low ADC. In addition, relatively well-differentiated malignant tumors containing a cartilaginous matrix (chondrosarcoma grade 1 or 2) typically have high ADC. For myxoid lesions, there is no significant difference of ADC values between benign myxoid tumors (myxoma) and malignant myxoid tumors or malignant tumors with a myxoid content (myxoid liposarcoma, myxofibrosarcoma) that also exhibit a high ADC.

7. Dynamic contrast-enhanced MR imaging should be systematically included in the images used to characterize a tumor. Early onset of contrast enhancement (<6 seconds), initial early enhancement at the periphery of the mass, and rapid progression of enhancement to an early plateau all favor malignancy (see Fig. 2-33). Absence of enhancement or late and diffuse enhancement favors a benign process. Notably, there exist important pitfalls. For instance benign peripheral nerve sheath tumors and deep fibromatoses typically show an early enhancement. At the opposite end of the spectrum of exceptions, some myxoid liposarcomas demonstrates a slow and progressive enhancement.

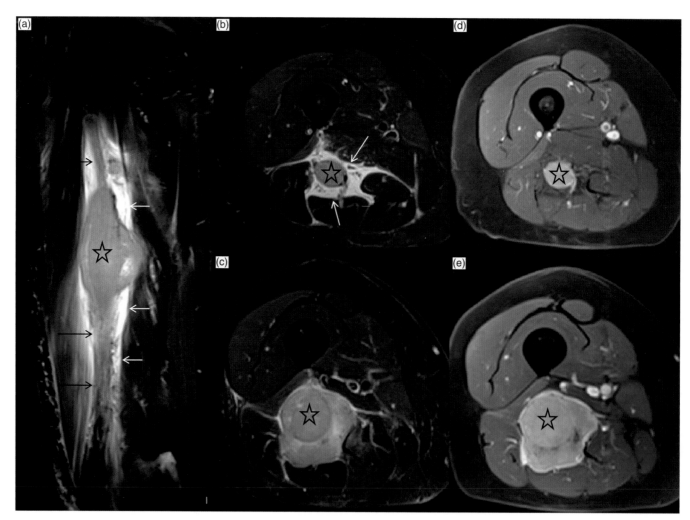

**Fig. 2-14.** Lymphoma of the sciatic nerve in a 71-year-old woman. (a, b, c) Coronal, axial fat-suppressed T2-weighted, and (d, e) axial post-contrast fat-suppressed T1-weighted MR images showing a thickened sciatic nerve (*black arrows*) entering and exiting a large fusiform soft tissue tumor (*stars*). Surrounding edema (*white arrows*).

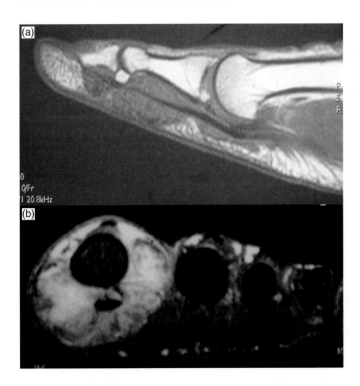

**Fig. 2-15.** Giant cell tumor of the tendon sheath of the flexor of the first toe. (a) Sagittal T1-weighted and (b) coronal fat-suppressed T2-weighted MR images showing a lobulated mass arising adjacent to the flexor tendon of the toe, heterogeneous on T1- and T2-weighted images.

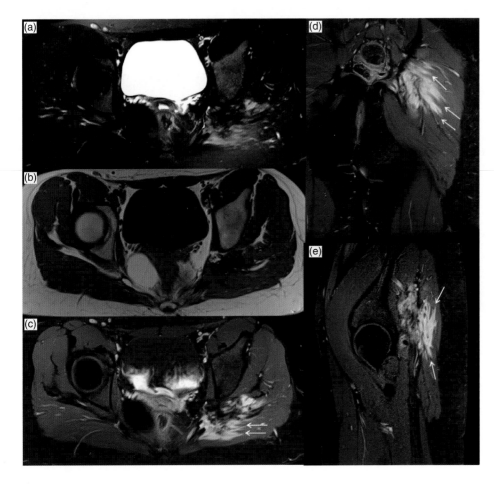

**Fig. 2-16.** Deep fibromatosis in a 15-year-old girl. (a) Axial fat-suppressed T2-weighted and (b) T1-weighted MR images; (c, d, e) axial, coronal, and sagittal post-contrast fat-suppressed T1-weighted MR images showing a deep infiltrative mass within the left gluteus muscles. The areas of markedly low signal intensity on T1- and T2-weighted images and the interdigitations (*arrows*) are highly suggestive of the diagnosis.

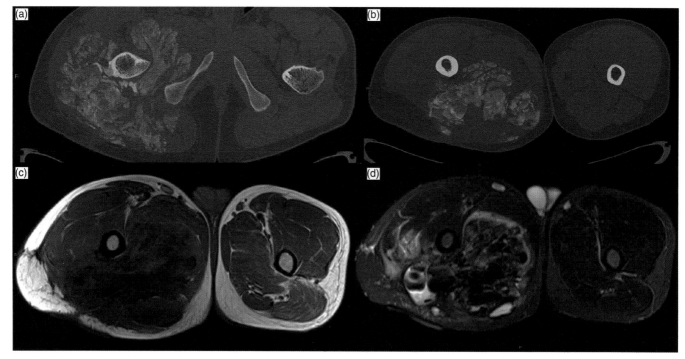

**Fig. 2-17.** Pseudotumoral calcinosis. (a, b) Axial reformatted CT images of the pelvis, and (c) axial T1-weighted and (d) axial fat-suppressed T2-weighted MR images showing large areas of calcium deposits in the soft tissues around the right hip and posterior thigh.

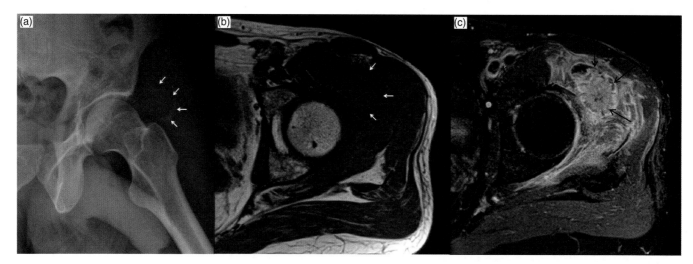

**Fig. 2-18.** Myositis ossificans of intermediate age in a 38-year-old male. Conventional radiograph and MR were obtained six to eight weeks after onset of pain, on the same day: (a) conventional radiograph shows a mass with a peripheral rim of mature bone (*arrows*). Axial T1-weighted MR images before (b) and after (c) contrast administration show a poorly defined mass (*arrows*) in the gluteus minimus, behind the tendon of the rectus femoral. The lesion is isointense to skeletal muscles on T1-weighted image. Curvilinear areas of decreased signal intensity at the periphery of the mass (*black arrows*) correspond to mineralization. Diffuse surrounding soft tissue edema.

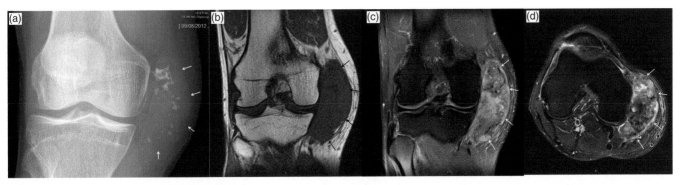

**Fig. 2-19.** Soft tissue chondroma in a 53-year-old man. (a) Anteroposterior radiograph of the right knee showing a medial soft tissue mass (*arrows*) containing cartilaginous calcifications. (b) Coronal T1-weighted and (c, d) coronal and axial fat-suppressed T2-weighted MR images showing a large soft tissue mass with a lobular architecture and areas of low signal intensity.

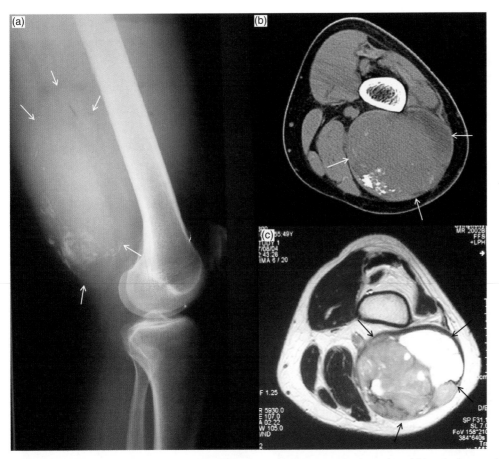

**Fig. 2-20.** Synovial sarcoma in the thigh of a 49-year-old man. (a) Conventional radiograph and (b) axial reformatted CT image showing a large soft tissue mass (*arrows*) in the posterior thigh. There are calcifications at the periphery of the mass. (c) T2-weighted MR image shows a heterogeneous mass with several signal intensities on T2, from very high (myxoid tissue) to very low (fibrous tissue, hemorrhage).

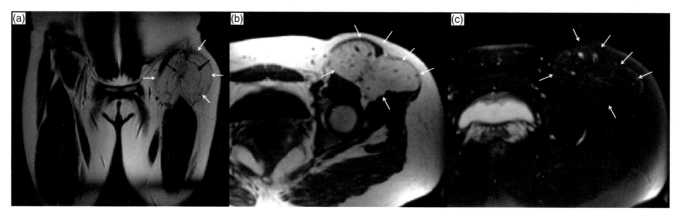

**Fig. 2-21.** Hibernoma. (a) Coronal fat-suppressed T2-weighted, (b) axial T1-weighted, and (c) axial fat-suppressed T2-weighted MR images showing a fat-containing mass. The signal of the fatty mass (*white arrows*) is not exactly that of the subcutaneous fat on T1- and fat-suppressed T2-weighted images ("brown fat"). Large serpiginous vessels (*black arrows*) are seen within the mass.

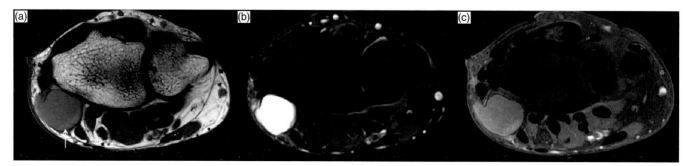

**Fig. 2-22.** Ganglia of the dorsal aspect of the wrist. (a) Axial T1-weighted, (b) axial fat-suppressed T2-weighted, and (c) axial post-contrast fat-suppressed T1-weighted MR images showing a cystic mass. The relatively high signal intensity on the T1-weighted image is in favor of a high protein content. There is also hemorrhage (*arrow*).

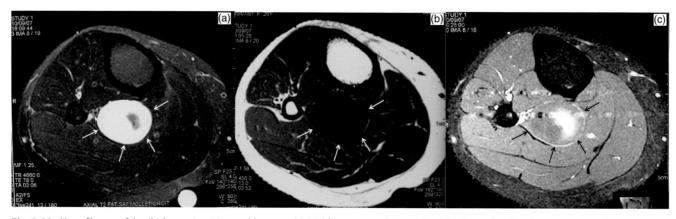

**Fig. 2-23.** Neurofibroma of the tibial nerve in a 26-year-old woman. (a) Axial fat-suppressed T2-weighted, (b) T1-weighted, and (c) post-contrast fat-suppressed T1-weighted MR images showing a mass located in an intermuscular space. There is a target sign on the T2-weighted image; it corresponds to a low signal intensity in the central part of the tumor (fibrous/densely cellular tissue), and high signal intensity peripherally (myxoid tissue). There is also a target sign in (b) and (c).

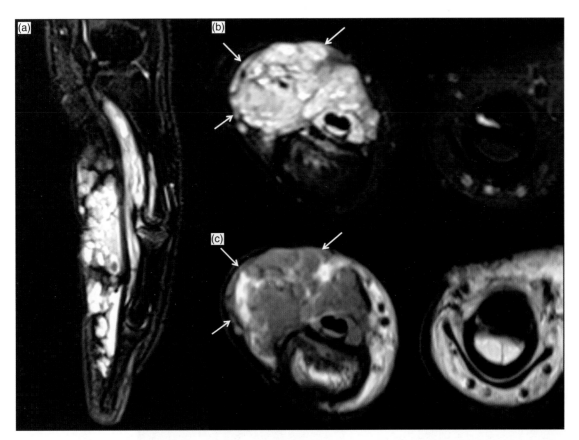

**Fig. 2-24.** Slow-flow vascular malformation of the fifth right finger. (a, b) Sagittal and axial fat-suppressed T2-weighted and (c) axial fat-suppressed T2-weighted MR images showing a soft tissue mass (*arrows*) composed of slow-flow vascular spaces. The signal intensity is hyperintense on the T1-weighted image.

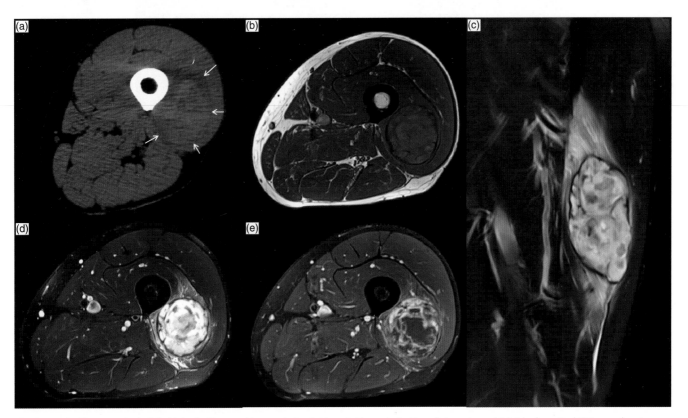

**Fig. 2-25.** Angiosarcoma in the left thigh of a 43-year-old man admitted at hospital for embolization of a hematoma. (a) Axial reformatted CT image showing a mass (*arrows*) in the rectus muscle with hyperdense foci corresponding to hemorrhage. In (b) axial T1-weighted, (c, d) sagittal and axial fat-suppressed T2-weighted MR images, the mass demonstrates areas of methemoglobin (hyperintense on the T1-weighted image) and a peripheral rim of hemosiderin (hypointense on all pulse sequences). (e) Axial post-contrast fat-suppressed T1-weighted MR image shows a central necrotic area.

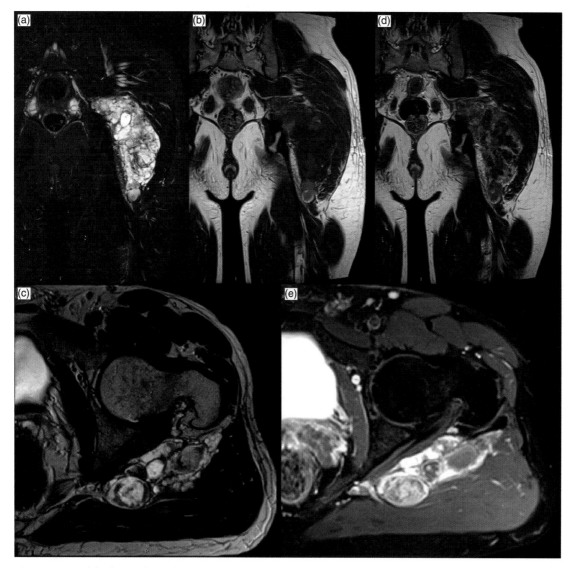

**Fig. 2-26.** Extraskeletal myxoid chondrosarcoma in a 42-year-old man. (a) Coronal fat-suppressed T2-weighted and (b) T1-weighted MR images, (c) axial T2-weighted, and (d, e) post-contrast T1-weighted MR images. The lesion is well defined, multilocular. On T1- and T2-weighted images, the signal intensity is heterogeneous. There are some myxoid and some hemorrhagic areas.

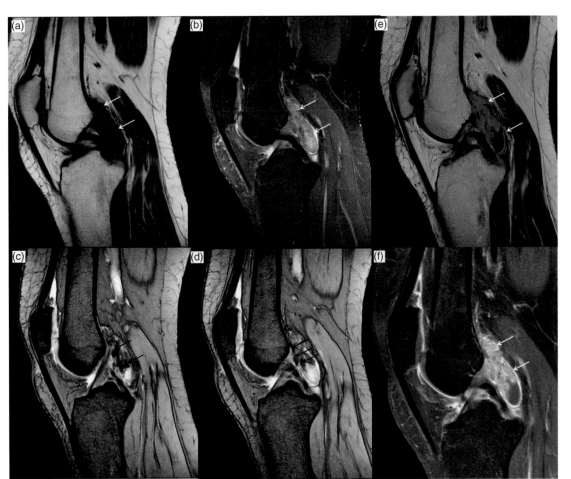

**Fig. 2-27.** Giant cell tumor of tendon sheath-diffuse type. (i.e., pigmented villonodular synovitis) in the knee of a 48-year-old woman. (a) Sagittal T1-weighted, (b) fat-suppressed T2-weighted, (c, d) T2*-weighted gradient-echo, and (e, f) post-contrast T1-weighted MR images showing a solid lesion (*white arrows*) behind the posterior cruciate ligament. Accentuated low signal intensity on T2*-weighted (*black arrows*) as compared with that on T2-weighted images is due to the presence of hemosiderin (susceptibility artefacts).

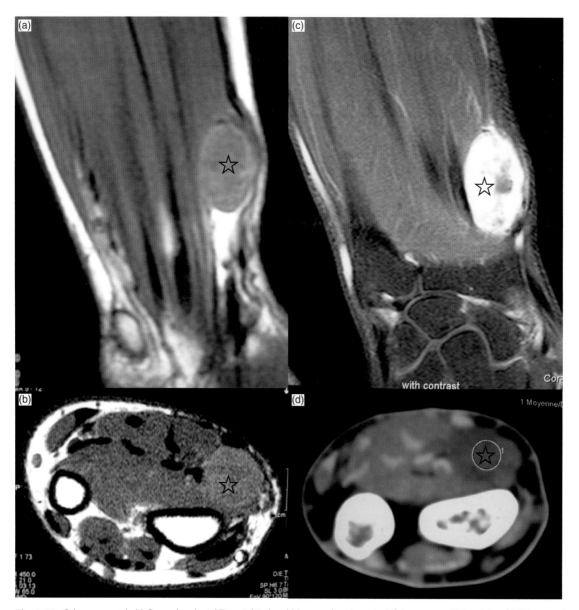

**Fig. 2-28.** Schwannoma. (a, b) Coronal and axial T1-weighted and (c) coronal post-contrast fat-suppressed T1-weighted MR images showing an intermuscular soft tissue mass that is hyperintense to skeletal muscle on T1-weighted MR images. The mass is hypodense to skeletal muscle on axial reformatted CT image (d). Myelin (lipids) contained in the tumor is partly responsible for the characteristics of signal intensity and density.

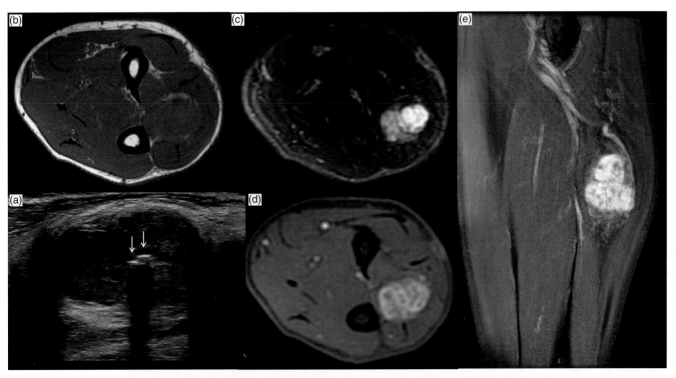

**Fig. 2-29.** Myoepithelioma of the left forearm in a 58-year-old male. (a) Ultrasonography, (B) axial T1-weighted, (c) axial fat-suppressed T2-weighted, and (d, e) post-contrast T1-weighted MR images showing a deep intermuscular mass with small calcifications (*white arrows in a*) and myxoid areas (*black arrows in c*).

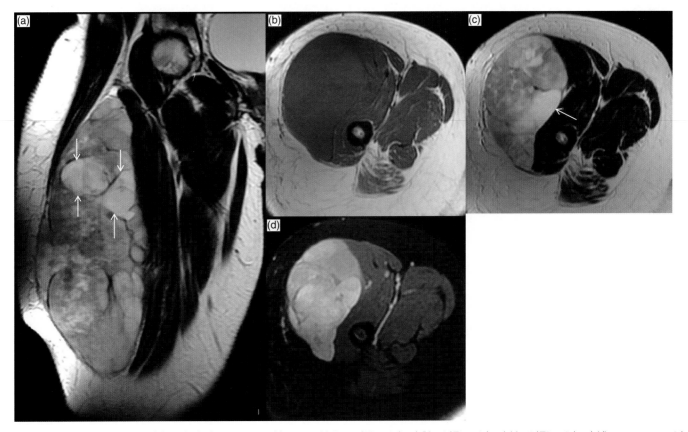

**Fig. 2-30.** Myxoid liposarcoma of the right thigh in a 42-year-old woman. (a) Coronal T2-weighted, (b) axial T1-weighted, (c) axial T2-weighted, (d) post-contrast axial T1-weighted MR images showing a deep, intermuscular soft tissue mass with myxoid areas (*arrows*). There is no fat visible on the T1-weighted image.

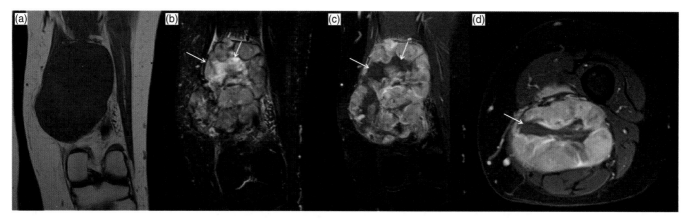

**Fig. 2-31.** Synovial sarcoma of the left thigh in a 73-year-old woman. (a) Coronal T1-weighted, (b) coronal fat-suppressed T2-weighted, and (c, d) post-contrast T1-weighted MR images showing a large intramuscular, lobulated soft tissue mass with necrotic areas (*arrows*).

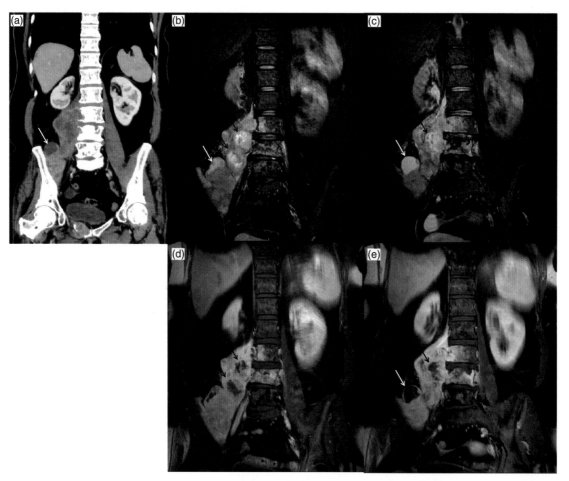

**Fig. 2-32.** Malignant peripheral nerve sheath tumor in a 55-year-old woman. (a) CT scan, (b, c) coronal fat-suppressed T2-weighted, and (d, e) coronal post-contrast T1-weighted MR images showing a large, right paravertebral soft tissue mass invading vertebral bodies and containing necrotic areas (*arrows*).

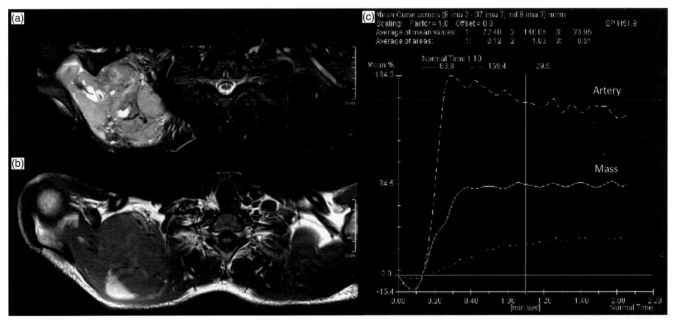

**Fig. 2-33.** Synovial sarcoma in a 27-year-old male. (a) Axial fat-suppressed T2-weighted and (b) axial T1-weighted MR images showing a huge heterogeneous mass of the right suprascapular fossa. (c) Dynamic contrast-enhanced curves: the dashed line corresponds to the artery, the solid line to the mass. The mass has an early enhancement and rapid progression of enhancement to an early plateau, in favor of malignancy.

## 3. What are the main diagnostic pitfalls?

In our experience, the main diagnostic errors in the radiologic diagnosis of soft tissue lesions are:

1. To misdiagnose a pseudocystic malignant tumor (myxoid liposarcoma, synovial sarcoma), especially when located in the vicinity of a joint, with a synovial cyst or a ganglia: always consider obtaining a gadolinium injection or an ultrasound examination.

2. To misdiagnose a bleeding tumor with a hematoma, especially in children: never accept the diagnosis of hematoma if there is no history of severe trauma; perform appropriate follow-up in doubtful cases.

3. To fail to recognize a myositis ossificans when MR imaging is the sole radiologic exam: always look at radiographs or CT exam when MR images show a large amount of edema. X-ray images will in fact demonstrate the characteristic ossifications after three weeks.

4. To fail to recognize an inflammatory reaction to calcium deposits when MR imaging is the sole radiologic exam: again always look at radiographs or CT exam when MR images show a large amount of edema.

5. To perform a biopsy without taking into account the surgical plan of a complete resection of the tumor. Such approach can affect the overall prognosis in case of a soft tissue sarcoma.

In conclusion, the diagnostic approach to pseudotumors and tumors of soft tissue is based on careful evaluation of both clinical data and imaging. The best strategy to reduce errors is to be systematic and to consider first the most common diagnoses. Key information includes age, past history, clinical context of occurrence, evolutionary pattern, unicity or multiplicity of lesions, the exact location and size of the lesion, and tissue composition. Radiologic criteria suggestive of malignancy need to be evaluated in the above-mentioned context.

## Chapter 2 Selected Key References

- Balach T, Stacy GS, Haydon RC. The clinical evaluation of soft tissue tumors. *Radiol Clin North Am.* 2011;**49**: 1185–96, vi.

- Calleja M, Dimigen M, Saifuddin A. MRI of superficial soft tissue masses: analysis of features useful in distinguishing between benign and malignant lesions. *Skeletal Radiol.* 2012;**41**:1517–24.

- Costa FM, Canella C, Gasparetto E. Advanced magnetic resonance imaging techniques in the evaluation of musculoskeletal tumors. *Radiol Clin North Am.* 2011;**49**:1325–58, vii–viii.

- Daniel A Jr, Ullah E, Wahab S, Kumar V Jr. Relevance of MRI in prediction of malignancy of musculoskeletal system—a prospective evaluation. *BMC Musculoskelet Disord.* 2009;**10**:125.

- Fayad LM, Jacobs MA, Wang X, Carrino JA, Bluemke DA. Musculoskeletal tumors: how to use anatomic, functional, and metabolic MR techniques. *Radiology.* 2012;**265**:340–56.

- Fayad LM, Mugera C, Soldatos T, Flammang A, del Grande F. Technical innovation in dynamic contrast-enhanced magnetic resonance imaging of musculoskeletal tumors: an MR angiographic sequence using a sparse k-space sampling strategy. *Skeletal Radiol.* 2013;**42**:993–1000.

- Hayashida Y, Hirai T, Yakushiji T, et al. Evaluation of diffusion-weighted imaging for the differential diagnosis of poorly contrast-enhanced and T2-prolonged bone masses: initial experience. *J Magn Reson Imaging.* 2006;**23**:377–82.

- Ilaslan H, Sundaram M. Advances in musculoskeletal tumor imaging. *Orthop Clin North Am.* 2006;**37**:375–391, vii.
- Kransdorf MJ, Murphey MD. *Imaging of Soft Tissue Tumors.* Philadelphia: W.B. Saunders Company; 1997. Chapter 2, Soft tissue tumors in a large referral population: prevalence and distribution of diagnoses by age, sex, and location; pp. 3–35.
- Kransdorf MJ, Murphey MD. Radiologic evaluation of soft-tissue masses: a current perspective. *AJR Am J Roentgenol.* 2000;**175**:575–87.
- Nagata S, Nishimura H, Uchida M, et al. Diffusion-weighted imaging of soft tissue tumors: usefulness of the apparent diffusion coefficient for differential diagnosis. *Radiat Med.* 2008;**26**:287–95.
- Papp DF, Khanna AJ, McCarthy EF, et al. Magnetic resonance imaging of soft-tissue tumors: determinate and indeterminate lesions. *J Bone Joint Surg Am.* 2007;**89** Suppl 3:103–15.
- Subhawong TK, Durand DJ, Thawait GK, Jacobs MA, Fayad LM. Characterization of soft tissue masses: can quantitative diffusion weighted imaging reliably distinguish cysts from solid masses? *Skeletal Radiol.* 2013;**42**: 1583–92.
- Thawait GK, Subhawong TK, Tatizawa Shiga NY, Fayad LM. "Cystic"-appearing soft tissue masses: what is the role of anatomic, functional, and metabolic MR imaging techniques in their characterization? *J Magn Reson Imaging.* 2014;**39**:504–11.
- van der Woude HJ, Verstraete KL, Hogendoorn PC, et al. Musculoskeletal tumors: does fast dynamic contrast-enhanced subtraction MR imaging contribute to the characterization? *Radiology.* 1998;**208**: 821–8.
- van Rijswijk CSP, Geirnaerdt MJA, Hogendoorn PCW, et al. Soft-tissue tumors: value of static and dynamic gadopentetate dimeglumine-enhanced MR imaging in prediction of malignancy. *Radiology.* 2004;**233**: 493–502.
- van Rijswijk CSP, Kunz P, Hogendoorn PCW, et al. Diffusion-weighted MRI in the characterization of soft-tissue tumors. *J Magn Reson Imaging.* 2002;**15**:302–7.
- Wu JS, Hochman MG. Soft-tissue tumors and tumorlike lesions: a systematic imaging approach. *Radiology.* 2009;**253**: 297–316.
- Yakushiji T, Oka K, Sato H, et al. Characterization of chondroblastic osteosarcoma: gadolinium-enhanced versus diffusion-weighted MR imaging. *J Magn Reson Imaging.* 2009;**29**:895–900.

# Principles of Local Therapy of Soft Tissue Neoplasms

Alessandro Gronchi MD

## Introduction

The surgical approach to adult soft tissue tumors has undergone significant changes over the past 10 years. A better understanding of the natural history of the different histologic subtypes, the importance of site, and the differing sensitivities to available drugs has opened the way to advances in the individualized treatment of most of them. The treatment strategy should ideally be planned at diagnosis and a decision for surgery be placed in the context of all other available therapies. The extent of surgery may vary broadly between the different histologic entities, and at times, surgery may be delayed or even omitted altogether. While surgery remains the standard and only potentially curative therapy in the management of localized soft tissue sarcomas (STSs) and gastrointestinal stromal tumors (GISTs), it is now postponed to a later line in desmoid fibromatosis (DF), if or until other available options fail. Although these three entities belong to the same overarching family of tumors, the natural histories, surgical principles, and sensitivity to locoregional and systemic therapies are completely different among them, and therefore they will be discussed separately.

## Surgery of Soft Tissue Sarcoma

Sarcomas usually present as solid masses. The periphery of the lesion is the most vital part of the mass. It is generally surrounded by a pseudocapsule of variable thickness consisting of compressed tumor cells embedded in a fibrovascular tissue, rarely associated with an inflammatory component, in continuity with the surrounding normal tissues. This is the reason why a simple excision, i.e., enucleation, cannot be curative, even if most sarcomas do not seem to infiltrate surrounding structures.

Indeed, sarcomas respect anatomic borders. Thus, the local anatomy influences tumor growth by setting natural barriers to their extension. In general, sarcomas take the path allowed by least-resistance anatomic planes and initially grow within the anatomic compartment in which they arose. Only at a later stage are the walls of that compartment violated (i.e., the cortex of a bone or the aponeurosis of a muscle), and the tumor breaks into another compartment. Soft tissue sarcomas may also arise between compartments (thus being extracompartmental) or in anatomic sites that are not walled off by anatomic barriers such as the intermuscular or subcutaneous planes. In the latter case, they remain extracompartmental and only at a later stage break into the adjacent compartment.

There are four basic types of excisions, depending on the relationship of the dissection plane to the surface of the tumor:

(1) An **intralesional** excision is performed within the tumor mass and results in removal of only a portion of it, so that macroscopic tumor is left behind. (2) In a **marginal** excision, the dissection plane crosses the pseudocapsule of the tumor. Such an excision may leave microscopic disease, and microscopic margins may be either positive or negative, depending on the type of tumor and surrounding tissues. (3) **Wide** excision entails removing the tumor with a cuff of circumferential healthy tissue. However, the adequate thickness of this cuff varies broadly according to the type of tissue. It should be of some centimeters along the longitudinal plane of the muscle. It can be 1 cm along the axial plane of the muscle. It can be a few millimeters, or even less, in proximity to tissues particularly resistant to tumor infiltration. These tissues are barriers because they tend to resist tumor invasion. They include muscular fascia, joint capsule, periosteum, epineurium, vascular adventitia, and peritoneum or pleura. If not infiltrated, the underlying structures can be safely preserved. If infiltrated, their removal should always be considered. (4) **Radical** resection implies removal of the tumor and the whole anatomic compartment in which it is located. Of course, a compartmental resection does not define per se the quality of surgical margins, because it can achieve a wide or a borderline margin, depending on how close the tumor is to the border of the compartment.

The quality of surgical margins is critical and ideally should always be evaluated by both the operating surgeon and the pathologist. The closest margin should be identified and extensively sampled. Microscopically, margins are defined as negative when the tumor edge is covered by at least 1 mm of healthy tissue or as positive when the tumor edge is covered by less than 1 mm of healthy tissue or is found at the inked surface.

In principle, the aim of surgery is to resect the tumor surrounded by healthy tissue and to avoid positive surgical margins. In fact, the risk of local failure doubles in case of positive margins, despite the use of postoperative radiation therapy (RT), with a subsequent impact on distant outcome and survival (Table 3A.1). While the initial prognosis mainly depends on the biology of the tumor, once a patient has "survived" the first period and the systemic risk dependent on tumor biology becomes weaker, the quality of surgery appears as the strongest prognosticator for outcome. Two factors can explain the impact of positive surgical margins on survival: a relatively slight increase in the risk of subsequent systemic spread in case of recurrence and a direct impact of local recurrence at some sites that may directly lead to death. In the case of pathologic positive margins, re-excision should

**Table 3A.1** Incidence of local recurrence, distant metastases, and death in major published series of extremities soft tissue sarcoma, according to microscopic surgical margins

| | 5-yr LR | | 5-yr DM | | 5-yr CSD | | 10-yr LR | | 10-yr DM | | 10-yr CSD | |
|---|---|---|---|---|---|---|---|---|---|---|---|---|
| | M + | M - | M + | M - | M + | M - | M + | M - | M + | M - | M + | M - |
| Trovik et al. (2000) | 36% | 18% | 28% | 28% | NR | NR | NR | NR | NR | NR | NR | NR |
| Zagars et al. (2003) | 36% | 12% | 25% | 28% | 31% | 25% | 44% | 14% | 33% | 33% | 39% | 34% |
| Stojadinovic et al. (2002) | 35% | 18% | 32% | 24% | 30% | 20% | NR | NR | NR | NR | NR | NR |
| Gronchi et al. (2010) | 26% | 10% | 20% | 21% | 29% | 16% | 30% | 12% | 24% | 24% | 38% | 19% |

**Legends:**
LR: incidence of local recurrence
DM: incidence of distant metastases
CSD: incidence of disease-specific death
M+: positive microscopic surgical margins
M–: negative microscopic surgical margins
NR: Not recorded

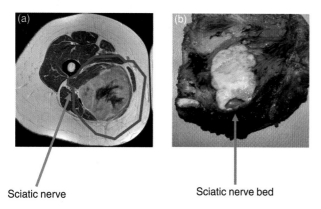

Sciatic nerve

Sciatic nerve bed

**Fig. 3A-1.** In tumors of the extremities, surgical resection involves surrounding soft tissues, mainly muscles, subcutaneous fat, and skin. Radiologic imaging (a) and surgical specimen (b).

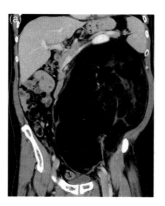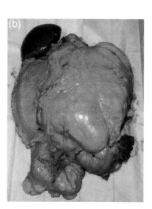

**Fig. 3A-2.** In the retroperitoneum, to reduce the risk of microscopically positive margins tumors should be resected en bloc with adjacent viscera even when not overtly involved. Radiologic imaging (a) and surgical specimen (b).

always be considered whenever feasible. This does not apply when a positive margin is planned in advance to preserve an important structure for function-sparing (i.e., a motor nerve), provided adequate RT is delivered (especially in the preoperative setting).

The same principles should be applied to tumors located outside the limbs and trunk wall, although wide margins may be more difficult to obtain and a careful balance between morbidity and chances of cure should always be made on a case-by-case basis.

The ability to reconstruct large defects by pedicled or free flaps; to restore function by replacing bone, vessels, and nerves; and to perform major visceral resections, whenever needed to improve quality of surgery, should be part of proper planning before the surgical procedure is undertaken. Therefore, a careful multidisciplinary approach is needed in all cases for proper treatment delivery.

In extremities and trunk walls, surgery basically implies the resection of surrounding soft tissues, mainly muscles,

subcutaneous fat, and skin (Fig. 3A-1). The necessity to cover the soft tissue loss by a flap transposition depends on several factors, such as the site and size of the defect, exposed structures (bone, vessels, nerves), functional restoring. Vessels, nerves, and bone are always resected when directly invaded/encased, while their resection has to be discussed on a case-by-case basis when their periostium, adventitia, epineurium are infiltrated without invasion of the underlying structure.

Similar principles apply to surgery of retroperitoneal sarcomas. In fact, unlike primary epithelial solid tumors, which are usually confined to a single organ and can generally be removed with resection of that organ, retroperitoneal STS commonly abuts multiple surrounding organs. Paralleling surgery in extremities, tumors should be systematically resected en bloc with surrounding tissues, which at this site are mainly the adjacent viscera, even when not overtly involved, to minimize the risk of microscopically positive margins (Fig. 3A-2) Indeed, not all uninvolved adjacent viscera/structures are routinely resected en bloc with the tumor. The objective is to

**Table 3A.2** Local recurrence-free survival and overall survival in major published series of retroperitoneal soft tissue sarcoma

| | Study period | Median FU | N. patients | Complete resection (%) | 5-yr LRFS | 5-yr OS |
|---|---|---|---|---|---|---|
| Tan et al., 2015 | 1982–2010 | 40 | 675 | 91 | 61 | 69 |
| Stoeckle et al., 2001 | 1980–1994 | 47 | 165 | 65 | 42 | 49 |
| Ferrario et al., 2003 | 1977–2001 | 41 | 79 | 99 | 43 | 65 |
| Hassan et al., 2004 | 1983–1995 | 36 | 97 | 78 | 56 | 51 |
| Lehnert et al., 2009 | 1998–2002 | 89 | 71 | 70 | 59 | 65 |
| **Gronchi et al., 2015** | 2002–2011 | 44 | 377 | 96 | 76 | 65 |

**Legends:**
FU: follow-up
N.: number
LRFS: local recurrence-free survival
OS: overall survival

Disease-specific survival, in bold: series of patients systematically resected by an extended approach.

achieve a wide microscopic margin along most surfaces, even by removing additional organs, while performing what is essentially a marginal excision along critical structures. In general, the ipsilateral kidney, colon, and mesocolon and at least a portion of the psoas can be safely and relatively easily resected without serious consequences. Resection of the pancreatic body and tail and spleen can usually be performed with a relatively low, short-term morbidity. Resection of other structures, including but not limited to the aorta, inferior vena cava, iliac vessels, femoral nerve, diaphragm, duodenum, head of the pancreas, uncinate process, liver, and bone (specifically, vertebral bodies), entails significant resections, with ensuing greater morbidity, so that it is not performed unless macroscopic invasion is documented. This extended approach has been systematically adopted only in recent years, with a significant improvement in local control in all patients and of survival in patients affected by low-/intermediate-grade sarcomas, whose outcome had been dominated by inoperable local recurrences (Table 3A.2).

Similar principles also apply, as long as it is feasible, to tumors at other sites (mediastinum, head, and neck), a systematic description of which goes beyond the scope of the present text.

Because the STS family is made up of at least 50 histologic subtypes, these general principles can be applied differently in selected subtypes, as follows.

## Atypical Lipomatous Tumor/Well-Differentiated Liposarcoma

This low-grade tumor, when arising in the extremity, has a relatively low rate of recurrence, may not recur for a relatively long interval, and has minimal or no risk of distant metastatic spread and death, unless dedifferentiation occurs. In fact, dedifferentiation in general entails a risk of metastatic spread as high as 20%, but in extremities, dedifferentiation develops only rarely (less than 5% of cases). In other words, a well-differentiated liposarcoma in extremities only occasionally poses a life threat. Furthermore, low-grade recurrent atypical lipomatous tumors (ALTs) may grow slowly for years. Therefore, such tumors can be resected with a modest positive margin, especially when preserving limb function is an issue. The same low-grade tumor, however, becomes a life-threatening disease when located at the retroperitoneum, even if lacking areas of dedifferentiation. In fact, as discussed, local control is an issue for retroperitoneal sarcomas, and patients often die of local regional failures without developing distant metastases. An extended surgical resection for well-differentiated liposarcoma located at this site is therefore recommended.

## Myxoid/Round Cell Liposarcoma

This tumor predominantly occurs in the extremities. It can be found even in the trunk, but almost always as a metastasis from a primary lesion located in the extremities. Pure myxoid liposarcoma rarely metastasizes, whereas the risk increases when a hypercellular component is present in more than 5% of the tumor. At variance with most other sarcomas, metastases can occur in the soft tissues, abdomen, mediastinum, and bone before affecting the lung. Chemotherapy and RT may be particularly active. Therefore, preoperative therapies, either by single or combined modalities, are often offered to reduce surgical morbidity and increase chances of cure.

## Dermatofibrosarcoma Protuberans

Dermatofibrosarcoma protuberans (DFSP) is a superficial tumor that infiltrates soft tissues far beyond the obvious margins of the lesion and can recur locally following inadequate resection. However, the more common variety of DFSP has no metastatic potential. The goal of surgery should be to achieve negative margins, often necessitating reconstruction by plastic surgery. When cosmetic/function preservation is an issue, limited positive margins may be accepted, and a wider resection postponed when there is a recurrence. Because DFSP is usually relatively superficial, resection of the underlying muscles is often unnecessary. In approximately 5–10% of patients with DFSP, the tumor presents as a more aggressive fibrosarcomatous variant (FS-DFSP), which may more often recur locally and potentially spread. These patients should be treated as are those having a "conventional" sarcoma, limited positive margins being only occasionally acceptable.

## Leiomyosarcoma

This sarcoma may arise from skin, soft tissues, visceral organs, or vessels and it is one of the most common histologic subtypes. The approach to skin leiomyosarcoma is easy, because the invasion of surrounding tissues is limited and the metastatic potential almost nil. On the contrary, deep-seated soft tissue leiomyosarcomas often present as large masses and have a systemic risk as high as 50%. An extended soft tissue en bloc resection with the mass is required. Adjuvant treatments are often discussed with the patient, although their impact on local and distant outcomes is limited. Gastrointestinal (GI) leiomyosarcomas are rare. They are treated by resection of the affected GI tract. Adjacent organs are resected only if directly infiltrated. They typically have a high metastatic risk and spread to the liver before other organs. Vascular leiomyosarcomas predominantly arise from veins and often abut outside the vessel extending in the soft tissues. The affected vascular tract should be resected en bloc with adjacent soft tissues. Intravascular tumor thrombi may be present and should be removed en bloc with the disease. Frozen margin specimens over the vessel should be taken to ensure free margins. The metastatic risk is significant, although a fraction of them may have a long natural history and can also be cured.

## Pleomorphic Liposarcoma, Unclassified Pleomorphic Sarcoma, Synovial Sarcoma

These tumors, although different from a histologic and biologic standpoint, are usually approached in the same manner. They predominantly affect the extremities and present as large and deeply located masses. They have a significant metastatic risk and are often treated by combined modalities. The surgical approach consists of the standard procedures described above.

## Myxofibrosarcoma

This malignant tumor, when located superficially, infiltrates through soft tissue (subcutaneous fat and investing fascia) far beyond the ostensible margins of the visible or palpable mass. When located intramuscularly, the extension of the infiltration tends to be limited by anatomic barriers, although it has a higher propensity to invade them as compared with other histologic subtypes. Myxofibrosarcoma most commonly arises in the extremities of elderly individuals. It demonstrates a 30% rate of local recurrence and a 16% rate of distant recurrence. Eventually, multiple local recurrences may lead to amputation. Therefore, it is critical to pursue aggressive local therapy. Wide surgical margins ($\geq 2$ cm beyond the clinical boundaries of the palpable mass in general and up to 4 cm for those that are superficial) should be the goal of surgery, which often requires complex wound closure or flap reconstruction by a plastic and reconstructive surgeon, as well as resection/reconstruction of vessels/nerves. Radiation therapy, either preoperatively or postoperatively (described below), may be considered.

## Malignant Peripheral Nerve Sheath Tumor

These tumors often arise from a major peripheral nerve, which can be identified macroscopically. They can occur sporadically or in the context of neurofibromatosis type 1 (NF1) syndrome. Malignant peripheral nerve sheath tumor is marked by an early propensity for distant metastases. When originating from a peripheral nerve, they also may spread along the nerve fibers proximally or distally. Wider margins at this level should be obtained (if possible, at least 4 cm of macroscopic healthy nerve) to limit locoregional failure, which eventually may reach the spinal cord. Frozen section intraoperative pathologic examination may help ensure the accomplishment of clear margins over the nerve stumps.

## Angiosarcoma

Management of primary and radiation-associated (secondary) angiosarcoma is challenging because of the multifocality of this disease. Angiosarcoma of the scalp is a particularly insidious malignancy. While radical surgery is possible (requiring complex flap reconstructions), it is not uncommon for patients to develop local recurrences immediately outside the margins of resection, even if the margins of the initial resection were widely negative, with or without radiation therapy. Angiosarcoma is sensitive to systemic chemotherapy and to radiation therapy. Because surgery is rarely curative, it should not be considered as the only treatment of choice, especially for scalp angiosarcoma. Surgery may be reserved for patients who are experiencing problems with local control (bleeding from a fungating tumor) or who only appear to have a solitary site of disease by both clinical examination and imaging while undergoing systemic therapy.

## Epithelioid and Clear Cell Sarcomas

Both these tumors tend to affect young adults and to occur in distal extremities. At variance with all other histologic subtypes, they may give rise to in-transit metastasis along the affected limb and to locoregional lymph node metastases. Accurate staging of the whole limb is mandatory, and sentinel lymph node biopsy should be considered as part of the routine approach to primary disease. Their sensitivity to conventional chemotherapy is at best limited. A more aggressive variant of epithelioid sarcoma, called proximal-type epithelioid sarcoma, tends to occur to the limb roots and the trunk. This variant behaves as a very aggressive sarcoma, having a high risk of hematogenous distant spread. Locoregional lymph nodes can be rarely involved. Its sensitivity to conventional chemotherapy is higher, but fast progression after response is often observed.

If a preoperative treatment is planned, the status of the disease must be carefully monitored.

## Radiation-Induced Sarcomas

Radiation-induced sarcomas are rare and include a variety of histologic subtypes, the most common of which are pleomorphic undifferentiated sarcoma, angiosarcoma, malignant peripheral nerve sheath tumor, and leiomyosarcoma. Along with the inherent characteristics of each histologic subtype, they are all marked by a high propensity to recur locally, given the difficulty in obtaining clear margins. In fact, it is very difficult to distinguish tumor infiltration of healthy tissues from radiation-induced changes around the tumor site. The lesion should be excised with as much surrounding tissue as possible. Often, if not always, this requires plastic surgery and liberal vascular-nerves resection and reconstruction. Systemic chemotherapy and re-irradiation are often considered, given the overall dismal prognosis.

## Surgery of Gastrointestinal Stromal Tumor

Gastrointestinal stromal tumors (GISTs) commonly arise in the stomach (50–70%), small intestine (25–35%), colon and rectum (5–10%), mesentery or omentum (7%), and esophagus (<5%).

In the past 12 years, the understanding and treatment of GISTs has witnessed remarkable advances because of two key developments: (1) the identification of constitutively active signals (oncogenic mutation of the c-KIT and platelet-derived growth factor alpha [PDGFRA] genes encoding receptor tyrosine kinases) and (2) the development of therapeutic agents that suppress tumor growth by specifically targeting and inhibiting this signal, resulting in improved outcomes (imatinib mesylate, sunitinib malate, and regorafenib). The advent of effective therapy has dramatically improved outcomes for patients with GIST. Nevertheless, surgery remains the only potentially curative therapy for patients with localized GIST.

In general, surgery is a wedge or segmental resection of the involved gastric or intestinal tract, with margins, which can be narrower than those required for an adenocarcinoma. Lymphadenectomy is not routinely required, because lymph nodes are rarely involved (in adult patients) and are thus resected only when they are clinically detectable. Sometimes, a more extensive resection (total gastrectomy for a large proximal gastric GIST, pancreaticoduodenectomy for a periampullary GIST, or abdominoperineal resection for a low rectal GIST) is needed.

Indeed, all GISTs greater than 2 cm in size should be resected when possible, as none of them can be considered "benign." The management of GISTs under 2 cm is more questionable. Although the low risk of progression of GISTs under 2 cm offers the possibility of a more conservative approach, a reliable mitotic index cannot be determined by biopsy or fine-needle aspiration (FNA), thus preventing the identification of those at higher risk. Therefore, both observation and resection for GISTs of 1 to 2 cm can well be considered, and the risks and benefits of one versus the other should

be discussed with the patient. Endoscopic resection of small gastric GISTs could be an option in these presentations. Risks of perforation may be low in highly experienced hands, although the decision is made on a case-by-case basis. Regardless of their size, any small GIST that is symptomatic (e.g., bleeding from erosions through the mucosa) or increases in size on serial follow-up should be resected.

Open or laparoscopic/laparoscopy-assisted resection of primary GISTs should be performed following standard oncologic principles. Although primary GISTs may demonstrate inflammatory adhesions to surrounding organs, true invasion is infrequent. The goal of surgery is a macroscopically complete en bloc excision. A macroscopically complete resection with negative or microscopically positive margins (R0 or R1 resection, respectively) is associated with a better prognosis than is a macroscopically incomplete resection (R2 resection). Available series have demonstrated that R1 resection patients are at no greater risk of local failure than are patients who undergo R0 resections, with or without adjuvant imatinib, so re-excision for a microscopically positive margin is rarely if ever indicated. One exception is rectal GIST, in which microscopically involved surgical margins appear to be associated with a higher risk of local failure and death. In general, though, local relapse after R0 surgery is very unlikely in GIST. In discussing margins with the patient and the pathologist, it is important to understand that most exophytic tumors are simply covered by a thin layer of peritoneum over a portion of the tumor, and thus it is not surprising that there is a high rate of peritoneal relapse even after R0/R1 surgery. Tumor rupture or violation of the tumor capsule during surgery is associated with a very high risk of recurrence, essentially equivalent to that of metastatic disease, and therefore should be avoided.

Given the extensive use of adjuvant therapy with imatinib in the high-risk populations and the activity of the drug, the use of preoperative imatinib should be considered before undertaking any major surgical procedure. This is particularly true for tumors located at critical sites, such as the esophagogastric junction, the duodenum, and the rectum (Fig. 3A-3), reducing the need for a complex operation. It may also be considered for large tumors at risk of rupture or for large tumors where tumor shrinkage may enable a minimally invasive approach. Retrospective single- and multiple-institution series as well as few prospective studies have shown how this approach is safe and able to minimize surgical morbidity. Neoadjuvant imatinib is currently recommended by all available guidelines whenever surgical morbidity is not considered to be minimal. The only drawback is the impossibility to calculate the risk of recurrence and therefore adapt the need of further adjuvant therapy, because the mitotic rate on the surgical specimen is inevitably influenced by the preoperative therapy. All patients who undergo neoadjuvant imatinib are therefore considered at high risk.

In the rare syndromic GIST (either succinate dehydrogenase [SDH]-deficient or NF1-related), tumors are often multifocal and confined either to the stomach (SDH-deficient GIST) or the small bowel (NF1-related GIST). The extent of surgery should be determined on a case-by-case basis, taking into

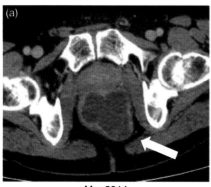 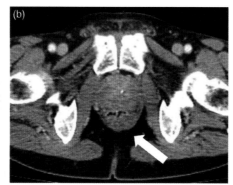

Mar 2014                    Feb 2015

**Fig. 3A-3.** The use of preoperative imatinib should be considered for tumors located at critical sites, such as the rectum, in order to achieve conservative surgery. Radiologic imaging of rectal GIST before (a) and after imatinib therapy (b).

account the risk of recurrence, the lack of benefit from available tyrosine kinase inhibitors (TKIs), and the actual behavior of the underlying disease.

## Surgery of Desmoid-Type Fibromatosis

Sporadic desmoid fibromatosis (DF) predominantly affects young adults, especially females, and although it may be observed in nearly every part of the body, it often involves the extremities (including pelvic and shoulder girdles), the trunk (i.e. abdominal wall), and the abdominal cavity (mainly within the mesentery or the pelvis). Familial adenomatous polyposis (FAP)-associated desmoids are predominantly located within the abdomen and have no gender predilection; the natural history is often complicated by previous surgery for FAP.

Historically, surgery (alone or in association with radiation therapy) was considered the mainstay of treatment, but was associated with considerable morbidity and high recurrence rates even after apparently adequate local treatment. The observation in more contemporary series that microscopic surgical margins were not significantly associated with higher local recurrence rate led to a reassessment of overall management, and preservation of function has now become the main priority. Furthermore, some patients experienced spontaneous stabilization or occasional regression of their tumors, even after multiple recurrences. Therefore, investigators proposed to further limit morbidity by considering an initial "wait and see" policy in all patients, including those with primary tumors, especially when surgery would have resulted in some functional loss.

In parallel with these observations, it became evident that DF is not a single disease but rather at least two entities quite different in behavior. Some DFs are marked by an indolent behavior and others can be locally aggressive, but predicting behavior is challenging. The more indolent tumors typically do not recur regardless of margins because of their natural tendency to regress or remain stable, whereas aggressive lesions do recur despite the adequacy of surgical resection and, of course, more commonly after margin-positive resections.

Several recent retrospective series have consistently shown progression-free survival rates of 60% at 5 years for patients managed with a front-line, conservative, "watchful waiting" approach. Although these initial observations demonstrate the potential safety of such an approach, it is important to emphasize that these patients remained under close observation, such that no patient was lost to follow-up and treatment plans could be altered if tumors progressed. Increase in size was usually mild and occurred in the first 2 years. Spontaneous regressions were also observed in as many as 20–30% of cases. There may be sites where regression is more common and observation may be safer (i.e., the abdominal wall). Nevertheless, regression has been observed at all sites. Therefore, it is reasonable to consider watchful waiting as an initial step when asymptomatic tumors are located at critical sites (i.e., mesentery), before undertaking subsequent treatments.

When the observational approach fails, surgery is still a valid option. When performed, surgical resection should be aimed at obtaining microscopic negative margins, although function preservation – especially for tumors located in the extremities and girdles – should always be taken into consideration and other alternatives, including radiation therapy, considered when appropriate. Furthermore, large sporadic mesenteric/retroperitoneal desmoid tumors may be treated by surgical resection just because of their size and possible related symptoms.

Therefore, in the absence of biologic prognostic factors capable of predicting the natural history of the disease, watchful waiting is a reasonable approach to minimize overtreatment and unnecessary morbidity in a subset of patients with desmoid tumors while secondarily also potentially limiting the costs of treatment.

Prospective observational studies are currently under way to validate these results and possibly shed more light on the biologic background of this intriguing disease (ClinicalTrials.gov Identifier: NCT01801176).

## Radiation Therapy

Radiation therapy is commonly used in soft tissue sarcoma and, occasionally, in desmoid-type fibromatosis either as an adjuvant or as a definitive treatment, although it is never used in localized GIST.

## Radiation Therapy of Soft Tissue Sarcoma

In general, limb-sparing surgery relies on the adjuvant administration of radiation therapy, to minimize risk of local recurrence, as demonstrated in two pivotal trials, one with brachytherapy and one with postoperative external beam radiotherapy (EBRT). Radiation therapy reduces the risk of local recurrence from greater than 30% to less than 10% in most series, but does not impact distant failure or overall survival.

External beam radiotherapy may be delivered preoperatively or postoperatively. When given preoperatively, the goal is to treat the margins to minimize the risk of recurrence, not necessarily to reduce the size of the tumor per se. A randomized comparison between preoperative and postoperative EBRT has been performed. There was no difference in local recurrence rates. Preoperative external beam radiotherapy was associated with a doubling in the rate of wound complications (35% vs. 17%), but with a lower rate of late complications and tissue fibrosis and better functional outcomes. The postoperative approach generally covers a larger field (including drain sites) and uses a higher dose than does the preoperative approach. This is particularly important in young adults of childbearing age with proximal thigh STS: preoperative EBRT may spare the gonads, whereas postoperative radiation may not.

Moreover, data from retrospective series suggest that the administration of preoperative radiation therapy minimizes the risk of limited close or positive margins. Therefore, whenever preservation of function is a goal and the tumor abuts critical structures, the administration of preoperative EBRT should be considered.

Brachytherapy may be delivered through after-loading catheters placed across the tumor bed at the end of surgery. Its goal is to deliver additional radiation to a close margin (including neurovascular structures) with minimal treatment to surrounding tissue, particularly when further external beam radiotherapy is no longer feasible. When the final pathologic margins are confirmed, the appropriate catheters may be loaded with radioactive seeds once or twice a day for a defined treatment period concentrated over the close margins. To minimize wound complications, catheters should not be loaded until at least postoperative day five. To minimize the risk of dislodging the catheters, any drains placed at the time of surgery should remain in place until the catheters have been removed.

Intraoperative radiation therapy (IORT) has also been studied in extremity STS, but it has failed to improve results of conventional external beam radiotherapy. It is therefore not routinely used in clinical practice.

Patients with small (<5 cm), superficial, well-circumscribed STS resected with a wide margin (>1 cm) of non-neoplastic tissue or a biologic barrier (fascia) may not require RT, provided that they can be reliably followed for local recurrence. The same may apply to low-grade tumors, independent of tumor location and size. Of note, high-grade myxoid liposarcoma and angiosarcoma are more sensitive to external beam radiotherapy than all other histologic subtypes. Therefore, this approach is more liberally used in patients affected by these histotypes, especially in the preoperative setting.

In retroperitoneal sarcomas (RPSs), the role of radiation therapy is controversial in the absence of phase III randomized controlled trial data. Whereas it unequivocally reduces the risk of local recurrence in patients with extremity STS, this has not been proved in RPS. Furthermore, the proximity of radiosensitive tissues and organs, such as the liver and small intestine, together with the large size of the radiation field, limits its utility. Those who utilize radiation therapy generally deliver it preoperatively, when the bulk of the tumor itself displaces uninvolved organs out of the radiation field. There is one ongoing randomized trial assessing the efficacy of preoperative RT in patients with RPS.

## Radiation Therapy of Desmoid-Type Fibromatosis

When surgery is performed, adjuvant radiation therapy can be considered. In general, in the case of R0 resections, there is no indication for postoperative radiotherapy. If, however, R1 or R2 resection status is achieved, patients should be monitored preferentially, as there is a lack of correlation between positive margins and local recurrence. Adjuvant radiotherapy may be an option for patients operated on for recurrent disease, especially if located at critical sites. The average desmoid fibromatosis patient is young, with an anticipated life expectancy of decades and can therefore be subject to late radiation-induced morbidity including secondary malignancies. Moreover, intra-abdominal localizations are not candidates for radiotherapy.

In the case of patients with symptomatic and/or progressive disease in whom surgery would result in significant morbidity and for whom medical therapy has failed, radiotherapy can be considered as a single-agent regimen.

Radiotherapy at a dose of 56 grays (Gy) in 28 once-daily fractions of 2 Gy has been shown to provide adequate local control in the majority of progressive patients. There is no statistically significant difference in local control between radiotherapy regimens above or below 56 Gy, but there is a significant increase in late radiation-related morbidity above 56 Gy. Local complete remissions are seen in 13.6–17% of cases, partial remissions and disease stabilization in 51–77.3% of cases, and local failures and/or recurrences in 18.5–32% of cases. However, the risk/benefit ratio must be discussed with the patient.

## Isolated Limb Perfusion

Isolated limb perfusion as a treatment modality is worth mentioning, as it is reserved for limb-threatening, soft tissue sarcomas and progressive extremity desmoid-type fibromatosis resistant to conventional treatments. This procedure involves placing vascular access catheters into the main artery and vein of the affected extremity and perfusing it with high-dose chemotherapy (usually melphalan) and tumor necrosis factor alpha (TNF-α) under hyperthermic conditions. Isolated limb perfusion is generally performed as an open procedure with cutdown directly onto the vessel and is delivered in the neoadjuvant setting.

Isolated limb perfusion with chemotherapy alone has uniformly failed in the treatment of unresectable extremity STSs. The addition of TNF-α to this treatment approach has proved to be critical in improving the outcome of locally advanced extremity STS.

Tumor necrosis factor alpha has both an early and a late effect; it enhances tumor-selective drug uptake during perfusion and also plays an essential role in the subsequent selective destruction of the tumor vasculature. These effects result in a high response rate, which translates into limb salvage in most cases. Several single institution reports have confirmed the safety and efficacy of this procedure.

## Chapter 3A Selected Key References

- Abraham JA, Weaver MJ, Hornick JL, Zurakowski D, Ready JE. Outcomes and prognostic factors for a consecutive case series of 115 patients with somatic leiomyosarcoma. *J Bone Joint Surg Am.* 2012;**94**(8):736–44.

- Aggarwal G, Sharma S, Zheng M, et al. Primary leiomyosarcomas of the gastrointestinal tract in the post-gastrointestinal stromal tumor era. *Ann Diagn Pathol.* 2012;**16**(6):532–40.

- Al Yami A, Griffin AM, Ferguson PC, et al. Positive surgical margins in soft tissue sarcoma treated with preoperative radiation: is a postoperative boost necessary? *Int J Radiat Oncol Biol Phys.* 2010;**77**:1191–7.

- Andreou D, Boldt H, Werner M, et al. Sentinel node biopsy in soft tissue sarcoma subtypes with a high propensity for regional lymphatic spread – results of a large prospective trial. *Ann Oncol.* 2013;**24**:1400–5.

- Anghileri M, Miceli R, Fiore M, et al. Malignant peripheral nerve sheath tumors: prognostic factors and survival in a series of patients treated at a single institution. *Cancer.* 2006;**107**:1065–74.

- Antonescu CR, Tschernyavsky SJ, Decuseara R, et al. Prognostic impact of P53 status, TLS-CHOP fusion transcript structure, and histological grade in myxoid liposarcoma: a molecular and clinicopathologic study of 82 cases. *Clin Cancer Res.* 2001;**7**:3977–87.

- Ballo MT, Zagars GK, Pollack A, et al: Desmoid tumor: prognostic factors and outcome after surgery, radiation therapy, or combined surgery and radiation therapy. *J Clin Oncol.* 1999;**17**:158–67.

- Baratti D, Pennacchioli E, Casali PG, et al. Epithelioid sarcoma: prognostic factors and survival in a series of patients treated at a single institution. *Ann Surg Oncol.* 2007;**14**:3542–51.

- Barnett CM, Corless CL, Heinrich MC. Gastrointestinal stromal tumors: molecular markers and genetic subtypes. *Hematol Oncol Clin North Am.* 2013;**27**: 871–88.

- Bonvalot S, Desai A, Coppola S, et al. The treatment of desmoid tumors: a stepwise clinical approach. *Ann Oncol.* 2012; **23** Suppl 10:x158–66.

- Bonvalot S, Eldweny H, Haddad V, et al. Extra-abdominal primary fibromatosis: aggressive management could be avoided in a subgroup of patients. *Eur J Surg Oncol.* 2008;**34**:462–8.

- Bonvalot S, Miceli R, Berselli M, et al. Aggressive surgery in retroperitoneal soft tissue sarcoma carried out at high-volume centers is safe and is associated with improved local control. *Ann Surg Oncol.* 2010;**17**:1507–14.

- Bonvalot S, Raut CP, Pollock RE, et al. Technical considerations in surgery for retroperitoneal sarcomas: position paper from E-Surge, a Master Class in Sarcoma Surgery, and EORTC–STBSG. *Ann Surg Oncol.* 2012;**19**:2981–91.

- Bonvalot S, Rivoire M, Castaing M, et al. Primary retroperitoneal sarcomas: a multivariate analysis of surgical factors associated with local control. *J Clin Oncol.* 2009;**27**:31–7.

- Bonvalot S, Ternes N, Fiore M, et al. Spontaneous regression of primary abdominal wall desmoids: more common than previously thought. *Ann Surg Oncol.* 2013; **20**:4096–102.

- Brunicardi FC, Andersen DK, Billiar TR, et al. Soft tissue sarcomas. In: Cormier JN, Gronchi A, Pollock RE, editors. *Schwartz's Principles of Surgery.* 10th ed. New York: McGraw-Hill Education; 2015.

- Bruno M, Carucci P, Repici A, et al. The natural history of gastrointestinal subepithelial tumors arising from muscularis propria: an endoscopic ultrasound survey. *J Clin Gastroenterol.* 2009;**43**:821–5.

- Cai H, Wang Y, Wu J, Shi Y. Dermatofibrosarcoma protuberans: clinical diagnoses and treatment results of 260 cases in China. *J Surg Oncol.* 2012;**105** (2):142–8.

- Callegaro D, Fiore M, Gronchi A. Personalizing surgical margins in retroperitoneal sarcoma. *Exp Rev Anticancer Ther.* 2015;**15**(5):553–67.

- Canter RJ, Qin LX, Maki RG, et al. A synovial sarcoma-specific preoperative nomogram supports a survival benefit to ifosfamide-based chemotherapy and improves risk stratification for patients. *Clin Cancer Res.* 2008;**14**:8191–7.

- Carneiro A, Francis P, Bendahl PO, et al. Indistinguishable genomic profiles and shared prognostic markers in undifferentiated pleomorphic sarcoma and leiomyosarcoma: different sides of a single coin? *Lab Invest.* 2009;**89**:668–75.

- Chung PW, Deheshi BM, Ferguson PC, et al. Radiosensitivity translates into excellent local control in extremity myxoid liposarcoma: a comparison with other soft tissue sarcomas. *Cancer.* 2009;**115**:3254–61.

- Colombo C, Miceli R, Collini P, et al. Leiomyosarcoma and sarcoma with myogenic differentiation: two different entities or two faces of the same disease? *Cancer.* 2012;**118**(21):5349–57.

- Colombo C, Miceli R, Le Péchoux C, et al. Sporadic extra abdominal wall desmoid-type fibromatosis: surgical resection can be safely limited to a minority of patients. *Eur J Cancer.* 2015;**51**(2):186–92.

- Colombo C, Randall RL, Andtbacka RH, Gronchi A. A new surgical perspective in soft tissue sarcoma (STS) management: more conservative in ESTS (extremity soft tissue sarcoma), more extended in RSTS (retroperitoneal soft tissue sarcoma). *Expert Rev Anticancer Ther.* 2012;**12**:1079–87.

- Dagan R, Indelicato DJ, McGee L, et al. The significance of a marginal excision after preoperative radiation therapy for soft tissue sarcoma of the extremity. *Cancer.* 2012;**118**(12):3199–207.

- Delaney TF. Radiation therapy: neoadjuvant, adjuvant, or not at all. *Surg Oncol Clinics N Am.* 2012 **21**:215–41.

- Demetri GD, Reichardt P, Kang YK, et al. on behalf of all GRID study investigators. Efficacy and safety of regorafenib for advanced gastrointestinal stromal tumours after failure of imatinib and sunitinib (GRID): an international, multicentre, randomised, placebo-controlled, phase 3 trial. *Lancet.* 2013;**381**:295–302.

- Demetri GD, van Oosterom AT, Garrett CR, et al. Efficacy and safety of sunitinib in patients with advanced gastrointestinal stromal tumour after failure of imatinib: a randomised controlled trial. *Lancet.* 2006;**368**:1329–38.

- Deroose JP, Eggermont AM, van Geel AN, et al. Long-term results of tumor necrosis factor alpha- and melphalan-based isolated limb perfusion in locally advanced extremity soft tissue sarcomas. *J Clin Oncol.* 2011;**29**:4036–44.

- Enneking WF, Spanier SS, Malawer MM. The effect of the anatomic setting on the results of surgical procedures for soft parts sarcoma of the thigh. *Cancer.* 1981;**47**(5):1005–22.

- ESMO / European Sarcoma Network Working Group. Gastrointestinal stromal tumors: ESMO Clinical Practice Guidelines for diagnosis, treatment and follow-up. *Ann Oncol.* 2014a;**25** Suppl 3: iii21–6.

- ESMO / European Sarcoma Network Working Group. Soft tissue and visceral sarcomas: ESMO Clinical Practice Guidelines for diagnosis, treatment and follow-up. *Ann Oncol.* 2014 b; **25** Suppl 3: iii102–12.

- Fayette J, Martin E., Piperno-Neumann S, et al. Angiosarcomas, a heterogeneous group of sarcomas with specific behavior depending on primary site: a retrospective study of 161 cases. *Ann Oncol.* 2007;**18**:2030–6.

- Ferrari A, Gronchi A, Casanova M, et al. Synovial sarcoma: a retrospective analysis of 271 patients of all ages treated at a single institution. *Cancer.* 2004;**01**: 627–34.

- Ferrario T, Karakousis CP. Retroperitoneal sarcomas: grade and survival. *Arch Surg.* 2003;**138**:248–51.

- Fiore M, Casali PG, Miceli R, et al. Prognostic effect of re-excision in adult soft tissue sarcoma of the extremities. *Ann Surg Oncol.* 2006;**13**:110–17.

- Fiore M, Colombo C, Locati P, et al. Surgical technique, morbidity, and outcome of primary retroperitoneal sarcoma involving inferior vena cava. *Ann Surg Oncol.* 2012;**19**:511–18.

- Fiore M, Grosso F, Lo Vullo S, et al. Myxoid/round cell and pleomorphic liposarcoma: prognostic factors and survival in a series of patients treated at a single institution. *Cancer.* 2007;**109**: 2522–31.

- Fiore M, Palassini E, Fumagalli E, et al. Preoperative imatinib mesylate for unresectable or locally advanced primary gastrointestinal stromal tumors (GIST). *Eur J Surg Oncol.* 2009;**35**:739–45.

- Fiore M, Rimareix F, Mariani L, et al. Desmoid-type fibromatosis: a front-line conservative approach to select patients for surgical treatment. *Ann Surg Oncol.* 2009;**16**:2587–93.

- Fletcher CD, Gustafson P, Rydholm A, Willén H, Akerman M. Clinicopathologic re-evaluation of 100 malignant fibrous histiocytomas: prognostic relevance of

subclassification. *J Clin Oncol.* 2001;**19**: 3045–50.

- Frankel TL, Chang AE, Wong SL. Surgical options for localized and advanced gastrointestinal stromal tumors. *J Surg Oncol.* 2011;**104**:882–7.

- Fury MG, Antonescu CR, Van Zee KJ, Brennan MF, Maki RG. A 14-year retrospective review of angiosarcoma: clinical characteristics, prognostic factors, and treatment outcomes with surgery and chemotherapy. *Cancer J.* 2005;**11**:241–7.

- Ghadimi MP, Liu P, Peng T, et al. Pleomorphic liposarcoma: clinical observations and molecular variables. *Cancer.* 2011;**117**:5359–69.

- Gill KR, Camellini L, Conigliaro R, et al. The natural history of upper gastrointestinal subepithelial tumors: a multicenter endoscopic ultrasound survey. *J Clin Gastroenterol.* 2009;**43**: 723–6.

- Giuliano AE, Eilber FR. The rationale for planned reoperation after unplanned total excision of soft tissue sarcomas. *J Clin Oncol.* 1985;**3**:1344–8.

- Gladdy RA, Qin LX, Moraco N, et al. Do radiation-associated soft tissue sarcomas have the same prognosis as sporadic soft tissue sarcomas? *J Clin Oncol.* 2010;**28**: 2064–9.

- Gladdy RA, Qin LX, Moraco N, et al. Predictors of survival and recurrence in primary leiomyosarcoma. *Ann Surg Oncol.* 2013; **20**:1851–7.

- Gronchi A, Bonvalot S, Le Cesne A, Casali PG. Resection of uninvolved adjacent organs can be part of surgery for retroperitoneal soft tissue sarcoma. *J Clin Oncol.* 2009;**27**:2106–7.

- Gronchi A, Casali PG, Mariani L, et al: Quality of surgery and outcome in extra-abdominal aggressive fibromatosis: a series of patients surgically treated at a single institution. *J Clin Oncol.* 2003;**21**: 1390–7.

- Gronchi A, Casali PG, Mariani L, et al. Status of surgical margins and prognosis in adult soft tissue sarcomas of the extremities: a series of patients treated at a single institution. *J Clin Oncol.* 2005;**23**:96–104.

- Gronchi A, Collini P, Miceli R, et al. Myogenic differentiation and histologic grading are major prognostic determinants in retroperitoneal liposarcoma. *Am J Surg Pathol.* 2015;**39**: 383–93.

- Gronchi A, Colombo C, Le Péchoux C, et al. Sporadic desmoid-type fibromatosis: a stepwise approach to a non-metastasising

neoplasm. A position paper from the Italian and the French Sarcoma Group. *Ann Oncol.* 2014;**25**:578–83.

- Gronchi A, Lo Vullo S, Colombo C, et al. Extremity soft tissue sarcoma in a series of patients treated at a single institution: the local control directly impacts survival. *Ann of Surg.* 2010;**251**:512–17.

- Gronchi A, Lo Vullo S, Fiore M, et al. Aggressive surgical policies in a retrospectively reviewed single-institution case series of retroperitoneal soft tissue sarcoma patients. *J Clin Oncol.* 2009;**27**:24–30.

- Gronchi A, Miceli R, Allard MA, et al. Personalizing the approach to retroperitoneal soft tissue sarcoma: histology specific patterns of failure and post-relapse outcome after primary extended resection. *Ann Surg Oncol.* 2015;**22**:1447–54.

- Gronchi A, Miceli R, Colombo C, et al. Primary extremity soft tissue sarcoma: outcome improvement over time at a single institution. *Ann Oncol.* 2011;**22**: 1675–81.

- Gronchi A, Miceli R, Colombo C, et al. Frontline extended surgery is associated with improved survival in retroperitoneal low-intermediate grade soft tissue sarcomas. *Ann Oncol.* 2012;**23**:1067–73.

- Gronchi A, Raut CP. The combination of surgery and imatinib in GIST: a reality for localized tumors at high risk, an open issue for metastatic ones. *Ann Surg Oncol.* 2012;**19**:1051–5.

- Gronchi A, Raut CP. Treatment of localized sarcomas. *Hematol Oncol Clin N Am.* 2013;**27**:921–38.

- Gronchi A, Strauss DC, Miceli R, et al. Variability in patterns of recurrence after resection of primary retroperitoneal sarcoma (RPS): a report on 1007 patients from the multi-institutional collaborative Transatlantic RPS Working Group. *Ann Surg.* 2016;**263**:1002–9.

- Gronchi A, Verderio P, De Paoli A, et al. Quality of surgery and neoadjuvant combined therapy in the ISG-GEIS trial on soft tissue sarcomas of limbs and trunk wall. *Ann Oncol.* 2013;**24**:817–23.

- Grosso F, Jones RL, Demetri GD, et al. Efficacy of trabectedin (ET-743) in advanced pre-treated myxoid liposarcomas. *Lancet Oncol.* 2007;**8**:595–602.

- Guadagnolo BA, Zagars GK, Ballo MT. Long-term outcomes for desmoid tumors treated with radiation therapy. *Int J Radiat Oncol Biol Phys.* 2008;**71**:441–7.

- Haglund KE, Raut CP, Nascimento AF, et al. Recurrence patterns and survival for patients with intermediate- and high-grade myxofibrosarcoma. *Int J Radiat Oncol Biol Phys.* 2012;**82**(1):361–7.

- Hassan I, Park SZ, Donohue JH, et al. Operative management of primary retroperitoneal sarcomas: a reappraisal of an institutional experience. *Ann Surg.* 2004;**239**:244–50.

- Hirota S, Isozaki K, Moriyama Y, et al. Gain of function mutations of c.kit in human gastrointestinal stroma tumors. *Science.* 1998;**279**: 577–80.

- Hocar O, Le Cesne A, Berissi S, et al. Clear cell sarcoma (malignant melanoma) of soft parts: a clinicopathologic study of 52 cases. *Dermatol Res Pract.* 2012;984–96.

- Hoffman A, Ghadimi MP, Demicco EG, et al. Localized and metastatic myxoid/ round cell liposarcoma: clinical and molecular observations. *Cancer.* 2013;**119**:1868–77.

- Hogg ME, Wayne JD. Atypical lipomatous tumor/well-differentiated liposarcoma: what is it? *Surg Oncol Clin N Am.* 2012;**21**:333–40.

- Hohenberger P, Ronellenfitsch U, Oladeji O, et al. Pattern of recurrence in patients with ruptured primary gastrointestinal stromal tumour. *Br J Surg.* 2010;**97**: 1854–9.

- Hornick JL, Dal Cin P, Fletcher CD. Loss of INI1 expression is characteristic of both conventional and proximal-type epithelioid sarcoma. *Am J Surg Pathol.* 2009;**33**:542–50.

- Janeway KA, Kim SY, Lodish M, et al. Defects in succinate dehydrogenase in gastrointestinal stromal tumors lacking KIT and PDGFRA mutations. *Proc Natl Acad Sci USA.* 2011;**108**:314–18.

- Joensuu H, Hohenberger P, Corless CL. Gastrointestinal stromal tumour. *Lancet.* 2013;**382**:973–83.

- Jones RL, Fisher C, Al-Muderis O, Judson IR. Differential sensitivity of liposarcoma subtypes to chemotherapy. *Eur J Cancer.* 2005;**41**:2853–60.

- Kamran SC, Howard SA, Shinagare AB, et al. Malignant peripheral nerve sheath tumors: prognostic impact of rhabdomyoblastic differentiation (malignant triton tumors), neurofibromatosis 1 status and location. *Eur J Surg Oncol.* 2013;**39**(1):46–52.

- Kasper B, Baumgarten C, Bonvalot S, et al. Management of sporadic desmoid-type fibromatosis: a European consensus approach based on patients' and professionals' expertise – a Sarcoma Patients EURONET (SPAEN) and European Organization for Research and Treatment of Cancer (EORTC) / Soft

Tissue and Bone Sarcoma Group (STBSG) initiative. *Eur J Cancer.* 2015; **51**: 127–36.

- Keus RB, Nout RA, Blay JY, et al. Results of a phase II pilot study of moderate dose radiotherapy for inoperable desmoid-type fibromatosis – an EORTC STBSG and ROG study (EORTC 62991–22998). *Ann Oncol.* 2013;**24**: 2672–6.

- Kilkenny JW, Bland KI, Copel EM. Retroperitoneal sarcoma: the University of Florida experience. *J Am Coll Surg.* 1996;**182**:329–39.

- Kolberg M, Høland M, Agesen TH, et al. Survival meta-analyses for >1800 malignant peripheral nerve sheath tumor patients with and without neurofibromatosis type 1. *Neuro Oncol.* 2013;**15**(2):135–47.

- Koontz MZ, Visser BM, Kunz PL. Neoadjuvant imatinib for borderline resectable GIST. *J Natl Compr Canc Netw.* 2012;**10**:1477–82.

- Lahat G, Dhuka AR, Hallevi H, et al. Angiosarcoma: clinical and molecular insights. *Ann Surg.* 2010;**251**: 1098–106.

- Lehnert T, Cardona S, Hinz U, et al. Primary and locally recurrent retroperitoneal soft-tissue sarcoma: local control and survival. *Eur J Surg Oncol.* 2009;**35**:986–93.

- Le Péchoux C, Musat E, Baey C, et al. Should adjuvant radiotherapy be administered in addition to front-line aggressive surgery (FAS) in patients with primary retroperitoneal sarcoma? *Ann Oncol.* 2013;**24**:832–7.

- Lev D, Kotilingam D, Wei C, et al. Optimizing treatment of desmoid tumors. *J Clin Oncol.* 2007;**25**(13): 1785–91.

- Lewis JJ, Boland PJ, Leung DH, et al. The enigma of desmoid tumors. *Ann Surg.* 1999;**229**:866–72.

- Lewis JJ, Leung D, Espat J, Woodruff JM, Brennan MF. Effect of re-excision in extremity soft tissue sarcoma. *Ann Surg.* 2000;**231**:655–63.

- Lindet C, Neuville A, Penel N, et al. Localised angiosarcomas: the identification of prognostic factors and analysis of treatment impact. A retrospective analysis from the French Sarcoma Group (GSF/GETO). *Eur J Cancer.* 2013;**49**:369–76.

- Lim YJ, Son HJ, Lee JS, et al. Clinical course of subepithelial lesions detected on upper gastrointestinal endoscopy. *World J Gastroenterol.* 2010;**16**: 439–44.

- Look Hong NJ, Hornicek FJ, Raskin KA, et al. Prognostic factors and outcomes of

patients with myxofibrosarcoma. *Ann Surg Oncol.* 2013;**20**:80–6.

- McBride SM, Raut CP, Lapidus M, et al. Locoregional recurrence after preoperative radiation therapy for retroperitoneal sarcoma: adverse impact of multifocal disease and potential implications of dose escalation. *Ann Surg Oncol.* 2013;**20**(7):2140–7.

- McCarter MD, Antonescu CR, Ballman KV, et al; American College of Surgeons Oncology Group (ACOSOG) Intergroup Adjuvant GIST Study Team. Microscopically positive margins for primary gastrointestinal stromal tumors: analysis of risk factors and tumor recurrence. *J Am Coll Surg.* 2012;**215**: 53–9.

- Miller SJ, Alam M, Andersen JS, et al. Dermatofibrosarcoma protuberans. *J Nat Compr Cancer Netw.* 2012;**10**:312–28.

- Moreau LC, Turcotte R, Ferguson P, et al. Myxoid/round cell liposarcoma (MRCLS) revisited: an analysis of 418 primarily managed cases. *Ann Surg Oncol.* 2012;**19**:1081–8.

- Mussi C, Collini P, Miceli R, et al. Prognostic impact of dedifferentiation in retroperitoneal liposarcoma: a series of patients surgically treated at a single institution. *Cancer.* 2008;**113**:1657–65.

- Mussi C, Schildhaus HU, Gronchi A, et al. Therapeutic consequences from molecular biology for GIST patients affected by neurofibromatosis type 1. *Clin Cancer Res.* 2008;**14**:4550–5.

- Mutter RW, Singer S, Zhang Z, Brennan MF, Alektiar KM. The enigma of myxofibrosarcoma of the extremity. *Cancer.* 2012;**118**(2):518–27.

- Nannini M, Biasco G, Astolfi A, Pantaleo MA. An overview on molecular biology of KIT/PDGFRA wild type (WT) gastrointestinal stromal tumours (GIST). *J Med Genet.* 2013;**50**:653–61.

- O'Donnell PW, Griffin AM, Eward WC, et al. The effect of the setting of a positive surgical margin in soft tissue sarcoma. *Cancer.* 2014;**120**:2866–75.

- O'Sullivan B, Davis AM, Turcotte R, et al. Preoperative versus postoperative radiotherapy in soft-tissue sarcoma of the limbs: a randomised trial. *Lancet.* 2002;**359**:2235–41.

- Pawlik TM, Pisters PW, Mikula L, et al. Long-term results of two prospective trials of preoperative external beam radiotherapy for localized intermediate- or high-grade retroperitoneal soft tissue sarcoma. *Ann Surg Oncol.* 2006;**13**(4):508–17.

- Pisters PW. Resection of some – but not all – clinically uninvolved adjacent viscera as part of surgery for retroperitoneal soft tissue sarcomas. *J Clin Oncol.* 2009;**27**:6–8.

- Pisters PW, O'Sullivan B, Maki RG. Evidence-based recommendations for local therapy for soft tissue sarcomas. *J Clin Oncol.* 2007;**25**(8):1003–38.

- Pisters PWT, Harrison LB, Leung DHY, et al. Long-term results of a prospective randomized trial of adjuvant brachytherapy in soft tissue sarcoma. *J Clin Oncol.* 1996;**14**:859–68.

- Raut CP, Swallow CJ. Are radical compartmental resections for retroperitoneal sarcomas justified? *Ann Surg Oncol.*2010; **17**:1481–4.

- Rutkowski P, Gronchi A, Hohenberger P, et al. Neoadjuvant imatinib in locally advanced gastrointestinal stromal tumors (GIST): the EORTC STBSG experience. *Ann Surg Oncol.* 2013;**20**:2937–43.

- Sakharpe A, Lahat G, Gulamhusein T, et al. Epithelioid sarcoma and unclassified sarcoma with epithelioid features: clinicopathological variables, molecular markers, and a new experimental model. *Oncologist.* 2011;**16**(4):512–22.

- Salas S, Dufresne A, Bui B, et al. Prognostic factors influencing progression-free survival determined from a series of sporadic desmoid tumors: a wait-and-see policy according to tumor presentation. *J Clin Oncol.* 2011;**29**: 3553–8.

- Sanfilippo R, Miceli R, Grosso F, et al. Myxofibrosarcoma: prognostic factors and survival in a series of patients treated at a single institution. *Ann Surg Oncol.* 2011;**18**:720–5.

- Sheth GR, Cranmer LD, Smith BD, Grasso-Lebeau L, Lang JE. Radiation-induced sarcoma of the breast: a systematic review. *Oncologist.* 2012;**17**(3):405–18.

- Sommerville SM, Patton JT, Luscombe JC, Mangham DC, Grimer RJ. Clinical outcomes of deep atypical lipomas (well-differentiated lipoma-like liposarcomas) of the extremities. *ANZ J Surg.* 2005;**75**:803–6.

- Stoeckle E, Coindre JM, Bonvalot S, et al. Prognostic factors in retroperitoneal sarcoma: a multivariate analysis of a series of 165 patients of the French Cancer Center Federation Sarcoma Group. *Cancer.* 2001;**92**:359–68.

- Stojadinovic A, Leung DHY, Hoos A, et al. Analysis of the prognostic significance of microscopic margins in 2084 localized primary adult soft tissue sarcomas. *Ann Surg.* 2002;**235**:424–34.

- Strauss DC, Hayes AJ, Thway K, et al. Surgical management of primary retroperitoneal sarcoma. *Br J Surg.* 2010;**101**: 520–3.

- Tan MC, Yoon SS. Surgical management of retroperitoneal and pelvic sarcomas. *J Surg Oncol.* 2015;**111**:553–61.

- Trovik CS, Bauer HC, Alvegard TA, et al. Surgical margins, local recurrence and metastasis in soft tissue sarcomas: 599 surgically-treated patients from the Scandinavian Sarcoma Group register. *Eur J Cancer.* 2000;**36**:710–16.

- van Broekhoven DLM, Deroose JP, Bonvalot S, et al. Isolated limb perfusion by tumor necrosis factor alpha and melphalan in patients with advanced aggressive fibromatosis. *Br J Surg.* 2014;**101**:1674–80.

- van Dalen T, Plooij JM, van Coevorden F, et al. Long-term prognosis of primary retroperitoneal soft tissue sarcoma. *Eur J Surg Oncol.* 2007;**33**:234–8.

- Verweij J, Casali PG, Zalcberg J, et al. Progression-free survival in gastrointestinal stromal tumours with high-dose imatinib: randomised trial. *Lancet.* 2004;**364**: 1127–34.

- Wang D, Zhang Q, Blanke CD, et al. Phase II trial of neoadjuvant/adjuvant imatinib mesylate for advanced primary and metastatic/recurrent operable gastrointestinal stromal tumors: long-term follow-up results of Radiation Therapy Oncology Group 0132. *Ann Surg Oncol.* 2012;**19**: 1074–80.

- Yang JC, Chang AE, Sindelar WF, et al. Randomized prospective study of the benefit of adjuvant radiation therapy in the treatment of soft tissue sarcomas of the extremity. *J Clin Oncol.* 1998;**16**:197–203.

- Zagars GK, Ballo MT, Pisters PW, et al: Surgical margins and re-excision in the management of patients with soft tissue sarcoma using conservative surgery and radiation therapy. *Cancer.* 2003;**97**: 2530–43.

# Medical Treatment of Adult Soft Tissue Sarcomas and Gastrointestinal Stromal Tumors

Paolo G. Casali MD

## Introduction

From a clinical point of view, sarcomas may be divided into adult soft tissue sarcomas (STSs), gastrointestinal stromal tumors (GISTs), "pediatric" sarcomas (osteosarcoma, Ewing sarcoma, rhabdomyosarcoma), and some rare adult bone sarcomas. By and large, one could say that two "revolutions" occurred with regard to the medical treatment of sarcomas. The first improved the cure rate of "pediatric" sarcomas from 10–20% (as achievable with local treatment alone) to more than 60%, thanks to the introduction of chemotherapy in the 1970s and 1980s. It is worth noting that Ewing sarcomas of soft tissues are included therein, because they should be treated in the same way as typical skeletal Ewing sarcoma (even when occurring in adulthood, as is more common for extraskeletal Ewing sarcoma). The second revolution significantly affected the prognosis of advanced GISTs and improved the relapse-free survival of localized GISTs, thanks to the introduction of molecularly targeted therapies beginning in 2000. A less striking evolution has been taking place in the past decades with regard to the medical treatment of STSs. In essence, it has to do with tailoring the medical therapy of STSs to their histologic subtypes. Indeed, medical oncologists had long approached all STSs uniformly, valuing the malignancy grade for their clinical choices, much less the histologic type. This includes both cytotoxic chemotherapy and the molecularly targeted therapies that are advancing in STS. Of course, the relevance of some histologic types may be clearly related to their defining molecular characteristics (e.g., dermatofibrosarcoma), and one may expect that in the future molecular factors will become more directly relevant as such. However, this will be unlikely to occur outside of classical histologic partitioning.

## Gastrointestinal Stromal Tumors

Among solid cancers, GISTs have become a model for patterns of efficacy of new molecularly targeted therapies. In fact, medical therapy of GIST is currently based entirely on molecularly targeted therapies directed toward *KIT* and *PDGFRA*. They have substantially improved overall survival in the advanced disease setting and have improved relapse-free survival, and to some extent even overall survival, in the localized disease setting.

The first molecularly targeted therapy used in GIST treatment has been imatinib, i.e., an anti-tyrosine kinase agent targeting both *KIT* and *PDGFRA*. Thus, its targeted mechanism of action exploits the alterations of these type III receptor tyrosine kinases, which are the result of gain-of-function mutations of the corresponding oncogenes. At the moment, two other anti-tyrosine kinase agents are standard treatment for advanced GIST beyond

imatinib: sunitinib and regorafenib. Both inhibit *KIT* and *PDGFRA*, but also exert a marked anti-angiogenic effect, so that their mechanism of action in GIST may be composite. All these are oral agents, conceived for prolonged treatment.

Indeed, imatinib displays an exceptional antitumor activity in the presence of most mutations of *KIT* and *PDGFRA*. A striking exception is the D842V mutation on exon 18 of *PDGFRA*, whereas mutations on exon 9 of *KIT* require higher-than-average doses of the drug. Wild-type (WT) GISTs are poorly responsive to imatinib, although they may be more sensitive to sunitinib and regorafenib. This predictive value of mutational analysis with regard to molecularly targeted treatments underlies its special relevance within pathologic diagnosis of GISTs. In addition, PDGFRA-mutated GISTs tend to give rise to less aggressive clinical entities, and the subsets of WT-GIST have distinct natural histories. Succinate dehydrogenase (SDH)-deficient WT-GISTs tend to occur at pediatric age, display a low degree of aggressiveness, may be multicentric within the stomach, and can involve regional lymph nodes, contrary to typical GIST. In WT-GIST related to type 1 neurofibromatosis, the primary site is the small bowel, again with possibly a multicentric extent of disease. Thus, mutational analysis is also a tool to stratify patients having natural histories diverging from typical KIT-mutated GIST. In brief, mutational analysis is important for medical oncologists not only for its predictive value in regard to responsiveness to targeted therapies, but also as a means to stratify patients who have an essentially different course of disease. It goes without saying that treatment choices, including those involving surgery in the localized and the advanced settings, may be radically different depending on the natural history of the disease and whether effective medical therapies are available.

Clinically, imatinib is standard treatment for advanced GIST patients (i.e., the metastatic or locally inoperable setting). The probability of response is very high in the presence of sensitive mutations. As illustrated in Chapter 4, tumor responses tend to occur rapidly and are marked by a myxoid degeneration of the tumor tissue, with apoptotic figures. This may translate into obvious tumor shrinkage of lesions, but sometimes tumor size does not change, or there may also be a degree of enlargement, even in the presence of a major pathologic tumor response. Radiologically, then, signs of altered tissue density may be more meaningful than changes in tumor size. Conversely, pathologic complete responses are rare, and nests of residual vital cells are often detectable in the periphery of lesions. This is the pathologic counterpart of the clinical need to continue medical therapy in order to maintain a tumor response. In fact, discontinuation of clinical studies showed that most patients with metastatic disease progress after stopping their therapy, in spite of any previous response. Indeed, it has still not been assessed whether this also applies to the minority of patients who become long-term, progression-free survivors (roughly 10% of metastatic GIST patients after 10 years of imatinib therapy). Although studies are planned to elucidate this, current standard treatment of metastatic GIST is to continue indefinitely medical therapy in all patients, as long as they are not progressing.

However, the main limiting factor of therapy with imatinib in advanced GIST is secondary resistance, i.e., the occurrence of secondary mutations to the same oncogene affected by primary mutations. They typically involve exons 13–14 or 17–18 of *KIT*, and the corresponding exons of *PDGFRA*, i.e., those encoding the ATP-binding pocket or the activation loop of the receptor. A simple mechanism of resistance may be that the drug can no longer be accommodated in the binding pocket of the receptor. Molecularly, the crucial finding has been that secondary mutations tend to be heterogeneous within the same patient. This means that different lesions, or even the same lesion, may harbor different secondary mutations. This limits the therapeutic potential of salvage therapies and undermines the predictive value of genotyping secondary progression with tumor biopsies. In fact, a secondary mutation found in one lesion may be accompanied by other mutations that go undetected. At the moment, standard second- and third-line molecularly targeted therapy is provided by sunitinib and regorafenib, with little room for any molecular prediction, though the two drugs differ in part with regard to their profile of sensitive secondary mutations. Tumor responses to second- and third-line molecularly targeted therapy tend to be less successful and prolonged than in first-line. Median progression-free survival to imatinib as a first-line agent is about 2 years, though with a high variability (as mentioned, with a low fraction of long-term, progression-free survivors). Intriguingly, re-challenging a progressing tumor with a previously employed anti-tyrosine kinase agent may be effective in some cases, at least for a while, probably because sensitive clones reexpand once the selective pressure of the drug had been removed. In a sense, this parallels the clinical observation of several "focal" progressions, i.e., patterns of progression that are limited to one or a few lesions, such that secondary resistance might spread progressively, not abruptly, in a proportion of cases. All this gives the impression of a kind of "liquid" resistance to targeted agents. New strategies to exploit available agents, and all future drugs, may be then envisaged, and the study of circulating DNA ("liquid biopsy") might be a tool to rationally drive rotation regimens and the like.

In the localized disease setting, imatinib has been extensively studied as an adjuvant to surgery in high-risk patients. Thus, a first requirement is to assess the risk of relapse. This is currently predicted by tumor size, tumor site, and the mitotic index, so that the latter is especially important to stratify patients eligible for an adjuvant treatment. Several prognostic scores are available. Probably the most useful are "heat maps," which incorporate both the mitotic index and tumor size as continuous variables, thus reducing the impact of small variations (whose meaning may be obviously amplified if one uses cut-off values, especially for the mitotic rate).

Currently, 3 years of imatinib treatment has become standard adjuvant therapy for high-risk GIST patients after complete surgery. It strikingly delays relapse, if this is due to occur, although the impression is that the cure rate is unlikely affected. However, a limited survival benefit has been demonstrated, which probably reflects the benefit of substantially delaying relapse in most patients. In other words, if, say, a patient receives 3 years of adjuvant imatinib, the risk of relapse is very low during the adjuvant period, whereas from 1 to 3 years after ending treatment, it will tend to return to the level it would have been without any adjuvant therapy. It is left to learn whether more prolonged adjuvant therapies, i.e., exceeding 3 years, may improve the potential of adjuvant imatinib therapy, with an impact on the cure rate or at least a more prolonged benefit in terms of occurrence of relapse. Of course, what matters is the behavior of secondary resistance in comparison with starting imatinib again in case of relapse after the end of a limited period of adjuvant therapy. In brief, currently adjuvant therapy is reserved to select those patients with a substantial risk of relapse and an imatinib-sensitive genotype, while the optimal duration of therapy is still a subject for clinical studies, and standard treatment is currently 3 years.

In the end, as of today, one could conclude that molecularly targeted agents are able to display a remarkable potential of disease control, and regression, if their target is present. However, both in the metastatic and in the localized disease setting, the chances of cure seem to be basically unaffected, owing to the preponderance of mechanisms of resistance. Substantially changing the potential of molecularly targeted therapies in the model of GIST would require improved capacities to cope with secondary resistance.

## Soft Tissue Sarcomas

Soft tissue sarcomas, the most incident group within the rare family of sarcomas, have an intermediate sensitivity to cytotoxic chemotherapy, which is mainly based on anthracyclines (adriamycin) and alkylating agents (ifosfamide) in the first-line medical treatment, and, in further-line treatment, on other cytotoxic agents, including trabectedin, dacarbazine, gemcitabine, and taxanes. Molecularly targeted agents, such as pazopanib, have been developed more recently in STS and have shown some efficacy. The activity of several such agents, whether cytotoxics or molecularly targeted drugs, is often confined to selected histologies.

In essence, chemotherapy is able to exert a palliative effect on the metastatic disease and to provide a distinct probability of cytoreduction in the locally advanced disease (which may be clinically useful, say, to achieve surgical resectability or conservative resectability, if they are precluded initially). In addition, following the large impact of adjuvant chemotherapy in osteosarcoma, Ewing sarcoma, and embryonal/alveolar rhabdomyosarcoma, chemotherapy has been extensively studied as an adjuvant to surgery in STS. When pooled, available clinical trials provide evidence in favor of a limited reduction in the risk of relapse of high-risk STS patients, but the conflicting nature of results across trials does not allow adjuvant chemotherapy to be considered as a standard. In high-risk patients, some preoperative treatment may help make surgery easier and/or improve surgical margins, so that chemotherapy may also be used with this intent (in addition to the conventional aim of all adjuvant therapies, i.e., decreasing the risk of relapse and improving survival). Preoperative chemotherapy can also be combined with radiation therapy, with further advantages in some cases (e.g., postoperative radiation therapy may be problematic after some reconstructive surgeries). In this regard, the interim analysis of a recent randomized trial showed that neoadjuvant full-dose chemotherapy with anthracyclines and ifosfamide was superior to a set of histology-driven regimens, thus providing randomized evidence of its efficacy. The trial was carried out in high-risk patients. If its results are confirmed, neoadjuvant chemotherapy may thus become standard treatment in the future for those STS patients with a substantial risk of relapse. Interestingly, tumor response may be difficult to assess in localized masses of STS, both radiologically and pathologically.

If resorted to, adjuvant or neoadjuvant chemotherapy is employed when the risk of relapse is high; therefore, risk assessment is crucial. Basically, risk of relapse in STS is currently estimated according to tumor size and tumor grading, meaning that tumor malignancy grade is fundamental for clinical decision making. This stresses the importance of a close collaboration between the pathologist and the clinician, especially for those presentations wherein a conventional grading system is not available. In other words, the biologic aggressiveness of the tumor, as perceived by the pathologist, is always a critical piece of information for the clinician, especially when the shortcomings of available classifications make it difficult to formally grade the tumor. Another crucial pathologic factor is the histologic subtype, because some subtypes have peculiar natural histories and/or specific patterns of chemosensitivity.

Indeed, in the past few years, there has been an increased perception of the selective activity of some cytotoxics, depending on histology. Thus, ifosfamide seems less active in leiomyosarcomas as compared with most other histologies, whereas it is more active in synovial sarcoma. Conversely, gemcitabine is markedly active in leiomyosarcoma and angiosarcoma. Taxanes are active in angiosarcoma. Trabectedin is mainly active in liposarcoma, leiomyosarcoma, and possibly synovial sarcoma. In myxoid liposarcoma, its mechanism of action seems to be related to the fusion transcript that marks this histology, and this justifies a magnitude of antitumor activity that is definitely higher than other histologies in which trabectedin works. Unfortunately, the reasons why the aforementioned cytotoxics exert different effects on different STS histologies are unknown. It goes without saying that the reasons for the selective activity of most cytotoxics in most cancers are poorly known as well, so that, in the end, what is seen in STS may just stress the diversity of STS as a variegated family of tumors.

Among molecularly targeted agents, imatinib is approved for dermatofibrosarcoma protuberans, in relation to its anti-PDGFB activity, given the fusion transcript of the disease. Dermatofibrosarcoma is obviously a mainly surgical disease, but there are rare instances in which a medical therapy may help. Imatinib is also active in fibrosarcomatous dermatofibrosarcoma, though the duration of response is shorter.

In dermatofibrosarcoma, imatinib works in a highly selective fashion, in a sense like it works in GIST. Currently, this has rarely been the case for most molecularly targeted agents that have shown efficacy in STS. Thus, pazopanib, an anti-tyrosine kinase agent with anti-angiogenic activity, is approved for STS, with the exception of liposarcomas, and seems to be active mainly in synovial sarcoma, leiomyosarcoma and possibly malignant peripheral nerve sheath tumor (MPNST), and other rare histologies, such as solitary fibrous tumors. However, its mechanism of action is less selective, or at least less understood. Indeed, the mechanism of action of similar agents may well differ from one histologic type to another, because similar agents may well display diverse efficacy in different histologies. This seems to be the case with anti-angiogenics such as pazopanib, sunitinib, and the like, which seem to function differently in different histologies both in vivo and in vitro.

Indeed, especially "rare" histologies, such as solitary fibrous tumors, alveolar soft part sarcoma, clear cell sarcoma, PEComas, and inflammatory myofibroblastic tumor, proved to be sensitive to some molecularly targeted agents. In a sense, many of these histologies are also "low-grade" entities. An explanation could well be that low-grade STS may be more likely to be more differentiated and thus more prone to be dependent on selective cellular pathways. This may be especially relevant with some translocation-related sarcomas. Then, on one side of the spectrum, we find agents such as imatinib in dermatofibrosarcoma (targeting PDGFB) or ALK-inhibitors in inflammatory myofibroblastic tumors, whose activity seems highly specific. Conversely, we find histologies that are sensitive to some anti-tyrosine kinase agents, such as sunitinib or pazopanib, which have a similar mechanism of action. It is true, however, that, say, sunitinib or pazopanib does not seem to work to the same extent in the same histologies (e.g., solitary fibrous tumor), though we fail to properly understand why. Then, there are some more "frequent" histologies within STS that might benefit from new agents under development, such as those targeting MDM2 or CDK4 in dedifferentiated liposarcoma. In the end, however, the model of GIST is that of a disease with a gain-of-function mutation of special pathogenetic relevance. In essence, this model has not been replicated in STS.

At the moment, immune therapies are used in several cancers and there is also interest in sarcomas. The rationale for their use may be manifold, including convincing demonstrations of an immune infiltrate in many sarcomas; the expression of cancer testis antigens in some histologies; the existence of a group of translocation-related sarcomas, with fusion transcripts of potential antigenic relevance; and, conversely, the existence of many sarcomas with a "complex" karyotype, resulting in a possibly higher mutational load; and the extensive use of cytotoxics and anti-tyrosine kinase agents as standard treatment of many sarcomas, as well as the extensive use of radiation therapy, which might be exploited as inducers of immune response. Indeed, there have been anecdotal demonstrations of efficacy of checkpoint inhibitors in some STS patients and of adoptive immune therapy in synovial sarcoma. Again, the main problem may well be the rarity of sarcomas, along with their diversity, so that any development of available or new immune agents, or immune treatment modalities, will probably need to be carried out through a series of patients according to histologies. In the end, this stresses the importance of pathology in STS even with medical options, such as immune therapies, that can function well across cancers.

There are several consequences, in the end. One is certainly that new methodologies to study rare cancers, not only sarcomas, are needed. Clinically speaking, another is that proper pathologic referral should be actively implemented in STS to optimize quality of pathologic diagnosis in a rare group of complex and variegated diseases. In addition, it is crucial that the pathologist and the clinical oncologist be part of a functional multidisciplinary tumor board, within which a smooth cross-discipline collaboration is allowed and the clinical decision is made by rationally taking into account all relevant diagnostic and clinical prognostic and predictive factors, including pathologic factors, and by aiming at a patient–physician shared decision making, often under conditions of uncertainty.

## Chapter 3B Selected Key References

- Benson C, Vitfell-Rasmussen J, Maruzzo M, et al. A retrospective study of patients with malignant PEComa receiving treatment with sirolimus or temsirolimus: the Royal Marsden Hospital experience. *Anticancer Res.* 2014;**34**:3663–8.

- Burgess M, Tawbi H. Immunotherapeutic approaches to sarcoma. *Curr Treat Options Oncol.* 2015;**16**:26.

- Butrynski JE, D'Adamo DR, Hornick JL, et al. Crizotinib in ALK-rearranged inflammatory myofibroblastic tumor. *N Engl J Med.* 2010;**363**:1727–33.

- Casali PG. Histology- and non-histology-driven therapy for treatment of soft tissue sarcomas. *Ann Oncol.* 2012;**23** Suppl 10:x167–9.

- Casali PG. Adjuvant chemotherapy for soft tissue sarcoma. *Am Soc Clin Oncol Educ Book.* 2015;**35**:e629–33.

- Casali PG, Bruzzi P, Bogaerts J, Blay JY; on behalf of the Rare Cancers Europe (RCE) Consensus Panel. Rare Cancers Europe (RCE) methodological recommendations for clinical studies in rare cancers: a European consensus position paper. *Ann Oncol.* 2015;**26**:300–306.

- Casali PG, Dei Tos AP, Gronchi A. Gastrointestinal stromal tumor. In: DeVita VT, Lawrence TS, Rosenberg SA, editors. *DeVita, Hellman, and Rosenberg's Cancer: Principles & Practice of Oncology.* 10th ed. Philadelphia: Wolters Kluwer; 2014.

- Casali PG, Le Cesne A, Poveda Velasco A, et al. Time to definitive failure to the first tyrosine kinase inhibitor in localized GI stromal tumors treated with imatinib as an adjuvant: a European Organisation for Research and Treatment of Cancer Soft Tissue and Bone Sarcoma Group intergroup randomized trial in collaboration with the Australasian Gastro-Intestinal Trials Group, UNICANCER, French Sarcoma Group, Italian Sarcoma Group, and Spanish Group for Research on Sarcomas. *J Clin Oncol.* 2015;**33**:4276–83.

- DeMatteo RP, Ballman KV, Antonescu CR, et al; American College of Surgeons Oncology Group (ACOSOG) Intergroup Adjuvant GIST Study Team. Adjuvant imatinib mesylate after resection of localised, primary gastrointestinal stromal tumour: a randomised, double-blind, placebo-controlled trial. *Lancet.* 2009;**373**:1097–104.

- Demetri GD, Jeffers M, Reichardt P, et al. Mutational analysis of plasma DNA from patients (pts) in the phase III GRID study of regorafenib (REG) versus placebo (PL) in tyrosine kinase inhibitor (TKI)-refractory GIST: Correlating genotype with clinical outcomes. *J Clin Oncol.* 2013;**31**: Suppl, abstr 10503 (meeting abstract)

- Demetri GD, Reichardt P, Kang YK, et al; GRID Study Investigators. Efficacy and safety of regorafenib for advanced gastrointestinal stromal tumours after failure of imatinib and sunitinib (GRID): an international, multicentre, randomised, placebo-controlled, phase 3 trial. *Lancet.* 2013;**381**:295–302.

- Demetri GD, van Oosterom AT, Garrett CR, et al. Efficacy and safety of sunitinib in patients with advanced gastrointestinal stromal tumour after failure of imatinib: a randomised controlled trial. *Lancet.* 2006;**368**:1329–38.

- Demetri GD, von Mehren M, Jones RL, et al. Efficacy and safety of trabectedin or dacarbazine for metastatic liposarcoma or leiomyosarcoma after failure of conventional chemotherapy: results of a phase III randomized multicenter clinical trial. *J Clin Oncol.* 2015 Sep;14:pii: JCO.2015.62.4734. [Epub ahead of print]

- D'Angelo SP, Tap WD, Schwartz GK, Carvajal RD. Sarcoma immunotherapy: past approaches and future directions. *Sarcoma.* 2014;**2014**:391967.

- D'Angelo SP, Shoushtari AN, Agaram NP, et al. Prevalence of tumor-infiltrating lymphocytes and PD-L1 expression in the soft tissue sarcoma microenvironment. *Hum Pathol.* 2015;**46**:357–65.

- Di Giandomenico S, Frapolli R, Bello E, et al. Mode of action of trabectedin in myxoid liposarcomas. *Oncogene.* 2014;**33**:5201–10.

- Frustaci S, Gherlinzoni F, De Paoli A, et al. Adjuvant chemotherapy for adult soft tissue sarcomas of the extremities and girdles: results of the Italian randomized cooperative trial. *J Clin Oncol.* 2001;**19**:1238–47.

- Gastrointestinal Stromal Tumor Meta-Analysis Group (MetaGIST). Comparison of two doses of imatinib for the treatment of unresectable or metastatic gastrointestinal stromal tumors: a meta-analysis of 1,640 patients. *J Clin Oncol.* 2010;**28**:1247–53.

- Gold JS, Gonen M, Gutierrez A, et al. Development and validation of a prognostic nomongram for recurrence-free survival after complete surgical resection of localized primary gastrointestinal stromal tumour: a retrospective analysis. *Lancet Oncol.* 2009;**10**:1045–52.

- Gronchi A, Colombo C, Le Péchoux C, et al; ISG and FSG. Sporadic desmoid-type fibromatosis: a stepwise approach to a non-metastasising neoplasm – a position paper from the Italian and the French Sarcoma Group. *Ann Oncol.* 2014;**25**:578–83.

- Gronchi A, Ferrari S, Quagliuolo V, et al. Histotype-tailored neoadjuvant chemotherapy versus standard chemotherapy in patients with high-risk soft-tissue sarcomas (ISG-STS 1001): an international, open-label, randomised, controlled, phase 3, multicentre trial. *Lancet Oncol.* 2017;**18**:812–22.

- Grosso F, Jones RL, Demetri GD, et al. Efficacy of trabectedin (ecteinascidin-743) in advanced pretreated myxoid liposarcomas: a retrospective study. *Lancet Oncol.* 2007;**8**:595–602.

- Heinrich MC, Maki RG, Corless CL, et al. Primary and secondary kinase genotypes correlate with the biological and clinical activity of sunitinib in imatinib-resistant gastrointestinal stromal tumor. *J Clin Oncol.* 2008;**26**:5352–9.

- Joensuu H. Risk stratification of patients diagnosed with gastrointestinal stromal tumors. *Hum Pathol.* 2008;**39**:1411–19.

- Joensuu H, Eriksson M, Sundby Hall K, et al. Adjuvant imatinib for high-risk GI stromal tumor: analysis of a randomized trial. *J Clin Oncol.* 2016;**34**:244–50.

- Joensuu H, Vehtari A, Riihimäki J, et al. Risk of gastrointestinal stromal tumour recurrence after surgery: an analysis of pooled population-based cohorts. *Lancet Oncol.* 2012;**13**:265–74.

- Judson I, Verweij J, Gelderblom H, et al; European Organisation and Treatment of Cancer Soft Tissue and Bone Sarcoma Group. Doxorubicin alone versus intensified doxorubicin plus ifosfamide for first-line treatment of advanced or metastatic soft-tissue sarcoma: a randomised controlled phase 3 trial. *Lancet Oncol.* 2014;**15**(4):415–23.

- Kang YK, Ryu MH, Yoo C, et al. Resumption of imatinib to control metastatic or unresectable gastrointestinal stromal tumours after failure of imatinib and sunitinib (RIGHT): a randomised, placebo-controlled, phase 3 trial. *Lancet Oncol.* 2013;**14**:1175–82.

- Maki RG, Wathen JK, Patel SR, et al. Randomized phase II study of gemcitabine and docetaxel compared with gemcitabine alone in patients with metastatic soft tissue sarcomas: results of sarcoma alliance for research through collaboration study 002 [corrected]. *J Clin Oncol.* 2007;**25**:2755–63.

- Miettinen M, Lasota J. Gastrointestinal stromal tumors: pathology and prognosis at different sites. *Semin Diagn Pathol.* 2006;**23**:70–83.

- Palassini E, Ferrari S, Verderio P, et al. Feasibility of preoperative chemotherapy with or without radiation therapy in localized soft tissue sarcomas of limbs and superficial trunk in the Italian Sarcoma Group/Grupo Español de Investigación en Sarcomas Randomized Clinical Trial: three versus five cycles of full-dose epirubicin plus ifosfamide. *J Clin Oncol.* 2015;**33**:3628–34.

- Patrikidou A, Chabaud S, Ray-Coquard I, et al; French Sarcoma Group. Influence of imatinib interruption and rechallenge on the residual disease in patients with advanced GIST: results of the BFR14 prospective French Sarcoma Group randomised, phase III trial. *Ann Oncol.* 2013;**24**:1087–93.

- Pautier P, Floquet A, Penel N, et al. Randomized multicenter and stratified phase II study of gemcitabine alone versus gemcitabine and docetaxel in patients with metastatic or relapsed leiomyosarcomas: a Federation Nationale des Centres de Lutte Contre le Cancer (FNCLCC) French Sarcoma Group Study (TAXOGEM study). *Oncologist.* 2012;**17**(9):1213–20.

- Pervaiz N, Colterjohn N, Farrokhyar F, et al. A systematic meta-analysis of randomized controlled trials of adjuvant chemotherapy for localized resectable soft-tissue sarcoma. *Cancer.* 2008;**113**:573–81.

- Postow MA, Callahan MK, Wolchok JD. Immune checkpoint blockade in cancer therapy. *J Clin Oncol.* 2015;**33**:1974–82.

- Ray-Coquard I, Blay JY, Italiano A, et al. Effect of the MDM2 antagonist RG7112 on the P53 pathway in patients with MDM2-amplified, well-differentiated or dedifferentiated liposarcoma: an exploratory proof-of-mechanism study. *Lancet Oncol.* 2012;**13**:1133–40.

- Robbins PF, Morgan RA, Feldman SA, et al. Tumor regression in patients with metastatic synovial cell sarcoma and melanoma using genetically engineered lymphocytes reactive with NY-ESO-1. *J Clin Oncol.* 2011;**29**:917–24.

- Rossi S, Miceli R, Messerini L, et al. Natural history of imatinib-naive GISTs: a retrospective analysis of 929 cases with long-term follow-up and development of a survival nomogram based on mitotic index and size as continuous variables. *Am J Surg Pathol.* 2011;**35**:1646–56.

- Rutkowski P, Gronchi A, Hohenberger P, et al. Neoadjuvant imatinib in locally advanced gastrointestinal stromal tumors (GIST): the EORTC STBSG experience. *Ann Surg Oncol.* 2013;**20**:2937–43.

- Sanfilippo R, Bertulli R, Marrari A, et al. High-dose continuous-infusion ifosfamide in advanced well-differentiated/dedifferentiated liposarcoma. *Clin Sarcoma Res.* 2014;**4**:16.

- Singer S, Tap WD, Crago AM, O'Sullivan B. Soft tissue sarcoma. In: DeVita VT, Lawrence TS, Rosenberg SA, editors. *DeVita, Hellman, and Rosenberg's Cancer: Principles & Practice of Oncology.* 10th ed. Philadelphia: Wolters Kluwer; 2014.

- Stacchiotti S, Marrari A, Dei Tos AP, Casali PG. Targeted therapies in rare sarcomas: IMT, ASPS, SFT, PEComa, and CCS. *Hematol Oncol Clin North Am.* 2013;**27**:1049–61.

- Stacchiotti S, Negri T, Libertini M, et al. Sunitinib malate in solitary fibrous tumor (SFT). *Ann Oncol.* 2012;**23**:3171–9.

- Stacchiotti S, Negri T, Zaffaroni N, et al. Sunitinib in advanced alveolar soft part sarcoma: evidence of a direct antitumor effect. *Ann Oncol.* 2011;**22**:1682–90.

- Stacchiotti S, Palassini E, Sanfilippo R, et al. Gemcitabine in advanced angiosarcoma: a retrospective case series analysis from the Italian Rare Cancer Network. *Ann Oncol.* 2012;**23**:501–8.

- Stacchiotti S, Pantaleo MA, Astolfi A, et al. Activity of sunitinib in extraskeletal myxoid chondrosarcoma. *Eur J Cancer.* 2014;**50**:1657–64.

- Stacchiotti S, Pantaleo MA, Negri T, et al. Efficacy and biological activity of imatinib in metastatic dermatofibrosarcoma protuberans (DFSP). *Clin Cancer Res.* 2016;**22**:938–46.

- Stacchiotti S, Verderio P, Messina A, et al. Tumor response assessment by modified Choi criteria in localized high-risk soft tissue sarcoma treated with chemotherapy. *Cancer.* 2012;**118**:5857–66.

- Tawbi HA, Burgess M, Bolejack V, et al. Pembrolizumab in advanced soft-tissue sarcoma and bone sarcoma (SARC028): a multicentre, two-cohort, single-arm, open-label, phase 2 trial. *Lancet Oncol.* 2017;**18**:1493–1501.

- van der Graaf WT, Blay JY, Chawla SP, et al; EORTC Soft Tissue and Bone Sarcoma Group; PALETTE study group. Pazopanib for metastatic soft-tissue sarcoma (PALETTE): a randomised, double-blind, placebo-controlled phase 3 trial. *Lancet.* 2012;**379**:1879–86.

- Verweij J, Casali PG, Zalcberg J, et al. Progression-free survival in gastrointestinal stromal tumours with high-dose imatinib: randomised trial. *Lancet.* 2004;**364**:1127–34.

- Wang WL, Conley A, Reynoso D, et al. Mechanisms of resistance to imatinib and sunitinib in gastrointestinal stromal tumor. *Cancer Chemother Pharmacol.* 2011;**67** Suppl 1:S15–24.

- Wang WL, Katz D, Araujo DM, et al. Extensive adipocytic maturation can be seen in myxoid liposarcomas treated with neoadjuvant doxorubicin and ifosfamide and pre-operative radiation therapy. *Clin Sarcoma Res.* 2012;**2**:25.

- Wardelmann E, Merkelbach-Bruse S, Pauls K, et al. Polyclonal evolution of multiple secondary KIT mutations in gastrointestinal stromal tumors under treatment with imatinib mesylate. *Clin Cancer Res.* 2006;**12**:1743–9.

# Intermediate Malignant and Malignant Tumors of Soft Tissue Featuring a Spindle Cell Morphology

Marta Sbaraglia MD and Angelo Paolo Dei Tos MD

## Introduction

Spindle cells are generally (and sometimes erroneously) regarded as the archetype of mesenchymal neoplasia. Not surprisingly, soft tissue sarcomas with spindle cell morphology most likely represent the largest group (approximately one-third) of all mesenchymal malignancies, and include lesions such as leiomyosarcoma or synovial sarcoma that rank among the most common sarcoma histotypes.

The morphologic approach to spindle cell sarcomas follows the same rules outlined in Chapter 1. The key to proper recognition is the variable combination of cell shape, pattern of growth, background, and type of vascularization. As an example, a superficial cellular spindle cell neoplasm organized in a herringbone pattern of growth most likely represents a fibrosarcomatous dermatofibrosarcoma protuberans, whereas a patternless spindle cell proliferation featuring cellular variation and a hemangiopericytoma-like vascular network almost certainly represents an example of solitary fibrous tumor. Unfortunately, significant morphologic overlap occurs, and therefore morphologic observation needs relatively often to be associated with immunohistochemical as well as molecular analysis. Furthermore, as exemplified by spindle cell melanoma and spindle cell carcinoma, a spindle cell malignancy does not per se identify a sarcoma. The main immunomorphologic and molecular features of spindle cell sarcomas are summarized in Table 4.1 and Table 4.2, respectively. It is important to mention the fact that, irrespective of very detailed immunohistochemical and molecular analysis, there remain cases in which a specific line of differentiation cannot be established. The latest WHO classification of soft tissue tumors has specifically addressed this issue, recognizing the existence of undifferentiated spindle cell sarcomas. In such cases, despite the difficulty in assigning a specific label, it is still relevant to annotate all the morphologic features that may predict aggressive behavior and may guide the clinical decision making. A further issue is represented by the fact that in lesions such as malignant peripheral nerve sheath tumor, both immunohistochemical and molecular analysis currently play a minor diagnostic role. This further underlines the actual value of traditional morphologic observation, on which all diagnostic conclusions should always be solidly rooted.

**Table 4.1** Immunophenotypic features of spindle cell sarcomas

| Sarcoma type | CD34 | SMA | Desmin | Myogenin | h-Cal | S100 | EMA | STAT6 | KIT | DOG1 | CK | MDM2 | TLE1 |
|---|---|---|---|---|---|---|---|---|---|---|---|---|---|
| DFSP/GCF | 100% | 5% focal | – | – | – | – | – | – | – | – | – | – | – |
| AFH | – | – | 50% | – | – | – | 50% | – | – | – | – | – | – |
| LGMS | – | – | – | – | – | – | – | – | – | – | – | – | – |
| GIST | 70% | 30% | 5% | – | 70% | – | – | – | 90% | 90% | 2% | – | – |
| LMS | 20% | >90% | 70% | – | 70% | – | 30% | – | – | – | 30% | – | – |
| SFT | 85% | – | – | – | – | – | – | >90% | – | – | – | – | 10% focal |
| SS | 10% | – | – | – | – | 30% | >80% | – | – | – | 60% | – | >90% |
| Infantile FS | – | 30% | – | – | – | – | – | – | – | – | – | – | – |
| MPNST | 5% | – | 5%* | 5%* | – | 30% | ** | – | – | – | ** | 70% focal | 10% focal |
| SC LPS | 40% | – | – | – | – | – | – | – | – | – | – | – | – |
| SC RMS | – | 70% | 100% | 100% | – | 5% | – | – | – | – | 5% | – | – |
| Intimal Sarcoma | – | 30% | 5% | – | – | – | – | – | – | – | – | 70% | – |

\* In malignant triton tumor
\*\* Positive in presence of epithelial differentiation

**Legends:**

DFSP/GCF: dermatofibrosarcoma protuberans/giant cell fibroblastoma

AFH: angiomatoid fibrous histiocytoma

LGMS: low-grade myofibroblastic sarcoma

GIST: gastrointestinal stromal tumor

LMS: leiomyosarcoma

SFT: solitary fibrous tumor

SS: synovial sarcoma

FS: fibrosarcoma

MPNST: malignant peripheral nerve sheath tumor

SC LPS: spindle cell liposarcoma

SC RMS: spindle cell rhabdomyosarcoma

**Table 4.2** Genetic aberrations occurring in spindle cell sarcomas

| Sarcoma type | Cytogenetic alterations | Molecular alterations |
| --- | --- | --- |
| DFSP/GCF | t(17;22)(q21.3;q13.1) | *COL1A1-PDGFB* |
| Angiomatoid fibrous histiocytoma | t(2;22)(q33;q12) | *EWSR1-CREB1* |
| | t(2;22)(q13;q12) | *EWSR1-ATF1* |
| | t(12;16)(q13;p11) | *FUS-ATF1* |
| Solitary fibrous tumor | Inversion of chromosome 12q13 | *NAB2-STAT6* |
| Synovial sarcoma | t(x;18)(p11;q11) | *SYT-SSX1* or *SSX2* or *SSX4* |
| Infantile fibrosarcoma | t(12;15)(p13;q26) | *ETV6-NTRK3* |
| Biphenotypic sinonasal sarcoma | t(2;4)(q35;q31.1) | *PAX3-MAML3* |
| Spindle cell rhabdomyosarcoma | | Amplification of *MYOD1* and *PIK3CA* |
| | | *NCOA2* gene rearrangement |
| Intimal sarcoma | 12q12-15 amplification | *MDM2* amplification |

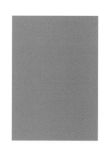

# Dermatofibrosarcoma Protuberans

## Definition and Epidemiology

Dermatofibrosarcoma protuberans (DFSP) represents a relatively common cutaneous spindle cell mesenchymal neoplasm characterized by locally aggressive clinical behavior. Morphologic progression to fibrosarcomatous DFSP (FS-DFSP) is observed in approximately 10–15% of cases and is associated with a moderate risk of developing distant metastases. Dermatofibrosarcoma protuberans occurs in a wide age range but predominates in young adults (peak incidence is in the third decade) and exhibits a slight male predominance.

## Clinical Presentation and Outcome

Dermatofibrosarcoma protuberans more frequently arises in the trunk and less frequently in the extremities and in the head and neck region. Interestingly, patients affected by adenosine deaminase-deficient severe combined immunodeficiency exhibit the tendency to develop multicentric DFSP in early childhood. Clinically, DFSP presents either as a plaque or as solitary or multiple nodules. The tumor exhibits high tendency to recur locally, whereas it almost never metastasizes unless it undergoes fibrosarcomatous change (FS-DFSP). The risk for distant metastases for FS-DFSP (mainly to the lungs) is estimated to be approximately 10–15%, whereas the rate of local recurrences overlaps with that of ordinary DFSP. In those exceptional cases featuring high-grade pleomorphic morphology, aggressive behavior is to be expected. Surgical excision with wide margins is the treatment of choice for both DFSP and FS-DFSP. The quality of the surgical treatment has a great impact over the clinical outcome. In fact, the likelihood of local recurrence after complete removal is less than 10%, whereas it is higher than 50% if the margins are positive. The use of Mohs surgery appears to reduce the risk of local recurrence by achieving higher rates of free surgical margins. Adjuvant radiotherapy, administered either before or after surgery, significantly reduces the risk of local recurrence in patients who have or who are likely to have close or positive margins. Imatinib mesylate, which is a potent inhibitor of several protein tyrosine kinases, including PDGFB, has proved to be effective in the treatment of DFSP, especially in patients with locally advanced disease or metastatic disease.

## Morphology and Immunophenotype

Macroscopically, the lesion may appear as an indurated plaque (Fig. 4-1) or as solitary or multiple nodules of variable size (Fig. 4-2). Microscopically, DFSP is composed of a remarkably uniform population of spindle cells arranged in short fascicles, relatively

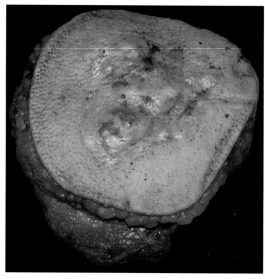

**Fig. 4-1.** Dermatofibrosarcoma protuberans. Grossly, the tumor appears as an indurate plaque of the skin.

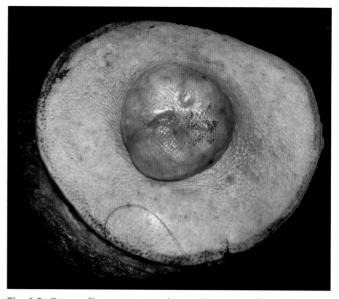

**Fig. 4-2.** Dermatofibrosarcoma protuberans. Macroscopically, a solitary nodule is shown.

often exhibiting a distinctive storiform pattern of growth (Fig. 4-3). The tumor diffusely infiltrates the subcutaneous fat extending along the fibrous septa and in between adipocytes, resulting in a

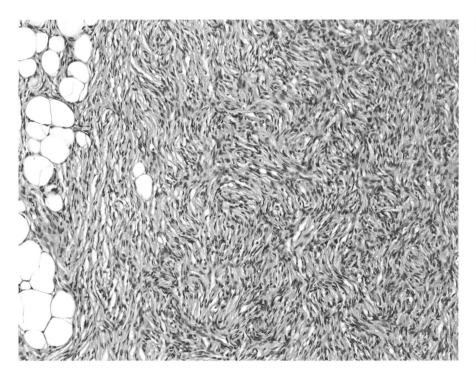

**Fig. 4-3.** Dermatofibrosarcoma protuberans. At low power, the tumor is composed of uniform spindle cells arranged in a storiform pattern of growth.

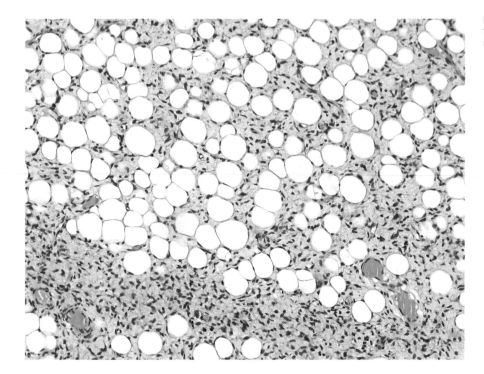

**Fig. 4-4.** Dermatofibrosarcoma protuberans. The tumor extensively infiltrates the subcutaneous fat, resulting in a honeycomb appearance.

distinctive honeycomb appearance (Fig. 4-4). The lesion is centered in the dermis, and early in the course of the disease there may be a narrow tumor-free zone (known as a "grenz zone") between the lesion and the epidermis. Neoplastic cells exhibit mild cytologic atypia, and mitotic activity is low to absent (Fig. 4-5). The superficial, subepidermal part of the lesion often tends to be remarkably hypocellular, to the extent that in small, superficial biopsies the presence of neoplastic cells may be overlooked (Figs. 4-6 and 4-7). Rarely, DFSP may feature prominent myxoid

change of the stroma that represents a potential source of diagnostic uncertainty (Figs. 4-8 and 4-9).

Approximately 10–15% of all DFSPs contains a fibrosarcomatous (FS-DFSP) component characterized by foci of increased cellularity (Fig. 4-10) and higher mitotic activity (often exceeding 10 mitoses/10 high power fields [HPF]), arranged in a distinctive fascicular, herringbone pattern of growth (Fig. 4-11). Fibrosarcomatous DFSP actually corresponds to the majority of the lesion that was classified in the past as adult fibrosarcoma. In

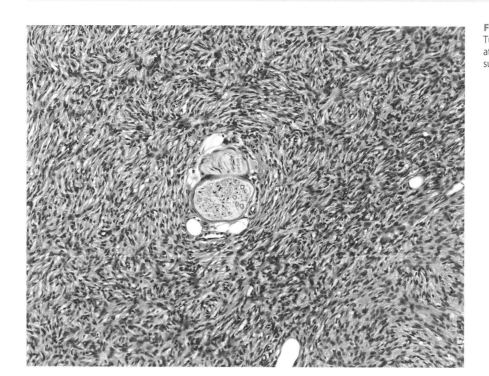

**Fig. 4-5.** Dermatofibrosarcoma protuberans. Tumor cells look uniform and exhibit mild cytologic atypia. A subcutaneous neural structure is surrounded by the neoplastic proliferations.

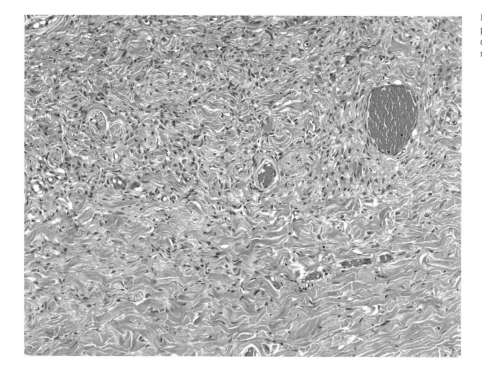

**Fig. 4-6.** Dermatofibrosarcoma protuberans. The presence of hypocellular areas that represent a diagnostic challenge are most often seen in the most superficial part of the lesion.

FS-DFSP, neoplastic cells maintain the typical monomorphism as well as limited cytologic atypia (Fig. 4-12). In extremely rare cases, morphologic progression to high-grade pleomorphic sarcoma can be observed (Fig. 4-13).

Approximately 3 to 5% of DFSPs feature the presence of melanin-containing cells, a condition that is also labeled eponymically as Bednar tumor (Fig. 4-14). Pigmented cells tend to be more numerous in the center of the lesion and may feature either a dendritic appearance or an oval shape devoid of cytoplasmic projections. Another subtle morphologic variation is represented by the presence of discrete bundles of smooth muscle actin-positive, eosinophilic myofibroblastic cells that are more often seen in FS-DFSP (Fig. 4-15). Immunohistochemically, DFSP shows diffuse positivity for CD34 (Fig. 4-16), whereas it is usually negative for S100 protein, actin, desmin, epithelial membrane antigen (EMA), and cytokeratin. CD34 positivity may be lost in fibrosarcomatous areas.

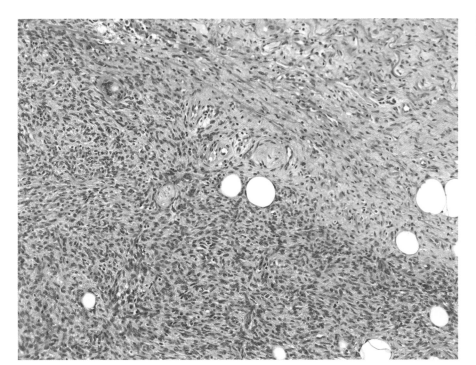

**Fig. 4-7.** Dermatofibrosarcoma protuberans. The transition from hypocellular to hypercellular areas is seen.

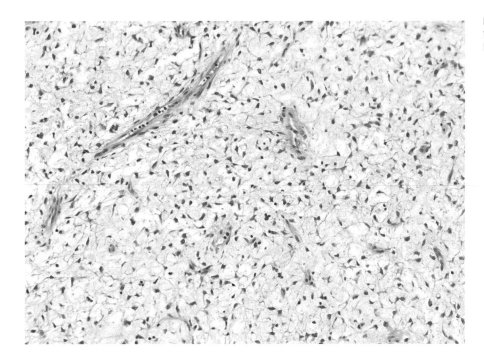

**Fig. 4-8.** Dermatofibrosarcoma protuberans. The tumor shows a relatively hypocellular neoplastic proliferation set in a myxoid stroma.

## Genetics

Cytogenetically, dermatofibrosarcoma protuberans most often shows the presence of ring chromosomes containing rearranged material from chromosomes 17 and 22 or, less frequently, an unbalanced der(22) t(17;22)(q21-23;q13). As a consequence, the collagen type I alpha 1 gene (*COL1A1*) becomes fused to the platelet-derived growth factor (PDGF) beta-chain gene (*PDGFB*). This rearrangement results in the deregulation of PDGF beta-chain expression and leads to continuous activation of the PDGF receptor beta (PDGFR-beta) protein tyrosine kinase, which promotes cell growth. PDGFB rearrangement is most often retained in both fibrosarcomatous areas as well as in the very rare "dedifferentiated" pleomorphic DFSP.

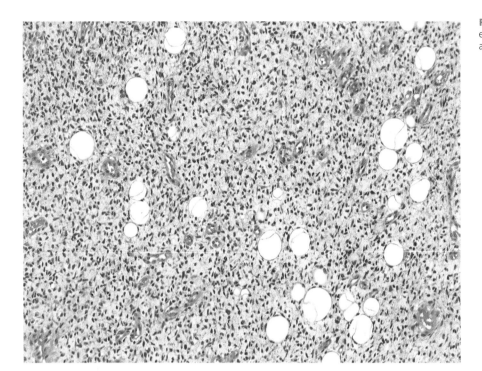

**Fig. 4-9.** Dermatofibrosarcoma protuberans. This example of myxoid DFSP exhibits greater cellularity and is associated with infiltration of adipose tissue.

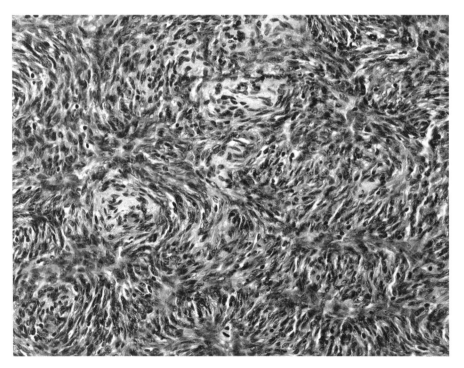

**Fig. 4-10.** Fibrosarcomatous dermatofibrosarcoma protuberans. The tumor is highly cellular and is composed of a uniform spindle cell population featuring mitotic figures. A storiform growth pattern is retained.

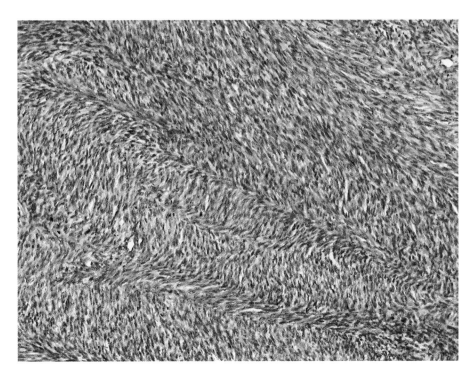

**Fig. 4-11.** Fibrosarcomatous dermatofibrosarcoma protuberans. The tumor cells are organized in long, intersecting fascicles that generate the distinctive "herringbone" growth pattern.

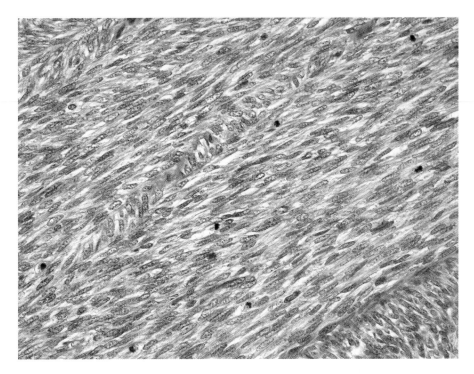

**Fig. 4-12.** Fibrosarcomatous dermatofibrosarcoma protuberans. Mitotic figures are numerous, often exceeding 10 mitoses/10HPF.

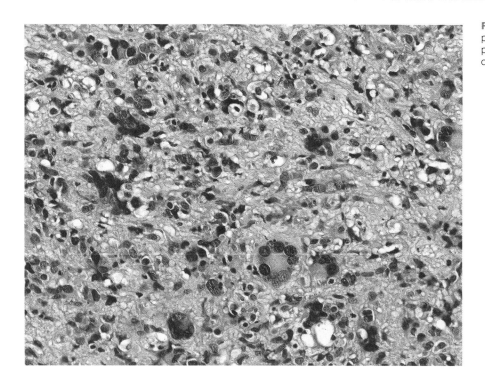

**Fig. 4-13.** Dedifferentiated dermatofibrosarcoma protuberans. Occasionally, morphologic progression to high-grade pleomorphic sarcoma can be observed.

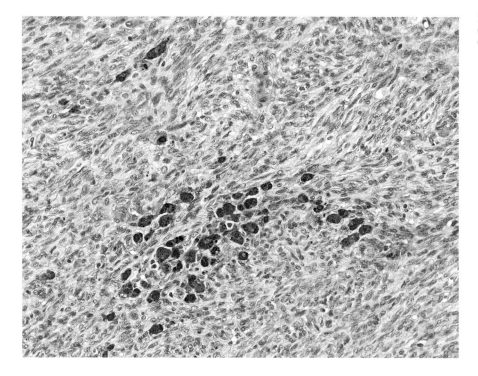

**Fig. 4-14.** Bednar tumor. Several cells containing granules of melanin pigment are scattered at the center of the tumor.

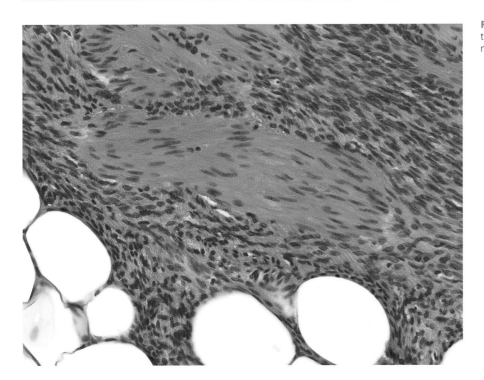

**Fig. 4-15.** Dermatofibrosarcoma protuberans. The tumor contains bundles of eosinophilic myofibroblastic cells.

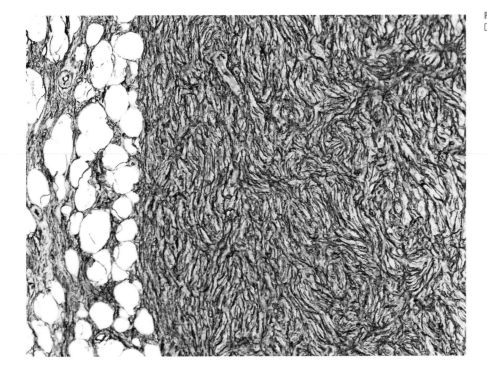

**Fig. 4-16.** Dermatofibrosarcoma protuberans. Diffuse CD34 immunopositivity is typically seen.

## Differential Diagnosis and Diagnostic Pitfalls

The main differential diagnosis of DFSP is with cellular benign fibrous histiocytoma. **Benign fibrous histiocytoma** in general represents the most frequent cutaneous mesenchymal lesion, and it is therefore worth briefly describing it here. This common lesion most often occurs in the dermis of the limbs and trunk of young adult and adult patients. Benign fibrous histiocytoma is not a reactive lesion, and as further proof of its neoplastic nature, a relatively specific genetic aberration represented by gene fusions involving either one of two protein kinase C genes (*PRKCB* and *PRKCD*) can be observed in a subset of cases. Clinical presentation and morphology are quite variable, to the extent that several variants are recognized. The **classic variant** (also commonly referred to as dermatofibroma) occurs in the limbs and the trunk of patients ranging from the third to fourth decade and shows a female predominance.

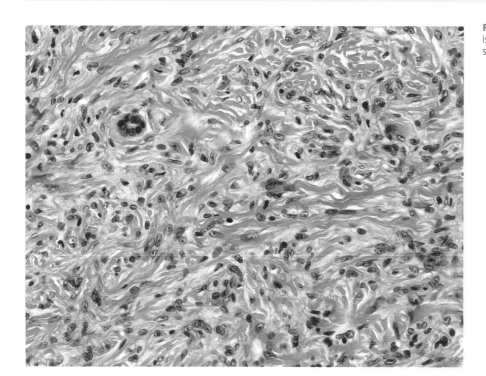

**Fig. 4-17.** Benign fibrous histiocytoma. The tumor is composed of a cytologically heterogeneous spindle cell population, set in a collagenous stroma.

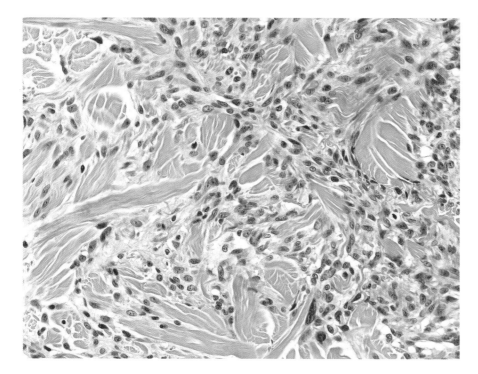

**Fig. 4-18.** Benign fibrous histiocytoma. Neoplastic cells are often associated with coarse collagenous bundles.

Typical lesions are composed of a remarkably polymorphous spindle cell proliferation (Fig. 4-17), most often associated with entrapment of collagen fibers (Fig. 4-18), epidermal hyperplasia with hyperpigmentation of the basal layer (Fig. 4-19), and the presence of a variable number (from numerous to none) of foamy histiocytes and Touton giant cells (Fig. 4-20). Immunohistochemically variable expression of CD68, CD163, and smooth muscle actin is observed. CD34 is most often negative; however, its expression can be observed in approximately 5% of cases. S100-positive dendritic cells can

be extremely numerous, potentially representing a source of diagnostic confusion with melanocytic or neural neoplasms. Dermatofibroma represents a benign lesion, and with the exceptions of the cellular, aneurysmal, and atypical subtypes, it recurs very rarely. Lung dissemination (impossible to predict) may occur occasionally but represents an extremely rare event. As mentioned, there exist several morphologic variants. The presence of abundant hemosiderin deposition identifies the **hemosiderotic** variant of benign fibrous histiocytoma (Fig. 4-21). The **ankle-type** variant (so-labeled because of its

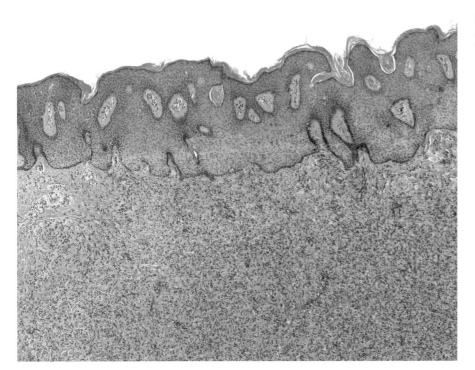

**Fig. 4-19.** Benign fibrous histiocytoma. The overlying epithelium typically appears hyperplastic with hyperpigmentation of the basal layer.

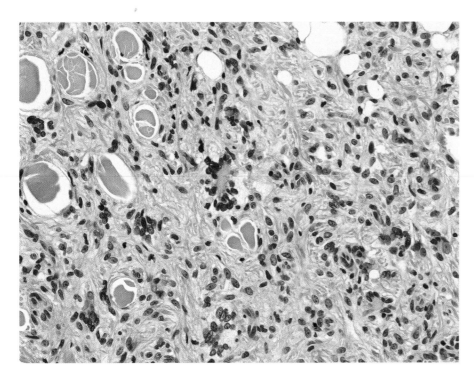

**Fig. 4-20.** Benign fibrous histiocytoma. The presence of foamy histiocytes and occasional Touton giant cells is relatively often observed.

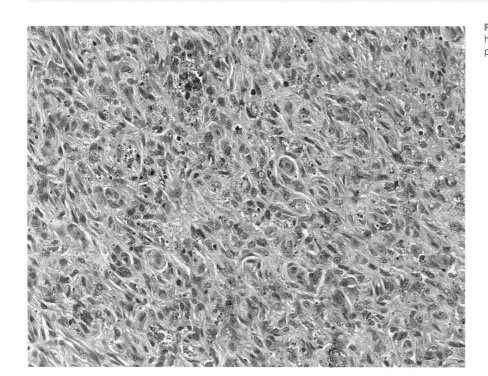

**Fig. 4-21.** Hemosiderotic benign fibrous histiocytoma. The tumor is characterized by the presence of abundant hemosiderotic pigment.

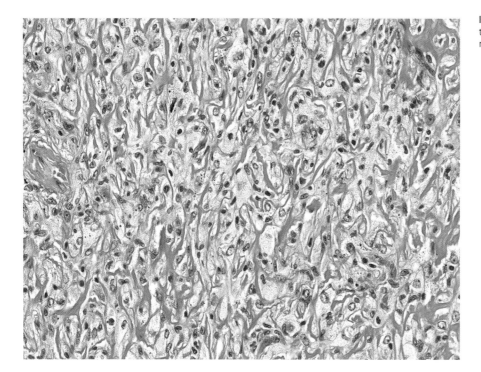

**Fig. 4-22.** Benign fibrous histiocytoma, "ankle-type." Numerous foamy histiocytes separated by refractile collagen fibers are typically observed.

tendency to occur around the ankle) is characterized by extensive lipidization as well as by the presence of distinctive refractile collagen fibers (Fig. 4-22). The **aneurysmal** variant, in addition to the presence of the conventional cell population of classic dermatofibroma, features the presence of variable amounts of pseudocystic spaces filled with blood and hemosiderin (Figs. 4-23 and 4-24). The most relevant clinical feature of aneurysmal fibrous histiocytoma is represented by the

tendency to recur locally in approximately 20% of cases. As mentioned in Chapter 7, **atypical dermatofibroma** represents the most challenging of all benign fibrous histiocytoma variants. Most cases arise in the limbs of young adults. Multifocal nuclear atypia that can be severe is seen in the context of an otherwise classic dermatofibroma (Figs. 4-25 and 4-26). An additional potential source of diagnostic uncertainty is the presence of brisk mitotic activity that can be associated with

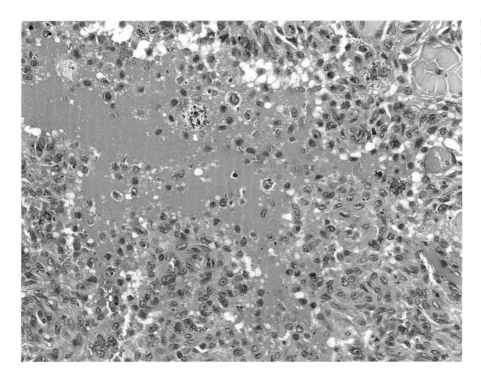

**Fig. 4-23.** Aneurysmal benign fibrous histiocytoma. The formation of microcystic spaces filled with amorphous eosinophilic fluid and hemosiderotic pigment represents a characteristic morphologic feature of this variant.

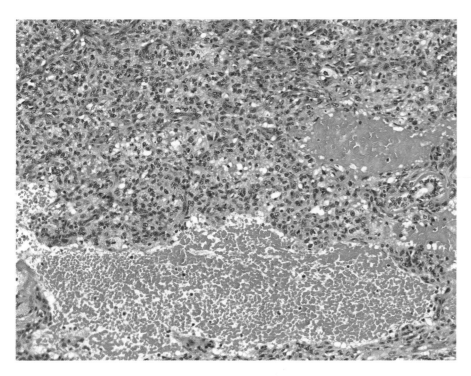

**Fig. 4-24.** Aneurysmal benign fibrous histiocytoma. In the context of the conventional cell population, erythrocyte-laden pseudovascular spaces are seen.

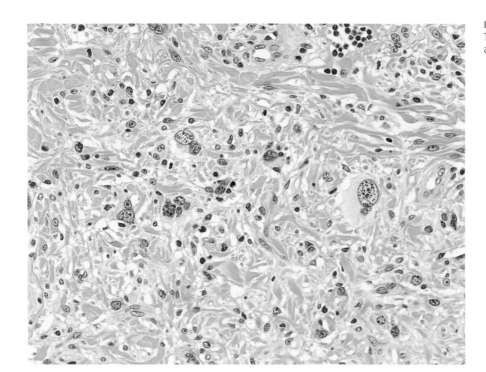

**Fig. 4-25.** Atypical benign fibrous histiocytoma. The tumor contains pleomorphic neoplastic cells associated with coarse collagen fibers.

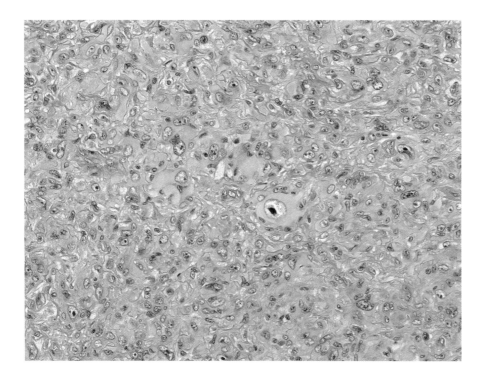

**Fig. 4-26.** Atypical benign fibrous histiocytoma. The presence of significant nuclear atypia may represent a major diagnostic challenge.

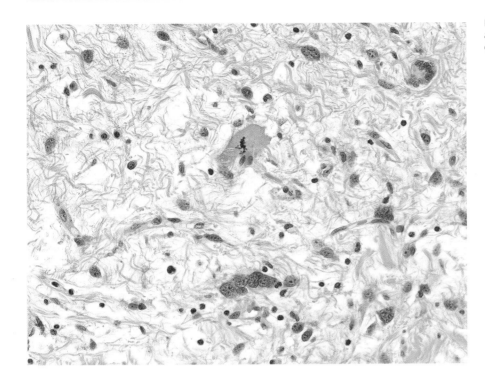

**Fig. 4-27.** Atypical benign fibrous histiocytoma. In addition to cytologic atypia, atypical mitotic figures can be observed.

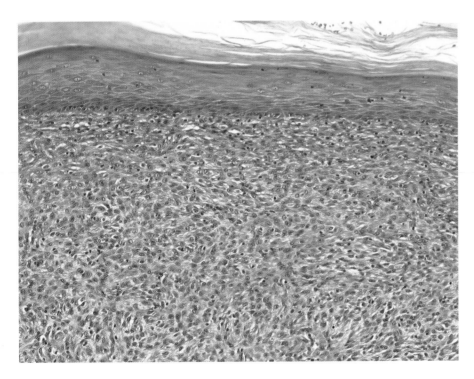

**Fig. 4-28.** Epithelioid benign fibrous histiocytoma. Neoplastic cells exhibit abundant cytoplasm and feature a distinctive epithelioid morphology.

atypical mitotic figures (Fig. 4-27). As mentioned, local recurrences are observed in approximately 20% of cases. Dermatofibroma may also rarely feature an epithelioid morphology that may be associated with EMA immunopositivity. **Epithelioid benign fibrous histiocytoma** most often exhibits a dome-shaped silhouette demarcated by an epithelial collarette (Fig. 4-28). Lesional cells feature striking epithelioid morphology as well as a solid pattern of growth (Fig. 4-29). Interestingly, rearrangement of the *ALK* gene is observed

in the majority of cases. This molecular characteristic would support the concept that epithelioid benign fibrous histiocytoma may actually be unrelated to the family of dermatofibroma.

Regarding the differential diagnosis with DFSP, all the above-mentioned variants are actually characterized by a distinctive cellular pleomorphism that contrasts with the morphologic uniformity that represents the diagnostic hallmark of DFSP. **Cellular benign fibrous histiocytoma** accounts for

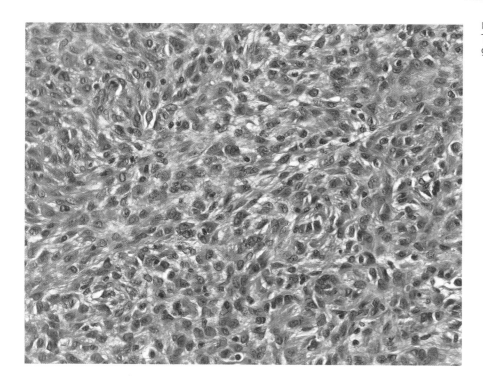

**Fig. 4-29.** Epithelioid benign fibrous histiocytoma. The tumor cells are organized in a solid pattern of growth.

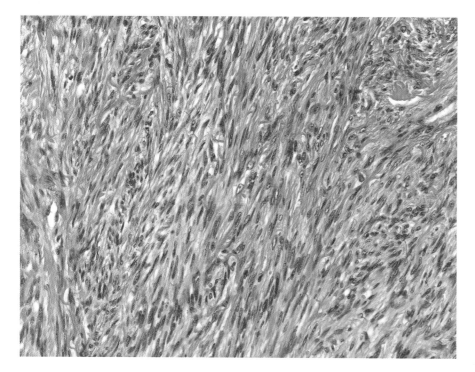

**Fig. 4-30.** Cellular benign fibrous histiocytoma. The tumor is composed of a more uniform spindle cell population that tends to grow in fascicles.

about 5% of all benign fibrous histiocytomas and is most often misdiagnosed as DFSP. Clinical presentation overlaps with that of classic variants; however, a male predominance is observed. Microscopically, in contrast to the other variants of fibrous histiocytomas, the cellular variant is composed of a relatively uniform spindle cell proliferation organized in a fascicular, somewhat myoid pattern of growth (Fig. 4-30). Such a cellular uniformity, along with the tendency to

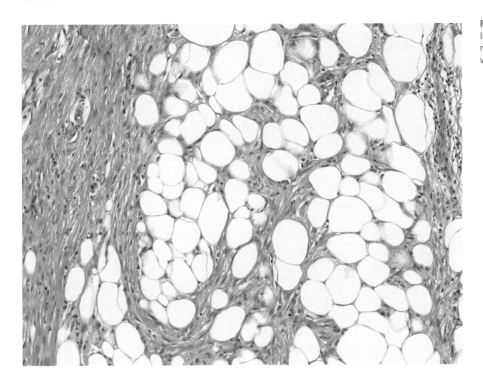

**Fig. 4-31.** Cellular benign fibrous histiocytoma. Infiltration of the subcutaneous fat is often seen and represents an overlapping morphologic feature with DFSP.

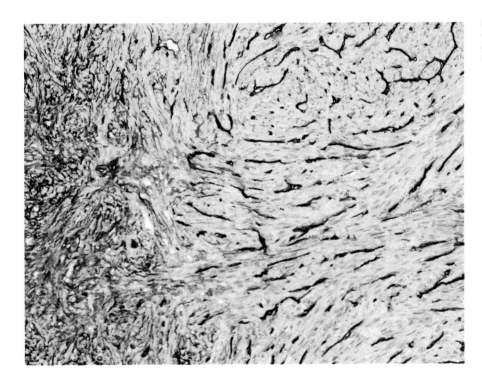

**Fig. 4-32.** Cellular benign fibrous histiocytoma. CD34 immunostaining shows the dermal fibroblasts displaced at the periphery of the lesion. Neoplastic cells are CD34 negative.

infiltrate at least focally the surrounding fat, represents the main morphologic feature that contributes to diagnostic confusion with DFSP (Fig. 4-31). Immunohistochemistry plays an important role in the differential diagnosis, because cellular benign fibrous histiocytoma (in stark contrast with DFSP) is most often (but not invariably) CD34 negative. Most often, CD34-positive dermal stroma cells are condensed at the periphery, with lesional cells being CD34 negative (Fig. 4-32). Cellular benign fibrous histiocytoma is characterized by a recurrence rate of approximately 20% that is independent of the quality of the surgical margins.

A final important issue is the fact that the benign fibrous histiocytomas can exceptionally metastasize. Even though this event is exceedingly rare, it represents a source of significant anxiety for pathologists. This phenomenon is chiefly observed with cellular, aneurysmal, and atypical variants. However, it must be clearly stated that there exist no morphologic features that can reliably predict systemic spread.

Another potential diagnostic challenge is the distinction between DFSP and **diffuse neurofibroma**. Neurofibromas represent the most common type of peripheral nerve sheath tumor. The vast majority occurs as sporadic cutaneous solitary lesions. Less often, multiple neurofibromas develop in the context of neurofibromatosis type 1 (NF1) syndrome (also known eponymically as von Recklinghausen disease). Cutaneous neurofibroma may present as either a localized or a diffuse lesion. Intraneural neurofibromas can be localized or plexiform. The most dramatic clinical presentation is represented by diffuse plexiform neurofibromas of soft tissue, capable of attaining massive sizes.

Microscopically, all variants of neurofibromas are composed of cytologically bland spindle cells, featuring scanty cytoplasm and harboring tapering or comma-shaped nuclei (Fig. 4-33). Neoplastic cells are set in a heterogeneous myxoid background harboring a variable amount of collagen fibers (Fig. 4-34). Solitary neurofibroma is well circumscribed but not capsulated. Diffuse neurofibroma (associated with NF1 syndrome in approximately 10% of cases) presents most often as an indurated, plaque-like superficial lesion, most often arising on the trunk of patients between the first and the third decade and having no sex predilection. Diffuse neurofibroma relatively often features areas of Meissner's differentiation and exhibits a tendency to infiltrate the adipose tissue with a "honeycomb" pattern of growth. This latter morphologic feature greatly contributes to diagnostic confusion with DFSP (Fig. 4-35). An extremely helpful diagnostic finding is represented by S100 immunopositivity (Fig. 4-36), which (in contrast to the diffuse staining observed in benign schwannomas) is seen in approximately half of all lesional cells. In fact, neurofibromas, in addition to S100-positive Schwann cells, are also composed of CD34-positive stromal cells and EMA-positive perineurial cells. Notably, DFSP is consistently negative for S100.

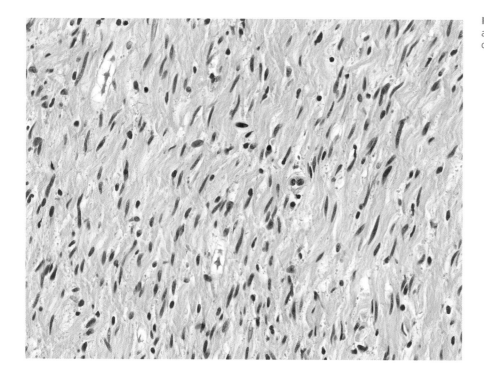

**Fig. 4-33.** Diffuse neurofibroma. The tumor cells are spindled, with tapering nuclei and scant, ill-defined cytoplasm.

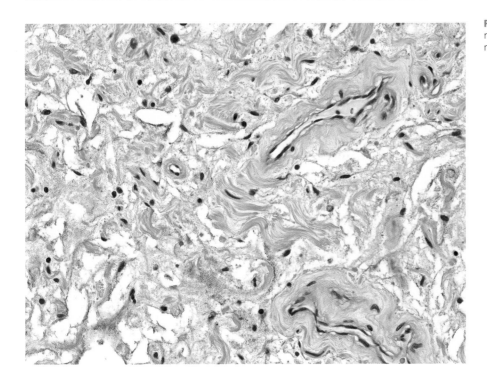

**Fig. 4-34.** Diffuse neurofibroma. The presence of a myxocollagenous background represents a typical morphologic feature of this lesion.

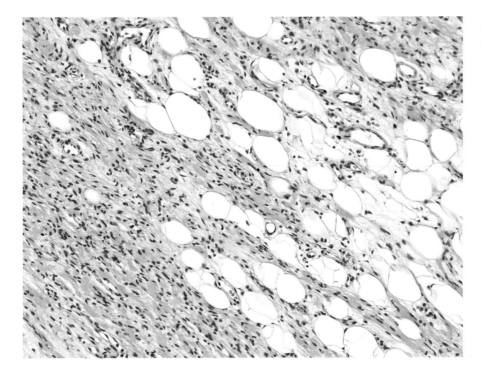

**Fig. 4-35.** Diffuse neurofibroma. Diffuse infiltration of fat can simulate the "honeycomb" appearance of DFSP.

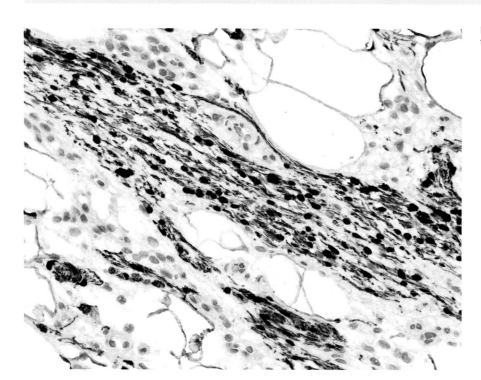

**Fig. 4-36.** Diffuse neurofibroma. The majority of tumor cells are immunopositive for S100.

### Key Points in Dermatofibrosarcoma Protuberans Diagnosis

- Occurrence in the superficial soft tissue of the trunk of young adults
- Monomorphous spindle cell proliferation
- Distinctive "honeycomb" infiltration of the subcutaneous fat
- Presence of *PDGFbeta* gene rearrangement
- Locally aggressive with no metastatic potential unless fibrosarcomatous change occurs

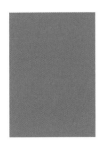

# Giant Cell Fibroblastoma

## Definition and Epidemiology

Giant cell fibroblastoma (GCF) is a locally aggressive, non-metastasizing mesenchymal lesion, currently considered a morphologic variant of DFSP that occurs primarily in children. Giant cell fibroblastoma occurs most often (but not exclusively) in the pediatric age-group and is characterized by male predominance.

## Clinical Presentation and Outcome

Most cases occur in the dermis and in the subcutaneous adipose tissues of the trunk, inguinal region, and axilla. More rarely, GCF may be observed in the extremities. Local recurrences are observed in approximately half of all patients; however, distant metastases have thus far not been reported. Wide surgical excision represents the treatment of choice.

## Morphology and Immunophenotype

Macroscopically, the lesion may appear as an indurated plaque or as solitary or multiple nodules of variable size. Microscopically, GCF features a spindle cell proliferation set in a myxocollagenous stroma (Fig. 4-37). As in DFSP, the most superficial part of the lesion tends to be remarkably hypocellular (Fig. 4-38). Morphology actually overlaps significantly with DFSP, including the presence of infiltration of the adipose tissue in a honeycomb pattern of growth (Fig. 4-39). The most distinctive feature of GCF is represented by the presence of pseudovascular, angiectoid spaces lined by multinucleated giant cells (Figs. 4-40 and 4-41). Areas of increased cellularity that can be associated with moderate pleomorphism are rarely seen (Fig. 4-42). Giant cell fibroblastoma exhibits an extremely infiltrative pattern of growth, with invasion of subcutaneous fat extending well beyond the main lesion (Fig. 4-43). Rarely, fibrosarcomatous areas can be observed. CD34 immunopositivity is observed in all cases. As further proof of the strict link between DFSP and GCF, hybrid lesions featuring aspects of both entities are rarely seen in adult patients.

## Genetics

Giant cell fibroblastoma harbors the same gene rearrangement of DFSP that fuses the collagen type I alpha 1 gene (*COL1A1*) on 17q21 with the platelet-derived growth factor (PDGF) beta-chain gene (*PDGFB*) on 22q13.

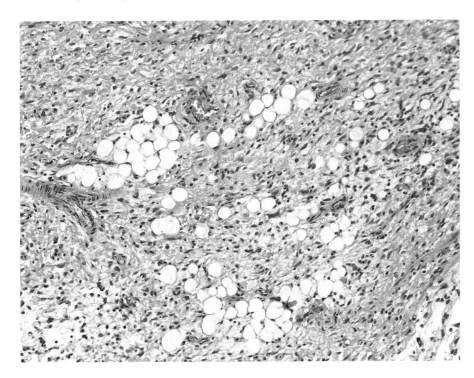

**Fig. 4-37.** Giant cell fibroblastoma. The tumor is composed of a spindle cell proliferation that tends to infiltrate the subcutaneous fat diffusely.

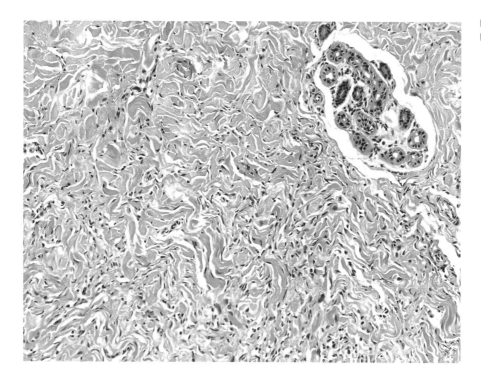

**Fig. 4-38.** Giant cell fibroblastoma. The superficial part of the lesion tends to be hypocellular.

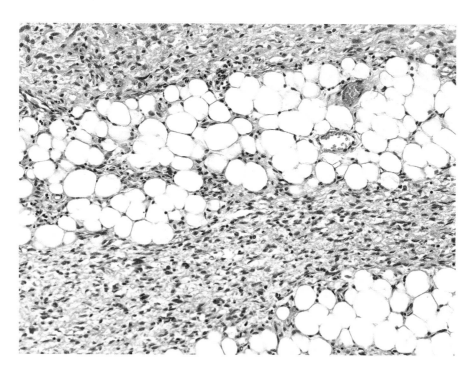

**Fig. 4-39.** Giant cell fibroblastoma. As in DFSP, adipose tissue infiltration generates a "honeycomb" appearance.

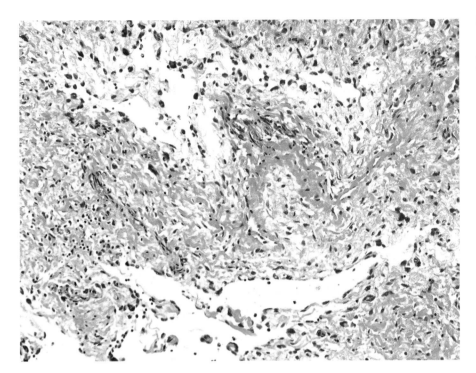

**Fig. 4-40.** Giant cell fibroblastoma. One of the most distinctive morphologic features is represented by the presence of pseudovascular, angiectoid spaces lined by multinucleated giant cells.

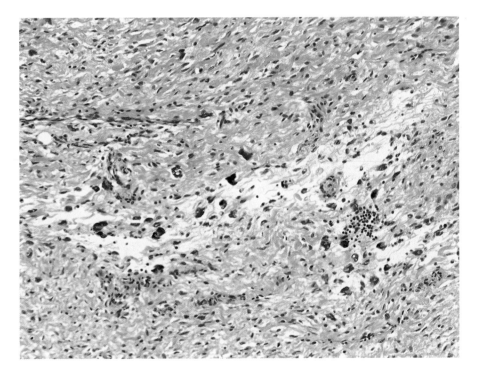

**Fig. 4-41.** Giant cell fibroblastoma. Giant cells feature hyperchromatic nuceli. By contrast, the surrounding spindle cell proliferation exhibits a relatively bland cytomorphology.

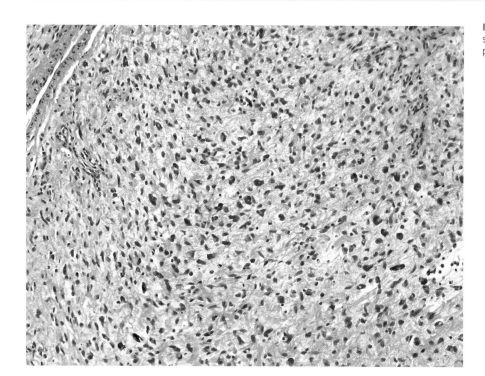

**Fig. 4-42.** Giant cell fibroblastoma. Rare cases show increased cellularity with multifocal pleomorphism.

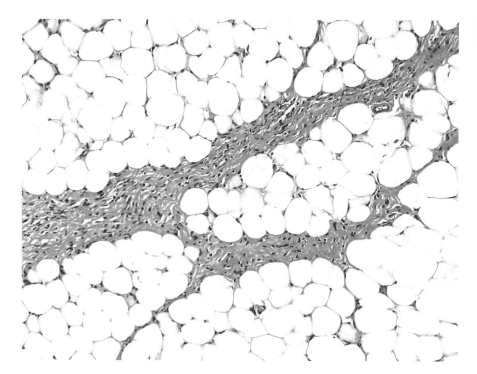

**Fig. 4-43.** Giant cell fibroblastoma. The tumor tends to infiltrate the subcutaneous fat well beyond the main lesion.

## Differential Diagnosis and Diagnostic Pitfalls

A relatively rare pediatric condition that may exhibit significant morphologic overlap with GCF is represented by **lipofibromatosis**. Lipofibromatosis represents a benign fibroblastic proliferation most often occurring in the superficial soft tissue of the limbs of newborns and children in their first year of life. Male predominance is generally observed. Lipofibromatosis is both grossly and microscopically poorly circumscribed and is composed of fascicles of spindle cells dispersed within lobules of mature fat (Fig. 4-44). Lesional cells are cytologically bland, and mitotic activity is low to absent (Fig. 4-45). At variance with GCF, diffuse effacement of adipose tissue is not observed. Immunohistochemically, lesional cells feature variable expression of smooth muscle actin and CD34. Lipofibromatosis is benign; however, non-destructive local recurrences are observed in approximately two-thirds of cases.

Another pediatric lesion that may enter the differential diagnosis is represented by **fibrous hamartoma of infancy**. First reported by Reye in 1956, fibrous hamartoma of infancy occurs most often in the superficial soft tissue of the axilla, shoulders, and trunk. A distinctive infiltrative pattern of growth is seen, and microscopically the key diagnostic feature is represented by the presence of a triphasic, organoid architecture (Fig. 4-46), that combines adipose tissue, fibrous tissue, and cellular islands of immature spindle cells set in a myxoid matrix (Fig. 4-47). The morphologic feature that may pose diagnostic difficulties with both lipofibromatosis and giant cell fibroblastoma is again represented by the tendency to infiltrate the surrounding adipose tissue (Fig. 4-48). Immunohistochemically, fibrous hamartoma of infancy exhibits variable expression of smooth muscle actin and desmin, most likely an expression of its myofibroblastic nature.

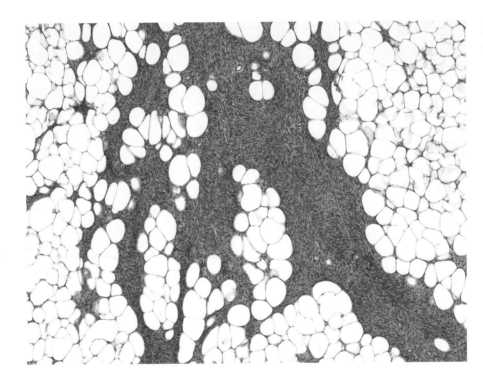

**Fig. 4-44.** Lipofibromatosis. The tumor is characterized by fascicles of spindle, non-atypical cells surrounded by mature adipocytic tissue.

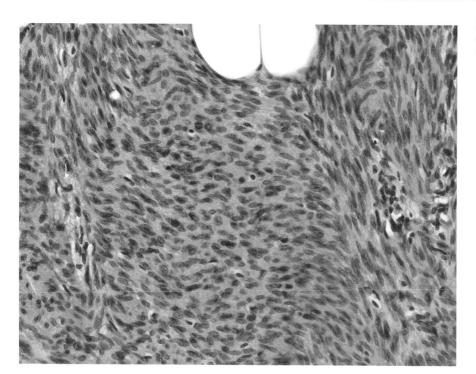

**Fig. 4-45.** Lipofibromatosis. Neoplastic cells are cytologically bland and mitotic activity is not observed.

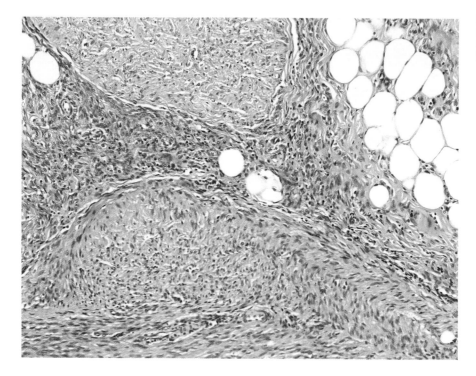

**Fig. 4-46.** Fibrous hamartoma of infancy. At low power, the distinctive "triphasic" morphology composed of fat, fibrous tissue, and islands of immature spindle cells is easily appreciated.

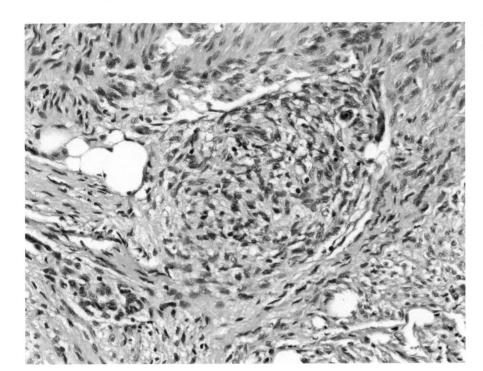

**Fig. 4-47.** Fibrous hamartoma of infancy. Fibrous tissue contains nodules of immature spindle cells set in a myxoid stroma.

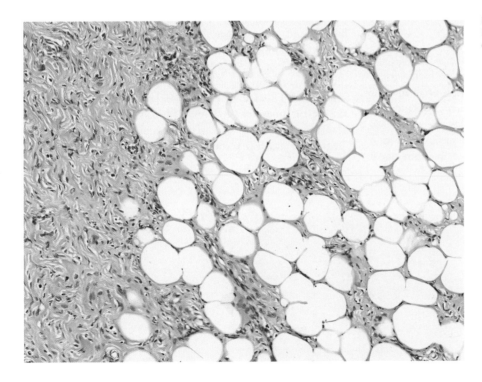

**Fig. 4-48.** Fibrous hamartoma of infancy. Extensive Infiltration of fat may generate diagnostic confusion with giant cell fibroblastoma.

### Key Points in Giant Cell Fibroblastoma Diagnosis

- Occurrence in the superficial soft tissue of the trunk of children
- Monomorphous spindle cell proliferation
- Distinctive "honeycomb" infiltration of the subcutaneous fat
- Presence of angiectoid spaces lined by multinucleated giant cells
- Presence of *PDGFbeta* gene rearrangement
- Locally aggressive with high rate of local recurrences but no metastatic potential

# Angiomatoid "Malignant" Fibrous Histiocytoma

## Definition and Epidemiology

Angiomatoid fibrous histiocytoma (AFH) represents an intermediate, rarely metastasizing lesion of unknown differentiation, not to be confused with aneurysmal fibrous histiocytoma (a variant of dermatofibroma). Angiomatoid fibrous histiocytoma occurs most frequently in children and young adults, with peak incidence at the second decade. Males and females are equally affected. Systemic signs such as pyrexia, anemia, or paraproteinemia are rarely observed and tend to disappear following removal of the lesion. The label "malignant" (introduced by Enzinger in 1979) has been abandoned because it has become broadly accepted that its metastatic potential has been overestimated.

## Clinical Presentation and Outcome

Angiomatoid fibrous histiocytoma most often occurs in the superficial soft tissues of the extremities, followed by the trunk and the head and neck region. Two-thirds of cases occur in areas wherein lymph nodes are normally present such as the inguinal and the supraclavicular regions. Rarely, AFH may be encountered at visceral sites such as the lungs. Local recurrence is observed in approximately 10% of cases. Metastatic spread to locoregional lymph nodes are observed in less than 2% of cases. Complete local excision is regarded as the standard therapeutic option.

## Morphology and Immunophenotype

Grossly, AFH is well circumscribed and multinodular, often showing cystic and hemorrhagic areas. A thick, fibrous pseudocapsule is usually present at the periphery of the lesion (Fig. 4-49) wherein a lymphoplasmacytic infiltrate is often observed (Fig. 4-50). Angiomatoid fibrous histiocytoma is composed of a multinodular proliferation of eosinophilic, "myoid" cells, featuring ovoid, uniform, plump nuclei and rather indistinct cytoplasmic borders (Fig. 4-51), and set in a collagenous background. Hemorrhagic areas (Fig. 4-52) and pseudovascular spaces containing a proteinaceous material can often be observed (Fig. 4-53). Stromal deposition of hemosiderin is also relatively common and is associated with the presence of hemosiderin-laden histiocytes (Fig. 4-54). Long-standing lesions may feature the presence of stromal fibrosis (Fig. 4-55). Cytologic atypia is very rare; however, occasional cases may exhibit "regressive" nuclear pleomorphism that is not associated with

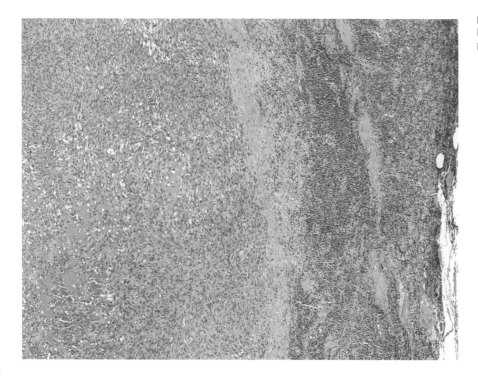

**Fig. 4-49.** Angiomatoid fibrous histiocytoma. At low power, the presence of thick, fibrous pseudocapsule is seen.

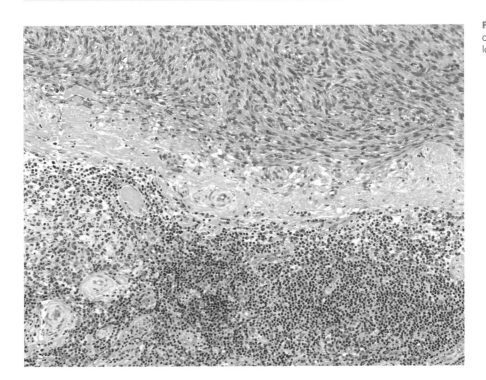

**Fig. 4-50.** Angiomatoid fibrous histiocytoma. Most often a dense lymphoplasmacytic infiltrate is located at the periphery of the lesion.

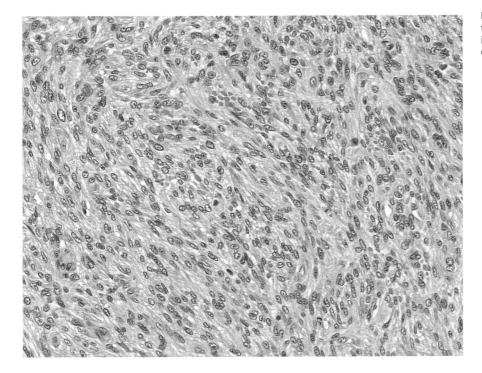

**Fig. 4-51.** Angiomatoid fibrous histiocytoma. The tumor cells contain ovoid, plump nuclei with inconspicuous nucleoli and scant, ill-defined cytoplasm.

aggressive behavior (Fig. 4-56). In some cases, neoplastic cells may acquire a distinctive epithelioid morphology (Figs. 4-57 and 4-58). Mitotic activity is generally low. Immunohistochemically, AFH exhibits desmin positivity in approximately 40% of cases (Fig. 4-59). EMA, muscle specific actin (not smooth muscle actin), CD99, and CD68 are also positive in less than half of the cases (Fig. 4-60).

## Genetics

Angiomatoid fibrous histiocytoma, similar to the much more aggressive clear cell sarcoma, is characterized by the presence of chromosome rearrangements leading to the formation of a *EWSR1-CREB1* fusion, and, more rarely, of a *EWSR1-ATF1* or a *FUS-ATF1* fusion.

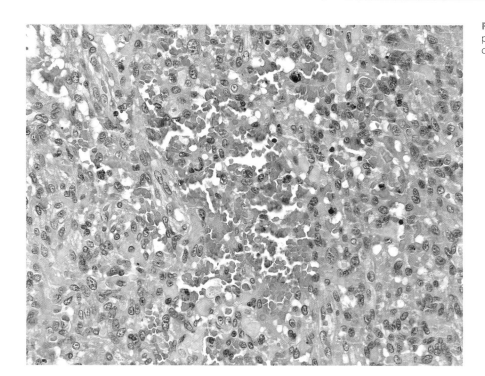

**Fig. 4-52.** Angiomatoid fibrous histiocytoma. The presence of hemorrhagic foci represents a relatively common morphologic feature.

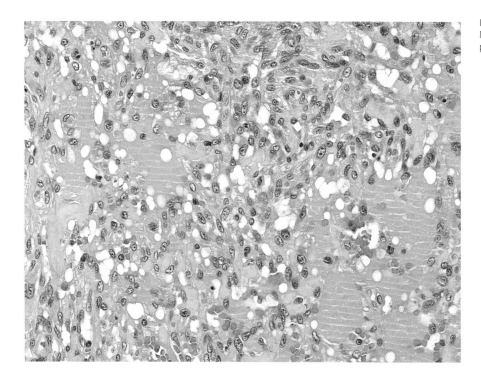

**Fig. 4-53.** Angiomatoid fibrous histiocytoma. Microcystic spaces filled with amorphous proteinaceous fluid are often seen.

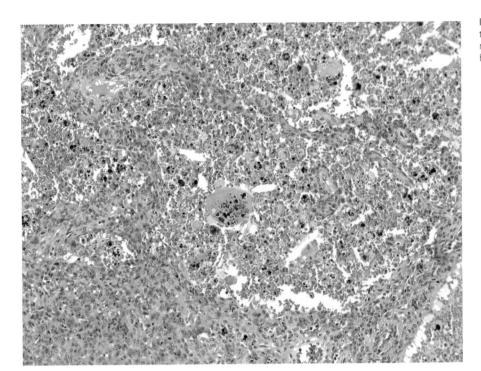

**Fig. 4-54.** Angiomatoid fibrous histiocytoma. The tumor contains hemorrhagic areas with multinucleated giant cells containing hemosiderotic pigment.

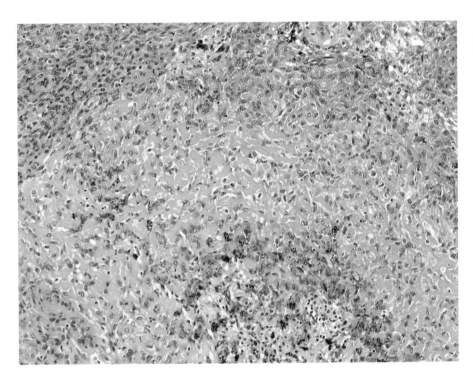

**Fig. 4-55.** Angiomatoid fibrous histiocytoma. Sometimes long-standing lesions present more extensive stromal fibrosis associated with hemosiderotic deposition.

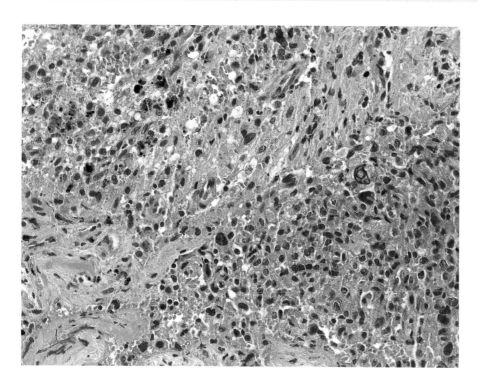

**Fig. 4-56.** Angiomatoid fibrous histiocytoma. Long-standing lesions may show multifocal regressive atypia.

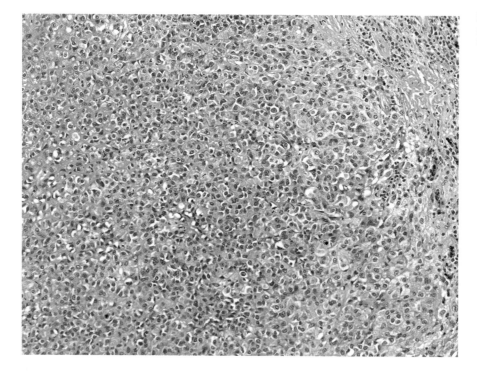

**Fig. 4-57.** Angiomatoid fibrous histiocytoma. The neoplastic cells may occasionally feature an epithelioid morphology.

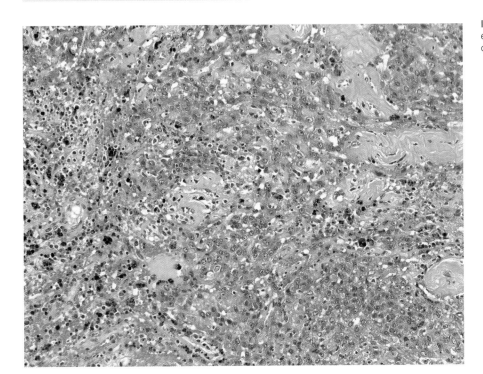

**Fig. 4-58.** Angiomatoid fibrous histiocytoma. An epithelioid cell proliferation is associated with a collagenous stroma and hemorrhagic foci.

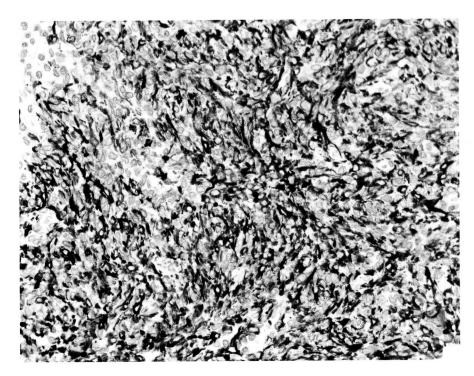

**Fig. 4-59.** Angiomatoid fibrous histiocytoma. Desmin immunopositivity is observed in approximately 40% of cases.

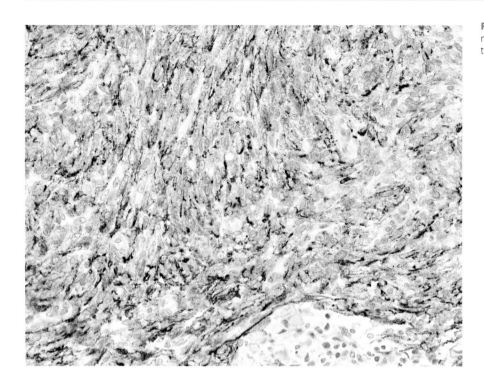

Fig. 4-60. Angiomatoid fibrous histiocytoma. The neoplastic cells are immunopositive for EMA in less than half of the cases.

## Differential Diagnosis and Diagnostic Pitfalls

The differential diagnosis includes **aneurysmal fibrous histiocytoma** and intranodal **Kaposi sarcoma**. Aneurysmal fibrous histiocytoma is actually at risk of being confused with angiomatoid "malignant" fibrous histiocytoma mainly because of the very similar label. As discussed previously, aneurysmal fibrous histiocytoma represents a variant of dermatofibroma typically centered in the dermis and featuring hemosiderin deposition associated with intralesional hemorrhage. At variance with AFH, expression of desmin is never observed.

Kaposi sarcoma is a human herpesvirus 8 (HHV-8)-induced cutaneous vascular proliferation and, in addition to the endemic form occurring at acral sites in elderly patients of Mediterranean descent, is most often seen in immunocompromised patients. Kaposi sarcoma can occur within lymph nodes and is composed of a rather monomorphous, hypercellular spindle cell proliferation, organized in intersecting fascicles and featuring moderate nuclear atypia associated with brisk mitotic activity (Fig. 4-61). Kaposi sarcoma is easily recognized on the basis of the expression of vascular markers (CD34 and CD31) as well as of nuclear expression of HHV-8 (Fig. 4-62).

In consideration of the peripheral inflammatory component somewhat mimicking a lymph node, AFH can be rarely misinterpreted as a metastatic lesion. Typical examples of AFH, however, lack cytologic atypia, and, most important, careful microscopic examination will reveal the absence of the subcapsular sinus.

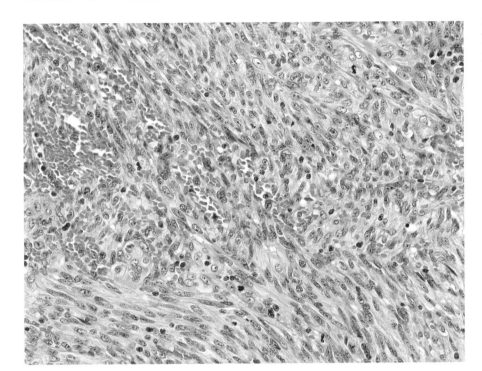

**Fig. 4-61.** Kaposi sarcoma. The tumor is composed of uniformly atypical spindle cells, organized in intersecting dense fascicles, with interposed red blood cells. The mitotic index is generally high.

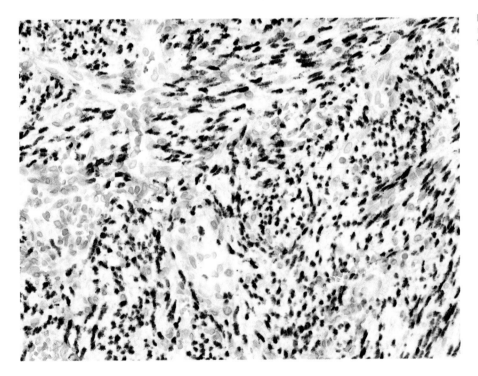

**Fig. 4-62.** Kaposi sarcoma. The presence of HHV-8 nuclear positivity represents a key diagnostic feature.

---

**Key Points in Angiomatoid Fibrous Histiocytoma Diagnosis**

- Occurrence in the superficial soft tissues of the extremities, trunk, and head and neck of children and young adults
- Uniform neoplastic cell proliferation featuring a myoid appearance.

- Desmin/EMA positivity in 40% of cases
- Presence of *EWSR1-CREB1*, *EWSR1-ATF1*, or *FUS-ATF1* fusion genes
- Indolent clinical course

# Low-Grade Myofibroblastic Sarcoma

## Definition and Epidemiology

Low-grade myofibroblastic sarcoma (LGMS) is a malignant mesenchymal myofibroblastic neoplasm superficially resembling desmoid fibromatosis. Low-grade myofibroblastic sarcoma occurs predominantly in adult patients, with a peak incidence in the fourth decade.

## Clinical Presentation and Outcome

Low-grade myofibroblastic sarcoma tends to exhibit a relatively broad anatomic distribution; however, up to 30% of cases appear to cluster in the soft tissue of the head and neck region, including the oral cavity and the larynx. The extremities and the abdominopelvic cavity represent less common sites of occurrence even if recent epidemiologic data would suggest higher incidence in the limbs. Low-grade myofibroblastic sarcoma is treated by surgical removal with wide margins. Local recurrences are observed in up to 50% of cases. Systemic spread to the lungs may occur, but it appears to be relatively rare.

## Morphology and Immunophenotype

Grossly, low-grade myofibroblastic sarcoma most often presents as a rather firm, white to tan mass, ranging between 1.5 and 20 cm in size (Fig. 4-63). Microscopically, it is composed of a spindle-shaped tumor cell proliferation, variably organized in a fascicular (Fig. 4-64) or whorled pattern of growth (Fig. 4-65), and set in a variably collagenous background. Neoplastic cells exhibit ill-defined pale or slightly basophilic cytoplasm. Nuclei are tapering with evenly distributed chromatin and small nucleoli (Fig. 4-66). Nuclear atypia is most often mild to moderate, and mitotic activity tends to be moderate. Nuclear pleomorphism can be occasionally seen in scattered

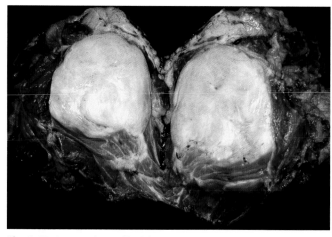

**Fig. 4-63.** Low-grade myofibroblastic sarcoma. Grossly, the tumor is most often represented by a firm, white to tan mass.

cells (Fig. 4-67). Small foci of necrosis may be present. Low-grade myofibroblastic sarcoma in most cases shows a distinctive infiltrative pattern of growth, sometimes with neoplastic cells distributing around individual skeletal muscle fibers, somewhat mimicking proliferative myositis (Fig. 4-68). The immunophenotype is very variable, with most cases showing a variable combination of smooth muscle actin (Fig. 4-69) and desmin positivity in up to 70% of cases. Approximately 30% of cases may exhibit nuclear expression of beta-catenin.

## Genetics

No specific recurrent genetic abnormalities have been reported so far.

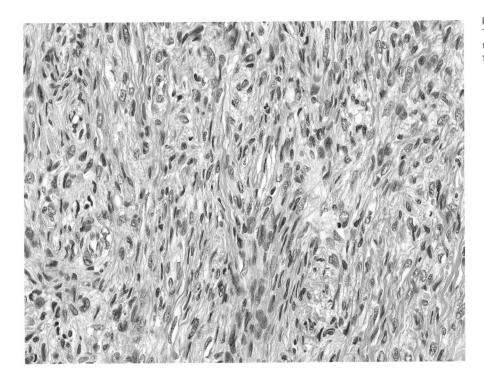

**Fig. 4-64.** Low-grade myofibroblastic sarcoma. The lesion is composed of spindle cells featuring mild to moderate atypia, organized in fascicles and set in a fibrous background.

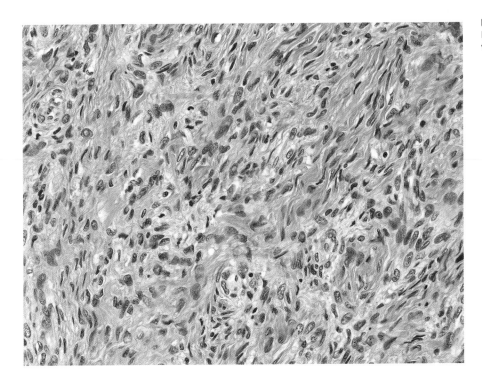

**Fig. 4-65.** Low-grade myofibroblastic sarcoma. Pattern of growth may vary from fascicular to whorled, as in this example.

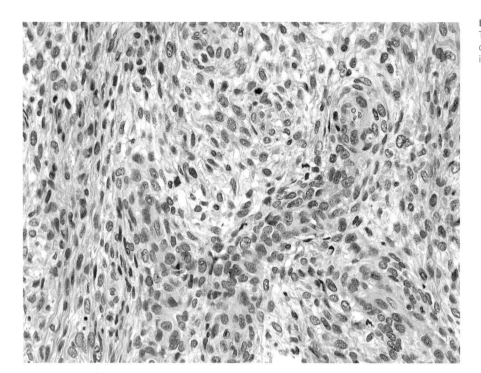

**Fig. 4-66.** Low-grade myofibroblastic sarcoma. The neoplastic cells exhibit tapering nuclei, evenly distributed chromatin, and small nucleoli with indistinct basophilic cytoplasm.

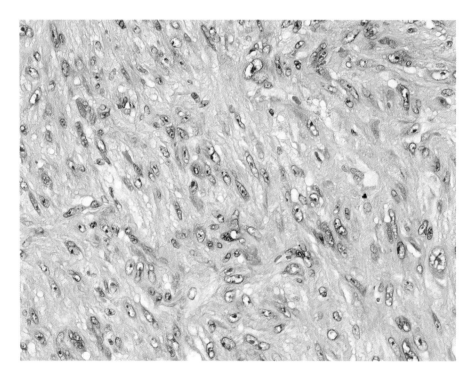

**Fig. 4-67.** Low-grade myofibroblastic sarcoma. Nuclear pleomorphism may be occasionally encountered.

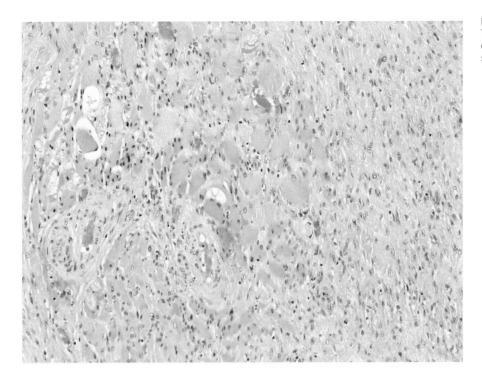

**Fig. 4-68.** Low-grade myofibroblastic sarcoma. The tumor typically features infiltrative margins with diffuse extension of neoplastic cells between skeletal muscle cells.

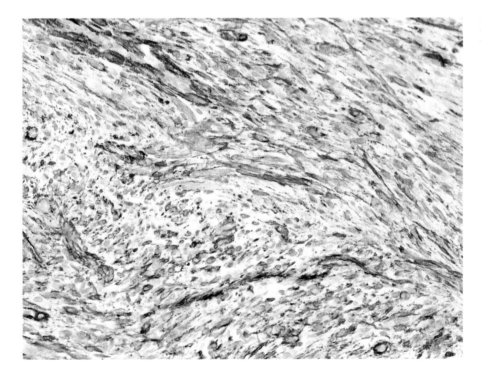

**Fig. 4-69.** Low-grade myofibroblastic sarcoma. Cytoplasmic staining for smooth muscle actin is frequently seen.

## Differential Diagnosis and Diagnostic Pitfalls

The differential diagnosis of LGMS is rather broad and includes a number of benign and malignant soft tissue neoplasms. **Nodular fasciitis** is discussed in more detail in Chapter 8 and represents a benign myofibroblastic lesion primarily occurring in the limbs of young adults. Not infrequently, however, it may occur in the head and neck region. Paradoxically, nodular fasciitis is more cellular and more mitotically active than low-grade myofibroblastic sarcoma. Main microscopic diagnostic clues are represented by a distinctive "cell culture" appearance, as well as by the absence of nuclear atypia.

**Myofibroma** is a benign myofibroblastic lesion and currently is regarded as part of a spectrum of perivascular neoplasms that include myopericytoma, angioleiomyoma, and glomus tumor. Myofibroma is characterized by bimodal occurrence in the pediatric age-group (from birth to 2 years) and in adults with a peak incidence in the fourth decade. Microscopically, they are characterized by a multinodular

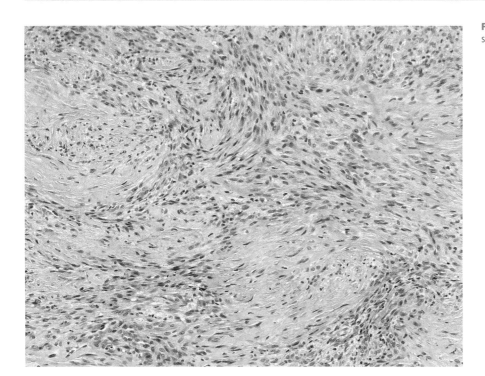

Fig. 4-70. Myofibroma. The tumor at low power shows a multinodular architecture.

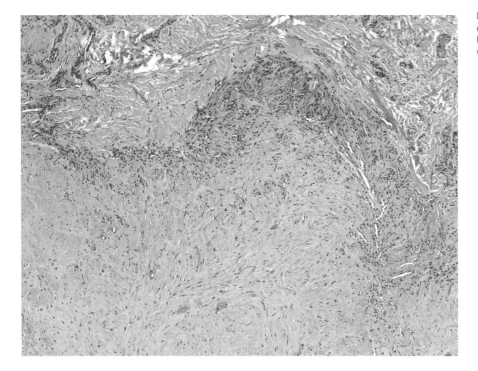

Fig. 4-71. Myofibroma. The tumor exhibits a distinctive biphasic appearance and is composed of hypercellular, immature peripheral areas merging with hypocellular myoid central areas.

pattern of growth (Fig. 4-70) as well as by a distinctive biphasic morphology (Fig. 4-71). Neoplastic modules are, in fact, composed of peripheral primitive hemangiopericytoma-like areas (Fig. 4-72), merging with areas composed of myoid spindle cells (Fig. 4-73). In some cases, myoid "maturation" predominates and the biphasic pattern can be lost (Fig. 4-74). The presence of hemangiopericytoma-like areas (along with occurrence in children) represents the rationale for the now-abandoned label "infantile hemangiopericytoma," currently replaced by "infantile myofibroma/myofibromatosis" (Fig. 4-75). Immunohistochemically, myofibroma expresses consistently smooth muscle actin (Fig. 4-76), h-caldesmon, and (in approximately 60% of cases) desmin. Myofibroma usually behaves in a benign fashion. The only exception is represented by those rare examples of pediatric cases in which multiple soft tissue, bone, and visceral locations are observed.

**Angioleiomyoma** represents the myogenic end of the spectrum of perivascular neoplasms and is one of the most

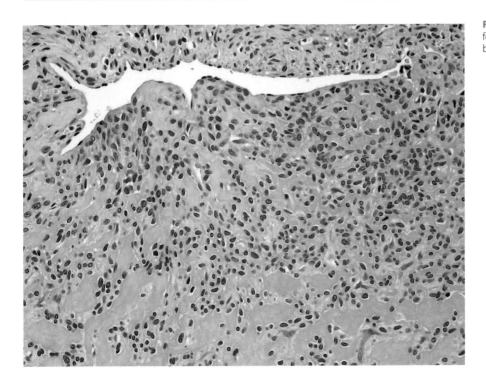

**Fig. 4-72.** Myofibroma. Immature areas typically feature the presence of hemangiopericytoma-like blood vessels.

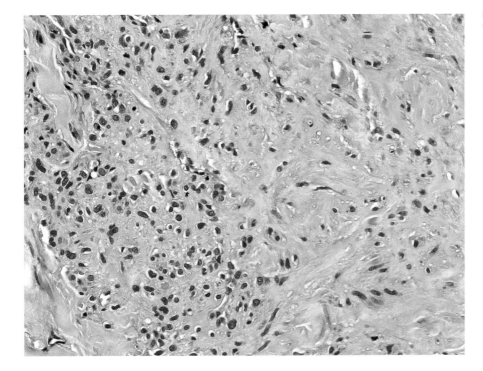

**Fig. 4-73.** Myofibroma. Immature areas merge with more mature, myoid areas.

common benign soft tissue lesions. Angioleiomyoma typically presents as a painful solitary nodule located in the subcutis of the limbs. Age range is broad and clinical behavior invariably benign. Morphologically, this lesion is composed of a cytologically bland, smooth muscle cell proliferation organized in a distinctive perivascular pattern of growth (Fig. 4-77). The abundance of blood vessels also contributes to the very characteristic morphology of angioleiomyoma (Fig. 4-78). At variance with leiomyoma of soft tissue, rare mitotic figures are

allowed and are not associated with aggressive behavior. Angioleiomyoma consistently expresses immunohistochemically smooth muscle actin, desmin, and h-caldesmon.

**Myopericytoma** also occurs predominantly in the dermis and the subcutis of the limbs of adult patients. Microscopically, myopericytoma is composed of a spindle cell proliferation featuring eosinophilic cytoplasm and plump nuclei, typically organized concentrically around blood vessels of various calibers (Figs. 4-79 and 4-80). Immunohistochemically, smooth

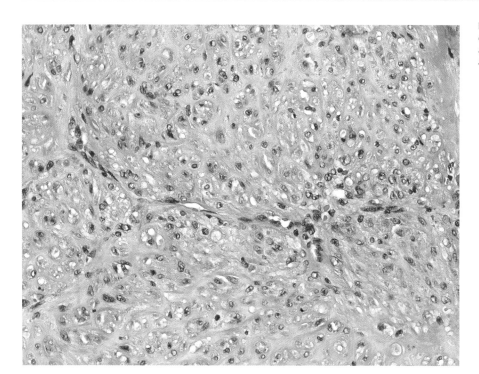

**Fig. 4-74.** Myofibroma. In rare cases, the tumor is composed almost exclusively of mature myoid cells and tends somewhat to lose the biphasic architecture.

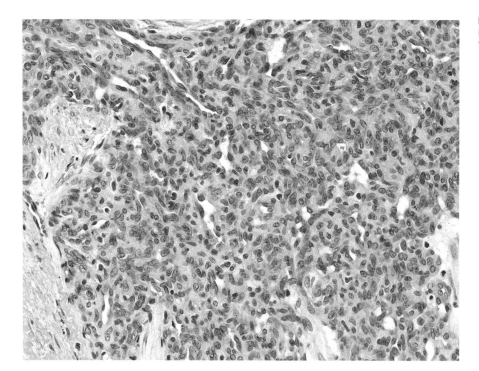

**Fig. 4-75.** Myofibroma. A closer view of the immature areas shows the distinctive "hemangiopericytoma-like" morphology.

muscle actin and h-caldesmon are consistently expressed, whereas desmin tends to be negative (Fig. 4-81). Cytologically, lesional cells are usually bland; however, rare cases may exhibit significant atypia that, in contrast to classic myopericytoma, which always pursues a benign course, may be associated with aggressive clinical behavior (Figs. 4-82 and 4-83). Interestingly, typical examples of myopericytoma are clearly described in the seminal paper on hemangiopericytoma written by Arthur Purdy Stout in 1942. As will be discussed later, this label has been temporarily abandoned; however, it

may well be that "hemangiopericytoma" will return in the future to replace the label "myopericytoma" and therefore fully recognize Dr. Stout's original description. Very recently, *PDGFRB* gene mutations have been detected in both myopericytoma and myopericytomatosis, a rare condition in which diffuse involvement of the dermis and the subcutis is observed. Interestingly, a novel *SRF-RELA* fusion has been reported within cellular examples of myopericytoma/myofibroma.

Another rare, benign myofibroblastic lesion that may be considered in the differential diagnosis is represented by

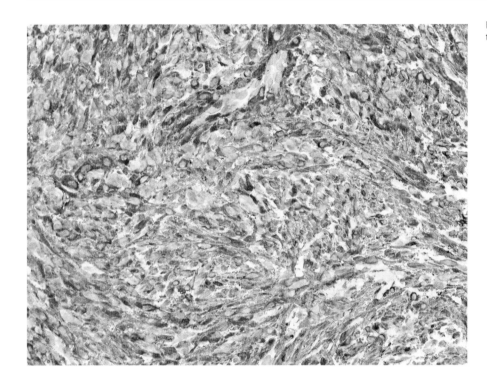

**Fig. 4-76.** Myofibroma. The neoplastic cells are typically immunopositive for smooth muscle actin.

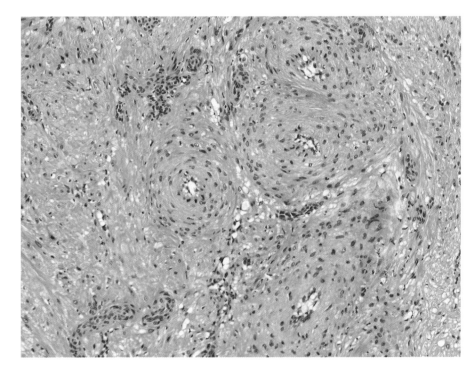

**Fig. 4-77.** Angioleiomyoma. The tumor is composed of cytologically bland smooth muscle cells organized in a distinctive perivascular pattern of growth. The abundant vascular component represents a major diagnostic clue.

**intranodal myofibroblastoma**. Intranodal myofibroblastoma is a benign myofibroblastic proliferation most often occurring in the inguinal lymph nodes and, more rarely, in the submandibular lymph nodes of middle-aged patients. Microscopically, the lesion is composed of a spindle cell proliferation centered in a lymph node (Fig. 4-84). Neoplastic cells feature non-atypical oval nuclei and palely eosinophilic cytoplasm (Fig. 4-85). A fascicular pattern of growth is most often observed, along with the presence of a variable number of eosinophilic fibrillary aggregates labeled "amianthoid fibers" (Fig. 4-86). Neoplastic cells sometimes seem to radiate from amianthoid fibers and may organize in palisades (Fig. 4-87). Paranuclear hyaline globules can be observed in approximately half of the cases. Immunohistochemically, neoplastic cells express diffusely smooth muscle actin.

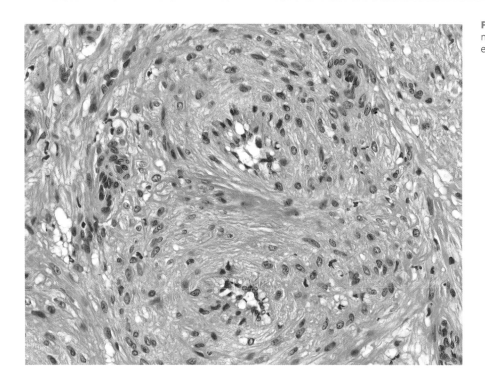

**Fig. 4-78.** Angioleiomyoma. The tumor cells have non-atypical, ovoid nuclei set in fibrillary, eosinophilic cytoplasm.

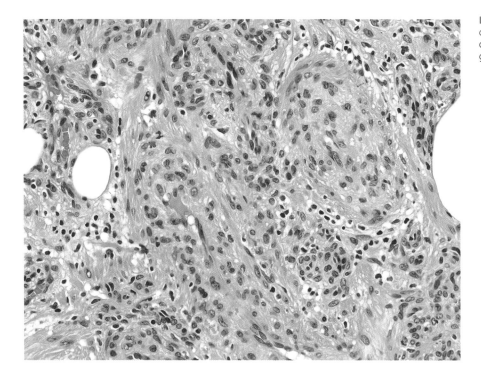

**Fig. 4-79.** Myopericytoma. The lesion is composed of a spindle cell proliferation organized in a distinctive perivascular, concentric pattern of growth.

**Desmoid fibromatosis** represents a locally aggressive but not metastasizing myofibroblastic tumor, discussed in more detail in Chapter 8, that may be difficult to distinguish from low-grade myofibroblastic sarcoma. Desmoid fibromatosis may overlap clinically with low-grade myofibroblastic sarcoma, as it may often arise in the shoulder girdle as well as in the head and neck region. Microscopically, desmoid fibromatosis most often lacks significant nuclear atypia; when compared with low-grade myofibroblastic sarcoma, desmoid fibromatosis is less cellular and less infiltrative, and proliferative activity is generally lower (Fig. 4-88). In addition, immunohistochemically tumor cells in fibromatosis stain focally positive for actin but only very infrequently for desmin. The fact that one-third of cases of low-grade myofibroblastic

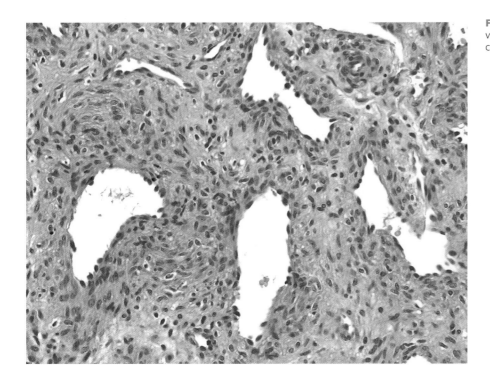

**Fig. 4-80.** Myopericytoma. Sometimes the blood vessels are more dilated. In this case, endothelial cells feature a "hobnail" appearance.

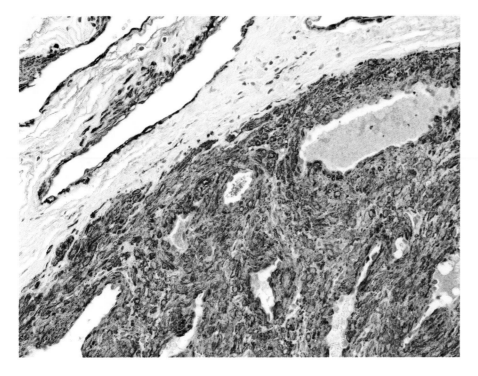

**Fig. 4-81.** Myopericytoma. Immunostaining for smooth muscle actin is diffusely positive.

sarcoma shows nuclear expression of beta-catenin (in the absence of *CTNNB1* gene mutations) certainly represents a major source of diagnostic confusion. At times, in particular when dealing with cases featuring increased cellularity as well as mitotic activity, molecular analysis of the *CTNNB1* gene may represent the only way to achieve a diagnosis of certainty.

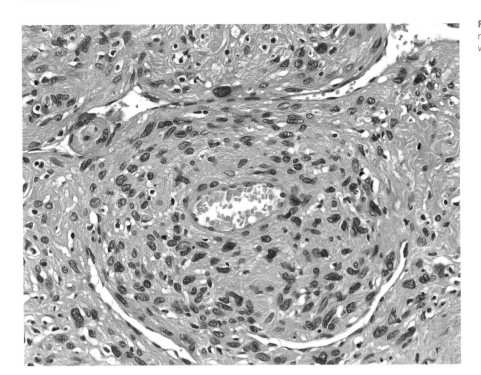

**Fig. 4-82.** Myopericytoma. In rare cases, multifocal nuclear atypia can be observed that may correlate with more aggressive behavior.

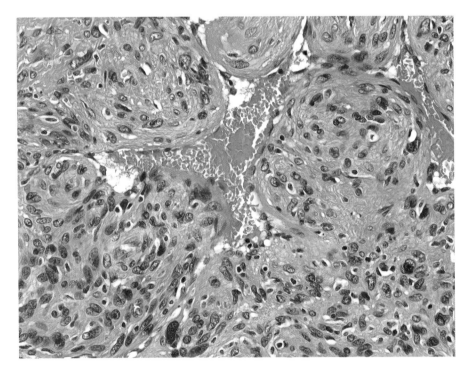

**Fig. 4-83.** Myopericytoma. Closer view of an atypical myopericytoma in which obvious nuclear pleomorphism is observed.

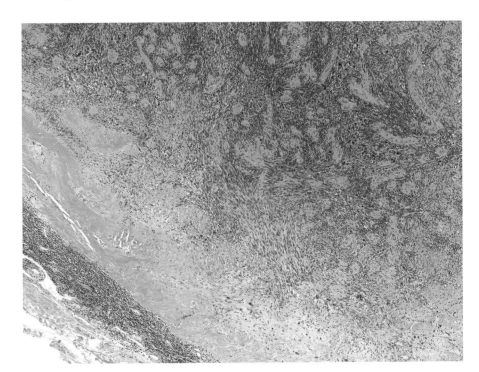

**Fig. 4-84.** Intranodal myofibroblastoma. Typically, this lesion is located in the center of a lymph node.

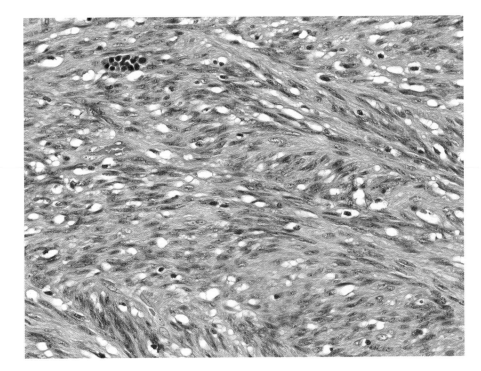

**Fig. 4-85.** Intranodal myofibroblastoma. The lesion is composed of a proliferation of cytologically bland, spindle cells featuring palely eosinophilic cytoplasm.

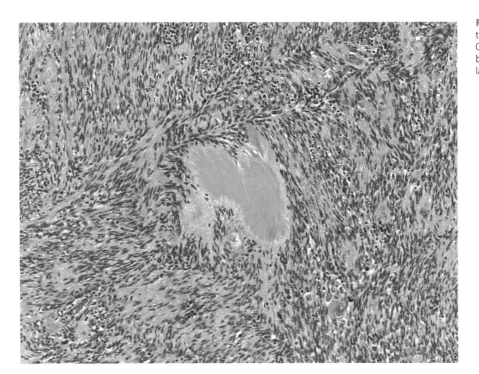

**Fig. 4-86.** Intranodal myofibroblastoma. The tumor cells are organized in intersecting fascicles. One of the most distinctive features is represented by the presence of eosinophilic fibrillary aggregates labeled "amianthoid fibers."

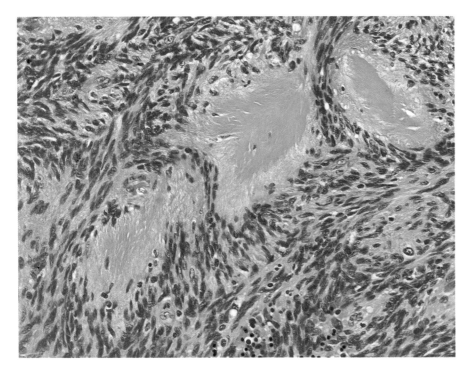

**Fig. 4-87.** Intranodal myofibroblastoma. High-power view of the lesion wherein tumor cells appear to radiate from the edge of the "amianthoid fibers."

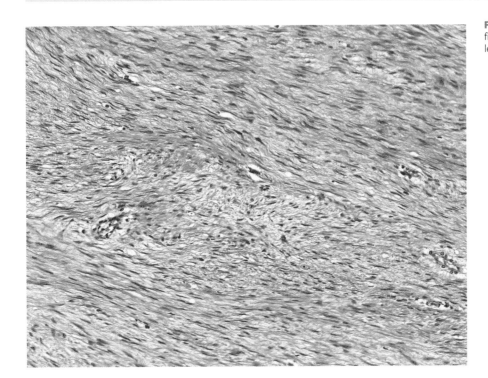

**Fig. 4-88.** Desmoid fibromatosis. Desmoid fibromatosis when compared with LGMS is usually less cellular, less atypical, and less infiltrative.

### Key Points in Low-Grade Myofibroblastic Sarcoma Diagnosis

- Occurrence in the head and neck region of adults
- Atypical spindle cell neoplasm somewhat resembling desmoid fibromatosis
- Variable expression of smooth muscle actin and desmin
- Locally aggressive with very rare metastatic spread

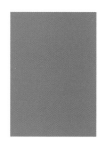

# Phosphaturic Mesenchymal Tumor

## Definition and Epidemiology

Phosphaturic mesenchymal tumor (PMT) represents an extremely rare spindle cell neoplasm associated with oncogenic osteomalacia caused by the secretion of fibroblastic growth factor 23 (FGF23) with consequent phosphaturia. Age range is very broad; however, PMT tends to occur most often in middle-aged adults, with a peak incidence between the fourth and fifth decade, and no sex predominance.

## Clinical Presentation and Outcome

Phosphaturic mesenchymal tumor occurs anywhere in the soft tissue of the limbs and the trunk. With the surgical excision of the lesion, phosphaturia disappears. Most PMTs behave in a benign fashion. In approximately 5 to 10% of cases there is local recurrence, and distant metastases are exceptional.

## Morphology and Immunophenotype

Microscopically, PMT is composed of a cytologic spindle cell proliferation set in fibrous stroma featuring hemangiopericytoma-like blood vessels (Fig. 4-89). A distinctive feature is represented by the presence of amorphous, "grungy" granular calcifications (Figs. 4-90 and 4-91) that may be associated with abundant osteoclast-like giant cells (Fig. 4-92). In rare cases, the presence of cartilaginous foci has been reported. Notably, in early lesions the distinctive calcifications may be focal or even absent. Mitotic activity tends to be very scarce and necrosis absent. Malignant change can exceptionally occur, most often following local recurrences, and is represented by progression to frankly sarcomatous, high-grade morphology. The expression of FGF23 can be demonstrated immunohistochemically in a subset of cases.

## Genetics

*FN1-FGFR1* and *FN1-FGF1* fusion genes have been recently reported in approximately half of the cases. The recently reported FN1-FGF1 chimeric protein may serve as a ligand that binds and activates FGFR1 to achieve an autocrine loop.

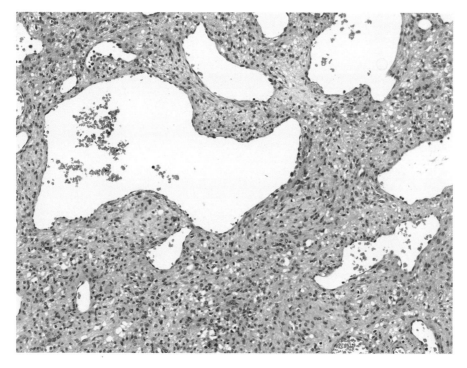

**Fig. 4-89.** Phosphaturic mesenchymal tumor. The tumor is characterized by the presence of hemangiopericytoma-like blood vessels.

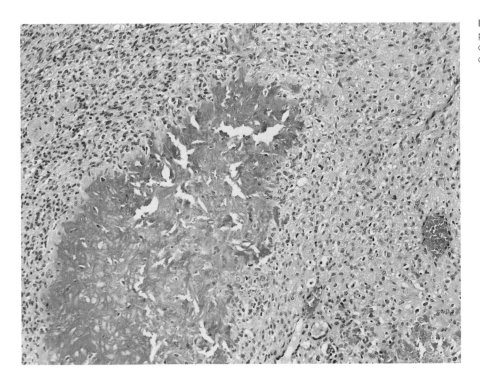

**Fig. 4-90.** Phosphaturic mesenchymal tumor. The presence of amorphous, "grungy" granular calcifications represents the most important diagnostic clue.

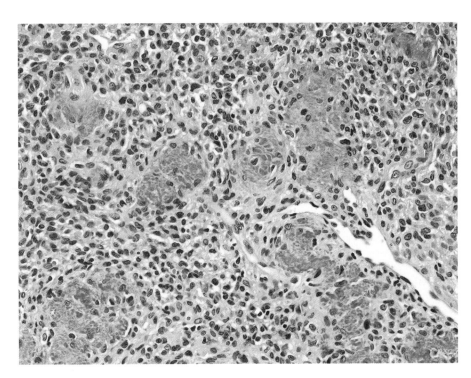

**Fig. 4-91.** Phosphaturic mesenchymal tumor. Sometimes the distinctive calcifications may be organized in smaller clusters.

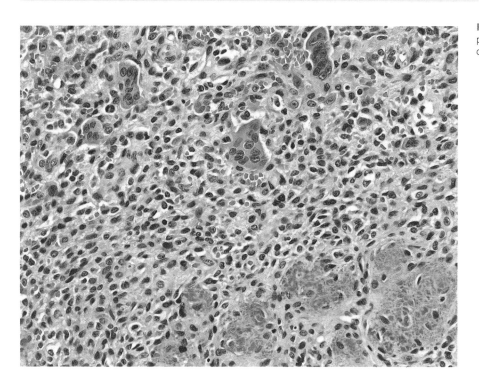

**Fig. 4-92.** Phosphaturic mesenchymal tumor. The presence of osteoclast-like multinucleated giant cells represents a common feature of the lesion.

## Differential Diagnosis and Diagnostic Pitfalls

In consideration of the prominent HPC-like vascular pattern, the differential diagnosis is primarily with solitary fibrous tumor. Solitary fibrous tumor frequently features the presence of a collagenized background; however, the absence of the distinctive calcified matrix as well as the presence of nuclear expression of STAT6 allow distinction in most cases.

### Key Points in Phosphaturic Mesenchymal Tumor Diagnosis

- Association with oncogenic osteomalacia and phosphaturia
- Spindle cell proliferation with hemangiopericytoma-like vascular network
- Presence of distinctive granular calcifications
- Expression of FGF23
- Most often benign clinical course

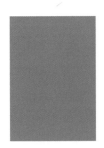

# Gastrointestinal Stromal Tumor (GIST)

## Definition and Epidemiology

Gastrointestinal stromal tumor (GIST) is a distinctive mesenchymal neoplasm exhibiting an almost absolute tropism for the gastrointestinal tract and possibly differentiating toward the interstitial cell of Cajal. Activating mutations of the KIT and PDGFRA genes are observed in approximately 80% of cases. Gastrointestinal stromal tumors occur at any age, but peak incidence is in the fifth and sixth decades. Males and females are equally affected. Annual incidence is estimated between 11 and 15 cases per million people. Pediatric GIST represents a clinically, genetically distinct group. Occurrence of submillimetric gastric GIST (so-called microGIST) seems to be remarkably common (according to surgical as well as autoptic series), as it is observed in approximately 20% of the general population. Fortunately, most of these lesions undergo regressive changes and calcification without progressing to a clinically meaningful lesion. GIST represents a fundamental, still unsurpassed model of molecularly targeted therapy for solid tumors.

## Clinical Presentation and Outcome

Gastrointestinal stromal tumors occur most commonly in the stomach (50–60%), followed by the small intestine (20–30%), the large bowel (5%), and the esophagus (5%). Rare cases occur primarily in the peritoneum. The risk of aggressive biologic behavior is assessed on the basis of size, mitotic activity, and anatomic site. Intraoperative tumor rupture increases the risk of abdominal dissemination dramatically (up to 90%). All these features have been variably assembled into several risk assessment schemes. Recently, a visual scheme based on heatmaps using size and mitotic counts as continuous variables was developed and is now gaining broad acceptance among clinicians (Fig. 4-93). Advanced and metastatic disease is currently treated with three lines of receptor tyrosine kinase (RTK) inhibitors (imatinib, sunitinib, and regorafenib) that block the activity of the mutated KIT of PDGFRA genes. Localized GIST is currently treated surgically, with high-risk patients undergoing adjuvant treatment with imatinib. The mutational status of KIT and PDGFRA predicts the response to RTK inhibitors and also assumes prognostic value.

Succinate dehydrogenase (SDH)-deficient GIST when compared with classic GIST appears to exhibit significant clinical differences. A tendency to occur (but not exclusively) in children and young adults is observed. Most cases occur in the stomach and, in stark contrast with classic GIST, exhibit a tendency to spread to the locoregional lymph nodes. With the exception of cases in the context of Carney-Stratakis syndrome, a female predominance is observed. Conventional risk assessment cannot be applied to SDH-deficient GIST; however, clinical behavior is distinctively indolent. Neurofibromatosis type 1–associated GISTs are typically multicentric, most often arise from the small bowel, and also have a rather indolent course.

## Morphology and Immunophenotype

Grossly, localized GIST presents as a localized mass of variable size (Fig. 4-94). It is well circumscribed, and the cut surface frequently shows foci of hemorrhage and/or necrosis (Fig. 4-95). Advanced disease most often presents as a main lesion associated with multiple peritoneal smaller nodules. Microscopically, the majority of cases can be classified into three broad categories: spindle cell type (70%), epithelioid type (20%), and mixed spindle and epithelioid cell type (10%). Importantly, GIST cytology does not have an impact over clinical outcome.

Spindle cell GIST is composed of a uniform eosinophilic spindle cell proliferation organized in short fascicles or in a short storiform growth pattern (Fig. 4-96). The neoplastic cells have a light eosinophilic cytoplasm, often with indistinct cell borders. Nuclei tend to be oval shaped and uniform in appearance, often with vesicular chromatin (Fig. 4-97). A peculiar albeit relatively infrequent feature, most often observed in gastric neoplasms, is represented by the presence of striking juxtanuclear cytoplasmic vacuoles (Fig. 4-98). In the past, this feature justified misinterpreting GIST as smooth muscle neoplasms (i.e., leiomyoblastoma). The presence of nuclear palisading is seen in a minority of cases and, as it is frequently observed in both smooth muscle and neural tumors, it may represent a potentially misleading histologic feature (Fig. 4-99). Microcystic stromal degeneration, fibrosis (Fig. 4-100), and stromal hemorrhage (Fig. 4-101) may represent a prominent feature in some cases.

Epithelioid GIST is composed of round-shaped cells exhibiting eosinophilic (Figs. 4-102 and 4-103) or clear cytoplasm (Fig. 4-104). Nuclei tend to be round to ovoid and uniform with vesicular chromatin (Fig. 4-105). In comparison with spindle cell GIST, tumor cells tend to exhibit a nested pattern of growth. Some cases may exhibit a striking "plasmacytoid" appearance (Fig. 4-106). Epithelioid GIST arise most often in the stomach and are frequently associated with PDGFRA gene mutations.

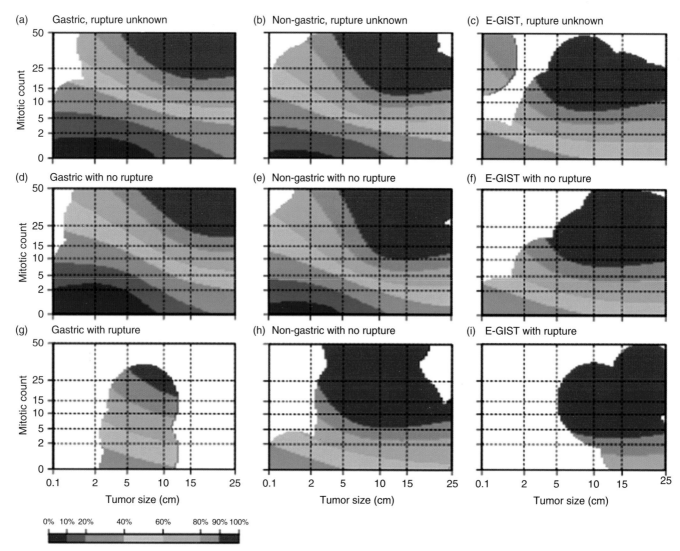

**Fig. 4-93.** Contour (heat) maps represent a visual tool for prediction of the risk of aggressive behavior in GIST.

Mixed cell type GIST may feature abrupt transition between spindle cell and epithelioid areas or, as an alternative, the two cell types may be intermingled (Fig. 4-107).

In approximately 10–20% of cases (of either spindle cell or epithelioid type), hyaline or fibrillary, brightly eosinophilic structures known as skeinoid fibers can be seen (Fig. 4-108). These structures appear to be composed of nodular tangles of collagen fibers and, typically, exhibit PAS positivity. Skenoid fibers seem to be more frequent in GIST arising in the small bowel wherein tumors also relatively often exhibit the tendency to show a nesting, paraganglioma-like growth pattern (Fig. 4-109). Prominent myxoid change is rarely seen (Fig. 4-110). Nuclear pleomorphism is not a typical feature of GIST; however, it can be observed in approximately 2% of cases (Fig. 4-111). Abrupt morphologic progression to high-grade pleomorphic sarcoma is rarely observed (so-called dedifferentiated GIST) (Fig. 4-112).

Succinate dehydrogenase-deficient GIST not only represents a clinically distinctive entity, but also shows relatively peculiar morphologic features. A distinctive multinodular pattern of growth is often seen (Fig. 4-113) that tends to be associated with a predominantly epithelioid morphology (Fig. 4-114). As mentioned, in contrast to classic GIST, lymph node metastases are seen relatively often (Fig. 4-115).

Even if there exist cases in which mitotic activity is remarkably high, in most GISTs it tends to be low. In fact, mitotic count (which represent a major prognostic determinant) is assessed on 50HPF or, as suggested more recently, on 5 mm$^2$. The latter approach has the advantage of overcoming inconsistencies arising from the use of a microscope with variable aperture of the oculars.

Not infrequently, pathologists are confronted with biopsies originating from post-treatment GIST. Depending on the level of response to RTK inhibitors, variable amounts of viable cells can be seen (Fig. 4-116). Often, most of the tissue can be merely represented by diffusely hyalinized fibrotic tissue (Fig. 4-117).

In consideration of current clinical as well as therapeutic implications, immunophenotypic analysis has gained a

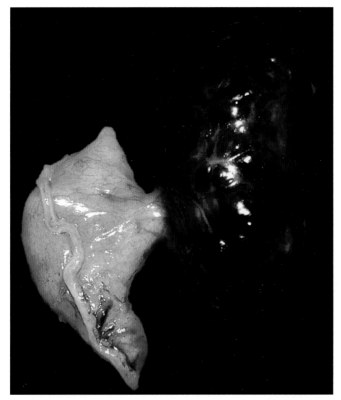

**Fig. 4-94.** Gastrointestinal stromal tumor. Grossly, this subserosal tumor is represented by an exophytic, peduncolated, well-circumscribed mass.

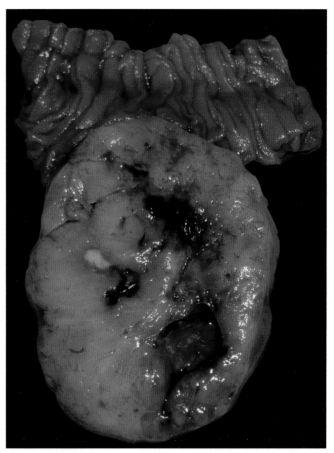

**Fig. 4-95.** Gastrointestinal stromal tumor. The cut surface appears fleshy, gray to tan, with foci of necrosis and hemorrhage.

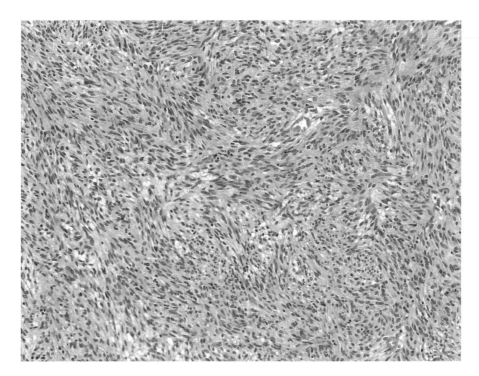

**Fig. 4-96.** Gastrointestinal stromal tumor. Spindle cell GIST is composed of a spindle cell proliferation featuring, in this case, a storiform pattern of growth.

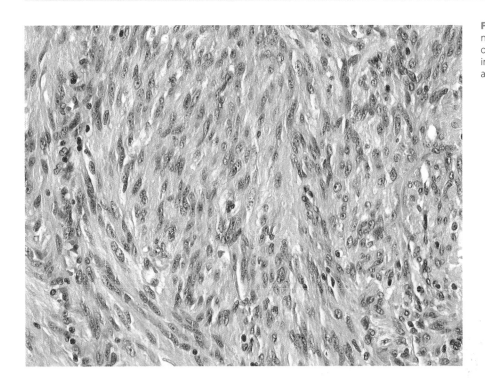

**Fig. 4-97.** Gastrointestinal stromal tumor. The neoplastic cells are characterized by mildly atypical ovoid nuclei with vesicular chromatin and inconspicuous nucleoli. The cytoplasm is ill-defined and indistinct and exhibits light eosinophilia.

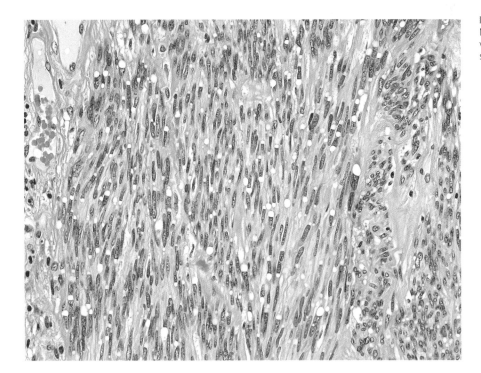

**Fig. 4-98.** Gastrointestinal stromal tumor. Numerous distinctive juxtanuclear cytoplasmic vacuoles are often seen in GIST arising in the stomach.

major diagnostic role. Most cases are KIT (CD117) immunoreactive; however, it has to be recognized that there exist lesions with typical cytoarchitectural features of GIST lacking KIT expression. This phenomenon occurs in 5–7% of cases overall and up to 18% of gastric GIST. A significant proportion of KIT-negative cases contains mutations of the *PDGFRA* gene and tends to exhibit an epithelioid morphology. The pattern of KIT expression is usually cytoplasmic and diffuse (Fig. 4-118); however, up to half of the cases will also show a dot-like accentuation of the staining (Fig. 4-119). More rarely, a dot-like pattern is seen in the absence of diffuse cytoplasmic staining. Approximately 50% of KIT-negative GIST actually express DOG1 (Fig. 4-120). In addition to KIT and DOG1, GIST frequently expresses CD34 in 60–70% of cases and smooth muscle actin in 30% of cases. Desmin and cytokeratin can be seen in less than 2% of

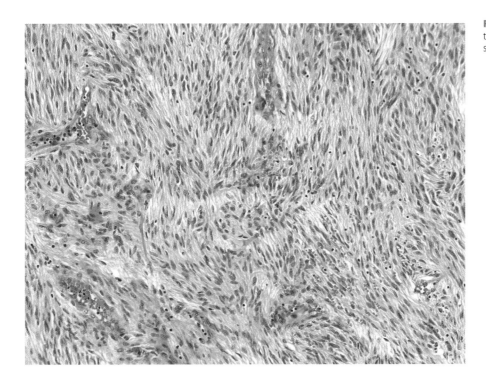

**Fig. 4-99.** Gastrointestinal stromal tumor. The tumor cells may feature palisading, somewhat simulating a neural neoplasm.

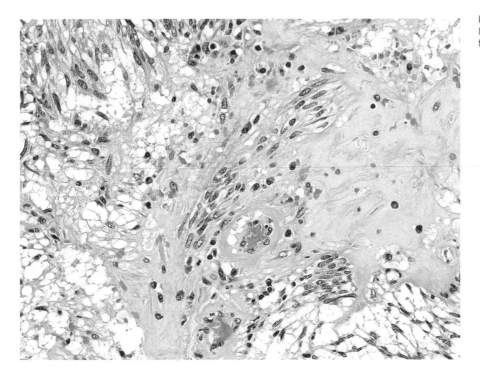

**Fig. 4-100.** Gastrointestinal stromal tumor. Multifocal, fibrous change of the stroma is frequently observed.

cases. SDHA and SDHB immunostaining is currently regarded as extremely helpful in recognizing SDH-deficient GIST. In fact, whatever the mutations of SDH, subunit loss of SDHB expression is seen (Fig. 4-121). On the other hand, loss of SDHA predicts the presence of mutations in the *SDHA* gene. Following therapy with RTK inhibitors, non-canonical immunophenotypes can be observed, such as diffuse expression of myogenic or epithelial differentiation markers.

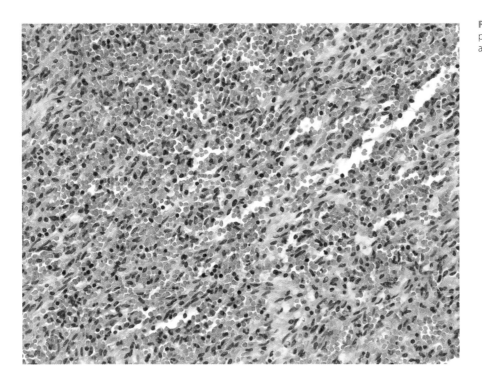

**Fig. 4-101.** Gastrointestinal stromal tumor. The presence of extravasated red blood cells represents a relatively common morphologic feature.

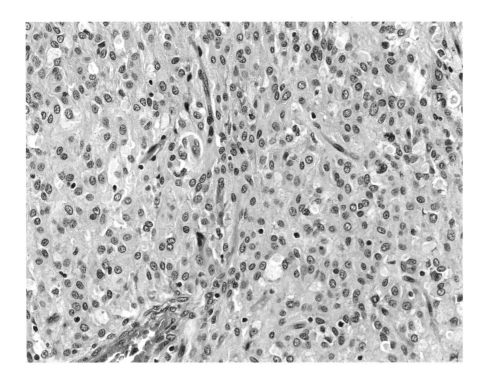

**Fig. 4-102.** Gastrointestinal stromal tumor. Epithelioid GIST is composed of epithelioid cells with round to oval nuclei harboring vesicular chromatin and small nucleoli. The cytoplasm appears eosinophilic.

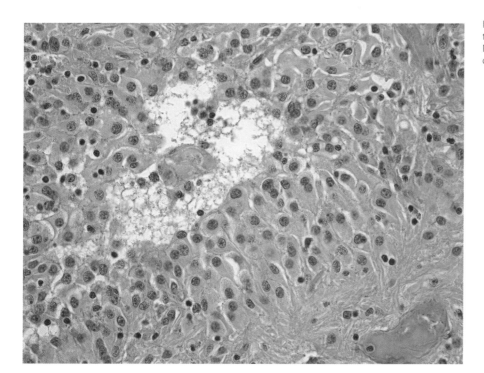

**Fig. 4-103.** Gastrointestinal stromal tumor. This tumor exhibits striking epithelioid morphology. Neoplastic cells herein exhibit well-defined cytoplasmic borders.

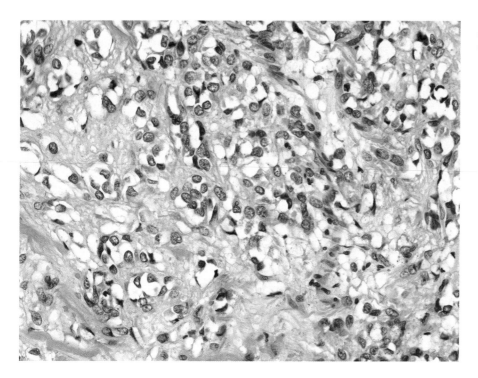

**Fig. 4-104.** Gastrointestinal stromal tumor. In epithelioid GIST, remarkable clearing of cytoplasm occasionally may be seen.

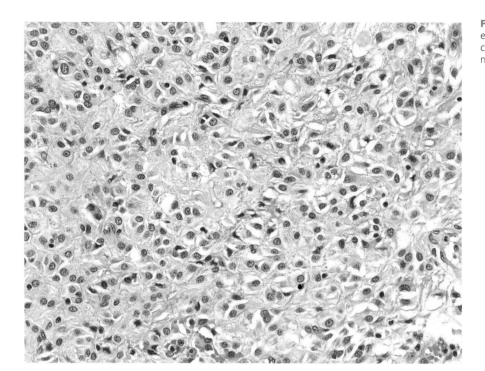

**Fig. 4-105.** Gastrointestinal stromal tumor. In epithelioid GIST, neoplastic cells tend to exhibit mild cytologic atypia, with round nuclei harboring small nucleoli.

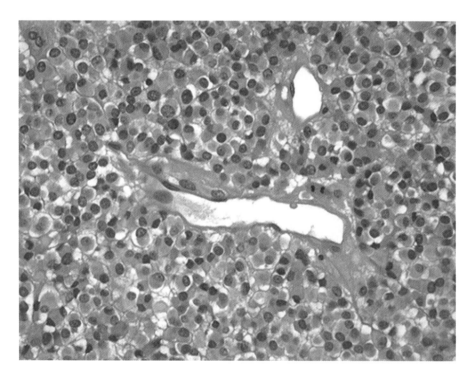

**Fig. 4-106.** Gastrointestinal stromal tumor. Rarely, epithelioid GIST may feature a striking plasmacytoid appearance.

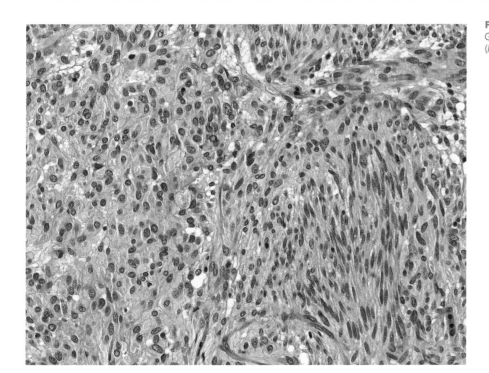

**Fig. 4-107.** Gastrointestinal stromal tumor. Mixed GIST is composed of a combination of epithelioid (*left*) and spindle (*right*) cells.

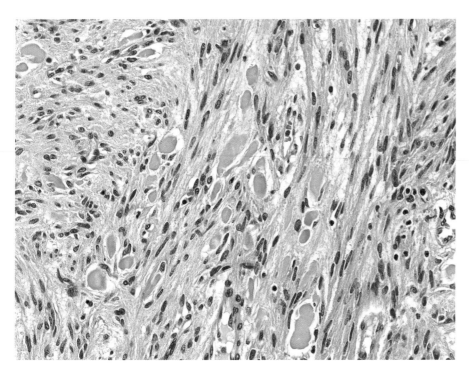

**Fig. 4-108.** Gastrointestinal stromal tumor. Fibrillary, brightly eosinophilic structures, so-called skenoid fibers, scattered throughout the tumor are seen.

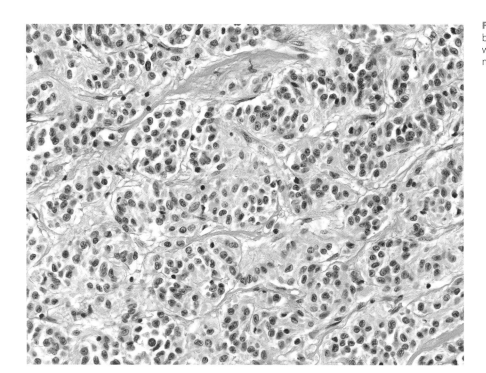

**Fig. 4-109.** Gastrointestinal stromal tumor. Small bowel GIST may associate epithelioid morphology with a nesting pattern of growth that may mimic a neuroendocrine neoplasm.

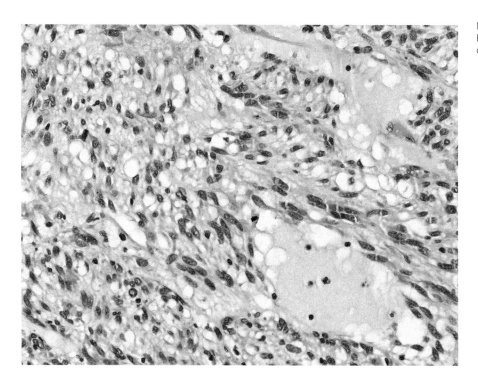

**Fig. 4-110.** Gastrointestinal stromal tumor. Prominent myxoid change of the stroma may be observed.

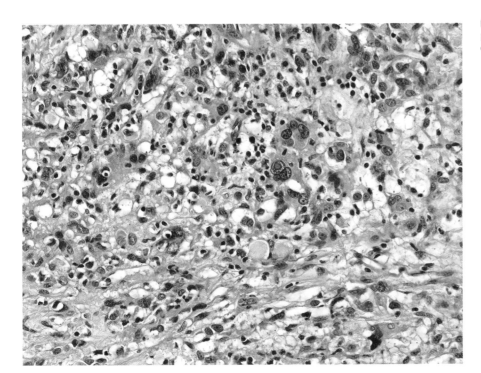

**Fig. 4-111.** Gastrointestinal stromal tumor. The presence of significant nuclear pleomorphism is observed very rarely.

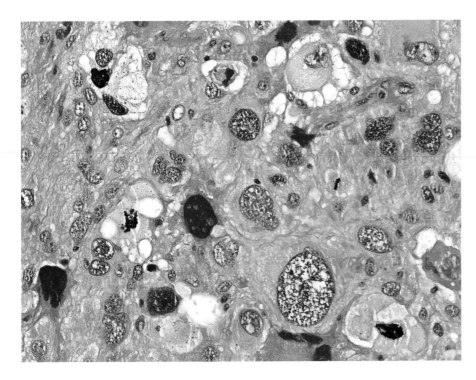

**Fig. 4-112.** Gastrointestinal stromal tumor. Dedifferentiated GIST is defined morphologically by the transition from conventional GIST to a high-grade pleomorphic sarcoma.

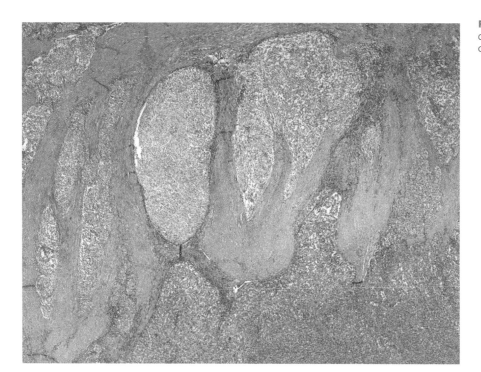

**Fig. 4-113.** Gastrointestinal stromal tumor. SDH-deficient gastrointestinal stromal tumor shows a characteristic multinodular pattern of growth.

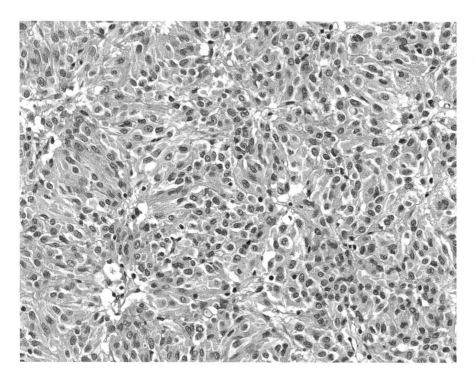

**Fig. 4-114.** Gastrointestinal stromal tumor. SDH-deficient gastrointestinal stromal tumor is composed predominantly of epithelioid cells often organized in nests.

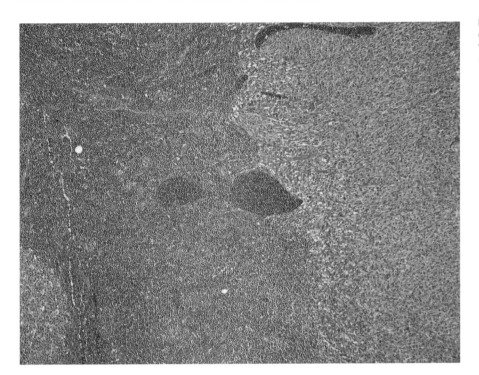

**Fig. 4-115.** Gastrointestinal stromal tumor. SDH-deficient gastrointestinal stromal tumors, at variance with classic types, relatively often feature metastatic spread to locoregional lymph nodes.

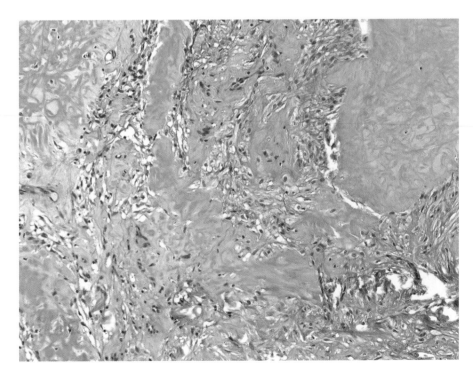

**Fig. 4-116.** Gastrointestinal stromal tumor. Following therapy with tyrosine kinase inhibitors, reduction of cellularity associated with hyalinized areas are observed.

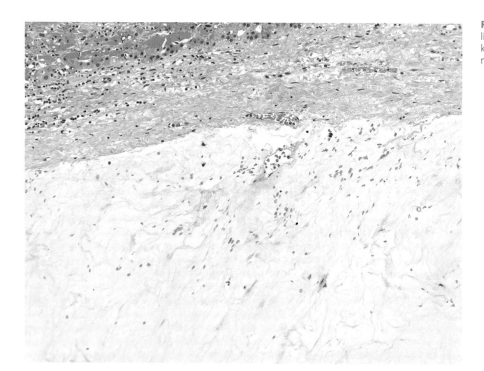

**Fig. 4-117.** Gastrointestinal stromal tumor. In this liver metastasis following therapy with tyrosine kinase inhibitors, tumor cells are totally replaced by myxohyaline tissue.

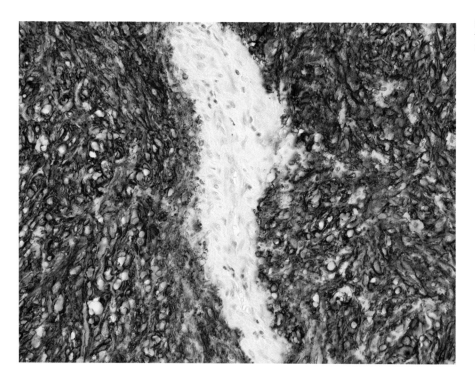

**Fig. 4-118.** Gastrointestinal stromal tumor. The tumor shows diffusely cytoplasmatic KIT immunopositivity.

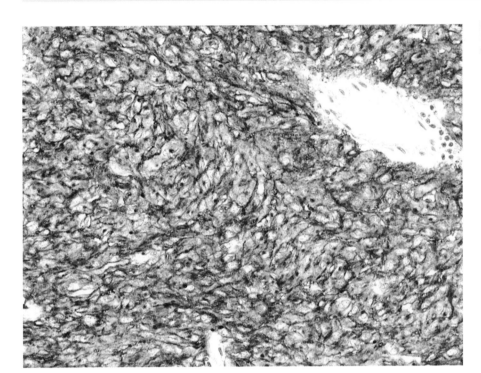

**Fig. 4-119.** Gastrointestinal stromal tumor. Dot-like accentuation of KIT immunostaining is observed.

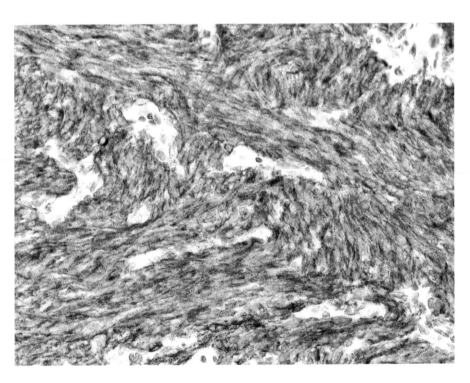

**Fig. 4-120.** Gastrointestinal stromal tumor. DOG1 strong cytoplasmatic immunopositivity is often identified.

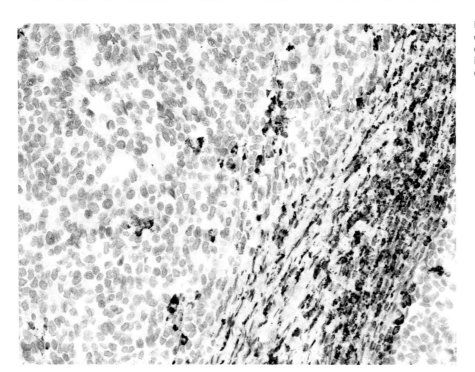

**Fig. 4-121.** Gastrointestinal stromal tumor. SDH-deficient gastrointestinal stromal tumor typically exhibits loss of cytoplasmic SDHB immunoexpression. Lymphocytes and endothelial cells represent the internal positive controls.

## Genetics

Molecularly, GIST represents a relatively heterogeneous and complex group of lesions. Gain-of-function mutations of the oncogenes located on chromosome 4 (4q12) encoding for the type III receptor tyrosine kinases KIT and PDGFRA can be found in approximately 80% of cases. With exceedingly rare exceptions, they are mutually exclusive and result in the constitutive activation of either KIT or PDGFRA. Normally, KIT and PDGFRA are activated by binding of their respective ligands, i.e., stem-cell factor and platelet-derived growth factor A. Downstream oncogenic signaling for both KIT and PDGFRA involves the RAS/MAPK and the PI3 K/AKT/mTOR pathways. Mutations can be deletions, insertions, and missense mutations involving exon 11 of the *KIT* gene (encoding for the juxtamembrane domain of the KIT receptor) in approximately 70% of GISTs; exon 9 of *KIT* (encoding for the extracellular domain of the receptor) in less than 10%; exon 13 and 17 of *KIT* (encoding for the intracellular ATP-binding pocket and activation loop domains, respectively) in a small subset of cases. Approximately 10% of GISTs harbor *PDGFRA* gene mutations involving exons 12, 14, and 18, with 70% being represented by the exon 18 D842V mutation. The D842V mutation is known for making GIST primarily resistant to currently available RTK inhibitors.

Approximately 10–15% of GIST is wild type for both *KIT* and *PDGFRA*. They represent a family of tumors with distinctive molecular pathogenesis and, to some extent, different natural histories. Their classification is rapidly evolving; however, at present one may identify (1) SDH-deficient GIST; (2) NF1-related GIST; and (3) others, including those with the *BRAF* V600E mutation. Approximately one-half of wild-type (WT)-GIST are marked by alterations involving the succinate dehydrogenase (SDH) complex, which plays a key role in the mitochondrial respiratory cell function. A group of them includes "pediatric" GIST and can be associated with the Carney triad, which, when full blown, is characterized by the concomitant occurrence of GIST, pulmonary chondromas, and paragangliomas. On the other hand, a group of SDH-deficient GISTs carries mutations of the SDHA, SDHB, or SDHC units of the SDH complex, and may be related to the Carney-Stratakis syndrome, a dominant autosomal disorder represented by association of GIST and paragangliomas. Wild-type GIST can occur in the context of NF1, wherein the mutation of the *NF1* gene leads to loss of neurofibromin and consequent activation of the RAS pathway. Finally, the remaining SDHB-positive WT-GISTs are probably a basketful of different conditions: Some were reported to have the V600E mutation of *BRAF* or, more rarely, *HRAS, NRAS, PIK3* mutations. Recent experience would indicate that a significant proportion of so-called quadruple-negative GIST exhibits *NF1* gene mutations that may be somatic or, more frequently, germline. As this happens in the absence of clinical evidence of type 1 neurofibromatosis, they possibly represent examples of subclinical forms of the syndrome. Using a massive parallel sequencing approach, an *ETV6-NTRK3* gene fusion has been recently detected in a quadruple-negative GIST. As WT-GIST tends not to be responsive to tyrosine kinase inhibitors (but keeping in mind that this alteration is very rare) molecular therapy targeting NTRK3 has already been successfully applied in the context of a clinical trial.

## Differential Diagnosis and Diagnostic Pitfalls

The differential diagnosis of GIST is rather broad and includes a wide variety of benign and malignant mesenchymal and non-mesenchymal tumors.

**Leiomyoma** and **leiomyosarcoma** outnumber GIST in the colon-rectum and in the esophagus but they can occur

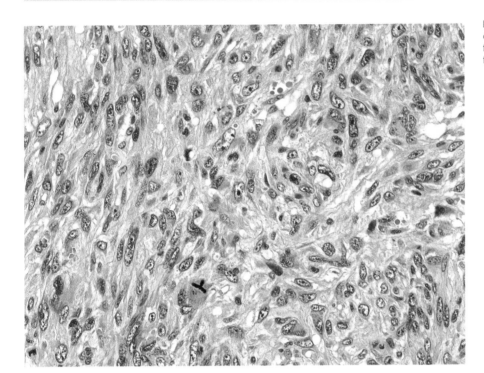

**Fig. 4-122.** Leiomyosarcoma. The tumor is composed of highly atypical spindle cells. Mitotic figures (including those that are atypical) are frequently encountered.

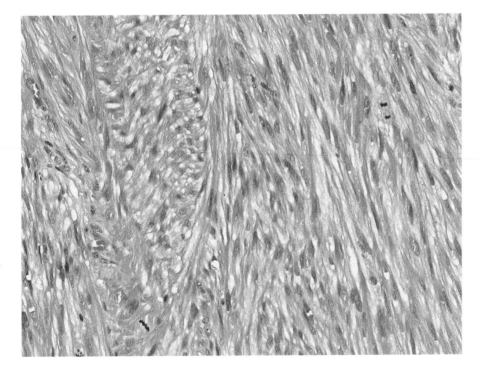

**Fig. 4-123.** Leiomyosarcoma. Well-differentiated leiomyosarcoma is typically composed of fascicles composed of spindle cells featuring cigar-shaped nuclei and eosinophilic cytoplasm. Several mitoses are seen.

anywhere along the gastrointestinal (GI) tract. Most cases occur in middle-aged patients, with a peak incidence in the fifth decade. Diagnosis is based on the presence of eosinophilic fibrillary cytoplasm variably associated with desmin, smooth muscle actin, and h-caldesmon positivity. Importantly, KIT is consistently negative, whereas DOG1 can be focally expressed. Leiomyosarcoma of the GI tract is most often a high-grade neoplasm (Fig. 4-122); however (particularly in the rectum), well-differentiated forms characterized by moderate cytologic atypia and low mitotic count can be observed (Fig. 4-123). Actually, detection of mitotic activity should always prompt consideration of malignancy. An important diagnostic pitfall is represented by the fact that the smooth muscle tumors of the GI tract may feature the presence of hyperplasia of interstitial cells of Cajal (Fig. 4-124).

As already discussed, both **schwannoma** and **reticular/microcystic schwannoma** may occur at a gastrointestinal location with relatively high frequency. Both entities are discussed

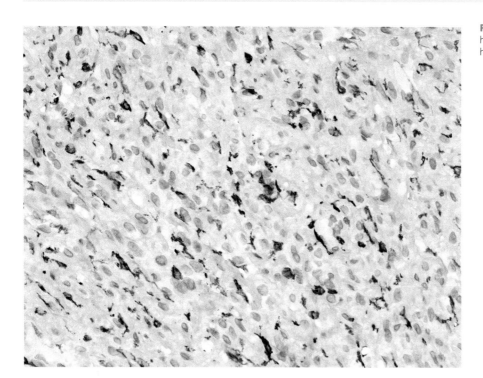

Fig. 4-124. Leiomyosarcoma. The tumor presents hyperplasia of interstitial cells of Cajal that are highlighted by KIT immunostain.

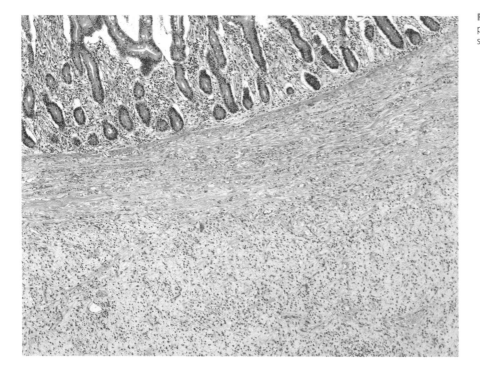

Fig. 4-125. Inflammatory fibroid polyps. At low power, the lesion is composed of a proliferation of spindle cells set in a fibromyxoid stroma.

in more detail elsewhere. In brief, schwannoma is composed of a well-circumscribed spindle cell population that in the GI tract tends to feature only "Antoni A" morphology. A frequent, helpful finding is represented by the presence of a chronic inflammatory infiltrate located at the periphery of the lesion. Microcystic/reticular schwannomas exhibit a very distinctive reticular pattern of growth associated with the presence of pseudocystic, mucin-laden spaces. Both lesions are KIT/DOG1 negative and diffusely express S100.

**Inflammatory fibroid polyps** represent large, benign, exophytic, at times peduncolated, stromal lesions typically arising in the GI tract. Approximately 80% of cases occur in the stomach, with a peak incidence in the sixth decade. Clinical presentation depends on the size of the lesion as well as on the anatomic site and may include gastrointestinal bleeding, obstruction, and intussusception. Surgical excision is curative, and local recurrence is never observed. Microscopically, inflammatory fibroid polyps are composed of a cytologically

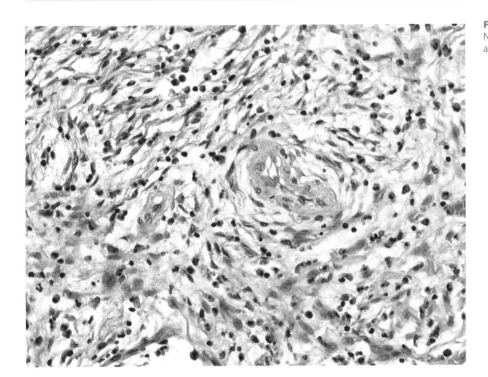

**Fig. 4-126.** Inflammatory fibroid polyps. Neoplastic cells are cytologically bland and associated with abundant eosinophils.

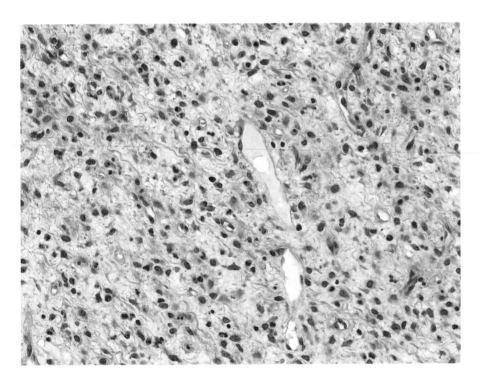

**Fig. 4-127.** Inflammatory fibroid polyps. The tumor cells harbor round to ovoid nuclei with small nucleoli and scant cytoplasm. Note the presence of fibrillary collagen and scattered eosinophils.

bland spindle cell proliferation set in a fibromyxoid stroma (Fig. 4-125) and associated with a variably prominent inflammatory infiltrate that may include abundant eosinophils (Fig. 4-126). Cellularity tends to be low but can be variable (Figs. 4-127 and 4-128). Immunohistochemically, fibroid polyps consistently express CD34 (Fig. 4-129) but are always KIT and DOG1 negative. Interestingly, a mutation of the exon 18 of the *PDGFRA* gene is observed in most cases.

**Plexiform angiomyxoid myofibroblastic tumor** (subsequently renamed "plexiform fibromyxoma") occurs almost

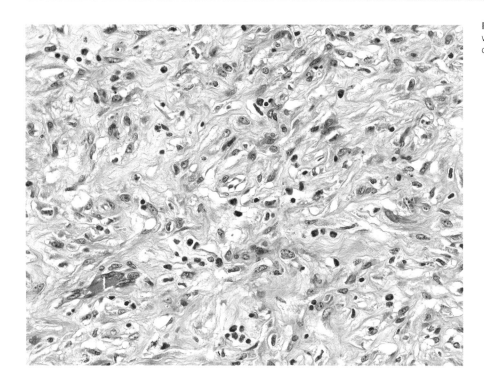

Fig. 4-128. Inflammatory fibroid polyps. Tumors with low cellularity tend to exhibit more abundant collagenous stroma.

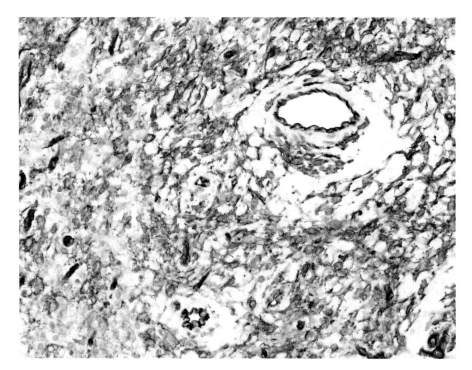

Fig. 4-129. Inflammatory fibroid polyps. Tumor cells showing CD34 diffuse immunopositivity.

exclusively in the gastric antrum of adult patients. No sex predilection is observed. The most common clinical presentation is anemia or hematemesis due to gastric bleeding. Morphologically, this lesion is composed of a multinodular proliferation (Fig. 4-130) of cytologically bland, uniform spindle cells, set in richly vascularized myxoid matrix (Figs. 4-131 and 4-132). Mitotic activity tends to be very low. Interestingly, intravascular extension of the tumors is seen relatively often, as is mucosal ulceration. Neoplastic cells variably express smooth muscle actin, h-caldesmon, and desmin and are invariably CD34 and KIT/DOG1 negative. Plexiform angiomyxoid myofibroblastic tumor is a benign lesion; however, it represents a potentially life-threatening condition because of the occurrence of fatal gastric hemorrhages. Interestingly, a recurrent translocation, t(11;12)(q11;q13), involving the long non-coding gene metastasis-associated lung adenocarcinoma transcript 1 (*MALAT1*) and the gene

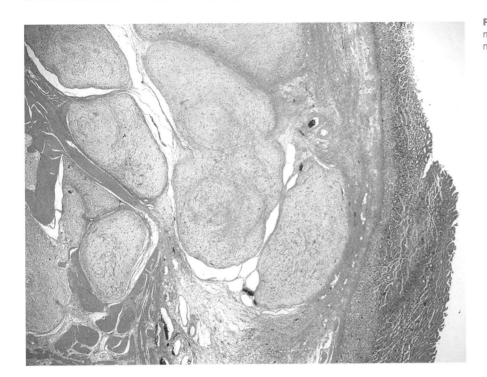

**Fig. 4-130.** Plexiform angiomyxoid myofibroblastic tumor. At low power, a striking multinodularity is observed.

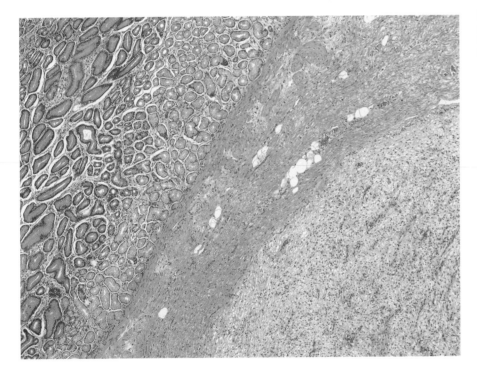

**Fig. 4-131.** Plexiform angiomyxoid myofibroblastic tumor. The neoplastic nodules are well demarcated and characterized by the presence of a richly vascularized stroma.

glioma-associated oncogene homologue 1 (*GLI1*) has been observed in a subset of these neoplasms.

**Mesenteric fibromatosis** belongs to the family of intra-abdominal fibromatoses and is discussed in Chapter 8. It occurs most often in the mesentery of the small bowel. In comparison with other subtypes of desmoid fibromatosis, higher cellularity can be seen as well as more prominent myxoid change of the matrix (Fig. 4-133). Nuclear expression of beta-catenin (associated with smooth muscle actin immuno-positivity) is extremely helpful in confirming the diagnosis. As

mentioned, nuclear expression of beta-catenin is related to mutations of either *CTNNB1* or *APC* genes, the latter being associated with familial adenomatous polyposis (FAP). An important diagnostic pitfall is represented by the fact that KIT positivity (not DOG1) can be seen in some cases and most likely represents a technical artifact due to excessive antigen retrieval.

Quite recently, it has become evident that the **glomus tumor**, in addition to arising in the preferred anatomic site represented by the superficial soft tissue, can also

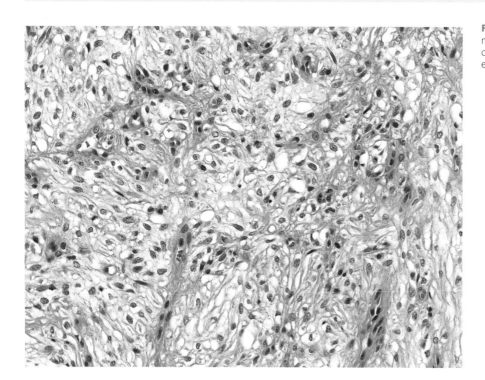

**Fig. 4-132.** Plexiform angiomyxoid myofibroblastic tumor. The tumor is composed of cytologically bland spindle cells with clear to eosinophilic cytoplasm.

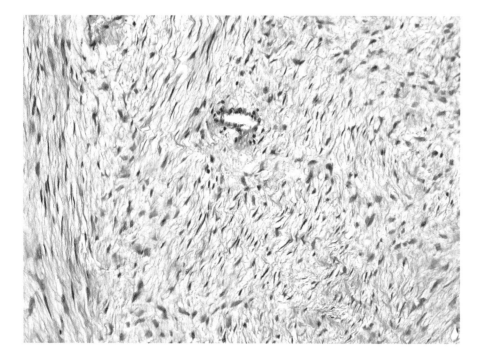

**Fig. 4-133.** Mesenteric fibromatosis. Intra-abdominal desmoids can exhibit higher cellularity. Neoplastic cells are set in a fibromyxoid stroma.

infrequently arise at visceral sites, particularly in the GI tract. The majority of lesions arise in the gastric antrum of adult patients, with a minority of cases arising in both the small and large bowels. Peak incidence in the sixth decade and a female predominance are observed. Microscopically, glomus tumor is composed of a remarkably uniform, epithelioid cell population (Fig. 4-134), featuring sharply defined cytoplasm, with round nuclei and small nucleoli (Fig. 4-135). Mitotic activity is low to absent, but quite commonly vascular invasion is seen. Immunohistochemically, most cases show immunopositivity for smooth muscle actin (Fig. 4-136) and h-caldesmon. Focal CD34 positivity can be observed in approximately one-third of cases. Consistent negativity for KIT and DOG1 is of great help in the differential diagnosis with epithelioid GIST. Glomus tumors of the GI tract are most often benign, with exceptional cases originating distant metastases. In consideration of the rarity, the criteria of malignancy developed for the soft tissue counterpart (deep seated; size greater than 2 cm; cytologic atypia; mitotic count exceeding 5 mitoses/50HPF) cannot be applied. Practically,

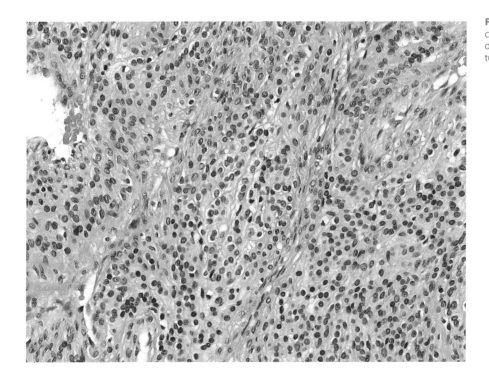

**Fig. 4-134.** Glomus tumor. Nests of epithelioid cells with round nuclei, small nucleoli, and well-defined eosinophilic cytoplasm characterize the tumor.

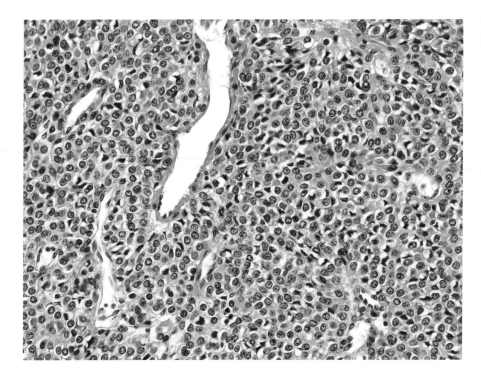

**Fig. 4-135.** Glomus tumor. The neoplastic cells grow around thin-walled, dilated, branching blood vessels.

the presence of cellular spindling as well as of overt nuclear atypia is strongly suspicious for malignancy.

**Dedifferentiated liposarcoma** occurs very frequently in the retroperitoneum and therefore may enter the differential diagnosis, particularly when mature adipocytic areas are scant or under-sampled. Diagnostic challenges can be even greater whenever dedifferentiated liposarcoma is not obviously pleomorphic and high grade, but instead features a low-grade morphology. The presence of MDM2 expression/amplification

(associated with negativity for both KIT and DOG1) represents an extremely helpful diagnostic finding.

**Synovial sarcoma** is increasingly recognized in the GI tract and is extensively discussed elsewhere in this chapter. Both monophasic and biphasic subtypes are encountered; however, it is the monophasic variant that possess the greatest diagnostic challenge. Morphologically, monophasic synovial sarcoma is distinctively more cellular, monomorphic, and mitotically active than GIST and often features the presence of a hemangiopericytoma-like vascularization. Immunohistochemically,

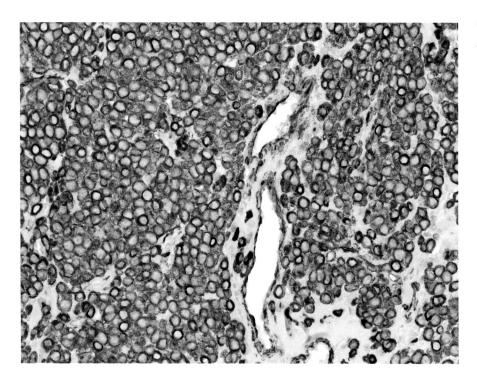

**Fig. 4-136.** Glomus tumor. Strong immunopositivity for smooth muscle actin is typically seen.

variable expression of EMA, TLE1, and cytokeratin is associated with negativity for KIT and DOG1. The presence of *SYT* gene rearrangements contrasts with the absence of mutations of both *KIT* and *PDGFRA*.

When dealing with epithelioid GIST, the differential diagnosis also includes non-mesenchymal malignancies. Infrequently, metastatic amelanotic melanoma can locate in the GI tract: Diagnostic confusion may be increased by the occurrence of KIT expression that, however, is associated with the expression of S100 and variable immunopositivity for melanoma markers. Neuroendocrine neoplasm may share with epithelioid GIST cellular uniformity as well as a nesting pattern of growth. Expression of cytokeratin along with chromogranin and synaptophysin are of great diagnostic help. Non-Hodgkin lymphoma may also occur in the GI tract and also

represents a source of diagnostic confusion; however, proper application of an immunophenotypic panel most often leads to the correct diagnosis.

### Key Points in Gastrointestinal Stromal Tumor Diagnosis

- Exclusive occurrence in the GI tract
- Spindle and/or epithelioid cytomorphology
- Immunohistochemical expression of KIT and/or DOG1
- SDHB loss in SDH-deficient GIST
- Mutations of *KIT* and *PDGFRA* genes observed in approximately 80% of cases
- Clinical behavior based on location, size, mitotic index, presence of intra-abdominal tumor rupture, and mutational status

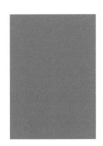

# Leiomyosarcoma

## Definition and Epidemiology

Leiomyosarcoma (LMS) represents a malignant mesenchymal neoplasm exhibiting morphologic and immunophenotypic features of smooth muscle differentiation. Leiomyosarcoma occurs predominantly in adult or elderly patients. Intra-abdominal LMS is more frequent in females, whereas LMS of the limbs and cutaneous LMS occur more frequently in males. Leiomyosarcoma rarely occurs in childhood, wherein it may arise in both viscera and in somatic soft tissues. Interestingly, visceral LMSs, particularly those arising in children, may be related to immunosuppression and etiologically linked to Epstein-Barr virus (EBV) infection.

## Clinical Presentation and Outcome

Leiomyosarcoma represents a relatively heterogeneous clinicopathologic entity: 45% of cases arise in the retroperitoneum, mesentery, and omentum and 35% occur in the deep soft tissue of the limbs. Cutaneous LMS accounts for approximately 15% of cases, whereas 5% originates in the inferior vena cava or other large veins. Leiomyosarcoma of external genitalia represents an additional category characterized by better prognosis. Anatomic location represents one of the major prognostic determinants. Intra-abdominal LMS frequently spreads to the lungs and liver and overall survival at 5 years is about 20–30%. In LMS of the deep soft tissue of the limbs, the overall survival at 5 years is approximately 60%. Cutaneous LMS, irrespective of morphology, tends to behave indolently, and distant metastases seem to be exceptional. A combination of radiotherapy and surgical excision is the therapeutic mainstay for localized disease. As discussed in Chapter 3, association with systemic therapy in high-grade LMS is often considered. Leiomyosarcoma of the GI tract is discussed in the context of the differential diagnosis of gastrointestinal stromal tumors (GIST). Immunocompromised patients may present with leiomyosarcomas that are associated with EBV infection. Multifocality with visceral involvement is most often seen. Clinical course is usually indolent and prognosis is primarily related to the underlying disorder. When dealing with leiomyosarcoma occurring in the superficial soft tissue (particularly in the head and neck region), patients should be investigated to exclude the presence of a primary tumor in the somatic deep soft tissue or in the retroperitoneum.

## Morphology and Immunophenotype

Grossly, leiomyosarcoma is typically fleshy with hemorrhage and necrosis varying according to the size of the neoplastic mass (Fig. 4-137).

Microscopically, LMS is relatively homogeneous independently from the site of origin. Well-differentiated lesions are characterized by fascicles composed of spindle cells containing oval, blunt-ended nuclei (Fig. 4-138) and distinctive eosinophilic fibrillary cytoplasm (Fig. 4-139). High-grade leiomyosarcoma features significant pleomorphism associated with numerous, often atypical mitotic figures (Fig. 4-140) and a variable amount of necrosis (Fig. 4-141). Variable cytoplasmic eosinophilia can represent the only morphologic clue of smooth muscle differentiation. Numerous morphologic variants exist, such as myxoid LMS (Fig. 4-142), epithelioid LMS (Fig. 4-143), giant cell-rich LMS (Fig. 4-144), and inflammatory LMS (Fig. 4-145). Epithelioid leiomyosarcoma is exceedingly rare. Immunohistochemically, approximately 70–80% of LMS stain with desmin (Fig. 4-146), whereas the vast majority will stain with smooth muscle actin (Fig. 4-147). h-Caldesmon is positive in approximately 60% of cases. Importantly, about 30% of LMSs may exhibit multifocal positivity for EMA and/or cytokeratin.

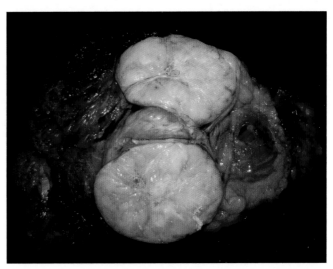

**Fig. 4-137.** Leiomyosarcoma. Grossly, the tumor appears as a deep-seated, well-circumscribed mass with a fleshy cut surface. Small foci of necrosis are seen.

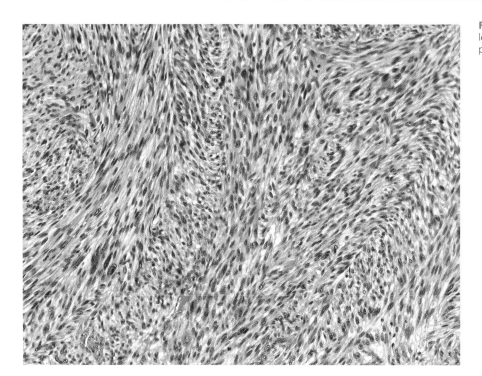

**Fig. 4-138.** Leiomyosarcoma. Well-differentiated leiomyosarcoma typically exhibits a fascicular pattern of growth.

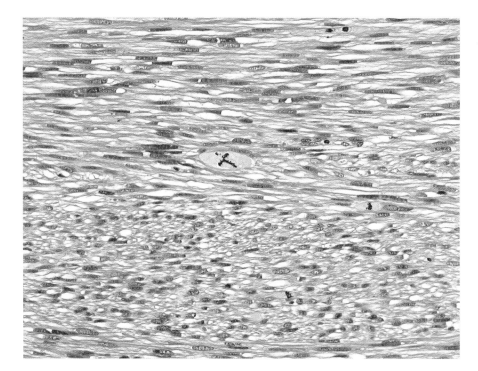

**Fig. 4-139.** Leiomyosarcoma. The tumor cells harbor blunt-ended nuclei and fibrillary, eosinophilic cytoplasm. Atypical mitotic figures are easily found.

## Genetics

Cytogenetically, LMS typically shows complex karyotypes with amplification, losses, and gains occurring in several chromosomes. Loss of RB1 and PTEN represents a comparatively common genetic event and is observed in up to 70% of cases.

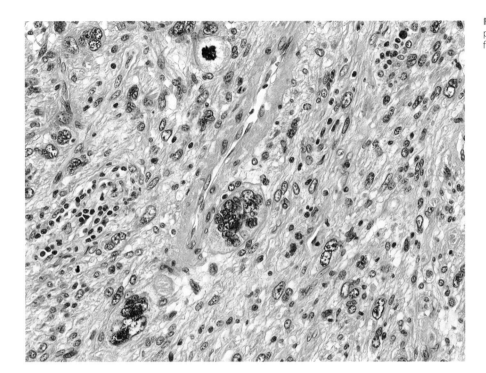

**Fig. 4-140.** Leiomyosarcoma. Diffuse pleomorphism associated with atypical mitotic figures is typically seen in high-grade lesions.

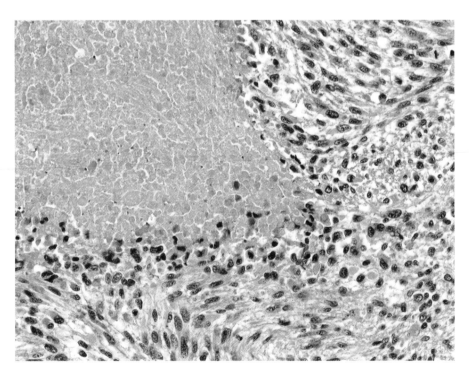

**Fig. 4-141.** Leiomyosarcoma. High-grade tumors often feature areas of coagulative necrosis.

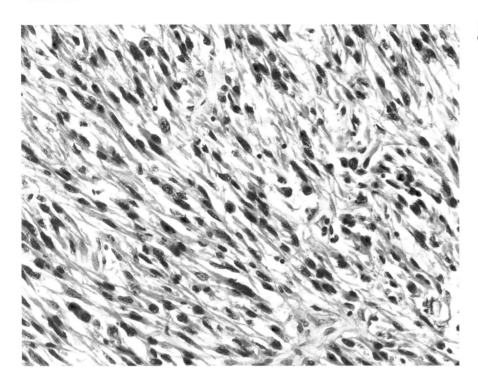

**Fig. 4-142.** Leiomyosarcoma. Diffuse myxoid change of the stroma can be infrequently seen.

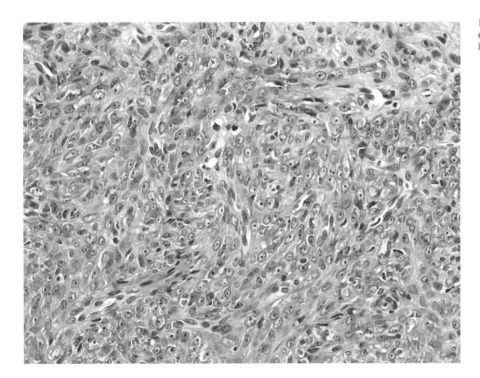

**Fig. 4-143.** Leiomyosarcoma. The presence of epithelioid morphology represents a rare finding in leiomyosarcoma.

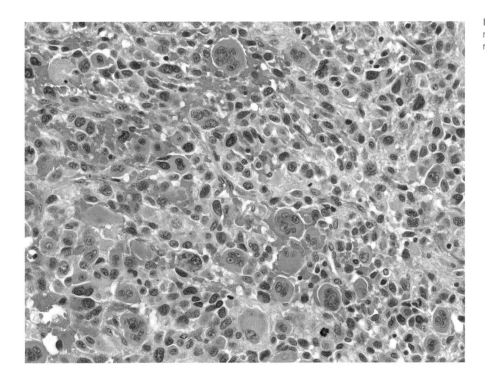

**Fig. 4-144.** Leiomyosarcoma. The presence of numerous osteoclast-like giant cells represents a relatively common morphologic finding.

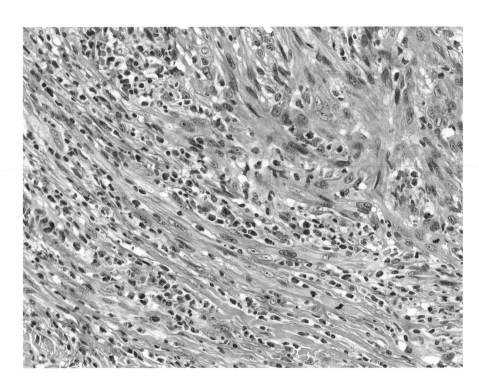

**Fig. 4-145.** Leiomyosarcoma. The presence of an abundant inflammatory infiltrate composed of eosinophils and lymphocytes is observed between neoplastic spindle cells.

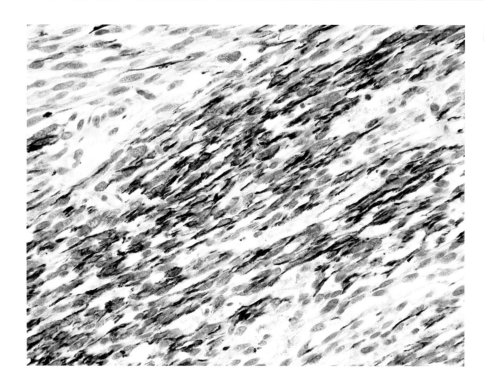

Fig. 4-146. Leiomyosarcoma. Desmin immunopositivity is often seen but can be focal.

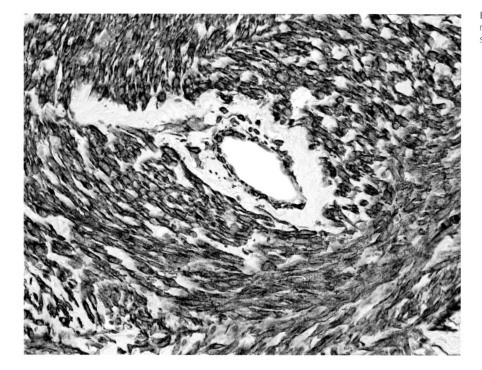

Fig. 4-147. Leiomyosarcoma. Diffuse smooth muscle actin immunopositivity is almost always seen.

## Differential Diagnosis and Diagnostic Pitfalls

One of the most important differential diagnoses is of leiomyoma of deep soft tissue. This lesion primarily occurs in the retroperitoneum, in the abdominal cavity, and in the inguinal region of adult females. Occurrence in the somatic soft tissue is comparatively very rare and may also occur in males. Diagnostic criteria depend on a rather complex combination of clinicopathologic features. Microscopically, most often neoplastic cells features eosinophilic fibrillary cytoplasm harboring elongated blunt-ended nuclei (Fig. 4-148). Cytologic atypia is minimal (Fig. 4-149); however, degenerative nuclear atypia (along with other changes such as cytologic degeneration, stroma hyalinization, and calcifications) can be observed in rare cases. Importantly, in this context, nuclear hyperchromasia does not represent per se a feature of malignancy. Mitotic count plays a key role, but threshold varies on the basis of anatomic locations. When dealing with smooth muscle lesions arising in

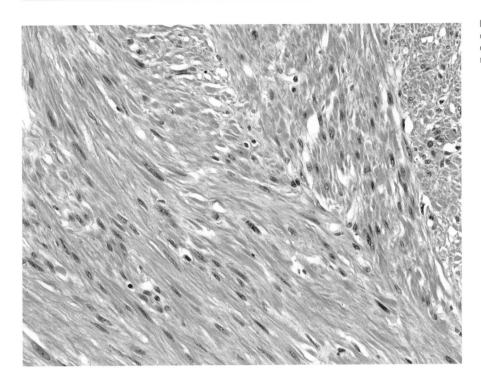

**Fig. 4-148.** Leiomyoma. The tumor is composed of cytologically bland spindle cells showing eosinophilic fibrillary cytoplasm and blunt-ended nuclei.

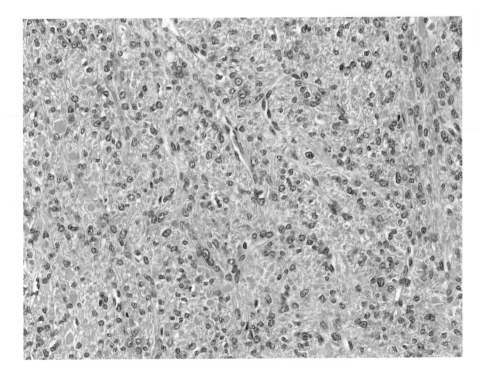

**Fig. 4-149.** Leiomyoma. A mild degree of nuclear atypia can be accepted in retroperitoneal leiomyoma.

the somatic soft tissue of the limbs, any mitotic activity (formally exceeding 1 mitosis/50HPF) is potentially correlated with malignant behavior. By contrast, in retroperitoneal smooth muscle neoplasms in females, whenever nuclear atypia is mild to absent, up to 10 mitoses/50HPF are allowed. Identical lesions may exceptionally occur in the retroperitoneum of male patients; however, in consideration of their rarity, application of the above-mentioned diagnostic criteria is not advised.

Differential diagnosis includes a variety of spindle cell sarcomas, which are all discussed in detail in this chapter: low-grade myofibroblastic sarcoma, malignant peripheral nerve sheath tumor (MPNST), and monophasic synovial sarcoma. Whatever the differential diagnosis, the most important morphologic clues in favor of leiomyosarcoma are represented by the presence of blunt-ended nuclei set in eosinophilic fibrillary cytoplasm. Both features are not present in either synovial sarcoma or MPNST. Myofibroblastic neoplasms tend to have tapering nuclei, and cytoplasm is amphophilic.

As discussed in Chapter 7, pleomorphic LMS needs to be separated from pleomorphic rhabdomyosarcoma. The presence of more intense cytoplasmic eosinophilia and, most important, the detection of nuclear expression of myogenin and/or MyoD1 (which most often tend to be very focal) represent key morphologic features in favor of pleomorphic rhabdomyosarcoma.

## Leiomyosarcoma of the Uterus

In consideration of its relative frequency, uterine leiomyosarcoma deserves a brief, separate discussion. This topic is generally covered in gynecologic pathology textbooks. However, increasingly mesenchymal malignancies of the gynecologic tract are drawing the attention of the sarcoma community.

Smooth muscle tumors of the uterus represent a fairly common group of lesions encompassing benign (leiomyomas represent by far the most common uterine neoplasm) and malignant lesions. Between these, there exists a rather blurred entity known as smooth muscle tumors of uncertain malignant potential (STUMP). The major current diagnostic challenge is in fact to distinguish leiomyosarcoma from leiomyoma; however, this task has been made difficult by two major issues: (1) The current definition of uterine leiomyosarcoma includes only high-grade lesions (which in a hypothetical, not validated, use of the French Federation of Cancer Centers Sarcoma Group [FNCLCC] grading system would qualify most lesions as grade 3), virtually denying the existence of low-grade leiomyosarcomas. (2) Even if it clearly stated that such a diagnosis should be rendered very rarely, the latest WHO classification has actually further broadened the STUMP category, resulting in a widespread (and sometimes irrational) use of the label. Practically, if necrosis is absent, multifocal atypia

is allowed only when mitotic activity is below 10 mitoses/10HPF. If necrosis is present, no atypia and no more than 10 mitoses/10HPF are allowed. As the definition of necrosis in smooth muscle tumors of the uterus is rather controversial, and the concept of atypia is unavoidably subjective, the label STUMP is increasingly used as a tool to minimize medical litigation. Obviously, there exists a strong need for more solid criteria, perhaps reconsidering retrospectively those STUMPs characterized by aggressive behavior on long-term follow-up.

Uterine leiomyosarcoma accounts for approximately 2% of uterine malignant tumors and exhibits a peak incidence in the fifth decade. It usually presents as a single fleshy mass but can be associated with multiple (usually smaller) leiomyomas. The criteria of malignancy for leiomyosarcoma were initially set up in the seminal paper of Bell, Kempson, and Hendrickson in 1994. It was a rather complex effort that emphasized the importance of three main morphologic parameters that, with several variations, are still in use: (1) presence of tumor (nonischemic) necrosis; (2) presence of nuclear atypia; (3) mitotic activity. As mentioned, whenever coagulative necrosis is present and mitotic activity exceeds 10 mitoses/10HPF, a diagnosis of leiomyosarcoma does not require the presence of nuclear atypia. In the absence of necrosis, the presence of any amount of moderate/severe nuclear atypia associated with more than 10 mitoses /10HPF is also in keeping with the diagnosis of leiomyosarcoma. As with somatic soft tissue tumors, morphology is most often spindled but epithelioid cell and myxoid variants exist. In both epithelioid (actually, most examples likely represent uterine PEComas) and myxoid uterine leiomyosarcoma, cut-offs for assessing mitotic activity are significantly lower (>3 mitoses/10HPF).

---

**Key Points in Leiomyosarcoma Diagnosis**

- Broad anatomic distribution: retroperitoneum, deep soft tissue of the limbs, skin, GI tract
- Predominant spindle morphology featuring eosinophilic fibrillary cytoplasm and blunt-ended nuclei
- Variable immunohistochemical expression of smooth muscle actin, desmin, and h-caldesmon
- Aggressive neoplasm; however, clinical behavior is dependent on anatomic location

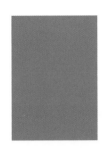

# Solitary Fibrous Tumor

## Definition and Epidemiology

Solitary fibrous tumor (SFT) represents a ubiquitous fibroblastic neoplasm showing a distinctive hemangiopericytoma-like vascular network. Age range is very broad; however, approximately 50% of cases are diagnosed between the fifth and the sixth decade. No sex predilection is observed. Solitary fibrous tumor encompasses a large majority of the once extremely popular mesenchymal lesion labeled with the now-abandoned term "hemangiopericytoma."

## Clinical Presentation and Outcome

Solitary fibrous tumor (SFT) has been first reported as a pleural-based lesion (localized benign mesothelioma). With time, it has become evident that SFT can arise anywhere in the somatic soft tissue, in the bone, in the meninges (formerly known as meningeal hemangiopericytoma), and in several visceral sites, including the peritoneal surface, mediastinum, retroperitoneum, upper respiratory tract, head and neck, and urogenital tract. Actually, pleural lesions account for less than one-third of all SFTs. The occurrence of systemic signs such as hypoglycemia and digital hippocratism has been rarely reported and is related to the production of insulin-like growth factors by neoplastic cells. The morphologic prediction of the clinical behavior of SFT seems to be a real challenge. Approximately 10% of cases behave aggressively. Metastases are most frequently observed in lungs, bone, and liver. Malignant behavior seems to be associated with the presence of cytologic atypia, increased cellularity, mitotic activity greater than 4 mitoses/10HPF, and necrosis; however, their absence does not exclude per se the possibility of an aggressive clinical course. As a consequence, we do not advise labeling any SFT as benign. Lesions deeply located (retroperitoneum, mediastinum, and pelvis) appear to behave more aggressively than do those arising in the somatic soft tissues of the limbs. Large size seems also to correlate with higher risk of aggressive behavior. Primary meningeal SFTs also appear to behave rather aggressively, with metastatic spread to the somatic soft tissue and even to the bone being, in fact, seen relatively often. Recently, several attempts have been made to identify factors predictive of aggressive behavior, including a risk assessment model based on evaluation of patient age, mitotic count, tumor size, and presence of necrosis that appears to provide good correlation with metastases-free survival rates (Table 4.3). The

**Table 4.3** Risk stratification model for solitary fibrous tumors

| Risk factor | Score |
|---|---|
| **Age** | |
| <55 | 0 |
| ≥55 | 1 |
| **Tumor size (cm)** | |
| <5 | 0 |
| 5 to <10 | 1 |
| 10 to <15 | 2 |
| ≥15 | 3 |
| **Mitotic figures (/10 high-power fields)** | |
| 0 | 0 |
| 1–3 | 1 |
| ≥4 | 2 |
| **Necrosis** | |
| <10% | 0 |
| ≥10% | 1 |
| **Risk class** | **Total score** |
| Low | 0–3 |
| Moderate | 4–6 |
| High | 6–7 |

(Reprinted by permission from Springer Nature: Demicco et al. Mod Pathol. 2017;30:1433–42)

use of systemic treatment is still a matter of debate; however, recent preclinical/clinical data would suggest potential benefit, at least in morphologically high-grade lesions.

## Morphology and Immunophenotype

Grossly, SFT is most often represented by a relatively well-circumscribed mass, with a white-gray cut surface, sometimes featuring myxoid degeneration, hemorrhage, and, very rarely, necrotic foci (Fig. 4-150). Intra-abdominal lesions tend to attain a large size.

Microscopically, classic SFT is well circumscribed (Fig. 4-151), characterized by a variably cellular spindle cell proliferation (often with a distinctive combination of hypocellular and hypercellular areas) (Figs. 4-152 and 4-153), organized in a short storiform (so-called patternless) pattern of growth (Fig. 4-154). A characteristic hemangiopericytoma-like vascular network, characterized by thin-walled, gaping, branching blood vessels, is almost invariably present (Fig. 4-155). In classic examples, neoplastic cells tend to exhibit mild atypia and are associated with abundant collagen (Fig. 4-156). Perivascular hyalinization is also frequently seen (Fig. 4-157). This latter feature can be extensive, to the extent that, rarely, SFT can mimic pleomorphic hyalinizing angiectatic tumor (Fig. 4-158). Rarely, SFT may present with extensive myxoid degeneration of the stroma, to the extent that the most typical morphologic picture is obscured (Fig. 4-159). Rare cases may exhibit an epithelioid rather than spindle cell morphology.

Malignant SFT refers to cases in which mitotic activity greater than 4 mitoses/10HPF is observed. Increased mitotic

activity is often associated with hypercellularity (Fig. 4-160), to the extent that the distinctive alternation between hypocellular and hypercellular areas may be lost. The presence of significant nuclear pleomorphism (Fig. 4-161) and necrosis,

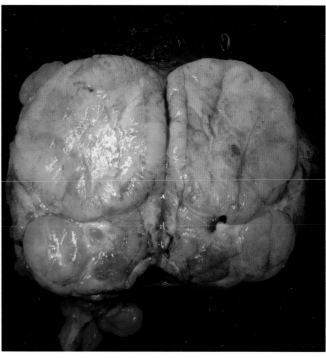

**Fig. 4-150.** Solitary fibrous tumor. Macroscopically, the tumor appears as a well-circumscribed mass, with a white-gray cut surface. Hemorrhagic and necrotic foci are seen.

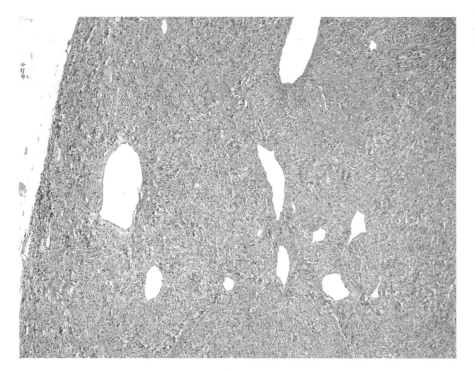

**Fig. 4-151.** Solitary fibrous tumor. At low power, the tumor appears well circumscribed. Prominent hemangiopericytoma-like vascularization is seen.

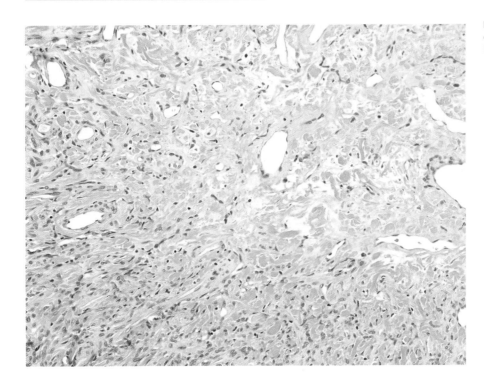

**Fig. 4-152.** Solitary fibrous tumor. The tumor is composed of a combination of hypocellular and hypercellular areas

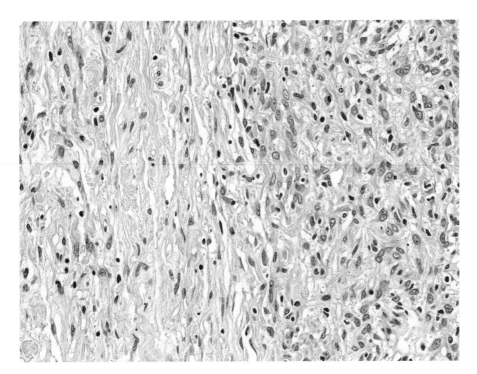

**Fig. 4-153.** Solitary fibrous tumor. High-power view of the transition from hypocellular to hypercellular areas.

even in the absence of high mitotic activity, should be regarded as unfavorable prognostic features. The neoplastic cell population may also lose the characteristic spindle cell morphology and assume a more epithelioid appearance. Dedifferentiated SFT represents the rarest variant and is characterized by an abrupt transition to high-grade, undifferentiated, most often pleomorphic morphology (Figs. 4-162 and 4-163). The dedifferentiated component may also exceptionally feature heterologous differentiation, most frequently rhabdomyoblastic.

Solitary fibrous tumor may rarely feature the presence of a variable amount of fat cells. This phenomenon has been

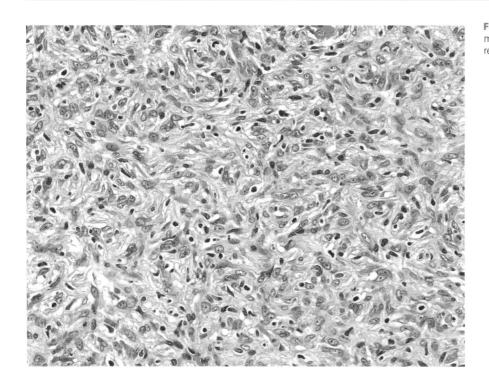

**Fig. 4-154.** Solitary fibrous tumor. Neoplastic cells most often exhibit a short storiform pattern, also referred to as "patternless" pattern of growth.

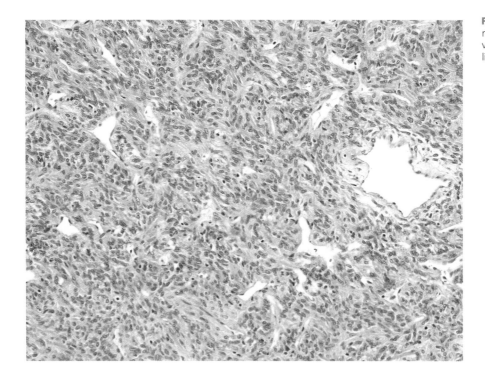

**Fig. 4-155.** Solitary fibrous tumor. The presence of numerous thin-walled, dilated, branching blood vessels results in the typical hemangiopericytoma-like appearance.

previously referred to as "lipomatous hemangiopericytoma"; however, it is now broadly accepted that this label merely identifies a morphologic variant of SFT, and these lesions are currently recognized under the term "fat-forming SFT" (Figs. 4-164 and 4-165). The same concept may apply to the entity known as **giant cell angiofibroma**, a lesion that tends to occur most often in the head and neck region (particularly in the orbit) and that features the presence of multinucleated giant cells (Fig. 4-166) that may be associated with the presence of angiectoid spaces. Whether giant cell angiofibroma merely represents a variant of SFT has long been a source of debate. Certainly giant cell angiofibroma seems to follow a remarkably indolent clinical behavior, but this may be related to anatomic site.

Immunohistochemically, SFT typically exhibits positivity for the ubiquitously expressed antigen CD34 (Fig. 4-167). Despite the fact that CD34 is expressed in a broad range of mesenchymal neoplasms, it must be underlined that in the

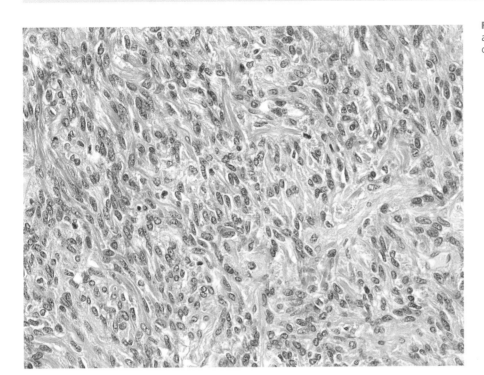

**Fig. 4-156.** Solitary fibrous tumor. The presence of abundant stromal collagen represents an extremely common finding.

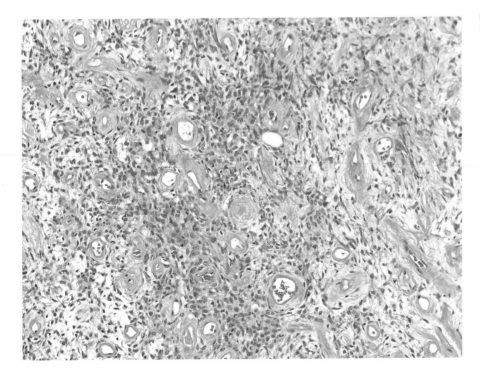

**Fig. 4-157.** Solitary fibrous tumor. Striking perivascular hyalinization is also frequently seen.

context of morphology it still retains great diagnostic value. A possible pitfall is represented by the fact that up to 5% of SFTs actually may be CD34 negative. CD99 as well as bcl2 are invariably expressed; however, their specificity is very limited, as is their diagnostic utility. Much greater diagnostic value is represented by nuclear expression of STAT6, which represents a fairly specific as well as sensitive new immunophenotypic marker (Fig. 4-168). Interestingly, a small subset of SFT exhibits nuclear immunopositivity for β-catenin. EMA, desmin, and S100 positivity may also be infrequently encountered.

## Genetics

Solitary fibrous tumor, independently from anatomic sites (pleura, meninges, or soft tissues), is characterized genetically by the presence of a *NAB2-STAT6* gene fusion. Normally, *NAB2* and *STAT6* represent adjacent genes on chromosome 12q13 and are transcribed in opposite directions. As an effect of chromosome inversion, *NAB2* and *STAT6* are fused and transcribed along the same direction. The *NAB2-STAT6* fusion induces the expression of EGFR1 target genes.

**161**

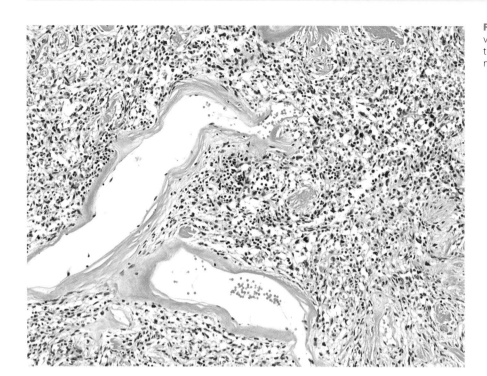

**Fig. 4-158.** Solitary fibrous tumor. Extreme vascular hyalinization is rarely seen, to the extent that a pleomorphic hyalinizing angiectatic tumor may be considered.

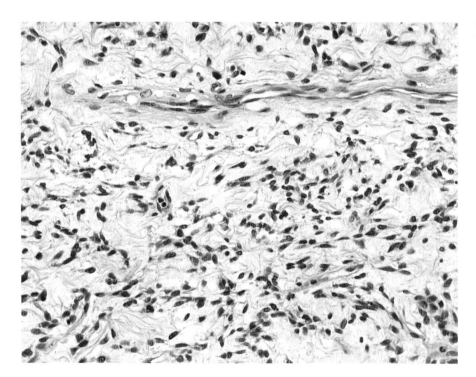

**Fig. 4-159.** Solitary fibrous tumor. In some cases, diffusely myxoid change of the stroma is seen.

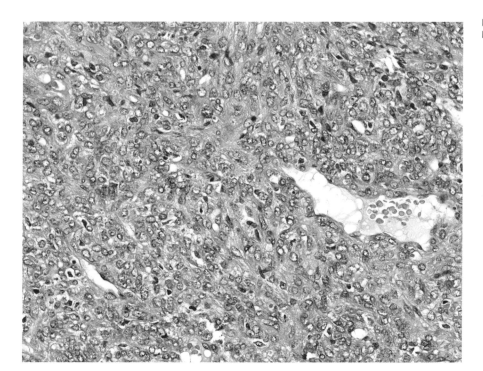

**Fig. 4-160.** Malignant solitary fibrous tumor. Increased cellularity is typically seen.

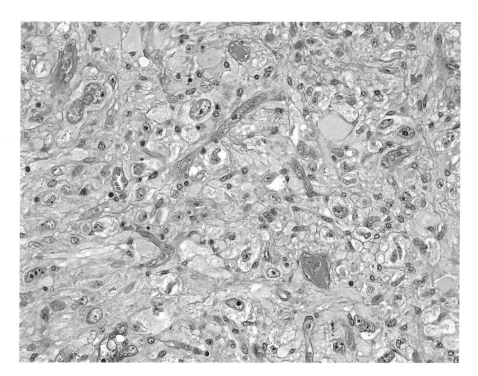

**Fig. 4-161.** Malignant solitary fibrous tumor. The presence of significant pleomorphism represents a relatively uncommon finding.

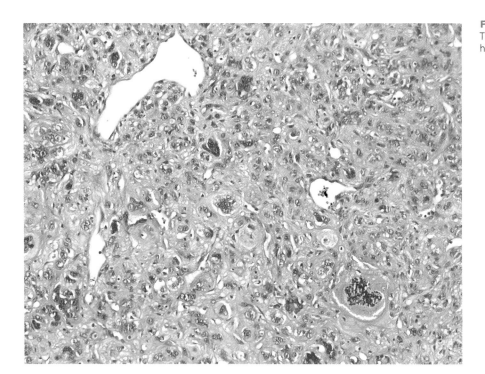

**Fig. 4-162.** Dedifferentiated solitary fibrous tumor. The dedifferentiated component is represented by high-grade undifferentiated pleomorphic sarcoma.

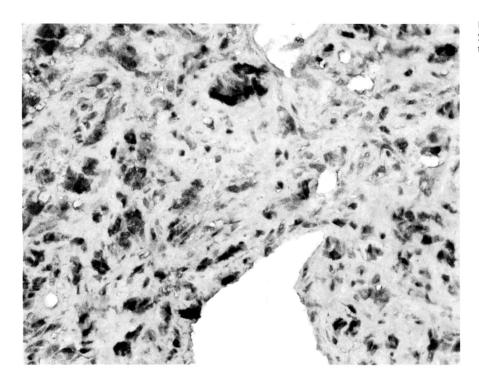

**Fig. 4-163.** Dedifferentiated solitary fibrous tumor. STAT6 nuclear immunopositivity is also retained in the dedifferentiated component of SFT.

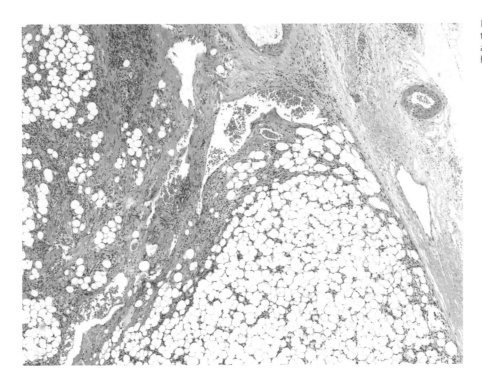

**Fig. 4-164.** Fat-forming solitary fibrous tumor. The tumor is composed of an admixture of spindle cell and mature adipocytes. Note the characteristic hemangiopericytoma-like vascular pattern.

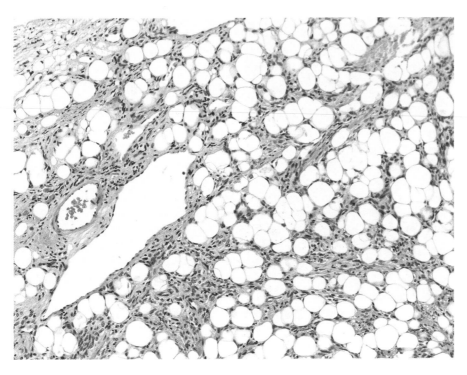

**Fig. 4-165.** Fat-forming solitary fibrous tumor. The characteristic admixture of fat tissue and classical tumor.

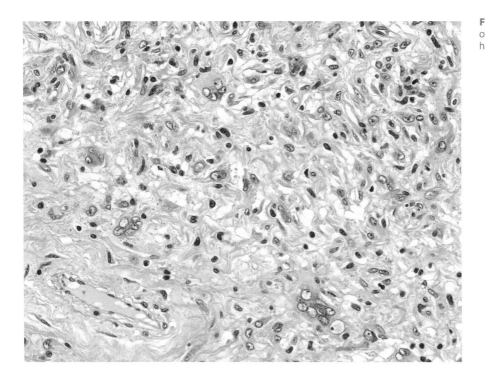

**Fig. 4-166.** Giant cell angiofibroma. The presence of multinucleated giant cells represents the hallmark of this variant of solitary fibrous tumor.

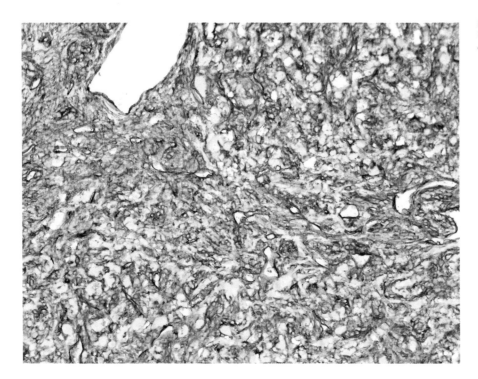

**Fig. 4-167.** Solitary fibrous tumor. CD34 immunopositivity is observed in the vast majority of cases.

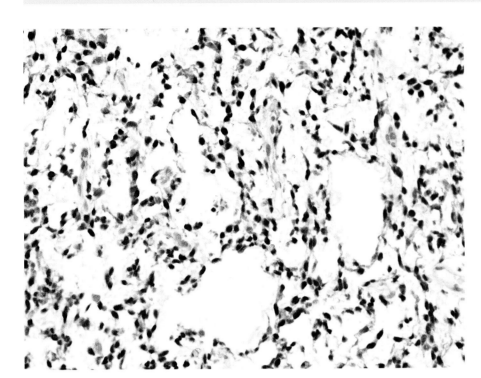

**Fig. 4-168.** Solitary fibrous tumor. Nuclear expression of STAT6 represents a major diagnostic clue.

## Differential Diagnosis and Diagnostic Pitfalls

There exists general agreement that recent cases of SFT have usually been grouped within the category of hemangiopericytoma. It is currently broadly accepted (and clearly stated in the latest WHO classification) that "hemangiopericytoma" is a term that has erroneously been used to encompass a wide variety of unrelated lesions sharing the presence of thin-walled blood vessels often exhibiting a "staghorn" configuration. This includes both benign lesions such as myofibroma/myofibromatosis and deep-seated benign fibrous histiocytoma, as well as malignant lesions such as synovial sarcoma, malignant peripheral nerve sheath tumors, mesenchymal chondrosarcoma, infantile fibrosarcoma, and endometrial stromal sarcoma. The use of the term "hemangiopericytoma" currently generates diagnostic confusion and its use is strongly discouraged.

Myofibroma/myofibromatosis has already been discussed in this chapter.

**Deep-seated fibrous histiocytoma** represents a benign (metastatic spread has been reported only exceptionally) mesenchymal lesion occurring in the deep subcutis (or, rarely, subfascially) of adults. Peak incidence is between the third and the fourth decade, with a male predominance. The limbs, followed by the head and neck region, represent the most common anatomic locations. Microscopically, deep-seated benign fibrous histiocytoma is composed of a spindle cell proliferation organized in a storiform pattern of growth (Fig. 4-169), often featuring a hemangiopericytoma-like vascular network (Fig. 4-170). At odds with classic variants of benign fibrous histiocytomas, the cell population tends to be uniform. However, one-third of cases may feature the presence of foamy histiocytes, chronic inflammatory cells, and osteoclast-like giant cells, therefore exhibiting a more heterogeneous morphologic picture. The potential diagnostic confusion with SFT is related not only to the presence of a hemangiopericytic morphology but also to the expression of CD34 (Fig. 4-171). STAT6 immunohistochemistry plays a key role in separating these two entities.

Another challenging differential diagnosis is represented by monophasic synovial sarcoma. Cellular examples of SFT may in fact exhibit significant morphologic overlap. Solitary fibrous tumor, however, does not exhibit the cytologic monomorphism of synovial sarcoma, is STAT6 +/EMA −, and never features rearrangements of the *SYT* gene.

Low-grade fibromyxoid sarcoma may exhibit some morphologic overlaps, particularly when dealing with core biopsies, wherein the distinctive HPC-like blood vessels can be easily overlooked. Diffuse positivity for MUC4 and negativity for STAT6/CD34 represent valuable immunophenotypic diagnostic clues.

When dealing with pleuropulmonary localization (either primary or metastatic) of SFT, a challenging differential diagnosis is with sarcomatoid malignant mesothelioma. History of exposure to asbestos, presence of pleural dissemination, greater cytologic atypia associated with an infiltrative pattern of growth, expression of cytokeratins (variably associated with expression of calretinin and WT1), and lack of STAT6 nuclear expression would strongly support the diagnosis of malignant mesothelioma.

167

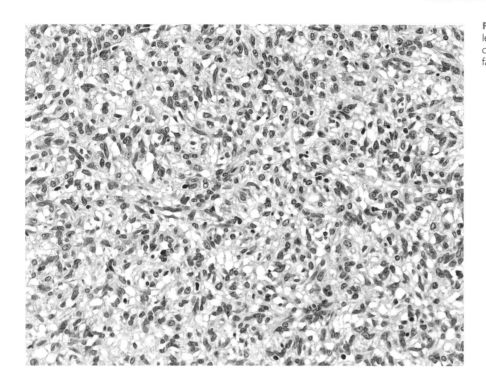

**Fig. 4-169.** Deep-seated fibrous histiocytoma. The lesion is composed of a cytologically bland spindle cell proliferation organized in short intersecting fascicles.

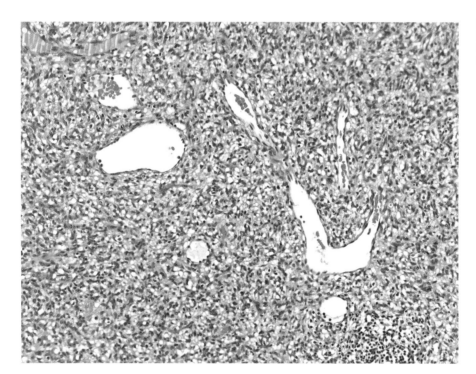

**Fig. 4-170.** Deep-seated fibrous histiocytoma. A hemangiopericytoma-like vascular network is often seen and determines some morphologic overlap with SFT.

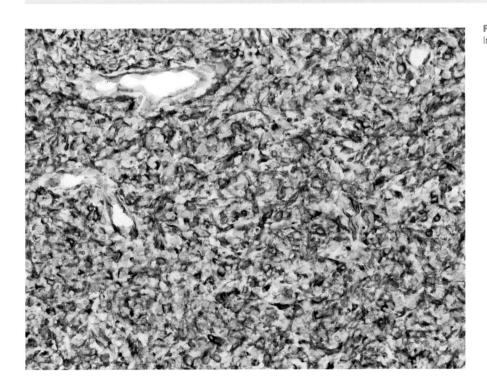

**Fig. 4-171.** Deep-seated fibrous histiocytoma. Immunopositivity for CD34 is often seen.

**Key Points in Solitary Fibrous Tumor Diagnosis**

- Ubiquitous fibroblastic spindle cell neoplasm
- Presence of hemangiopericytoma-like vascular pattern
- Spindle cell proliferation featuring variation of cellularity
- Immunohistochemical expression of CD34 and STAT6
- Presence of *NAB2-STAT6* gene fusion
- Aggressive behavior associated with increased mitotic activity

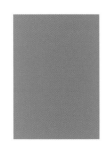

# Synovial Sarcoma

## Definition and Epidemiology

Synovial sarcoma is a mesenchymal malignant spindle cell neoplasm, featuring variable epithelial differentiation, including gland formation, and harbors a specific chromosomal translocation, t(X;18) (p11;q11), producing a *SYT-SSX* fusion gene. Synovial sarcoma accounts for approximately 15% of all soft tissue sarcomas. It can occur at any age; however, peak incidence is between the first and third decade. A male predominance (male-to-female ratio is 2:1) is observed. Synovial sarcoma represents the most common malignant non-rhabdomyosarcomatous soft tissue sarcoma in children and adolescents. It is currently recognized that synovial sarcoma is wholly unrelated to normal synovium; however, because this label identifies a very distinctive clinicopathologic entity (and a meaningful alternative does not exist), it has been retained to avoid further confusion.

## Clinical Presentation and Outcome

Synovial sarcoma most often occurs in the soft tissues of the lower extremities (especially around the knee and ankle), followed by the trunk, the head and neck region (including larynx and hypopharynx), and the mediastinum. Even if typical of soft tissues, synovial sarcoma is also described at visceral sites, such as the lungs (wherein it represents by far the most common mesenchymal malignancy) and pleura, the gastrointestinal tract, and the kidney. Exceptionally, synovial sarcoma can arise primarily in bone. Approximately 30% of synovial sarcomas feature the presence of irregular calcifications that can be visualized radiographically. Because the tumor tends to grow slowly, symptoms (which may include pain) can be present for quite a while before the diagnosis is made. Up to 50% of cases of synovial sarcoma metastasize, with the lungs, the locoregional lymph nodes, and the bone representing the most common sites of systemic spread. Systemic spread to the lungs represents the most common cause of death. Overall, survival at 5 years is about 60% but drops to 30% at 10 years with no significant difference between monophasic and biphasic subtypes. FNCLCC grading, less than 10 mitoses/10HPF, absence of necrosis, absence of poorly differentiated areas, pediatric age, size less than 5 cm, presence of stromal calcifications, and complete surgery all represent favorable prognostic factors. Surgical resection in association with adjuvant radiotherapy and/or ifosfamide-based chemotherapy represents the mainstays of treatment. Following the publication of large retrospective studies that have led to contradicting results, the

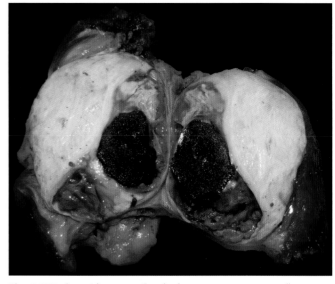

**Fig. 4-172.** Synovial sarcoma. Grossly, the tumor appears as a well-circumscribed, deep-seated mass. The cut surface is gray to tan, with a blood-filled cystic space.

existence of a prognostic role of the different molecular transcripts remains controversial.

## Morphology and Immunophenotype

Grossly, synovial sarcoma tends to be multinodular and well circumscribed, and relatively often features blood-filled cystic spaces (Fig. 4-172). Size is very variable and ranges from 1 to 10 cm. Poorly differentiated synovial sarcoma typically shows hemorrhagic areas and abundant necrosis.

Microscopically, synovial sarcoma is further classified based on morphology into three main subtypes: (1) monophasic spindle cell synovial sarcoma; (2) biphasic synovial sarcoma; and (3) poorly differentiated synovial sarcoma.

Monophasic spindle cell synovial sarcoma is composed of a cytologically uniform spindle cell population, organized in cellular sheets and fascicles, and set in a variably collagenous background (Fig. 4-173). In approximately half of the cases, synovial sarcoma features the presence of pseudocystic spaces often filled with blood. Extravasated erythrocytes are also frequently seen (Fig. 4-174). Even if not specific for synovial sarcoma, numerous mast cells are often encountered. Prominent palisading is sometimes observed, therefore mimicking a neural neoplasm

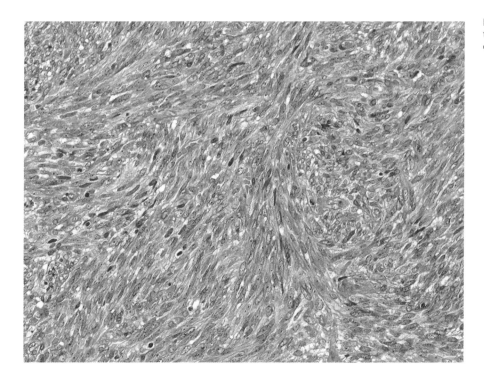

**Fig. 4-173.** Monophasic synovial sarcoma. The tumor is composed of a uniformly atypical spindle cell population, organized in intersecting fascicles.

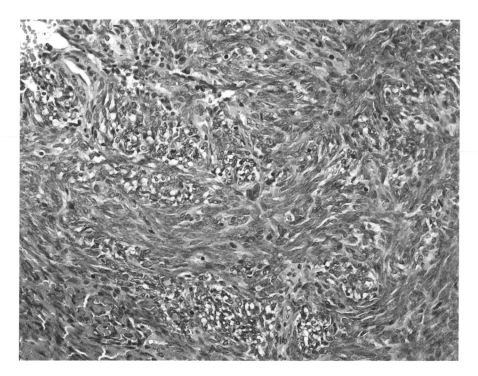

**Fig. 4-174.** Monophasic synovial sarcoma. Intratumoral stromal hemorrhage is frequently seen.

(Fig. 4-175). The amount of collagen is extremely variable and most often is organized in a distinctive pericellular distribution (Fig. 4-176). In approximately 60% of cases, a distinctive hemangiopericytoma-like vascularization is seen, represented by dilated, thin-walled blood vessels often assuming a branching, "staghorn" configuration (Fig. 4-177). Extensive stromal hyalinization with calcifications (Fig. 4-178), myxoid changes that at times can become extensive (Fig. 4-179), bone metaplasia, and, rarely, chondroid changes can be variably observed. Even if cellular monomorphism represents one of the key morphologic features of synovial sarcoma, marked nuclear pleomorphism is very rarely encountered (Figs. 4-180 and 4-181). Most often, synovial sarcoma exhibits high cellularity; however, there exist examples of monophasic spindle cell lesions that may feature a less cellular spindle cell population and that represent a major diagnostic challenge (Fig. 4-182).

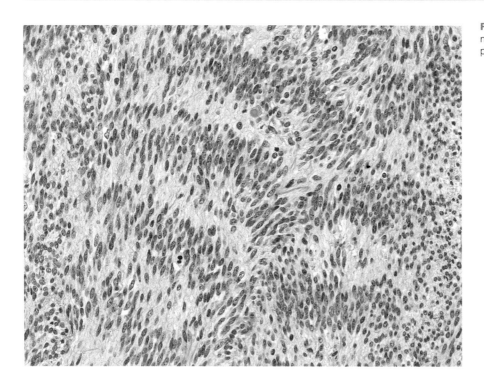

Fig. 4-175. Monophasic synovial sarcoma. The neoplastic cells are sometimes organized in palisades, mimicking a neural neoplasm.

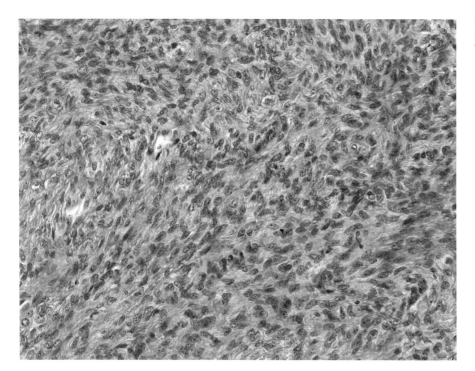

Fig. 4-176. Monophasic synovial sarcoma. The presence of pericellular collagen represents a common morphologic feature.

Biphasic synovial sarcoma is defined by the presence of variable amounts of epithelial differentiation in context with a spindle cell component that exhibits the same morphologic features of monophasic spindle cell synovial sarcoma (Fig. 4-183). Epithelial differentiation may be full blown with formation of true glandular structures (Fig. 4-184), or be less obvious and represented by a solid cluster of plump, epithelioid neoplastic cells (so-called incipient epithelial differentiation) (Fig. 4-185).

Very rare examples of synovial sarcoma featuring a predominant epithelial differentiation have been reported; however, experience is rather limited.

The poorly differentiated variant (which is associated with more aggressive behavior) accounts for approximately 20% of all synovial sarcomas and may exhibit three main cytomorphologies: large cell, spindle cell, and round cell. Most often, poorly differentiated areas are associated with conventional monophasic or biphasic synovial sarcoma;

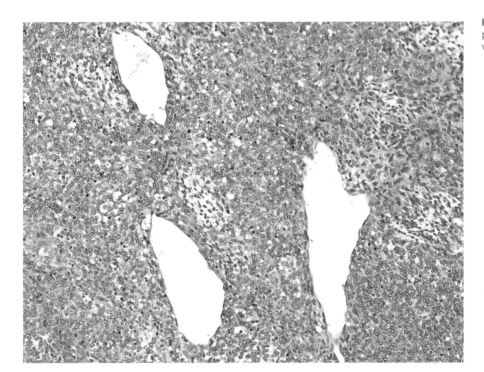

**Fig. 4-177.** Monophasic synovial sarcoma. The presence of a hemangiopericytoma-like vascularization is seen relatively often.

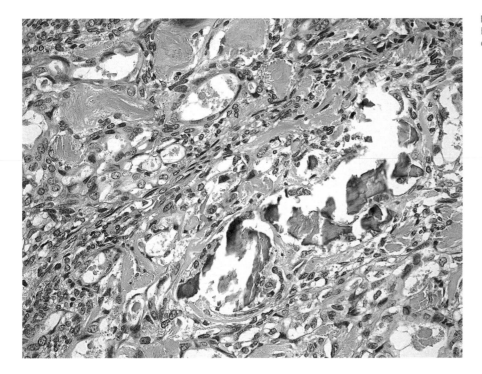

**Fig. 4-178.** Monophasic synovial sarcoma. Extensive stromal hyalinization associated with calcifications is seen.

however, there exist cases in which only a poorly differentiated morphology is seen. The round cell variant is by far the most frequent and shows significant morphologic overlap with other small round cell sarcomas, particularly with Ewing sarcoma (Fig. 4-186). Spindle cell, poorly differentiated synovial sarcoma, when compared with the conventional monophasic, shows a less uniform cell population featuring multifocal nuclear atypia and numerous mitoses (Fig. 4-187).

Synovial sarcoma shows variable immunoreactivity for EMA (Fig. 4-188) and cytokeratins (Fig. 4-189). EMA is by far more sensitive to cytokeratins and is particularly helpful with poorly differentiated synovial sarcoma wherein cytokeratin tends to be negative in up to 60%

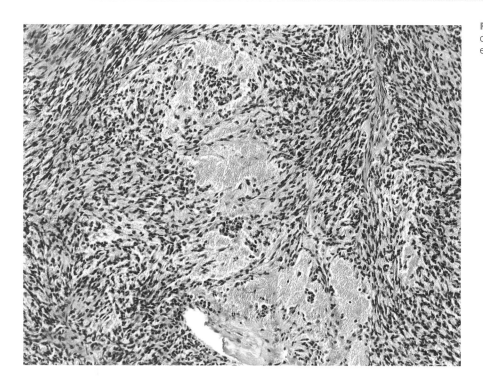

**Fig. 4-179.** Monophasic synovial sarcoma. Rarely, diffuse myxoid change of the stroma can be encountered.

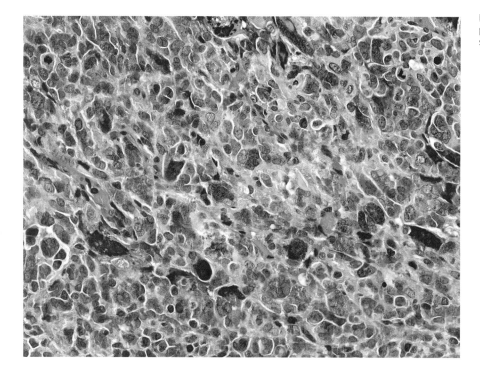

**Fig. 4-180.** Monophasic synovial sarcoma. The presence of significant nuclear pleomorphism is seen extremely rarely.

of cases. Epithelial marker staining is particularly helpful in detecting biphasic synovial sarcoma featuring incipient epithelial differentiation. CD99 immunopositivity is also seen in most cases; however, the pattern of staining tends to be diffuse, with most contrasting with the thick-membrane decoration typically observed in Ewing sarcoma. Immunoreactivity for S100 protein (up to 30% of cases), smooth muscle actin, and calponin is also reported. TLE1 represents a recently discovered transcription factor that

appears to be a rather sensitive (albeit not entirely specific) new diagnostic marker (Fig. 4-190). TLE1 immunopositivity can also be seen in MPNST; however, in contrast to synovial sarcoma, its intensity is weaker and expression is limited to a minority of neoplastic cells. Multifocal loss of INI1 is observed in approximately one-third of cases. Recently, it has been shown that NY-ESO-1 (New York Esophageal Squamous Cell Carcinoma: a cancer/testis antigen encoded by the *CTAG 1* gene) is

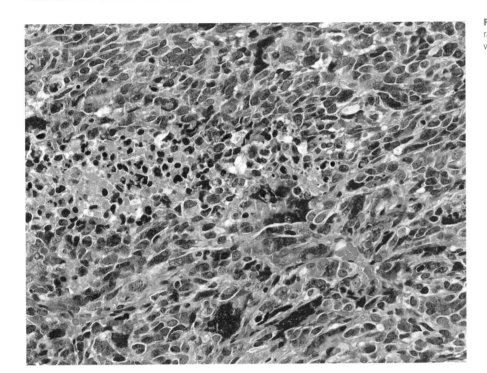

**Fig. 4-181.** Monophasic synovial sarcoma. In this rare example, cytologic pleomorphism is associated with focal necrosis.

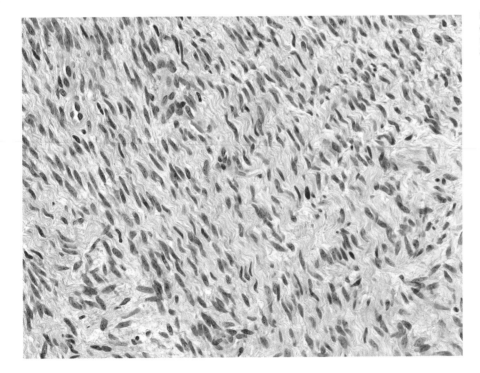

**Fig. 4-182.** Monophasic synovial sarcoma. A major diagnostic challenge is represented by cases showing relative hypocellularity and bland cytologic atypia.

strongly and diffusely expressed in approximately two-thirds of synovial sarcomas, but only rarely in other spindle cell mesenchymal lesions. Beyond its role in patient selection for targeted therapy (clinical trials using a T-cell receptor [TCR]-based targeted therapy against NY-ESO-1 are ongoing), NY-ESO-1 immunopositivity may be diagnostically useful for distinguishing synovial sarcoma from other mimics.

## Genetics

Synovial sarcoma is characterized by the presence of a specific translocation, t(X;18) (p11;q11), that fuses the *SYT* gene from chromosome 18 with the *SSX1* (in about two-thirds of cases), *SSX2* (in about one-third of cases), or *SSX4* (in rare cases) gene from the X chromosome, generating fusion transcripts. Rare cases of both SYT/SSX1 and SYT/SSX2 fusion transcripts have been described. As both SYT and SSX do not contain DNA

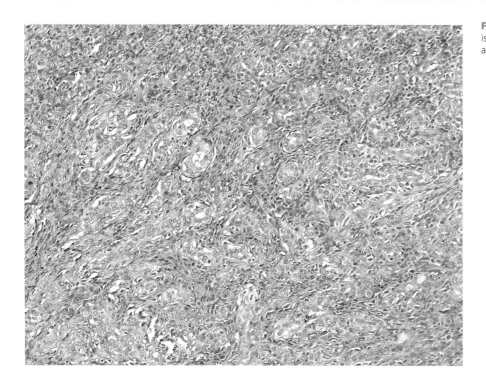

**Fig. 4-183.** Biphasic synovial sarcoma. The tumor is composed of a spindle cell proliferation associated with an epithelial component.

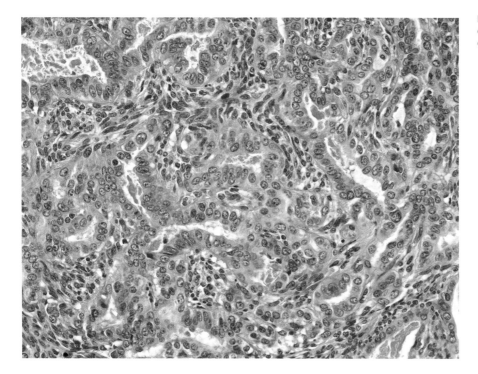

**Fig. 4-184.** Biphasic synovial sarcoma. The epithelial differentiation may be represented by true glandular structures.

binding domains, the oncogenic effect of the chimeric protein is exerted through epigenetic mechanisms. The SYT/SSX1 variant is reported to be associated with the biphasic variant. The association of SYT/SSX1 with reduced metastasis-free survival in localized tumors was not confirmed in all series, and the prognostic relevance of the fusion gene typing is still uncertain. Molecular analysis appears to be of greatest diagnostic value when dealing with poorly differentiated lesions or with tumors arising at visceral sites.

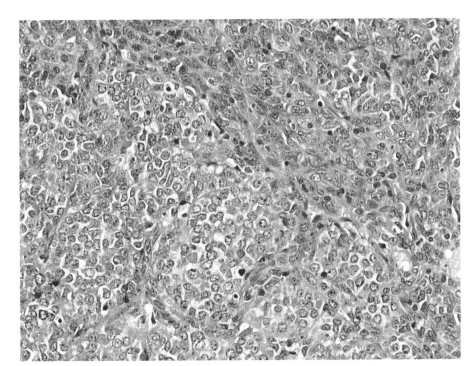

**Fig. 4-185.** Biphasic synovial sarcoma. The epithelial component may be represented by a solid cluster of plump, epithelioid neoplastic cells. This morphologic aspect is also called "incipient epithelial differentiation."

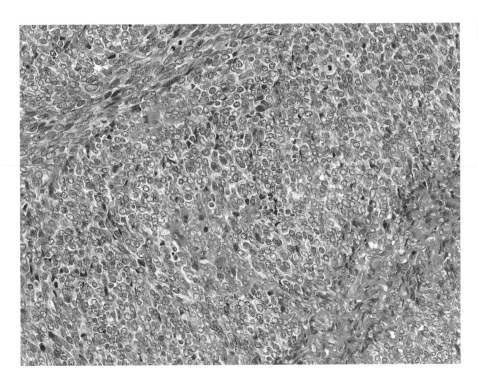

**Fig. 4-186.** Synovial sarcoma. Poorly differentiated tumors may exhibit a round cell morphology.

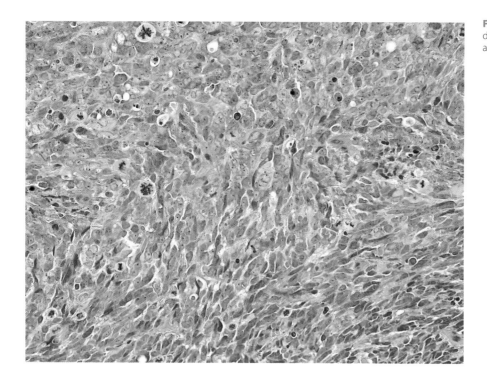

**Fig. 4-187.** Synovial sarcoma. Spindle cell, poorly differentiated forms exhibit greater nuclear atypia and remarkably brisk mitotic activity.

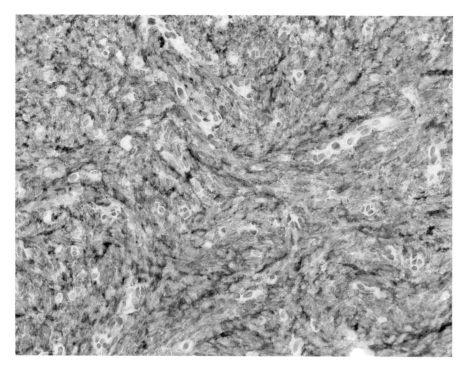

**Fig. 4-188.** Synovial sarcoma. Immunopositivity for EMA is almost always seen.

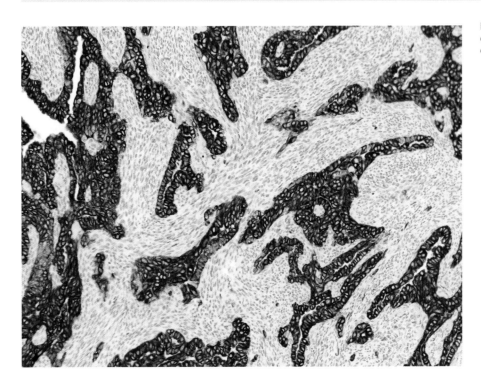

**Fig. 4-189.** Biphasic synovial sarcoma. Expression of cytokeratin is usually stronger in the epithelial component.

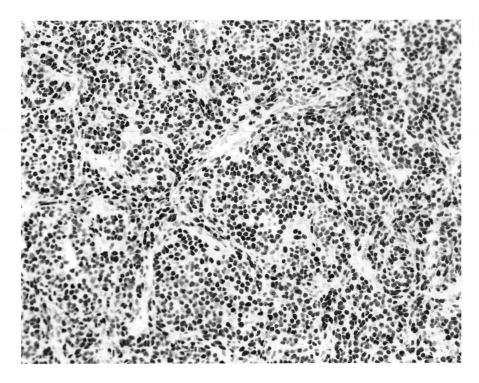

**Fig. 4-190.** Synovial sarcoma. TLE1 nuclear immunopositivity represents a valuable confirmatory finding.

## Differential Diagnosis

The differential diagnosis is rather broad, and some of the main differential diagnoses (i.e., solitary fibrous tumor, leiomyosarcoma, malignant peripheral nerve sheath tumor) are discussed in detail in this chapter.

In brief, solitary fibrous tumor is recognized on the basis of a richer hemangiopericytoma-like vascular pattern, more prominent stromal collagen, distinctive alternation between hypocellular and hypercellular areas, and nuclear expression of STAT6. However, both hypercellular SFT and hypocellular synovial sarcoma can represent a major diagnostic challenge. Molecular analysis to establish the presence of *SYT* gene rearrangement at times represents the safest way to achieve a firm diagnosis.

Leiomyosarcoma typically exhibits distinctive fibrillary eosinophilia of cytoplasm associated with cigar-shaped nuclei. Variable expression of desmin, smooth muscle actin, and h-caldesmon represents a consistent immunophenotypic feature that has never been observed in synovial sarcoma. In this context, the fact that leiomyosarcoma can variably express cytokeratin should not represent a major diagnostic problem.

Malignant peripheral nerve sheath tumor exhibits a less monomorphous spindle cell population characterized by variation (with perivascular accentuation) of cellularity. Immunopositivity of S100 is rather useless, as can be seen in both MPNST and synovial sarcoma. As mentioned, TLE1 can also be misleading, as its expression can also be seen (albeit weaker and in a minority of neoplastic cells) in MPNST. Even if morphology allows separation, in most cases there exist situations such as MPNST with epithelial differentiation wherein only molecular confirmation of *SYT* gene rearrangement can provide a diagnosis of certainty.

Synovial sarcoma may feature the presence of hyalinized collagen that may somewhat overlap morphologically with malignant osteoid. Extraskeletal osteosarcoma, however, is most often highly pleomorphic and characterized by diffuse nuclear expression of SATB2. A major caveat is that focal SATB2 immunopositivity may be seen in those examples of synovial sarcoma featuring bone metaplasia.

Poorly differentiated round cell synovial sarcoma may show significant morphologic overlap with Ewing sarcoma. Diagnostic confusion may be enhanced by the fact that CD99 can be diffusely positive in both entities. The pattern of staining is, however, different (more diffuse in synovial sarcoma with much less evident membrane reinforcement). The presence of *EWSR1* and *SYT* gene rearrangement in Ewing sarcoma and synovial sarcoma, respectively, also represents an extremely helpful diagnostic finding.

---

**Key Points in Synovial Sarcoma Diagnosis**

- Occurrence in the limbs of young adults
- Uniform spindle cell proliferation (monophasic variant)
- Variable epithelial differentiation (biphasic variant)
- Cystic change relatively common
- Expression of epithelial differentiation markers and TLE1
- Presence of *SYT* gene rearrangement
- Aggressive clinical behavior

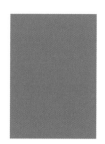

# Infantile Fibrosarcoma

## Definition and Epidemiology

Congenital, infantile, or juvenile fibrosarcoma is a rare spindle cell malignancy characterized by a favorable prognosis, with a low rate of distant metastases and a high long-term survival rate. Infantile fibrosarcoma accounts for about 10% of soft tissue malignancies in the pediatric age-group, with most cases occurring in the first 5 years of life, with a slight male predominance. The entity known as "congenital mesoblastic nephroma" is currently regarded as its renal counterpart.

## Clinical Presentation and Outcome

Infantile fibrosarcoma occurs most commonly in the extremities, the upper extremities being more often affected than the lower. The next most common site of involvement is the head and neck region, followed by the trunk. Tumor mass can attain a very large size. The standard treatment for infantile fibrosarcoma has been wide surgical excision. In consideration of the exquisite chemosensitivity, neoadjuvant chemotherapy may be useful in reducing the size of these tumors before surgical excision. Distant metastases occur in only 5 to 10% of cases (usually to the lungs), and 5-year survival may be higher than 90%. However, local recurrence rates have been reported to range between 17 and 43%. Overall mortality appears to be reduced to 5% of cases.

## Morphology and Immunophenotype

Infantile fibrosarcoma is typically large and may generate superficial ulcerations that are often associated with bleeding. Grossly, the cut surface is firm, fleshy, and gray-white. Focal cystic change may be observed. Microscopically, most tumors are highly cellular and composed of uniform oval- to spindle-shaped cells with hyperchromatic nuclei separated by variable amounts of collagen (Fig. 4-191), often arranged in long fascicles. A herringbone pattern somewhat similar to that of FS-DFSP can be seen (much more rarely than commonly believed) in some lesions (Fig. 4-192), as it is a prominent hemangiopericytoma-like vascular pattern (Fig. 4-193). Rarely, infantile fibrosarcoma may feature a more epithelioid cell population (Fig. 4-194). Mitotic rate is variable but tends to be quite high. Zonal necrosis is relatively frequent. Some lesions may present multiple myxoid foci that may be associated with the presence of foci of chronic inflammation (Fig. 4-195). Multifocal hemorrhage can be seen (Fig. 4-196). Most often, infantile fibrosarcoma is well circumscribed; however, there exist cases in which infiltration of surrounding adipose tissue can be seen (Fig. 4-197). Unfortunately, no specific tumor markers have been identified for infantile fibrosarcoma. Immunohistochemically, these tumors are diffusely positive for vimentin and may occasionally contain actin- and desmin-positive cells, most likely related to partial myofibroblastic differentiation.

## Genetics

Infantile fibrosarcoma is genetically related to congenital mesoblastic nephroma, and most cases present a recurrent chromosomal rearrangement of t(12;15)(p13;q25), resulting in the gene fusion ETV6-NTRK3 (ETS variant gene 6; neurotrophic tyrosine kinase receptor type 3). Other nonrandom changes are represented by trisomies of chromosomes 8, 11, 17, and 20. Interestingly, the same genetic aberration is also seen in myeloid leukemia, secretory breast carcinoma, post-radiation papillary thyroid carcinoma, and even in GIST. This fact further underlines the importance of evaluating molecular genetic findings in context with morphology. It has recently been shown that pediatric spindle cell sarcomas exhibiting significant morphologic overlap with infantile fibrosarcoma but lacking NTRK3 gene rearrangements harbor novel SEPT7-BRAF and TPM3-NTRK1 gene fusion. In the same series, a EML4-NTRK3 chimeric gene has been detected in one case.

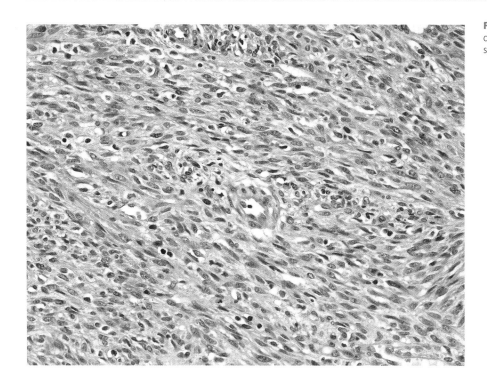

**Fig. 4-191.** Infantile fibrosarcoma. The tumor is densely cellular and composed of relatively uniform spindle cells set in a variably collagenous stroma.

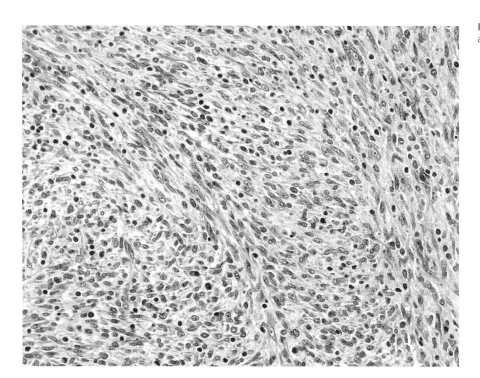

**Fig. 4-192.** Infantile fibrosarcoma. The tumor cells are organized in long intersecting fascicles.

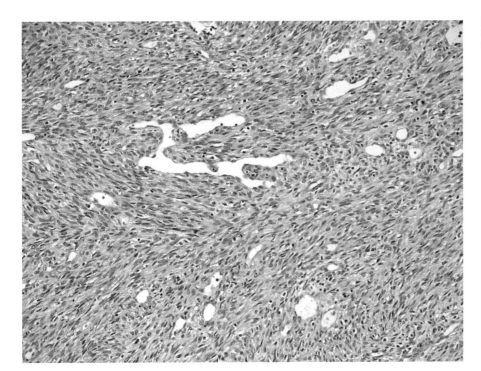

**Fig. 4-193.** Infantile fibrosarcoma. The presence of a hemangiopericytoma-like vascular pattern is seen relatively often.

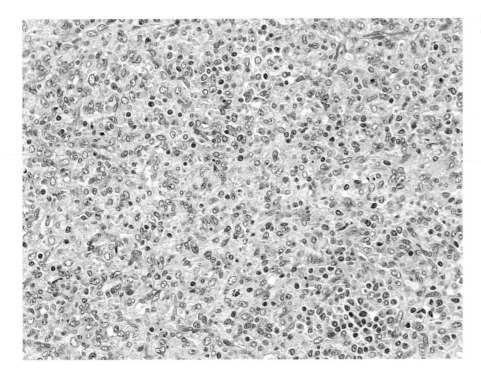

**Fig. 4-194.** Infantile fibrosarcoma. Rare cases are composed of a more epithelioid cell population.

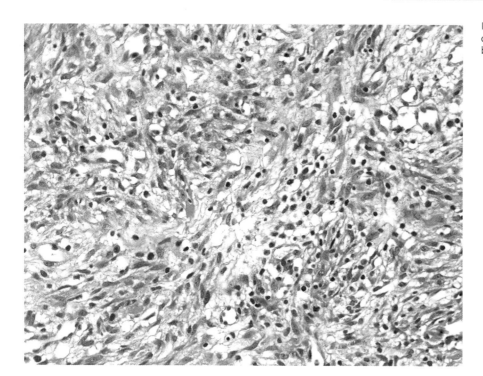

**Fig. 4-195.** Infantile fibrosarcoma. Myxoid change of the stroma and foci of chronic inflammation may be occasionally observed.

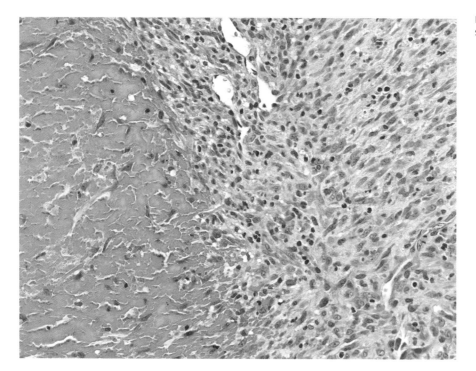

**Fig. 4-196.** Infantile fibrosarcoma. Multifocal stromal intratumoral hemorrhage can be seen.

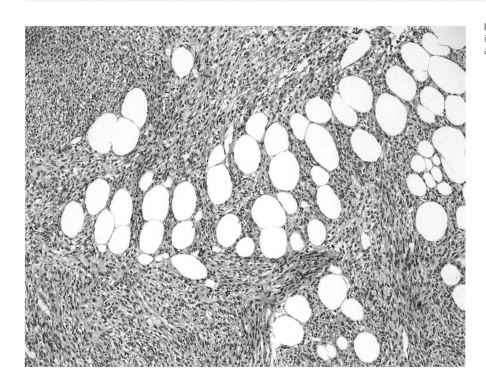

**Fig. 4-197.** Infantile fibrosarcoma. The tumor may infiltrate the surrounding adipose tissue, resulting in a honeycomb appearance.

## Differential Diagnosis and Diagnostic Pitfalls

Infantile fibrosarcoma needs to be distinguished from other spindle cell lesions of the soft tissues. First, infantile fibrosarcoma has a number of histologic features that overlap with desmoid fibromatosis, making it difficult to distinguish between the lesions. In general, infantile fibrosarcoma is more cellular, has a higher mitotic activity, and lacks nuclear expression of beta-catenin.

Spindle cell rhabdomyosarcoma may also be difficult to distinguish from infantile fibrosarcoma. As discussed in more detail later in this chapter, it occurs more frequently in the paratesticular region and in the head and neck, and neoplastic cells, in addition to a distinctive cytoplasmic eosinophilia, are consistently positive for desmin, myogenin, and MyoD1.

Leiomyosarcoma is extremely rare in the pediatric age-group (unless it is associated with immunodeficiency-associated EBV infection). Most cases are reported as low grade and display typical smooth muscle features, such as interwoven fascicles of spindle cells with cigar-shaped nuclei and eosinophilic, fibrillary cytoplasm.

Inflammatory myofibroblastic sarcoma is discussed in detail in Chapter 9. In brief, neoplastic spindle cells tend to be associated with a variably prominent inflammatory infiltrate and, particularly in the pediatric age-group, most often exhibit rearrangement of the *ALK* gene.

Monophasic synovial sarcoma is uncommon in infancy. Here neoplastic cells have plumper nuclei and express epithelial markers (EMA and cytokeratins) and TLE1, and the *SYT-SSX* fusion transcript can be identified.

Malignant peripheral nerve sheath tumor (MPNST) is also regarded as extremely uncommon in children. A significant proportion of lesion diagnoses as such actually represent examples of plexiform cellular schwannoma. Neoplastic cells show wavy nuclei and are characterized by a distinctive alternation between hypercellular and hypocellular zones, most often with perivascular accentuation of cellularity.

### Key Points in Infantile Fibrosarcoma Diagnosis

- Occurrence in the limbs of newborns and young children
- Uniform spindle cell proliferation
- Presence of *ETV6* gene rearrangement
- Indolent clinical behavior
- Exquisite chemosensitivity

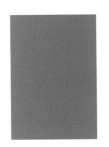

# Malignant Peripheral Nerve Sheath Tumor

## Definition and Epidemiology

Malignant peripheral nerve sheath tumor (MPNST) represents a spindle cell sarcoma showing morphologic features of nerve sheath differentiation, not necessarily arising from a peripheral nerve. Malignant peripheral nerve sheath tumor occurs from the third to the sixth decade and is regarded as very rare in the pediatric population. The association with neurofibromatosis type 1 (von Recklinghausen disease) is observed in approximately half of the cases. The lifetime risk for an NF1 patient of developing MPNST ranges between approximately 2 and 10%. In NF1-associated tumors, peak incidence is in the third decade, whereas in sporadic MPNST peak incidence occurs in the fourth decade. Male predominance is observed in NF1-associated lesions, whereas a female predominance is reported in those that are sporadic. More than one-third of cases arise from a plexiform neurofibroma in the context of NF1 syndrome. Exceptionally, MPNST has been reported arising from benign schwannoma, ganglioneuroma, and pheochromocytoma. In 10% of patients, a history of previous irradiation is reported. Notably, the term "malignant mesenchymoma" has now been abandoned, based on the fact they most often represent examples of MPNST (less often, dedifferentiated liposarcoma) with heterologous differentiation.

## Clinical Presentation and Outcome

Malignant peripheral nerve sheath tumor most often presents as slow-growing masses. The limbs, the trunk, and the retroperitoneum are among the most commonly affected anatomic sites, followed by the head and neck region. Neurofibromatosis type 1–associated MPNST tends to arise in the context of a nerve or of a pre-existing neurofibroma. When MPNST arises from a peripheral nerve, the sciatic nerve is the most frequently affected. Approximately 10% of cases occur on the site of previous irradiation. Overall survival at 5 years seems to be affected by clinical presentation, being approximately 50% in sporadic cases, 25% in NF1 patients, and 15% in post-irradiation cases. Striated muscle heterologous differentiation is associated with a 10%, 5-year overall survival. The presence of angiosarcomatous heterologous differentiation represents a most aggressive morphologic feature and is associated with 100% mortality at 5 years. Metastatic spread to the lungs represents the most frequent cause of death. From a therapeutic standpoint, complete surgery represents the mainstay. Systemic therapy can also be applied in association, even if MPNST is generally regarded as a rather refractory histotype.

## Morphology and Immunophenotype

Grossly, MPNST usually attains a large size. Foci of necrosis and hemorrhage are quite common (Fig. 4-198), as it is an infiltrative rather than expansive growth pattern. It can be associated with a pre-existing neural lesion (Fig. 4-199).

Microscopically, a spindle cell proliferation organized in long fascicles is seen (Fig. 4-200). Cell nuclei are most often wavy and irregularly shaped (Fig. 4-201). The presence of significant variation in cellularity represented by the transition from hypercellular to myxoid areas represents a relatively common morphologic finding (Figs. 4-202 and 4-203). Rarely, MPNST may feature a herringbone pattern of growth somewhat mimicking fibrosarcomatous DFSP (Fig. 4-204). A distinctive circling and clustering of neoplastic cells around blood vessels is often seen (Fig. 4-205) and is more rarely associated with invasion of the wall with intrusion in the lumen (Fig. 4-206). As discussed in Chapter 7, overt pleomorphism may be observed, but it represents a rare event. Palisading represents a relatively rare finding and is actually more often seen in synovial sarcoma and leiomyosarcoma. As mentioned, MPNST, in contrast to most sarcomas, may diffusely infiltrate around the surrounding soft tissues (Fig. 4-207). In approximately 10–15% of cases, heterologous differentiation is observed. Such a phenomenon appears to be more common in NF1 patients. The heterologous component can be osteogenic (Fig. 4-208), chondrosarcomatous (Fig. 4-209), angiosarcomatous (Fig. 4-210), or epithelial (Fig. 4-211), but most often it is rhabdomyosarcomatous (so-called malignant triton tumor) (Figs. 4-212 and 4-213).

As mentioned, most examples of MPNST are high grade; however, low-grade MPNST does exist and represents tumor progression occurring in a pre-existing benign neural lesion, most often a plexiform neurofibroma in the context of NF1 syndrome. The presence of multifocal nuclear atypia and increased cellularity per se do not represent sufficient criteria of malignancy, and a diagnosis of atypical neurofibroma seems to be appropriate in these cases (Fig. 4-214). However, whenever those morphologic features are associated with any mitotic activity, a diagnosis of low-grade MPNST should be made (Fig. 4-215). Recently, a consensus conference focusing on NF1-associated neurofibromatous tumor proposed a set of morphologic criteria to separate neurofibroma from low-grade MPNST. Also introduced was the category of "atypical neurofibromatous tumor of uncertain malignant potential" (ANTUMP), which at best underlines the intrinsic difficulty

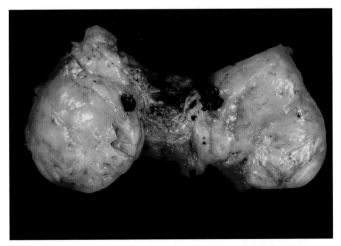

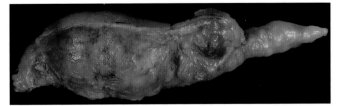

**Fig. 4-199.** Malignant peripheral nerve sheath tumor. In this case the tumor is associated with a pre-existing neural lesion (plexiform neurofibroma).

**Fig. 4-198.** Malignant peripheral nerve sheath tumor. Grossly, the tumor appears as a voluminous deep-seated mass featuring necrosis and hemorrhagic foci.

in correlating morphology with clinical behavior in this context.

Immunophenotypically, MPNST expresses S100 protein in approximately half the cases; however, immunoreactivity is usually limited to a fraction of neoplastic cells (Fig. 4-216). Glial fibrillary acidic protein (GFAP) positivity is also observed in less than one-third of cases. Malignant peripheral nerve sheath tumors with glandular differentiation, in addition to expression of EMA and cytokeratins, often features expression of neuroendocrine markers such as chromogranin A. EMA immunoreactivity may also be observed, and it is generally regarded as possible evidence of perineural differentiation. Nuclear expression of SOX10 seems to be associated with

MPNST, even if the sensitivity is less than optimal. Very recently, it has been shown that the loss of expression of H3K27me3 appears to be fairly specific to MPNST.

## Genetics

Cytogenetically, MPNST is characterized by the occurrence of non-specific complex chromosome aberrations. At the molecular level, NF1 deletions are often observed in both the NF1 and non-NF1 groups. NF1 normally encodes neurofibromin, a protein that negatively regulates the Ras/Raf/MAPK pathway by promoting accelerated degradation of Ras-GTP. Net gain of distal 17q material (involving topoisomerase-II alpha as well as other genes) has been reported that correlates with aggressive behavior. It has recently been shown that the inactivation of the polycomb regressive complex 2 (PRC2) can be observed in up to 90% of MPNST. This molecular event is determined by the occurrence of inactivating mutations of either *SUZ12* or *EED1* genes. As mentioned, *PRC2* inactivation results in a loss of the histone H3K27 trimethylation (H3K27me3) that can be detected by immunohistochemistry.

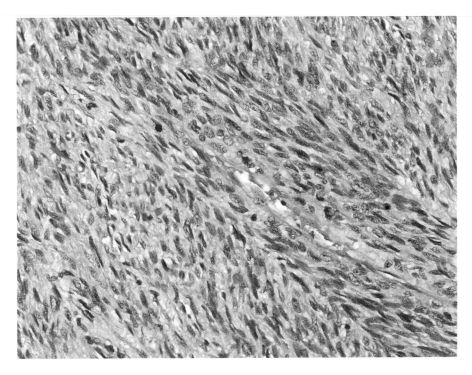

**Fig. 4-200.** Malignant peripheral nerve sheath tumor. The tumor is composed of a hypercellular spindle cell proliferation organized in long fascicles.

**187**

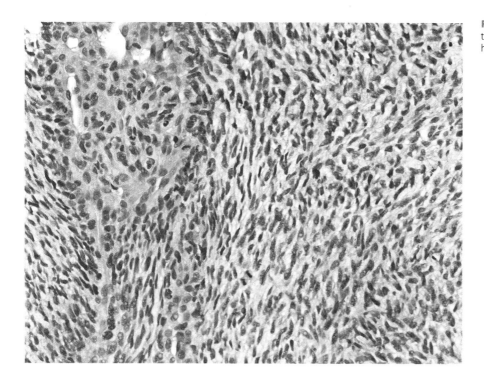

**Fig. 4-201.** Malignant peripheral nerve sheath tumor. The neoplastic cells contain wavy and hyperchromatic nuclei.

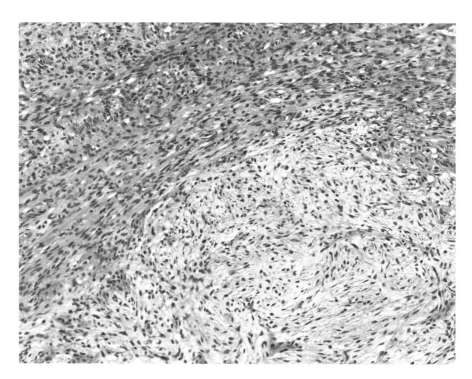

**Fig. 4-202.** Malignant peripheral nerve sheath tumor. The presence of a variation of cellularity shown by a transition from hypercellular to hypercellular myxoid areas is a common morphologic finding.

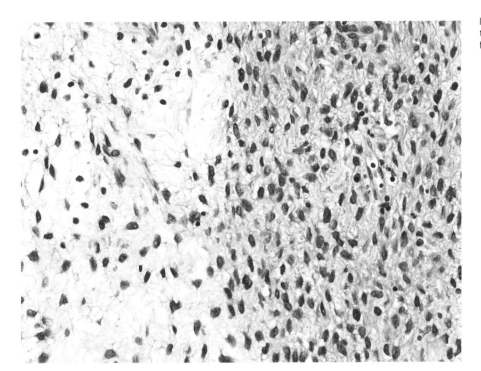

**Fig. 4-203.** Malignant peripheral nerve sheath tumor. High-power view showing the transition from hypercellular to hypocellular areas.

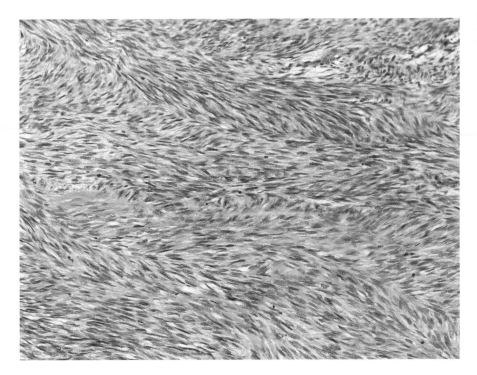

**Fig. 4-204.** Malignant peripheral nerve sheath tumor. In some cases, a herringbone pattern of growth can be observed.

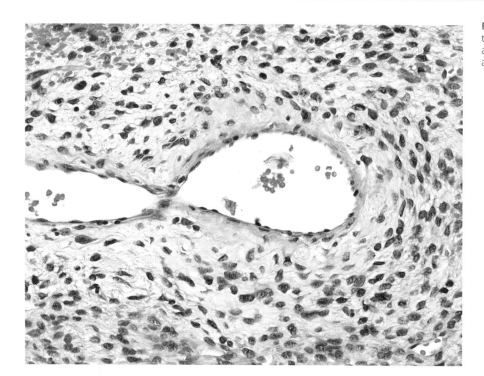

**Fig. 4-205.** Malignant peripheral nerve sheath tumor. Circling and clustering of neoplastic cells around blood vessels are often seen and represent an important diagnostic clue.

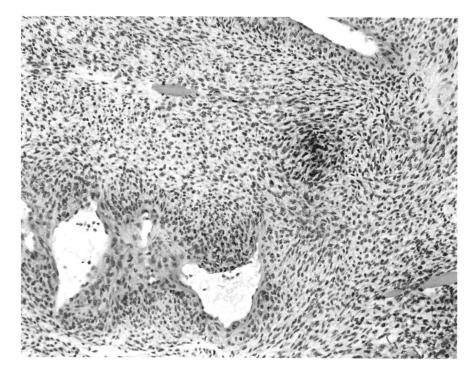

**Fig. 4-206.** Malignant peripheral nerve sheath tumor. The neoplastic cells are clustered around blood vessels and tend to infiltrate the vessel wall.

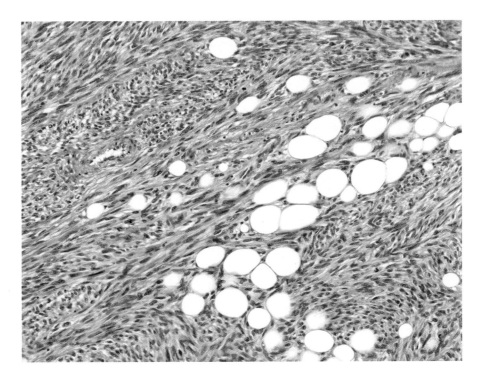

**Fig. 4-207.** Malignant peripheral nerve sheath tumor. The tumor infiltrates the surrounding soft tissues.

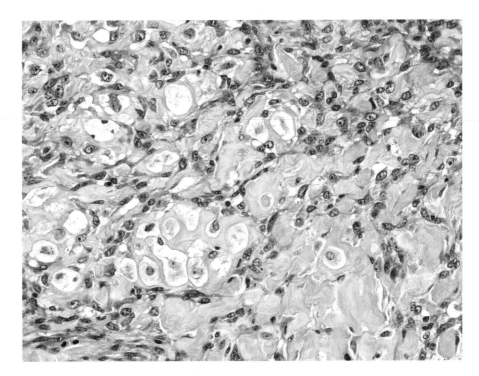

**Fig. 4-208.** Malignant peripheral nerve sheath tumor. The tumor presents foci of osteogenic heterologous differentiation.

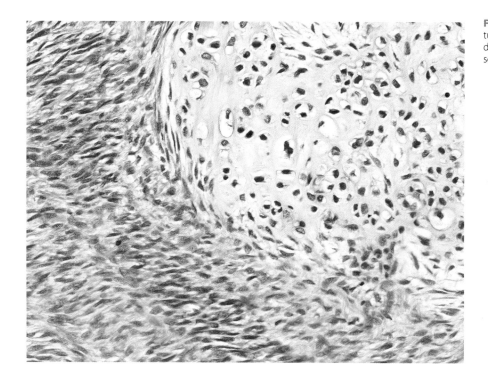

**Fig. 4-209.** Malignant peripheral nerve sheath tumor. In the tumor, an area of cartilaginous differentiation with features of chondrosarcoma is seen.

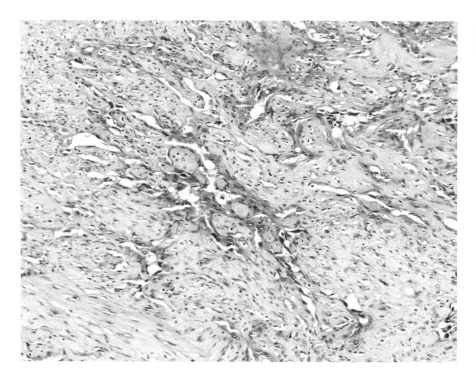

**Fig. 4-210.** Malignant peripheral nerve sheath tumor. Rarely, the heterologous component is represented by angiosarcoma and confers extreme clinical aggressiveness.

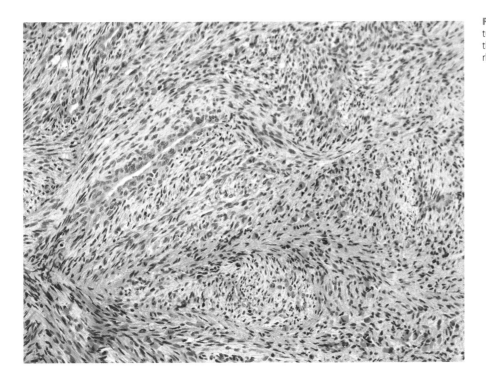

**Fig. 4-211.** Malignant peripheral nerve sheath tumor. This tumor presents epithelial differentiation that is associated with the presence of rhabdomyoblasts.

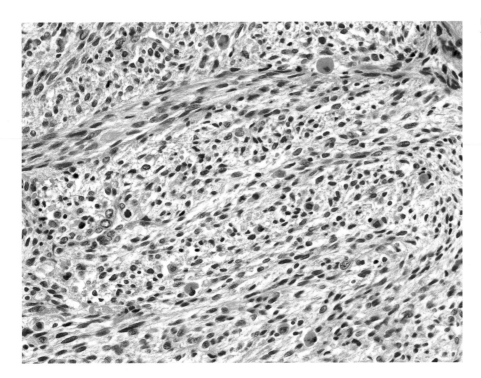

**Fig. 4-212.** Malignant peripheral nerve sheath tumor. The presence of rhabdomyoblastic heterologous differentiation identifies the so-called malignant triton tumor.

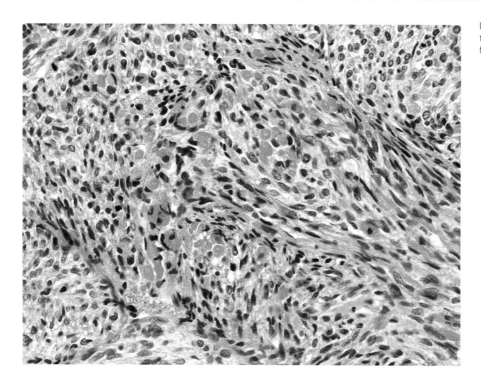

**Fig. 4-213.** Malignant peripheral nerve sheath tumor. High-power view of malignant triton tumor featuring abundant rhabdomyoblasts.

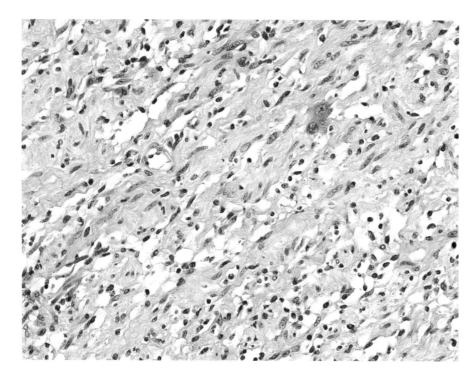

**Fig. 4-214.** Atypical neurofibroma. The tumor is composed of spindle cells with multifocal nuclear pleomorphism. No significant mitotic activity is detected.

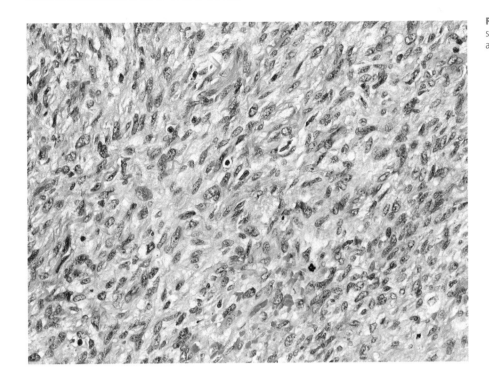

**Fig. 4-215.** Low-grade malignant peripheral nerve sheath tumor presents moderate cellular atypia associated with increased mitotic activity.

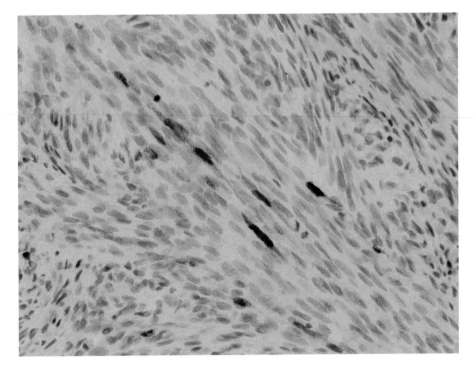

**Fig. 4-216.** Malignant peripheral nerve sheath tumor. S100 immunopositivity is generally limited to a small fraction of neoplastic cells.

## Differential Diagnosis and Diagnostic Pitfalls

One of the most important diagnostic pitfalls is represented by **cellular schwannoma**. First reported by Woodruff in 1981, this variant of benign schwannoma characteristically originates along the paravertebral region (most often in the mediastinum, retroperitoneum, and pelvis). Grossly, cellular schwannoma is typically well circumscribed (Fig. 4-217). Morphologically, cellular schwannoma is composed of a mitotically active spindle cell proliferation, featuring a predominant Antoni-A growth pattern (Fig. 4-218). Blood vessels very often exhibit a distinctive hyalinization (Fig. 4-219), which rarely represents a predominant morphologic feature (Fig. 4-220). Variable numbers of macrophages are seen, along with lymphocytic infiltrates typically located at the periphery of the lesion (Fig. 4-221). Cellular schwannoma, because of high cellularity, possible focal degenerative atypia, and significant mitotic activity (generally less than 4 mitoses/10HPF, but this can be significantly higher), is often mistaken for a sarcoma (approximately 30% according to the original Woodruff series). At variance with MPNST, cellular schwannoma is always well circumscribed, diffusely expresses S100 (Fig. 4-222), and features a variable amount of EMA-positive perineurial cells at the periphery. A small subset of cellular schwannoma exhibits a plexiform morphology and seems to occur predominantly in the pediatric age-group.

Among malignant lesions, the differential diagnosis includes leiomyosarcoma and monophasic synovial sarcoma. As repeatedly mentioned, leiomyosarcoma is distinguished by the presence of morphologic findings (blunt-ended nuclei harbored by eosinophilic fibrillary cytoplasm) as well as by the expression of smooth muscle markers. Synovial sarcoma is ruled out on the basis of the expression of epithelial differentiation markers (EMA and cytokeratin) and also by the

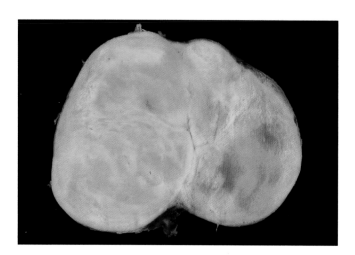

**Fig. 4-217.** Cellular schwannoma. Grossly, the tumor is always a well-circumscribed, firm mass.

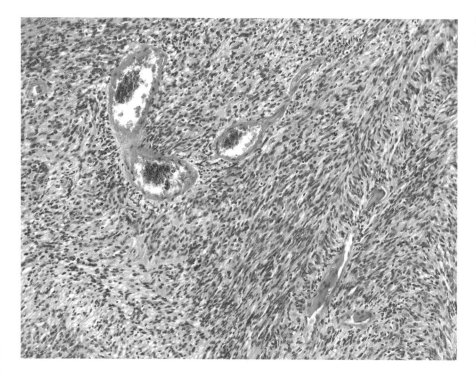

**Fig. 4-218.** Cellular schwannoma. A densely cellular spindle cell proliferation organized in long fascicles is seen.

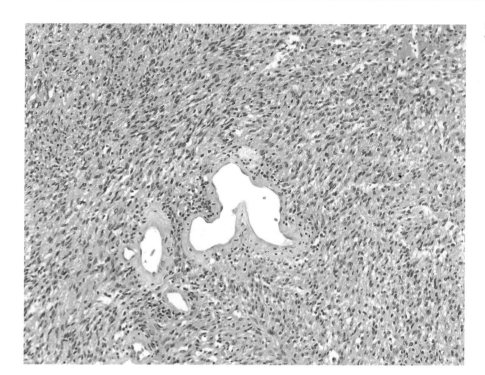

**Fig. 4-219.** Cellular schwannoma. Blood vessels with distinctive hyalinization of the wall are seen.

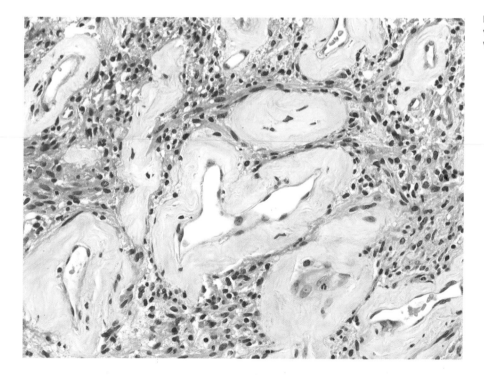

**Fig. 4-220.** Cellular schwannoma. High-power view showing extensive hyalinization of the vessel wall.

presence of the t(X;18) specific chromosome translocation. Molecular genetics may prove particularly helpful in distinguishing biphasic synovial sarcoma from MPNST showing glandular heterologous differentiation. Data reporting the presence of *SYT* rearrangement in MPNST (and even in benign neurofibroma) have proved false, a result of technical failure. Malignant triton tumor (MPNST with heterologous rhabdomyoblastic differentiation) needs to be separated from spindle cell rhabdomyosarcoma and dedifferentiated liposarcoma with striated muscle differentiation. In spindle cell rhabdomyosarcoma, positivity for desmin is usually diffuse and not multifocal, as in MPNST. In dedifferentiated liposarcoma, MDM2 amplification represents a consistent molecular alteration that plays a major diagnostic role.

A recently described malignant lesion that enters the differential diagnosis is represented by the so-called **biphenotypic**

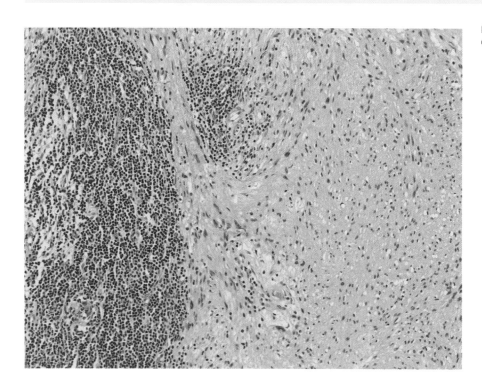

**Fig. 4-221.** Cellular schwannoma. Very often, a rim of lymphocytes is seen at the periphery of the lesion.

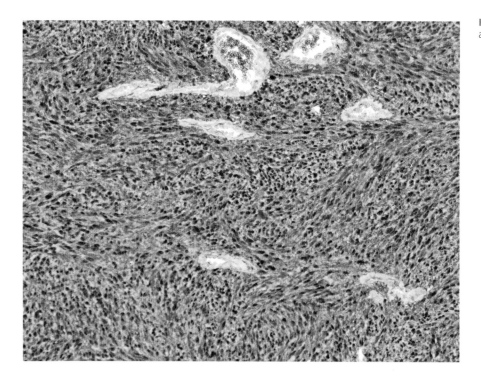

**Fig. 4-222.** Cellular schwannoma. The tumor cells are diffusely immunopositive for S100.

**sinonasal sarcoma** (BNS). Biphenotypic sinonasal sarcoma represents a low-grade spindle cell sarcoma characterized by dual myogenic and neural differentiation, occurring in the sinonasal region of adult patients. Female predominance is reported. Morphologically, BNS is composed of a cellular, cytologically uniform spindle cell proliferation (Fig. 4-223), which exhibits a distinctive infiltrative pattern of growth (Fig. 4-224). Immunohistochemically, most cases co-express S100 (Fig. 4-225) and smooth muscle actin (Fig. 4-226). Genetically, BNS is characterized by the presence of a translocation, t(2;4)(q35; q31.1), that fuses the *PAX3* and *MAML3* genes. A *PAX3-NCOA1* fusion has been recently reported in rare examples featuring rhabdomyoblastic differentiation. Most patients experience local recurrences; however, distant spread has not been reported thus far.

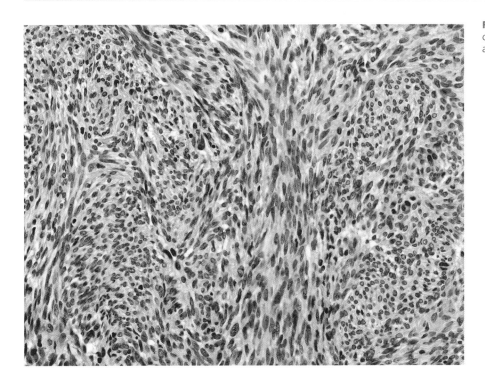

**Fig. 4-223.** Biphenotypic sinonasal sarcoma is composed of a cellular, cytologically uniform, atypical spindle cell proliferation.

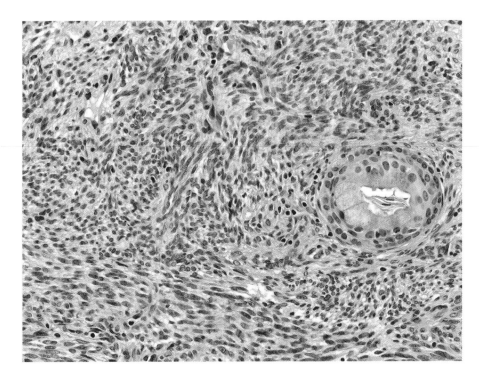

**Fig. 4-224.** Biphenotypic sinonasal sarcoma. The tumor is characterized by a distinctive infiltrative pattern of growth. A residual normal glandular structure is seen.

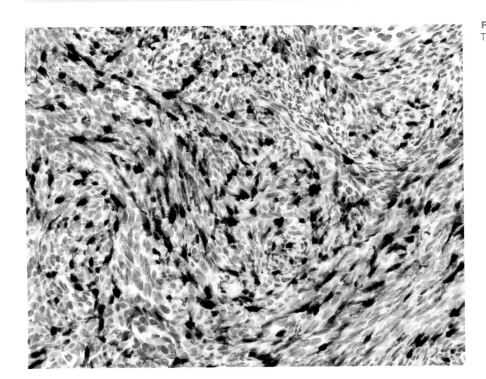

**Fig. 4-225.** Biphenotypic sinonasal sarcoma. Tumor cells show multifocal S100 immunopositivity.

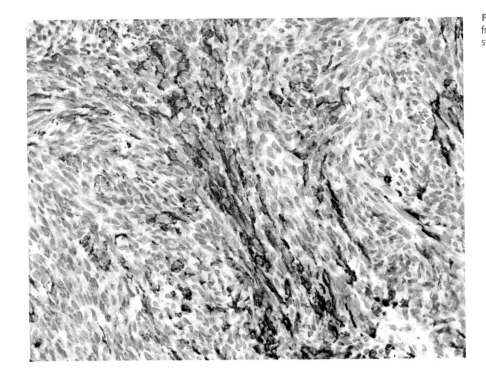

**Fig. 4-226.** Biphenotypic sinonasal sarcoma. A fraction of neoplastic cell exhibits positivity for smooth muscle actin.

### Key Points in Malignant Peripheral Nerve Sheath Tumor Diagnosis

- Occurrence in the limbs, the trunk, and the retroperitoneum
- Association with NF1 syndrome in 50% of cases
- Possible association with a peripheral nerve or a pre-existing benign neural tumor
- Hypercellular spindle cell proliferation with perivascular accentuation of cellularity
- Presence of heterologous differentiation
- Aggressive clinical behavior

# Spindle Cell Liposarcoma

## Definition and Epidemiology

A spindle cell low-grade malignancy is associated with the presence of lipoblasts. Spindle cell liposarcoma represents the rarest variant of WD liposarcoma, accounting for approximately 2% of cases and occurring almost exclusively in adults. Spindle cell liposarcoma is a synonym for the recently suggested term "atypical spindle cell lipomatous tumor."

## Clinical Presentation and Outcome

Spindle cell liposarcoma exhibits an anatomic distribution comparable to that of the other WD liposarcoma subtypes; however, a tendency to be more superficial and to involve the subcutis was observed initially and confirmed by the observation of a larger number of cases. The extremities and the trunk are among the most commonly affected anatomic sites. The clinical course seems to be rather indolent. A 20% local recurrence rate is observed, with dedifferentiation being observed only exceptionally. No metastatic potential is reported.

## Morphology and Immunophenotype

The main morphologic feature of spindle cell liposarcoma is the presence of a relatively bland spindle cell proliferation reminiscent of a neural neoplasm set in a fibrous and/or myxoid background (Fig. 4-227) and associated with an atypical lipomatous component, which usually includes lipoblasts (Fig. 4-228). Multifocal nuclear atypia is most often seen; however, overt pleomorphism is not part of the typical morphology (Fig. 4-229). Immunohistochemically, variable expression of CD34 is seen, whereas MDM2 is most often negative.

## Genetics

Spindle cell liposarcoma does not exhibit *MDM2/CDK4* gene amplification and probably represents a genetically distinct subtype of well-differentiated liposarcoma. Monosomy of chromosome 7 has been reported.

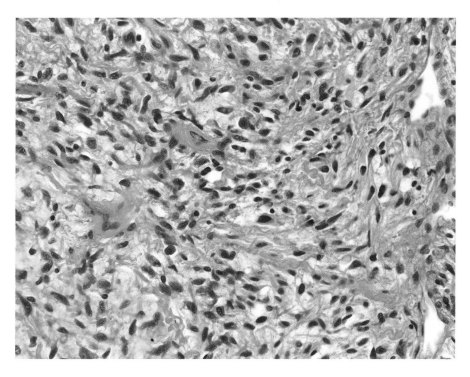

**Fig. 4-227.** Spindle cell liposarcoma. The tumor is composed of atypical spindle cells set in a fibromyxoid background.

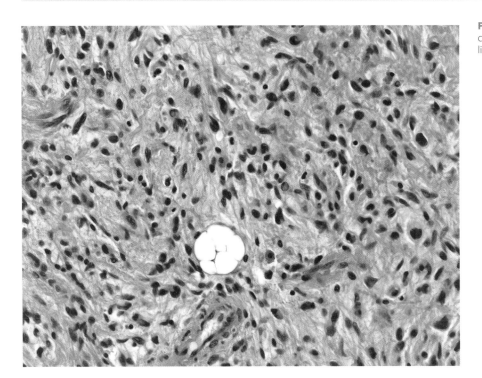

**Fig. 4-228.** Spindle cell liposarcoma. In the context of the tumor, an isolated multivacuolated lipoblast is seen.

## Differential Diagnosis and Diagnostic Pitfalls

The differential diagnosis of spindle cell liposarcoma includes spindle cell lipomas, neural lesions (primarily neurofibromas), and DFSP. Spindle cell lipomas most often occur in the superficial soft tissue of the head and neck area of middle-aged patients. Microscopically, these feature a variable combination of mature adipocytes and spindle cells. Major diagnostic clues are represented by the absence of cytologic atypia (with the notable exception of pleomorphic lipoma) as well as the presence of coarse, eosinophilic collagen bundles. Neurofibromas all express S100 immunopositivity and never feature the presence of lipoblasts. The expression of CD34 may represent a potential source of diagnostic confusion with DFSP; however, spindle cell liposarcoma is better circumscribed and

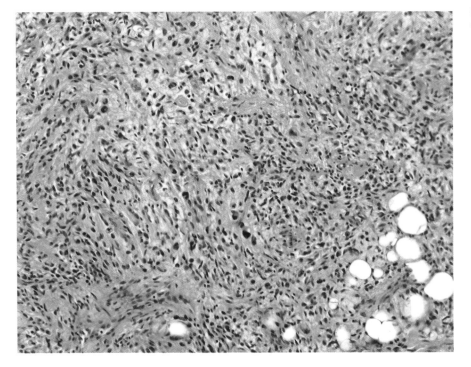

**Fig. 4-229.** Spindle cell liposarcoma. The presence of focal nuclear atypia can be seen relatively often.

cytologically less homogeneous than DFSP; it never features "honeycomb" infiltration of fat; and it does not harbor rearrangements of the *PDGFB* gene. Low-grade dedifferentiated liposarcoma represents a major source of diagnostic confusion; however, it most often arises in the retroperitoneum (wherein spindle cell liposarcoma is exceedingly rare) and consistently exhibits MDM2 over-expression/amplification.

**Key Points in Spindle Cell Liposarcoma Diagnosis**

- Occurrence in the superficial soft tissue of adults
- Spindle cell proliferation associated with the presence of lipoblasts
- No expression/amplification of MDM2
- Indolent clinical behavior with no metastatic potential

# Spindle Cell and Sclerosing Rhabdomyosarcoma

## Definition and Epidemiology

Spindle cell rhabdomyosarcoma and sclerosing rhabdomyosarcoma represent rare distinct (but somewhat related) subtypes of rhabdomyosarcoma (RMS) that may occur in both children and adults. Originally considered variants of embryonal rhabdomyosarcoma, it has become evident that these entities have no clear relationship with embryonal rhabdomyosarcoma and alveolar rhabdomyosarcoma. A male predominance is reported.

## Clinical Presentation and Outcome

Spindle cell rhabdomyosarcoma occurs predominantly in the paratesticular region (about 30% of cases), followed by the head and neck, orbit, and retroperitoneum. In adults, it most commonly involves non-paratesticular sites. Sclerosing rhabdomyosarcoma may also occur in both children and adults and most often arises in the limbs and in the head and neck region. Pediatric forms of spindle cell rhabdomyosarcoma tend to pursue a rather indolent clinical course, with a 95% 5-year survival. However, this is not true in adults. Recent data would suggest that the type of genetic aberration correlates with outcome. In particular, fusion-positive spindle cell rhabdomyosarcomas seem to behave indolently, whereas those that are *MyoD1* mutated tend to be aggressive, most often with fatal outcome despite multimodal therapy.

## Morphology and Immunophenotype

Grossly, spindle cell and sclerosing RMS forms a firm, fibrous mass with a tan-yellow, whorled, and lobular cut surface, somewhat resembling a leiomyoma. Microscopically, it is characterized by densely arrayed whorls and/or fascicles of elongated spindle cells (Fig. 4-230), resembling smooth muscle cells but with more intense cytoplasmic eosinophilia (Fig. 4-231). Contrary to common belief, cytoplasmic cross striations can be seen only exceptionally. Neoplastic cells exhibit positive immunoreactivity for both desmin and myogenin (Fig. 4-232).

Sclerosing rhabdomyosarcoma is composed of a highly infiltrative spindle cell proliferation set in a variable amount of heavily collagenized stroma (Figs. 4-233, 4-234, and 4-235). Immunohistochemically, sclerosing rhabdomyosarcoma features multifocal positivity for desmin and most often very

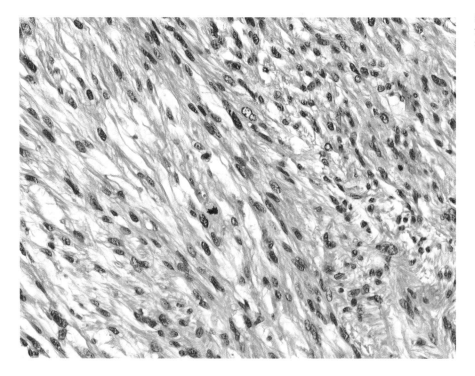

**Fig. 4-230.** Spindle cell rhabdomyosarcoma. The tumor is composed of mitotically active, atypical spindle cells organized in long fascicles.

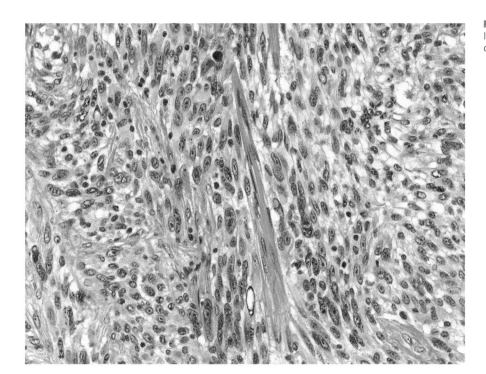

**Fig. 4-231.** Spindle cell rhabdomyosarcoma. Intense eosinophilia of cytoplasm is very often observed.

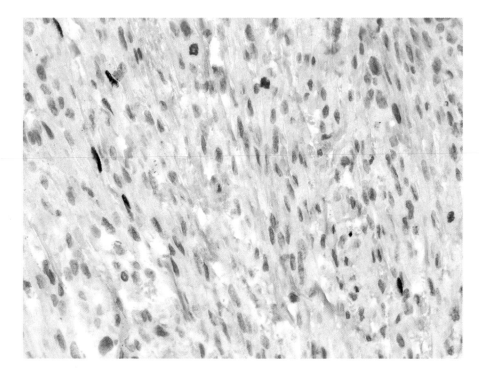

**Fig. 4-232.** Spindle cell rhabdomyosarcoma. Myogenin nuclear immunopositivity is present in scattered neoplastic cells.

limited nuclear expression of myogenin. By contrast, MyoD1 expression tends to be strong and diffuse. Smooth muscle actin is also seen in approximately half of the cases.

## Genetics

Recurrent somatic mutations of the *MyoD1* gene with or without *PIK3CA* mutations seem to represent a distinctive molecular feature of adult spindle cell/sclerosing rhabdomyosarcoma. In addition, a sclerosing phenotype seems to be associated with concomitant *MyoD1/PIK3CA* mutations. More recently, it has been shown that pediatric cases exhibit the presence of *NCOA2* gene rearrangements that may fuse with *SRF, TAED1*, and *VGLL2* genes. Alternatively, *VGLL2* has been shown to fuse with *CITED2*.

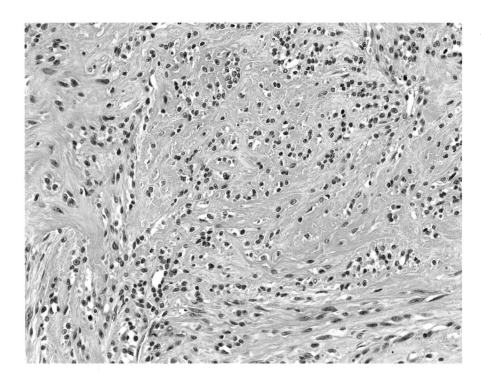

**Fig. 4-233.** Sclerosing rhabdomyosarcoma. The tumor is composed of a spindle cell proliferation set in a densely sclerotic stroma.

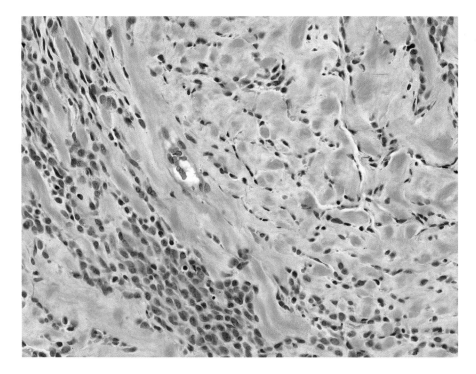

**Fig. 4-234.** Sclerosing rhabdomyosarcoma. At high power, the neoplastic cells look entrapped in the sclerotic stroma.

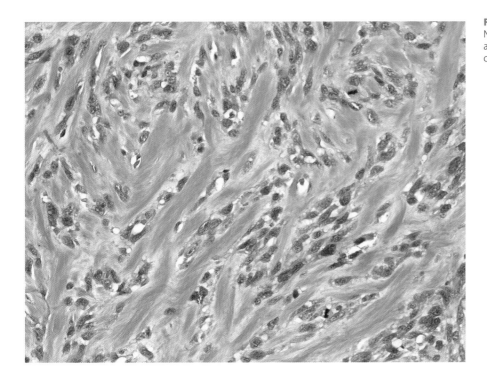

**Fig. 4-235.** Sclerosing rhabdomyosarcoma. Neoplastic cells exhibit cytoplasmic eosinophilia and are set in a sclerotic stroma featuring coarse collagen bundles.

## Differential Diagnosis and Diagnostic Pitfalls

Spindle cell rhabdomyosarcoma, particularly when dealing with adult patients, needs to be separated from leiomyosarcoma, MPNST with heterologous rhabdomyoblastic differentiation, spindle cell carcinoma, and spindle cell melanoma.

The cytoplasm of spindle cell rhabdomyosarcoma tends to be more homogeneously eosinophilic, lacking the distinct fibrillarity of leiomyosarcoma. Immunopositivity for myogenin and/or MyoD1 represents a key diagnostic feature. Spindle cell "sarcomatoid" carcinoma also enters the differential diagnosis. The presence of adjacent epidermal dysplasia, along with expression of keratins and p63, represents valuable diagnostic findings. Spindle cell melanoma can be quite challenging; however, the presence of a junctional malignant component as well as of S100 immunopositivity plays a key diagnostic role. Importantly, all common melanoma markers such as HMB45 or Melan-A tend to be consistently negative in spindle cell melanoma.

The presence of a dense sclerotic matrix in sclerosing rhabdomyosarcoma generates potential diagnostic confusion with both sclerosing epithelioid fibrosarcoma and extraskeletal osteosarcoma. Epithelioid sclerosing fibrosarcoma exhibits a striking epithelioid morphology, often associated with cytoplasmic clearing. Most important, strong MUC4 immunopositivity is seen in most cases and is associated with negativity for myogenic markers. Extraskeletal osteosarcoma most often tends to be more pleomorphic and exhibits strong nuclear expression of SATB2, which is never seen in sclerosing rhabdomyosarcoma.

---

**Key Points in Spindle Cell/Sclerosing Rhabdomyosarcoma Diagnosis**

- Occurrence in the soft tissue of children and adults
- Hypercellular spindle cell neoplasm featuring cytoplasmic eosinophilia
- Presence of densely sclerotic stroma in the sclerosing subtypes
- Immunohistochemical expression of desmin, myogenin, and MYoD1
- Complex genetic profile that includes mutations of *MYOD1* and *PIK3CA* in adults and *NCOA2* gene rearrangement
- Indolent clinical behavior in children
- Aggressive neoplasm in adult patients

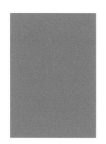

# Intimal Sarcoma

## Definition and Epidemiology

Intimal sarcoma represents a highly aggressive, extremely rare malignant mesenchymal neoplasm exhibiting exquisite tropism for the large blood vessels of the systemic and pulmonary circulation. Peak incidence is in the fourth decade for pulmonary lesion and in the sixth decade in the case of aortic location. A slight female predominance is reported for pulmonary intimal sarcomas, but not observed in cases occurring in the aorta.

## Clinical Presentation and Outcome

Intimal sarcoma represents an aggressive lesion with extremely poor overall survival, and with early metastatic spread. Patients with pulmonary location most often die within 2 years of diagnosis. Patients presenting with aortic location have a mean survival of 8 months.

## Morphology and Immunophenotype

Grossly, intimal sarcoma most often presents as an endoluminal polypoid mass. Microscopically, it is composed of a hypercellular spindle cell proliferation (Fig. 4-236) featuring an extremely variable degree of nuclear atypia from moderate (Fig. 4-237) to high (Figs. 4-238 and 4-239). Mitotic activity is often high, and areas of necrosis can be found. The presence of heterologous differentiation (primarily rhabdomyosarcomatous, chondrosarcomatous, and osteosarcomatous) has been reported. Rare cases may exhibit significant nuclear pleomorphism. Immunohistochemically, intimal sarcoma variably expresses smooth muscle actin, and a minority of cases also exhibit desmin immunopositivity. Importantly, MDM2 nuclear expression is observed in up to 70% of cases (Fig. 4-240).

## Genetics

Intimal sarcoma is characterized genetically by amplification of the 12q12-15 chromosome region, wherein the *MDM2*, *CDK4*, and *GLI* genes map. In addition, amplification of the *PDGFRA* and *KIT* genes has been reported. *MDM2* amplification seems to be fairly specific for intimal sarcomas, as other cardiac sarcomas (even those overexpressing MDM2 immunohistochemically) such as undifferentiated spindle cell and pleomorphic sarcomas never show copy number alterations of MDM2 locus.

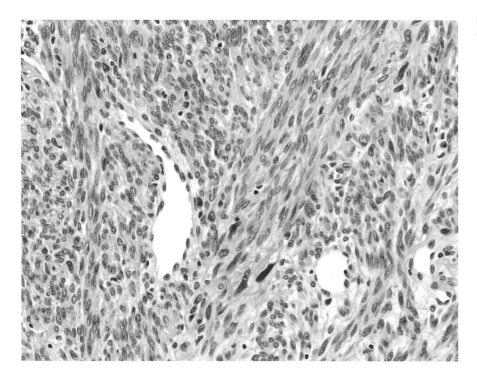

**Fig. 4-236.** Intimal sarcoma. The tumor is composed of a hypercellular, atypical spindle cell proliferation.

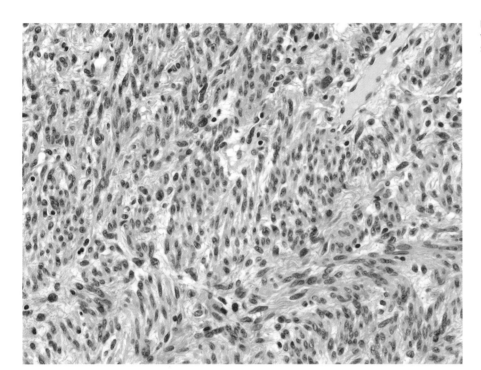

**Fig. 4-237.** Intimal sarcoma. Nuclear atypia is variable. In this example, moderately atypical spindle cells are seen.

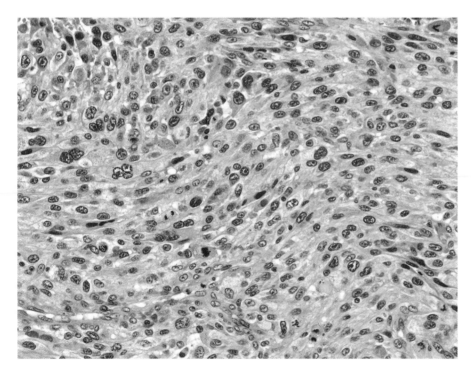

**Fig. 4-238.** Intimal sarcoma. In this example, severe atypia in neoplastic cells is seen.

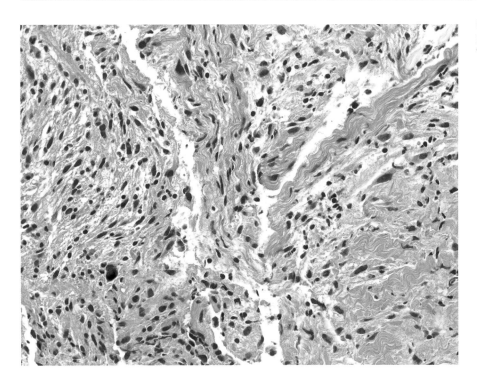

**Fig. 4-239.** Intimal sarcoma. Nuclear pleomorphism is associated with a more collagenous stroma.

## Differential Diagnosis and Diagnostic Pitfalls

Intimal sarcoma may closely mimic leiomyosarcoma. However, the distinctive fibrillary eosinophilia of the cytoplasm is not present. In addition, MDM2 overexpression/amplification are almost never seen in leiomyosarcoma. In consideration of its very peculiar anatomic location, spindle cell angiosarcoma certainly needs to be considered in the differential diagnosis. However, expression of vascular markers such as CD31 and ERG represents extremely helpful diagnostic features.

**Key Points in Intimal Sarcoma Diagnosis**

- Occurrence in the large blood vessels of the systemic and pulmonary circulation
- Hypercellular, variably atypical spindle cell proliferation
- Overexpression/amplification of MDM2
- Aggressive clinical behavior with early metastatic spread

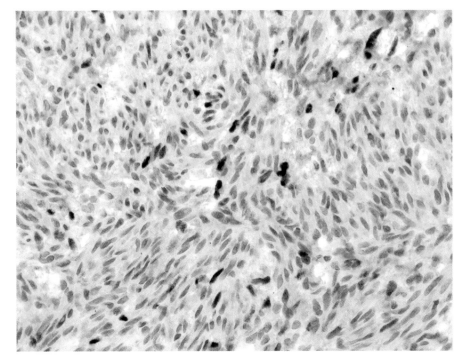

**Fig. 4-240.** Intimal sarcoma. Nuclear expression of MDM2 is seen. This is associated with *MDM2* gene amplification.

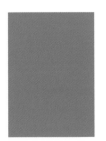

# Undifferentiated Spindle Cell Sarcoma

The 2013 WHO classification strongly emphasizes the fact that a number of sarcomas do not fit under any specific label. This is also true for spindle sarcomas that rarely (up to 5% of cases) totally lack any morphologic, immunophenotypic, or molecular distinctive feature. Undifferentiated spindle sarcoma most often exhibits a fascicular pattern of growth and may be either low or high grade (Figs. 4-241 and 4-242). A significant proportion may be associated with a previous history of radiation therapy, a clinical presentation that is almost always associated with high-grade morphology and aggressive clinical behavior. In the past, most of these cases were grouped within the category of fibrosarcoma. "Fibrosarcoma" underwent a profound conceptual evolution and currently this term is used to define very specific clinicopathologic entities (i.e., fibrosarcomatous DFSP; myxofibrosarcoma, sclerosing epithelioid fibrosarcoma). The use of fibrosarcoma as a surrogate label for undifferentiated spindle cell sarcoma should be discontinued.

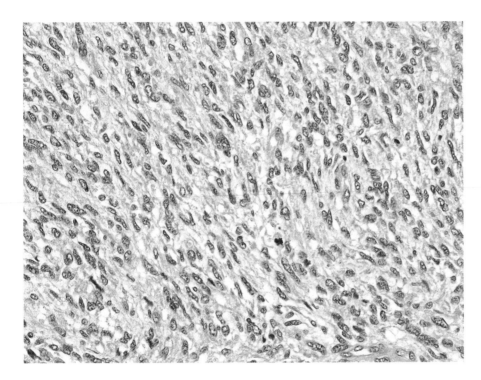

**Fig. 4-241.** Undifferentiated spindle cell sarcoma. A moderately atypical spindle cell neoplasm is seen. Mitotic activity is easily detected.

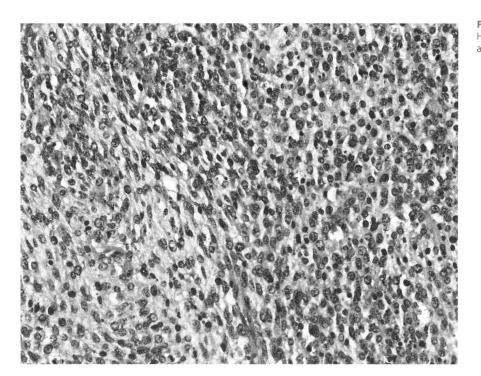

**Fig. 4-242.** Undifferentiated spindle cell sarcoma. Hypercellularity, severe atypia, and high mitotic activity are typically seen in high-grade lesions.

## Chapter 4 Selected Key References

### Dermatofibrosarcoma Protuberans and Its Differential Diagnosis

- Abbott JJ, Erickson-Johnson M, Wang X, Nascimento AG, Oliveira AM. Gains of COL1A1-PDGFB genomic copies occur in fibrosarcomatous transformation of dermatofibrosarcoma protuberans. *Mod Pathol.* 2006;19:1512–18.
- Abbott JJ, Oliveira AM, Nascimento AG. The prognostic significance of fibrosarcomatous transformation in dermatofibrosarcoma protuberans. *Am J Surg Pathol.* 2006;30:436–43.
- Calonje E, Fletcher CD. Aneurysmal benign fibrous histiocytoma: clinicopathological analysis of 40 cases of a tumour frequently misdiagnosed as a vascular neoplasm. *Histopathology.* 1995;26:323–31.
- Calonje E, Fletcher CD. Myoid differentiation in dermatofibrosarcoma protuberans and its fibrosarcomatous variant: clinicopathologic analysis of 5 cases. *J Cutan Pathol.* 1996;23:30–6.
- Calonje E, Mentzel T, Fletcher CD. Cellular benign fibrous histiocytoma. Clinicopathologic analysis of 74 cases of a distinctive variant of cutaneous fibrous histiocytoma with frequent recurrence. *Am J Surg Pathol.* 1994;18:668–76.

- Doyle LA, Fletcher CD. Metastasizing "benign" cutaneous fibrous histiocytoma: a clinicopathologic analysis of 16 cases. *Am J Surg Pathol.* 2013;37:484–95.
- Doyle LA, Mariño-Enriquez A, Fletcher CD, Hornick JL. ALK rearrangement and overexpression in epithelioid fibrous histiocytoma. *Mod Pathol.* 2015;28:904–12.
- Fiore M, Miceli R, Mussi C, et al. Dermatofibrosarcoma protuberans treated at a single institution: a surgical disease with a high cure rate. *J Clin Oncol.* 2005;23:7669–75.
- Kaddu S, McMenamin ME, Fletcher CD. Atypical fibrous histiocytoma of the skin: clinicopathologic analysis of 59 cases with evidence of infrequent metastasis. *Am J Surg Pathol.* 2002;26:35–46.
- McArthur GA, Demetri GD, van Oosterom A, et al. Molecular and clinical analysis of locally advanced dermatofibrosarcoma protuberans treated with imatinib: Imatinib Target Exploration Consortium Study B2225. *J Clin Oncol.* 2005;23:866–73.
- Mentzel T, Beham A, Katenkamp D, Dei Tos AP, Fletcher CD. Fibrosarcomatous ("high-grade") dermatofibrosarcoma protuberans: clinicopathologic and immunohistochemical study of a series of 41 cases with emphasis on prognostic significance. *Am J Surg Pathol.* 1998;22:576–87.
- Mentzel T, Schärer L, Kazakov DV, Michal M. Myxoid dermatofibrosarcoma

protuberans: clinicopathologic, immunohistochemical, and molecular analysis of eight cases. *Am J Dermatopathol.* 2007;29:443–8.
- Reimann JD, Fletcher CD. Myxoid dermatofibrosarcoma protuberans: a rare variant analyzed in a series of 23 cases. *Am J Surg Pathol.* 2007;31:1371–7.
- Singh Gomez C, Calonje E, Fletcher CD. Epithelioid benign fibrous histiocytoma of skin: clinico-pathological analysis of 20 cases of a poorly known variant. *Histopathology.* 1994;24:123–9.
- Stacchiotti S, Astolfi A, Gronchi A, et al. Evolution of dermatofibrosarcoma protuberans to dfsp-derived fibrosarcoma: an event marked by epithelial-mesenchymal transition-like process and 22q loss. *Mol Cancer Res.* 2016;14:820–9.
- Stacchiotti S, Pantaleo MA, Negri T, et al. Efficacy and biological activity of imatinib in metastatic dermatofibrosarcoma protuberans (DFSP). *Clin Cancer Res.* 2016;22:837–46
- Takahira T, Oda Y, Tamiya S, et al. Detection of COL1A1-PDGFB fusion transcripts and PDGFB/PDGFRB mRNA expression in dermatofibrosarcoma protuberans. *Mod Pathol.* 2007;20:668–75.
- Terrier-Lacombe MJ, Guillou L, Maire G, et al. Dermatofibrosarcoma protuberans, giant cell fibroblastoma, and hybrid lesions in children: clinicopathologic

comparative analysis of 28 cases with molecular data. A study from the French Federation of Cancer Centers Sarcoma Group. *Am J Surg Pathol.* 2003;**27**:27–39.

- Woodruff JM. Pathology of the major peripheral nerve sheath neoplasms. *Monogr Pathol.* 1996;**38**:129–61.

# Giant Cell Fibroblastoma and Its Differential Diagnosis

- Al-Ibraheemi A, Martinez A, Weiss SW, et al. Fibrous hamartoma of infancy: a clinicopathologic study of 145 cases, including 2 with sarcomatous features. *Mod Pathol.* 2017;**30**:474–85.

- Dymock RB, Allen PW, Stirling JW, Gilbert EF, Thornbery JM. Giant cell fibroblastoma. A distinctive, recurrent tumor of childhood. *Am J Surg Pathol.* 1987;**11**:263–71.

- Enzinger FM. Fibrous hamartoma of infancy. *Cancer.* 1965 Feb;**18**:241–8.

- Fetsch JF, Miettinen M, Laskin WB, Michal M, Enzinger FM. A clinicopathologic study of 45 pediatric soft tissue tumors with an admixture of adipose tissue and fibroblastic elements, and a proposal for classification as lipofibromatosis. *Am J Surg Pathol.* 2000;**24**: 1491–500.

- Fletcher CD. Giant cell fibroblastoma of soft tissue: a clinicopathological and immunohistochemical study. *Histopathology.* 1988;**13**:499–508.

- Fletcher CD, Powell G, van Noorden S, McKee PH. Fibrous hamartoma of infancy: a histochemical and immunohistochemical study. *Histopathology.* 1988 Jan;**12**(1):65–74.

- Jha P, Moosavi C, Fanburg-Smith JC. Giant cell fibroblastoma: an update and addition of 86 new cases from the Armed Forces Institute of Pathology, in honor of Dr. Franz M. Enzinger. *Ann Diagn Pathol.* 2007;**11**:81–8.

- Shmookler BM, Enzinger FM, Weiss SW. Giant cell fibroblastoma. A juvenile form of dermatofibrosarcoma protuberans. *Cancer.* 1989;**64**:2154–61.

# Angiomatoid "Malignant" Fibrous Histiocytoma

- Antonescu CR, Dal Cin P, Nafa K, et al. EWSR1-CREB1 is the predominant gene fusion in angiomatoid fibrous histiocytoma. *Genes Chromosomes Cancer.* 2007;**46**:1051–60.

- Calonje E, Fletcher CD. Aneurysmal benign fibrous histiocytoma: clinicopathological analysis of 40 cases of a tumour frequently misdiagnosed as a vascular neoplasm. *Histopathology.* 1995;**26**:323–31.

- Costa MJ, Weiss SW. Angiomatoid malignant fibrous histiocytoma. A follow-up study of 108 cases with evaluation of possible histologic predictors of outcome. *Am J Surg Pathol.* 1990;**14**:1126–32.

- Enzinger FM. Angiomatoid malignant fibrous histiocytoma: a distinct fibrohistiocytic tumor of children and young adults simulating a vascular neoplasm. *Cancer.* 1979;**44**:2147–57.

- Fanburg-Smith JC, Miettinen M. Angiomatoid "malignant" fibrous histiocytoma: a clinicopathologic study of 158 cases and further exploration of the myoid phenotype. *Hum Pathol.* 1999;**30**:1336–43.

- Fletcher CD. Angiomatoid "malignant fibrous histiocytoma": an immunohistochemical study indicative of myoid differentiation. *Hum Pathol.* 1991;**22**:563–8.

- Rossi S, Szuhai K, Ijszenga M, et al. EWSR1-CREB1 and EWSR1-ATF1 fusion genes in angiomatoid fibrous histiocytoma. *Clin Cancer Res.* 2007;**13**:7322–8.

- Schaefer IM, Fletcher CD. Myxoid variant of so-called angiomatoid "malignant fibrous histiocytoma": clinicopathologic characterization in a series of 21 cases. *Am J Surg Pathol.* 2014;**38**:816–23.

- Thway K, Nicholson AG, Wallace WA, et al. Endobronchial pulmonary angiomatoid fibrous histiocytoma: two cases with EWSR1-CREB1 and EWSR1-ATF1 fusions. *Am J Surg Pathol.* 2012;**36**:883–8.

- Thway K, Stefanaki K, Papadakis V, Fisher C. Metastatic angiomatoid fibrous histiocytoma of the scalp, with EWSR1-CREB1 gene fusions in primary tumor and nodal metastasis. *Hum Pathol.* 2013;**44**:289–93.

- Weinreb I, Rubin BP, Goldblum JR. Pleomorphic angiomatoid fibrous histiocytoma: a case confirmed by fluorescence in situ hybridization analysis for EWSR1 rearrangement. *J Cutan Pathol.* 2008;**35**:855–60.

# Low-Grade Myofibroblastic Sarcoma and Its Differential Diagnosis

- Allen PW. Nodular fasciitis. *Pathology.* 1972 Jan;**4**(1):9–26.

- Antonescu CR, Sung YS, Zhang L, Agaram NP, Fletcher CD. Recurrent SRF-RELA fusions define a novel subset of cellular myofibroma/myopericytoma: a potential diagnostic pitfall with sarcomas with myogenic differentiation. *Am J Surg Pathol.* 2017;**41**:677–84.

- Beham A, Badve S, Suster S, Fletcher CD. Solitary myofibroma in adults: clinicopathological analysis of a series. *Histopathology.* 1993;**22**:335–41.

- Chan JY, Gooi Z, Wong EW, et al. Low-grade myofibroblastic sarcoma: A population-based study. *Laryngoscope.* 2017;**127**:116–12.

- Fletcher CD, Stirling RW. Intranodal myofibroblastoma presenting in the submandibular region: evidence of a broader clinical and histological spectrum. *Histopathology.* 1990;**16**:287–93.

- Gronchi A, Colombo C, Le Péchoux C, et al. Sporadic desmoid-type fibromatosis: a stepwise approach to a non-metastasising neoplasm – a position paper from the Italian and the French Sarcoma Group. *Ann Oncol.* 2014;**25**:578–83.

- Hung YP, Fletcher CDM. Myopericytomatosis: clinicopathologic analysis of 11 cases with molecular identification of recurrent PDGFRB alterations in myopericytomatosis and myopericytoma. *Am J Surg Pathol.* 2017;**41**:1034–104.

- Le Guellec S, Soubeyran I, Rochaix P, et al. CTNNB1 mutation analysis is a useful tool for the diagnosis of desmoid tumors: a study of 260 desmoid tumors and 191 potential morphologic mimics. *Mod Pathol.* 2012;**25**:1551–8.

- McMenamin ME, Fletcher CD. Malignant myopericytoma: expanding the spectrum of tumours with myopericytic differentiation. *Histopathology.* 2002;**41**:450–60.

- Mentzel T, Calonje E, Nascimento AG, Fletcher CD. Infantile hemangiopericytoma versus infantile myofibromatosis. Study of a series suggesting a continuous spectrum of infantile myofibroblastic lesions. *Am J Surg Pathol.* 1994;**18**:922–30.

- Mentzel T, Dei Tos AP, Sapi Z, Kutzner H. Myopericytoma of skin and soft tissues: clinicopathologic and immunohistochemical study of 54 cases. *Am J Surg Pathol.* 2006;**30**:104–13.

- Mentzel T, Dry S, Katenkamp D, Fletcher CD. Low-grade myofibroblastic sarcoma: analysis of 18 cases in the spectrum of myofibroblastic tumors. *Am J Surg Pathol.* 1998;**22**:1228–38.

- Suster S, Rosai J. Intranodal hemorrhagic spindle-cell tumor with "amianthoid" fibers. Report of six cases of a distinctive mesenchymal neoplasm of the inguinal region that simulates Kaposi's sarcoma. *Am J Surg Pathol.* 1989;**13**:347–57.
- Weiss SW, Gnepp DR, Bratthauer GL. Palisaded myofibroblastoma. A benign mesenchymal tumor of lymph node. *Am J Surg Pathol.* 1989;**13**:341–6.

## Phosphaturic Mesenchymal Tumor

- Bahrami A, Weiss SW, Montgomery E, et al. RT-PCR analysis for FGF23 using paraffin sections in the diagnosis of phosphaturic mesenchymal tumors with and without known tumor induced osteomalacia. *Am J Surg Pathol.* 2009;**33**:1348–54.
- Folpe AL, Fanburg-Smith JC, Billings SD, et al. Most osteomalacia-associated mesenchymal tumors are a single histopathologic entity: an analysis of 32 cases and a comprehensive review of the literature. *Am J Surg Pathol.* 2004;**28**:1–30.
- Lee JC, Jeng YM, Su SY, et al. Identification of a novel FN1-FGFR1 genetic fusion as a frequent event in phosphaturic mesenchymal tumour. *J Pathol.* 2015;**235**:539–45.
- Lee JC, Su SY, Changou CA, et al. Characterization of FN1-FGFR1 and novel FN1-FGF1 fusion genes in a large series of phosphaturic mesenchymal tumors. *Mod Pathol.* 2016;**29**:1335–46.
- Salassa RM, Jowsey J, Arnaud CD. Hypophosphatemic osteomalacia associated with "nonendocrine" tumors. *N Engl J Med.* 1970;**283**:65–70.

## Gastrointestinal Stromal Tumor (GIST) and Its Differential Diagnosis

- Antonescu CR, Romeo S, Zhang L, et al. Dedifferentiation in gastrointestinal stromal tumor to an anaplastic KIT-negative phenotype: a diagnostic pitfall: morphologic and molecular characterization of 8 cases occurring either de novo or after imatinib therapy. *Am J Surg Pathol.* 2013;**37**:385–92.
- Boikos SA, Pappo AS, Killian JK, et al. Molecular subtypes of KIT/PDGFRA wild-type gastrointestinal stromal tumors: a report from the National Institutes of Health Gastrointestinal Stromal Tumor Clinic. *JAMA Oncol.* 2016;**2**:922–8.
- Brenca M, Rossi S, Polano M, et al. Transcriptome sequencing identifies ETV6-NTRK3 as a gene fusion involved in GIST. *J Pathol.* 2016;**238**:543–9.
- Corless CL, Schroeder A, Griffith D, et al. PDGFRA mutations in gastrointestinal stromal tumors: frequency, spectrum and in vitro sensitivity to imatinib. *J Clin Oncol.* 2005;**3**:5357–64.
- Dei Tos AP. The reappraisal of GIST: from Stout to the KIT revolution. *Virchows Arch.* 2003;**443**:421–428.
- Demetri GD, Reichardt P, Kang YK, et al. Efficacy and safety of regorafenib for advanced gastrointestinal stromal tumours after failure of imatinib and sunitinib (GRID): an international, multicentre, randomised, placebo-controlled, phase 3 trial. *Lancet.* 2013;**381**:295–302.
- Demetri GD, van Oosterom AT, Garrett CR, et al. Efficacy and safety of sunitinib in patients with advanced gastrointestinal stromal tumour after failure of imatinib: a randomised controlled trial. *Lancet.* 2006;**14**;368:1329–38.
- Fletcher CD, Berman JJ, Corless C, et al. Diagnosis of gastrointestinal stromal tumors: A consensus approach. *Hum Pathol*, 2002;**33**:459–65.
- Folpe AL, Fanburg-Smith JC, Miettinen M, Weiss SW. Atypical and malignant glomus tumors: analysis of 52 cases, with a proposal for the reclassification of glomus tumors. *Am J Surg Pathol.* 2001;**25**:1–12.
- Gasparotto D, Rossi S, Polano M, et al. Quadruple-negative GIST is a sentinel for unrecognized neurofibromatosis type 1 syndrome. *Clin Cancer Res.* 2017;**23**:273–82.
- Heinrich MC, Corless CL, Blanke CD, et al. Molecular correlates of imatinib resistance in gastrointestinal stromal tumors. *J Clin Oncol.* 2006;**24**:4764–74.
- Heinrich MC, Corless CL, Duensing A, et al. PDGFRA activating mutations in gastrointestinal stromal tumors. *Science.* 2003;**299**:708–10.
- Hirota S, Isozaki K, Moriyama Y, et al. Gain-of-function mutations of c-kit in human gastrointestinal stromal tumors. *Science.* 1998;**279**:577–80.
- Janeway KA, Kim SY, Lodish M, et al. Defects in succinate dehydrogenase in gastrointestinal stromal tumors lacking KIT and PDGFRA mutations. *Proc Natl Acad Sci U S A.* 2011;**108**:314–18.
- Joensuu H, Roberts PJ, Sarlomo-Rikala M, et al. Effect of the tyrosine kinase inhibitor STI571 in a patient with a metastatic gastrointestinal stromal tumour. *N Engl J Med.* 2001;**344**:1052–6.
- Joensuu H, Vehtari A, Riihimäki J, et al. Risk of recurrence of gastrointestinal stromal tumour after surgery: an analysis of pooled population-based cohorts. *Lancet Oncol.* 2012;**13**:265–74.
- Kay S, Callahan WP Jr, Murray MR, Randall HT, Stout AP. Glomus tumors of the stomach. *Cancer.* 1951;**4**:726–36.
- Kindblom L-G, Remotti HE, Aldenborg F, Meis-Kindblom JM. Gastrointestinal pacemaker cell tumor (GIPACT): gastrointestinal stromal tumors show phenotypic characteristics of the interstitial cells of Cajal. *Am J Pathol.* 1998;**152**:1259–69.
- Lasota J, Wang ZF, Sobin LH, Miettinen M. Gain-of-function PDGFRA mutations, earlier reported in gastrointestinal stromal tumors, are common in small intestinal inflammatory fibroid polyps. A study of 60 cases. *Mod Pathol.* 2009;**22**:1049–56.
- Liegl B, Bennett MW, Fletcher CD. Microcystic/reticular schwannoma: a distinct variant with predilection for visceral locations. *Am J Surg Pathol.* 2008;**32**:1080–7.
- Makhlouf HR, Ahrens W, Agarwal B, et al. Synovial sarcoma of the stomach: a clinicopathologic, immunohistochemical, and molecular genetic study of 10 cases. *Am J Surg Pathol.* 2008;**32**:275–81.
- Mason EF, Hornick JL. Conventional risk stratification fails to predict progression of succinate dehydrogenase-deficient gastrointestinal stromal tumors: a clinicopathologic study of 76 cases. *Am J Surg Pathol.* 2016;**40**:1616–21.
- Matyakhina L, Bei TA, McWhinney SR, et al. Genetics of Carney triad: recurrent losses at chromosome 1 but lack of germline mutations in genes associated with paragangliomas and gastrointestinal stromal tumors. *J Clin Endocrinol Metab.* 2007;**92**:2938–43
- Miettinen M, Felisiak-Golabek A, Wang Z, Inaguma S, Lasota J. GIST manifesting as a retroperitoneal tumor: clinicopathologic immunohistochemical, and molecular genetic study of 112 cases. *Am J Surg Pathol.* 2017;**41**:577–85.
- Miettinen M, Furlong M, Sarlomo-Rikala M, et al. Gastrointestinal stromal tumors, intramural leiomyomas, and leiomyosarcomas in the rectum and anus: a clinicopathologic, immunohistochemical, and molecular

genetic study of 144 cases. *Am J Surg Pathol.* 2001;**25**:1121–33.

- Miettinen M, Lasota J. Gastrointestinal stromal tumors: review on morphology, molecular pathology, prognosis, and differential diagnosis. *Arch Pathol Lab Med.* 2006;**130**:1466–78.

- Miettinen M, Makhlouf HR, Sobin LH, Lasota J. Plexiform fibromyxoma: a distinctive benign gastric antral neoplasm not to be confused with a myxoid GIST. *Am J Surg Pathol.* 2009;**33**:1624–32.

- Miettinen M, Sarlomo-Rikala M, Sobin LH, Lasota J. Gastrointestinal stromal tumors and leiomyosarcomas in the colon: a clinicopathologic, immunohistochemical, and molecular genetic study of 44 cases. *Am J Surg Pathol.* 2000;**24**:1339–52.

- Miettinen M, Wang ZF, Lasota J. DOG1 antibody in the differential diagnosis of gastrointestinal stromal tumors: a study of 1840 cases. *Am J Surg Pathol.* 2009;**33**:1401–8.

- Novelli M, Rossi S, Rodriguez-Justo M, et al. DOG1 and CD117 are the antibodies of choice in the diagnosis of gastrointestinal stromal tumours. *Histopathology.* 2010;**57**:259–70.

- Pasini B, McWhinney SR, Bei T, et al. Clinical and molecular genetics of patients with the Carney-Stratakis syndrome and germline mutations of the genes coding for the succinate dehydrogenase subunits SDHB, SDHC, and SDHD. *Eur J Hum Genet.* 2008;**16**:79–88.

- Romeo S, Rossi S, Acosta Marín M, at al. Primary synovial sarcoma (SS) of the digestive system: a molecular and clinicopathological study of fifteen cases. *Clin Sarcoma Res.* 2015;**5**:7.

- Rossi S, Gasparotto D, Miceli R, et al. KIT, PDGFRA, and BRAF mutational spectrum impacts on the natural history of imatinib-naive localized GIST: a population-based study. *Am J Surg Pathol.* 2015;**39**:922–30.

- Rossi S, Gasparotto D, Toffolatti L, et al. Molecular and clinicopathologic characterization of gastrointestinal stromal tumors (GISTs) of small size. *Am J Surg Pathol.* 2010;**34**:1480–91.

- Rossi S, Miceli R, Messerini L, et al. Natural history of imatinib-naive GISTs: a retrospective analysis of 929 cases with long-term follow-up and development of a survival nomogram based on mitotic index and size as continuous variables. *Am J Surg Pathol.* 2011;**35**:1646–56.

- Rubin BP, Heinrich MC, Corless CL. Gastrointestinal stromal tumour. *Lancet.* 2007;**369**:1731–41.

- Spans L, Fletcher CD, Antonescu CR, et al. Recurrent MALAT1-GLI1 oncogenic fusion and GLI1 up-regulation define a subset of plexiform fibromyxoma. *J Pathol.* 2016;**239**:335–43.

- Takahashi Y, Shimizu S, Ishida T, et al. Plexiform angiomyxoid myofibroblastic tumor of the stomach. *Am J Surg Pathol.* 2007;**31**:724–8.

- Wagner AJ, Remillard SP, Zhang YX, et al. Loss of expression of SDHA predicts SDHA mutations in gastrointestinal stromal tumors. *Mod Pathol.* 2013;**26**:289–94.

- West RB, Corless CL, Chen X, et al. The novel marker, DOG1, is expressed ubiquitously in gastrointestinal stromal tumors irrespective of KIT or PDGFRA mutation status. *Am J Pathol.* 2004;**165**:107–13.

## Leiomyosarcoma

- Bell SW, Kempson RL, Hendrickson MR. Problematic uterine smooth muscle neoplasms. A clinicopathologic study of 213 cases. *Am J Surg Pathol.* 1994;**18**:535–58.

- Dei Tos AP, Maestro R, Doglioni C, et al. Tumor suppressor genes and related molecules in leiomyosarcoma. *Am J Pathol.* 1996;**148**:1037–45.

- De Sain Aubain Somerhausen N, Fletcher CDM. Leiomyosarcoma of soft tissue in children: clinicopathologic analysis of 20 cases. *Am J Surg Pathol.* 1999;**23**:755–63.

- Deyrup AT, Lee VK, Hill CE, et al. Epstein-Barr virus-associated smooth muscle tumors are distinctive mesenchymal tumors reflecting multiple infection events: a clinicopathologic and molecular study of 29 tumors from 19 patients. *Am J Surg Pathol.* 2006;**30**:75–82.

- Fletcher CD, Kilpatrick SE, Mentzel T. The difficulty in predicting behavior of smooth-muscle tumors in deep soft tissue. *Am J Surg Pathol.* 1995;**19**:116–17.

- Kilpatrick SE, Mentzel T, Fletcher CD. Leiomyoma of deep soft tissue. Clinicopathologic analysis of a series. *Am J Surg Pathol.* 1994;**18**:576–82.

- Mandhal N, Fletcher CDM, Dal cin P, et al. Comparative cytogenetic study of spindle cell and pleomorphic leiomyosarcoma of soft tissue: a report from the CHAMP study group. *Cancer Genet Cytogenet.* 2000;**116**:66–73.

- Massi D, Franchi A, Alos L, et al. Primary cutaneous leiomyosarcoma: clinicopathological analysis of 36 cases. *Histopathology.* 2010;**56**:251–62.

- Mentzel T, Calonje E, Fletcher CD. Leiomyosarcoma with prominent osteoclast-like giant cells. Analysis of eight cases closely mimicking the so-called giant cell variant of malignant fibrous histiocytoma. *Am J Surg Pathol.* 1994;**18**:258–65.

- Merchant W, Calonje E, Fletcher CD. Inflammatory leiomyosarcoma: a morphological subgroup within the heterogeneous family of so-called inflammatory malignant fibrous histiocytoma. *Histopathology.* 1995;**27**:525–32.

- Miettinen M. Smooth muscle tumors of soft tissue and non-uterine viscera: biology and prognosis. *Mod Pathol.* 2014;**27** Suppl 1:S17–29.

- Oda Y, Miyajima K, Kawaguchi K, et al. Pleomorphic leiomyosarcoma: clinicopathologic and immunohistochemical study with special emphasis on its distinction from ordinary leiomyosarcoma and malignant fibrous histiocytoma. *Am J Surg Pathol.* 2001;**25**:1030–8.

- Rubin BP, Fletcher CD. Myxoid leiomyosarcoma of soft tissue: an underrecognized variant. *Am J Surg Pathol.* 2000;**24**:927–36.

- Wile AG, Evans HL, Romsdhal MM. Leiomyosarcoma of soft tissue a clinicopathologic study. *Cancer.* 1981;**48**:1022–32.

## Solitary Fibrous Tumor and Its Differential Diagnosis

- Chan JKC. Solitary fibrous tumor – everywhere, and a diagnosis in vogue. *Histopathology.* 1997;**31**:568–76.

- Chilosi M, Facchetti F, Dei Tos AP, et al. Bcl-2 expression in pleural and extrapleural solitary fibrous tumours. *J Pathol.* 1997;**181**:362–7.

- Chmielecki J, Crago AM, Rosenberg M, et al. Whole-exome sequencing identifies a recurrent NAB2-STAT6 fusion in solitary fibrous tumors. *Nat Genet.* 2013 **45**:131–2.

- Collini P, Negri T, Barisella M, et al. High-grade sarcomatous overgrowth in solitary fibrous tumors: a clinicopathologic study of 10 cases. *Am J Surg Pathol.* 2012;**36**:1202–15.

- Dei Tos AP, Seregard S, Calonje E, et al. Giant cell angiofibroma. A distinctive orbital tumor in adults. *Am J Surg Pathol.* 1995;**19**:1286–93.

- Demicco EG, Park MS, Araujo DM, et al. Solitary fibrous tumor: a clinicopathological study of 110 cases and proposed risk assessment model. *Mod Pathol.* 2012;**25**:1298–306.

- Demicco EG, Wagner MJ, Maki RG, et al. Risk assessment in solitary fibrous tumors: validation and refinement of a risk stratification model. *Mod Pathol.* 2017;**30**:1433–42.
- de Saint Aubain Somerhausen N, Rubin BP, Fletcher CDM. Myxoid solitary fibrous tumor: a study of seven cases with emphasis on differenttial diagnosis. *Mod Pathol.* 1999;**12**:463–71.
- Dorfman DM, To K, Dickersin GR, et al. Solitary fibrous tumor of the orbit. *Am J Surg Pathol.* 1994;**18**:281–7.
- Doyle LA, Fletcher CD. Predicting behavior of solitary fibrous tumor: are we getting closer to more accurate risk assessment? *Ann Surg Oncol.* 2013;**20**:4055–6.
- Doyle LA, Vivero M, Fletcher CD, Mertens F, Hornick JL. Nuclear expression of STAT6 distinguishes solitary fibrous tumor from histologic mimics. *Mod Pathol.* 2014;**27**:390–5.
- England DM, Hochholzer L, McCarthy MJ. Localized benign and malignant fibrous tumors of the pleura. A clinicopathologic review of 223 cases. *Am J Surg Pathol.* 1989;**13**:640–58.
- Fritchie KJ, Jin L, Rubin BP, et al. NAB2-STAT6 gene fusion in meningeal hemangiopericytoma and solitary fibrous tumor. *J Neuropathol Exp Neurol.* 2016;**75**:263–71.
- Gengler C, Guillou L. Solitary fibrous tumour and haemangiopericytoma: evolution of a concept. *Histopathology.* 2006;**48**:63–74.
- Gleason BC, Fletcher CD. Deep "benign" fibrous histiocytoma: clinicopathologic analysis of 69 cases of a rare tumor indicating occasional metastatic potential. *Am J Surg Pathol.* 2008;**32**:354–62.
- Gold JS, Antonescu CR, Hajdu C, et al. Clinicopathologic correlates of solitary fibrous tumors. *Cancer.* 2002;**15**:1057–68.
- Goodlad J, Fletcher CDM. Solitary fibrous tumor arising at unusual sites: analysis of series. *Histopathology.* 1991;**19**:515–22.
- Guillou L, Gebhard S, Coindre JM, et al. Lipomatous hemangiopericytoma: a fat containing variant of solitary fibrous tumor? *Hum Pathol.* 2000a;**31**:1108–15.
- Guillou L, Gebhard S, Coindre JM, et al. Orbital and extraorbital giant cell angiofibroma: a giant cell rich variant of solitary fibrous tumor? *Am J Surg Pathol.* 2000b;**24**:971–9.
- Hanau CA, Miettinen M. Solitary fibrous tumor: histological and immunohistochemical spectrum of benign and malignant variants presenting at different sites. *Hum Pathol.* 1995;**26**:440–9.
- Lee JC, Fletcher CD. Malignant fat-forming solitary fibrous tumor (so-called "lipomatous hemangiopericytoma"): clinicopathologic analysis of 14 cases. *Am J Surg Pathol.* 2011;**35**:1177–85.
- Mentzel T, Bainbridge TC, Katenkamp D. Solitary fibrous tumor: clinicopathological, immunohistochemical, and ultrastructural analysis of 12 cases arising in soft tissues, nasal cavity and nasopharynx, urinary bladder and prostate. *Virchows Arch.* 1997;**430**:445–53.
- Mosquera JM, Fletcher CD. Expanding the spectrum of malignant progression in solitary fibrous tumors: a study of 8 cases with a discrete anaplastic component is this dedifferentiated SFT? *Am J Surg Pathol.* 2009;**33**:1314–21.
- Ng TL, Gown AM, Barry TS, et al: Nuclear beta-catenin in mesenchymal tumors, *Mod Pathol.* 2005;**18**:68–74.
- Nielsen GP, O'Connell JX, Dickersin GR. Solitary fibrous tumor of soft tissue: A report of 15 cases, including 5 malignant examples with light microscopic, immunohistochemical, and ultrastructural data. *Mod Pathol.* 1997;**10**:1028–37.
- Robinson DR, Wu YM, Kalyana-Sundaram S, et al. Identification of recurrent NAB2-STAT6 gene fusions in solitary fibrous tumor by integrative sequencing. *Nat Genet.* 2013;**45**:180–5.
- Schweizer L, Koelsche C, Sahm F, et al. Meningeal hemangiopericytoma and solitary fibrous tumors carry the NAB2-STAT6 fusion and can be diagnosed by nuclear expression of STAT6 protein. *Acta Neuropathol.* 2013;**125**:651–8.
- Stacchiotti S, Saponara M, Frapolli R, et al. Patient-derived solitary fibrous tumour xenografts predict high sensitivity to doxorubicin/dacarbazine combination confirmed in the clinic and highlight the potential effectiveness of trabectedin or eribulin against this tumour. *Eur J Cancer.* 2017;**76**:84–92.
- Suster S, Nascimento AG, Miettinen M, Sickel JZ, Moran CA. Solitary fibrous tumors of soft tissue. A clinicopathologic and immunohistochemical study of 12 cases. *Am J Surg Pathol.* 1995;**19**:1257–66.
- Vallat-Decouvelaere AV, Dry SM, Fletcher CDM. Atypical and malignant solitary fibrous tumors in extrathoracic locations: evidence of their comparability to intra-thoracic tumors. *Am J Surg Pathol.* 1998;**22**:1501–11.
- van Houdt WJ, Westerveld CM, Vrijenhoek JE, et al. Prognosis of solitary fibrous tumors: a multicenter study. *Ann Surg Oncol.* 2013 Dec;**20**(13):4090–5.
- Westra WH, Grenko RT, Epstein J. Solitary fibrous tumor of the lower urogenital tract: a report of five cases involving the seminal vesicles, urinary bladder, and prostate. *Hum Pathol.* 2000;**31**:63–8.
- Witkin GB, Rosai J. Solitary fibrous tumor of the mediastinum. A report of 14 cases. *Am J Surg Pathol.* 1989;**13**:547–57.
- Yang EJ, Howitt BE, Fletcher CD, Nucci MR. Solitary fibrous tumor of the female genital tract: a clinicopathologic analysis of 25 cases. *Histopathology.* 2017 Nov 6.

## Synovial Sarcoma

- Antonescu C, Leung DH, Dudas M, et al. Alterations of cell cycle regulators in localized synovial sarcoma: A multifactorial study with prognostic implications. *Am J Pathol.* 2000;**156**:977–83.
- Bégueret H, Galateau-Salle F, Guillou L, et al. Primary intrathoracic synovial sarcoma: a clinicopathologic study of 40 t(X;18)-positive cases from the French Sarcoma Group and the Mesopath Group. *Am J Surg Pathol.* 2005;**29**:339–46.
- Bianchi G, Sambri A, Righi A, et al. Histology and grading are important prognostic factors in synovial sarcoma. *Eur J Surg Oncol.* 2017;**43**:1733–9.
- Clark J, Rocques PG, Crew AJ, et al. Identification of novel genes, SYT and SSX, involved in the t(X;18)(p11.2;q11.2) translocation found in human synovial sarcoma. *Nat Genet.* 1994;**7**:502–7.
- Crew AJ, Clark J, Fisher C, et al. Fusion of SYT to two genes, SSX1 and SSX2, encoding proteins with homology to the Kruppel-associated box in human synovial sarcoma. *EMBO J.* 1995;**14**:2333–40.
- Dei Tos AP, Dal Cin P, Sciot R, et al. Synovial sarcoma of the larynx and hypopharynx. *Ann Othol Rhinol Laryngol.* 1998;**107**:1080–5.
- Dei Tos AP, Wadden C, Calonje E. Immunohistochemical demonstration of p30/32MIC2 (CD99) in synovial sarcoma. A potential cause of diagnostic confusion. *Appl Immunohistochem.* 1995;**3**:168–73.
- Fisher C, Folpe AL, Hashimoto H, Weiss SW. Intra-abdominal synovial sarcoma: a clinicopathological study. *Histopathology.* 2004;**45**:245–53.
- Fligman I, Lonardo F, Jhanwar SC, et al. Molecular diagnosis of synovial sarcoma

and characterization of a variant SYT-SSX2 fusion transcript. *Am J Pathol.* 1995;**147**:1592–9.

- Folpe AL, Schmidt RA, Chapman D, Gown AM. Poorly differentiated synovial sarcoma. Immunohistochemical distinction from primitive neuroectodermal tumors and high grade malignant peripheral nerve sheath tumors. *Am J Surg Pathol.* 1998;**22**:673–82.

- Guillou L, Benhattar J, Bonichon F, et al. Histologic grade, but not SYT-SSX fusion type, is an important prognostic factor in patients with synovial sarcoma: a multicenter, retrospective analysis. *J Clin Oncol.* 2004;**22**:4040–50.

- Guillou L, Wadden C, Kraus MD, et al. S-100 protein reactivity: in synovial sarcomas: A potentially frequent diagnostic pitfall. Immunohistochemical analysis of 100 cases. *Appl Immunohistochem.* 1996;**4**:167–75.

- Hartel PH, Fanburg-Smith JC, Frazier AA, et al. Primary pulmonary and mediastinal synovial sarcoma: a clinicopathologic study of 60 cases and comparison with five prior series. *Mod Pathol.* 2007;**20**:760–9.

- Kawai A, Woodruff J, Healey JH, et al. SYT-SSX gene fusion as a determinant of morphology and prognosis in synovial sarcoma. *N Engl J Med.* 1998;**338**:153–60.

- Krane JF, Bertoni F, Fletcher CD. Myxoid synovial sarcoma: an underappreciated morphologic subset. *Mod Pathol.* 1999;**12**:456–62.

- Lai JP, Robbins PF, Raffeld M, et al. NY-ESO-1 expression in synovial sarcoma and other mesenchymal tumors: significance for NY-ESO-1-based targeted therapy and differential diagnosis. *Mod Pathol.* 2012;**25**:854–8.

- Lewis JJ, Antonescu, CR, Leung DH, et al. Synovial sarcoma: A multivariate analysis of prognostic factors in 112 patients with primary localized tumors of the extremity. *J Clin Oncol.* 2000;**18**:2087–94.

- Majeste RM, Beckman EN. Synovial sarcoma with an overwhelming epithelial component. *Cancer.* 1988;**61**:2527–31.

- Robbins PF, Morgan RA, Feldman SA, et al. Tumor regression in patients with metastatic synovial cell sarcoma and melanoma using genetically engineered lymphocytes reactive with NY-ESO-1. *J Clin Oncol.* 2011;**29**:917–24.

- Shipley J, Crew J, Birdsall S, et al. Interphase fluorescence in situ hybridization and reverse transcription polymerase chain reaction as a diagnostic aid for synovial sarcoma. *Am J Pathol.* 1996;**148**:559–67.

- Spurrell EL, Fisher C, Thomas JM, et al. Prognostic factors in advanced synovial sarcoma: an analysis of 104 patients treated at the Royal Marsden Hospital. *Ann Oncol.* 2005;**16**:437–44.

- Suster S, Moran CA. Primary synovial sarcomas of the mediastinum: a clinicopathologic, immunohistochemical, and ultrastructural study of 15 cases. *Am J Surg Pathol.* 2005;**29**:569–78.

- Terry J, Saito T, Subramanian S, et al. TLE1 as a diagnostic immunohistochemical marker for synovial sarcoma emerging from gene expression profiling studies. *Am J Surg Pathol.* 2007;**31**:240–6.

- Van de Rijn M, Barr, FG, Collins MH, Xiong QB, Fisher C. Absence of SYT-SSX fusion products in soft tissue tumors other than synovial sarcoma. *Am J Clin Pathol.* 1999;**112**:43–9.

- Van de Rijn M, Barr, FG, Xiong QB, et al. Poorly differentiated synovial sarcoma. An analysis of clinical, pathologic, and molecular genetic features. *Am J Surg Pathol.* 1999;**23**:106–12.

## Infantile Fibrosarcoma

- Chung EB, Enzinger FM. Infantile fibrosarcoma. *Cancer.* 1976;**38**:729–39.

- Coffin CM, Dehner LP. Fibroblastic-myofibroblastic tumors in children and adolescents: a clinicopathologic study of 108 examples in 103 patients. *Pediatr Pathol.* 1991;**11**:569–88.

- Coffin CM, Jaszcz W, O'Shea PA, Dehner LP. So-called congenital-infantile fibrosarcoma: does it exist and what is it? *Pediatr Pathol.* 1994;**14**:133–50.

- Dal Cin P, Brock P, Casteels-Van Daele M, et al. Cytogenetic characterization of congenital or infantile fibrosarcoma. *Eur J Pediatr.* 1991;**150**:579–81.

- Kao YC, Fletcher CDM, Alaggio R, et al. Recurrent BRAF gene fusions in a subset of pediatric spindle cell sarcomas: expanding the genetic spectrum of tumors with overlapping features with infantile fibrosarcoma. *Am J Surg Pathol.* 2018;**42**:28–38.

- Knezevich SR, Garnett MJ, Pysher TJ, et al. ETV6-NTRK3 gene fusions and trisomy 11 establish a histogenetic link between mesoblastic nephroma and congenital fibrosarcoma. *Cancer Res.* 1998;**58**:5046–8.

- Knezevich SR, McFadden DE, Tao W, Lim JF, Sorensen PH. A novel ETV6-NTRK3 gene fusion in congenital fibrosarcoma. *Nat Genet.* 1998;**18**:184–7.

- Mandahl N, Heim S, Rydholm A, Willen H, Mitelman F. Nonrandom numerical chromosome aberrations (+8, +11, +17, +20) in infantile fibrosarcoma. *Cancer Genet Cytogenet.* 1989;**40**:137–9.

- Rubin BP, Chen CJ, Morgan TW, et al. Congenital mesoblastic nephroma t(12;15) is associated with ETV6-NTRK3 gene fusion: cytogenetic and molecular relationship to congenital (infantile) fibrosarcoma. *Am J Pathol.* 1998;**153**:1451–8.

- Sheng WQ, Hisaoka M, Okamoto S, et al. Congenital-infantile fibrosarcoma. A clinicopathologic study of 10 cases and molecular detection of the ETV6-NTRK3 fusion transcripts using paraffin-embedded tissues. *Am J Clin Pathol.* 2001;**115**: 348–55.

- Soule EH, Pritchard DJ. Fibrosarcoma in infants and children: a review of 110 cases. *Cancer.* 1977;**40**:1711–21.

## Malignant Peripheral Nerve Sheath Tumor (MPNST) and Its Differential Diagnosis

- Brooks JSJ, Freeman M, Enterline HT. Malignant "triton" tumors. Natural history and immunohistochemistry of nine new cases with literature review. *Cancer.* 1985;**55**:2543–9.

- Ch'ng ES, Hoshida Y, Iizuka N, et al. Composite malignant pheochromocytoma with malignant peripheral nerve sheath tumour: a case with 28 years of tumour-bearing history. *Histopathology.* 2007;**51**:420–2.

- D'Agostino AN, Soule EH, Miller RH. Primary malignant neoplasms of nerves (malignant neurilemmomas) in patients without manifestations of multiple neurofibromatosis (von Recklinghausen's disease). *Cancer.* 1963a;**16**:1003–14.

- D'Agostino AN, Soule EH, Miller RH. Sarcomas of peripheral nerves and somatic soft tissues associated with multiple neurofibromatosis (von Recklinghausen's disease). *Cancer.* 1963b;**16**:1015–27.

- Daimaru Y, Hashimoto H, Enjoji M. Malignant "triton" tumors: a clinicopathologic and immunohistochemical study of nine cases. *Hum Pathol.* 1984;**15**:768–78.

- Ducatman BS, Scheithauer BW, Piepgras DG, Reiman HM, Ilstrup DM. Malignant peripheral nerve sheath tumors. A clinicopathologic study of 120 cases. *Cancer.* 1986;**57**:215–26.

- Ferner RE. Neurofibromatosis 1 and neurofibromatosis 2: a twenty first century perspective. *Lancet Neurol.* 2007 **6**:340–51.

- Fritchie KJ, Jin L, Wang X, et al. Fusion gene profile of biphenotypic sinonasal sarcoma: an analysis of 44 cases. *Histopathology.* 2016;**69**:930–6.

- Ghosh BC, Gosh L, Huvos AG, et al. Malignant schwannoma. A clinicopathologic study. *Cancer.* 1973;**31**:184–90

- Guccion JG, Enzinger FM. Malignant schwannoma associated with von Recklinghausen's neurofibromatosis. *Virchows Arch [A].* 1979;**383**:43–57.

- Huang SC, Ghossein RA, Bishop JA, et al. Novel PAX3-NCOA1 fusions in biphenotypic sinonasal sarcoma with focal rhabdomyoblastic differentiation. *Am J Surg Pathol.* 2016;**40**:51–9.

- King AA, Debaun MR, Riccardi VM, et al. Malignant peripheral nerve sheath tumors in neurofibromatosis 1. *Am J Med Genet.* 2000;**93**:388–92.

- Lewis JT, Oliveira AM, Nascimento AG, et al. Low-grade sinonasal sarcoma with neural and myogenic features: a clinicopathologic analysis of 28 cases. *Am J Surg Pathol.* 2012;**36**:517–25.

- Miettinen MM, Antonescu CR, Fletcher CDM, et al. Histopathologic evaluation of atypical neurofibromatous tumors and their transformation into malignant peripheral nerve sheath tumor in patients with neurofibromatosis 1-a consensus overview. *Hum Pathol.* 2017;**67**:1–10.

- Schaefer IM, Fletcher CD, Hornick JL. Loss of H3K27 trimethylation distinguishes malignant peripheral nerve sheath tumors from histologic mimics. *Mod Pathol.* 2016;**29**:4–13.

- Sorensen SA, Mulvihill JJ, Nielsen A. Long-term follow-up of von Recklinghausen neurofibromatosis. Survival and malignant neoplasms. *N Eng J Med.* 1986;**314**:1010–15.

- Wang X, Bledsoe KL, Graham RP, et al. Recurrent PAX3-MAML3 fusion in biphenotypic sinonasal sarcoma. *Nat Genet.* 2014;**46**:666–8.

- Wong WJ, Lauria A, Hornick JL, et al. Alternate PAX3-FOXO1 oncogenic fusion in biphenotypic sinonasal sarcoma. *Genes Chromosomes Cancer.* 2016;**55**:25–9.

- Woodruff JM, Godwin TA, Erlandson RA, Susin M, Martini N. Cellular schwannoma: a variety of schwannoma sometimes mistaken for a malignant tumor. *Am J Surg Pathol.* 1981;**5**:733–44.

- Woodruff JM, Perino G. Non germ cell or teratomatous malignant tumors showing additional rhabdomyoblastic differentiation, with emphasis on the malignant Triton tumor. *Semin Diagn Pathol.* 1994;**11**:69–81.

## Spindle Cell Liposarcoma

- Creytens D, Mentzel T, Ferdinande L, et al. "Atypical" pleomorphic lipomatous tumor: a clinicopathologic, immunohistochemical and molecular study of 21 cases, emphasizing its relationship to atypical spindle cell lipomatous tumor and suggesting a morphologic spectrum (atypical spindle cell/pleomorphic lipomatous tumor. *Am J Surg Pathol.* 2017;**41**:1443–55.

- Creytens D, van Gorp J, Savola S, et al. Atypical spindle cell lipoma: a clinicopathologic, immunohistochemical, and molecular study emphasizing its relationship to classical spindle cell lipoma. *Virchows Arch.* 2014;**465**:97–108.

- Dei Tos AP, Mentzel T, Newman PL, Fletcher CD. Spindle cell liposarcoma, a hitherto unrecognized variant of liposarcoma. Analysis of six cases. *Am J Surg Pathol.* 1994;**18**:913–21.

- Mariño-Enriquez A, Nascimento AF, Ligon AH, Liang C, Fletcher CD. Atypical spindle cell lipomatous tumor: clinicopathologic characterization of 232 cases demonstrating a morphologic spectrum. *Am J Surg Pathol.* 2017;**41**:234–44.

## Spindle Cell and Sclerosing Rhabdomyosarcoma

- Alaggio R, Zhang L, Sung YS, et al. A molecular study of pediatric spindle and sclerosing rhabdomyosarcoma: identification of novel and recurrent VGLL2-related fusions in infantile cases. *Am J Surg Pathol.* 2016;**40**:224–35.

- Cavazzana AO, Schmidt D, Ninfo V, et al. Spindle cell rhabdomyosarcoma. A prognostically favorable variant of rhabdomyosarcoma. *Am J Surg Pathol.* 1992;**16**:229–35.

- Kohsaka S, Shukla N, Ameur N, et al. A recurrent neomorphic mutation in MYOD1 defines a clinically aggressive subset of embryonal rhabdomyosarcoma associated with PI3 K-AKT pathway mutations. *Nat Genet.* 2014;**46**:595–600.

- Mosquera JM, Sboner A, Zhang L, et al. Recurrent NCOA2 gene rearrangements in congenital/infantile spindle cell rhabdomyosarcoma. *Genes Chromosomes Cancer.* 2013;**52**:538–50.

- Nascimento AF, Fletcher CD. Spindle cell rhabdomyosarcoma in adults. *Am J Surg Pathol.* 2005;**29**:1106–13.

- Szuhai K, de Jong D, Leung WY, Fletcher CD, Hogendoorn PC. Transactivating mutation of the MYOD1 gene is a frequent event in adult spindle cell rhabdomyosarcoma. *J Pathol.* 2014;**23**:300–7.

## Intimal Sarcoma

- Dewaele B, Floris G, Finalet-Ferreiro J, et al. Coactivated platelet-derived growth factor receptor{alpha} and epidermal growth factor receptor are potential therapeutic targets in intimal sarcoma. *Cancer Res.* 2010;**70**:7304–14.

- Neuville A, Collin F, Bruneval P, et al. Intimal sarcoma is the most frequent primary cardiac sarcoma: clinicopathologic and molecular retrospective analysis of 100 primary cardiac sarcomas. *Am J Surg Pathol.* 2014;**38**:461–9.

- Sebenik M, Ricci A Jr, DiPasquale B, et al. Undifferentiated intimal sarcoma of large systemic blood vessels: report of 14 cases with immunohistochemical profile and review of the literature. *Am J Surg Pathol.* 2005;**29**: 1184–93.

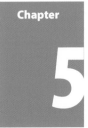

# Soft Tissue Sarcomas with Epithelioid Morphology

Marta Sbaraglia MD and Angelo Paolo Dei Tos MD

## Introduction

Epithelioid morphology refers to resemblance to epithelial cells. Epithelioid cells usually feature a polygonal shape and exhibit abundant cytoplasm. These can show variable growth patterns as solid, nesting, sheet-like, cord-like, or glandular-like.

Epithelioid mesenchymal tumors form a heterogeneous as well as rare (they account for approximately 5–10% of sarcomas) group of lesions, which sometimes exhibit overlapping morphology, and therefore represent a major diagnostic challenge. They also tend to share a variable immunophenotypic expression of epithelial differentiation markers (namely, cytokeratins and epithelial membrane antigens [EMAs]), which, in unexperienced hands, may be a source of further difficulty (Table 5.1). In fact, in addition to mesenchymal malignancies, the differential diagnosis includes metastatic carcinoma, metastatic melanoma, epithelioid malignant mesothelioma, and large cell variants of non-Hodgkin lymphoma. Molecular genetics may be of diagnostic help in selected histologies (Table 5.2).

This chapter will focus on mesenchymal malignancies predominatly composed of epithelioid cells, including those lesions of which an epithelioid variant is clearly identified. Admittedly, lesions such as pseudomyogenic hemangioendothelioma and myoepitheliomas can exhibit either a spindle or an epithelioid cell morphology (or a combination of both). Their allocation in this chapter is justified, considering the challenges in differential diagnosis.

**Table 5.1** Key immunohistochemical features of sarcoma with epithelioid morphology

| | Pankeratin | CD31 | ERG | S100 | Loss of INI1 | EMA | HMB45 | MelanA | TFE3 | Desmin | SMA | Myogenin | ALK |
|---|---|---|---|---|---|---|---|---|---|---|---|---|---|
| ES | >90% | – | 40% | – | >90% | >90% | – | – | – | – | – | – | – |
| Myoepith-elioma | 80% | – | – | 90% | 20% | 60% | – | – | – | 10% | 30% | – | – |
| EHE | 30% focal | 100% | 100% | – | – | rare | – | – | – | – | – | – | – |
| EAS | 30% | 100% | 100% | – | – | rare | – | – | – | – | – | – | – |
| PEHE | 100% | 50% | >90% | – | – | – | – | – | – | – | – | – | – |
| E-MPNST | 20% | – | – | 100% | 60% | 30% | – | – | – | – | – | – | – |
| Clear cell sarcoma | – | – | – | 100% | – | – | 70% | 60% | – | – | – | – | – |
| ASPS | – | – | – | – | – | – | – | – | >90% | – | – | – | – |
| PEComa | – | – | – | Rare | – | – | > 90% | >50% | 5% | 25% | 80% | – | – |
| MRT | 80% | – | – | – | 100% | 50% | – | – | – | – | – | – | – |
| E-RMS | Rare/focal | – | – | Rare/focal | – | – | – | – | – | >90% | 10% | 100% | – |
| E-IMT | – | – | – | – | – | – | – | – | – | 90% | 80% | – | 100% |

**Legends:**

ES: epithelioid sarcoma

EHE: epithelioid hemangioendothelioma

EAS: epithelioid angiosarcoma

PEHE: pseudomyogenic hemangioendothelioma

E-MPNST: epithelioid malignant peripheral nerve sheath tumor

ASPS: alveolar soft part sarcoma

MRT: Malignant rhabdoid tumor

E-RMS: epithelioid rhabdomyosarcoma

E-IMT: epithelioid inflammatoty myofibroblastic tumor

**Table 5.2** Genetic features of sarcomas with epithelioid morphology

| Histotype | Cytogenetic alteration | Molecular alterations |
| --- | --- | --- |
| Epithelioid sarcoma | Unknown | Inactivation of *SMARCB1* |
| Malignant rhabdoid tumor | Deletion or translocation on 22q; inactivating mutations; monosomia 22 | Loss of *SMARCB1* |
| Malignant myoepithelioma | t(6;22) (q21;q12)<br>t(19;22) (q13;q12)<br>t(1;22) (q23;q12)<br>t(12;22) (q13;q12)<br>t(9;22) (q33;q12)<br>t(1;16) (p34;p11) | *EWSR1-POU5F1*<br>*EWSR1-ZNF444*<br>*EWSR1-PBX1*<br>*EWSR1-ATF1*<br>*EWSR1-PBX3*<br>*FUS-KLF17* |
| Pseudomyogenic hemangioendothelioma | t(7;19)(q22;q13) | *SERPINE1-FOSB* |
| Epithelioid hemangioendothelioma | t(1;3) (p36;q25)<br>t(11;X) (q22;p11) | *WWTR1-CAMTA1*<br>*YAP1-TEF3* |
| Epithelioid angiosarcoma | Complex | Upregulation of vascular-specific receptor |
| E-MPNST | Unknown | inactivation *INI1* |
| Clear cell sarcoma | t(12;22) (q13;q12)<br>t(2;22) (q33;q12) | *EWSRR1-ATF1*<br>*EWSR1-CREB1* |
| Sclerosing epithelioid fibrosarcoma | t(7;16) (q33;p11)<br>t(11;16) (p11;p11)<br>t(11;22) (p11;q12) | *FUS-CREB3L2*<br>*FUS-CREB3L1*<br>*EWSR1-CREB3L1* |
| Alveolar soft part sarcoma | t(X;17) (p11;q25) | *ASPL-TFE3* |
| PEComa | Deletion 16p<br>Translocation xp11 | Lost *TSC2*<br>*TFE3* rearrangement |
| Epithelioid pleomorphic liposarcoma | Complex | Unknown |
| Epithelioid gastrointestinal stromal tumor (GIST) | Monosomies and deletions | *KIT* or *PDGFRA* mutation; minority of cases *BRAF*, *RAS*, SDH, *NF1* mutation |
| Epithelioid myxofibrosarcoma | Complex | *NF1* aberration (rare) |
| Epithelioid leiomyosarcoma | Complex | Defects in *TP53*, *FANCA*, or *ATM* |
| Epithelioid rhabdomyosarcoma | Complex | Alteration on *TP53*, *RB1*, *RAS* |
| Epithelioid inflammatory myofibroblastic sarcoma | t(2;2)(p23;q13) | *RANBP2-ALK* |

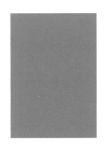

# Epithelioid Sarcoma

## Definition and Epidemiology

First reported in 1970 by Franz Enzinger, the classic variant of epithelioid sarcoma (ES) is a very rare (it accounts for no more than 2% of soft tissue sarcomas) distinctive sarcoma of uncertain differentiation, characterized by a predominantly epithelioid cytomorphology. Two main variants of epithelioid sarcoma are currently recognized: classical or conventional type (C-ES) and proximal type (P-ES). Classical ES occurs in adolescents and young adults (peak incidence being in the second decade) and predominates in males. Proximal ES occurs in middle-aged adults (median age 40) and often pursues a more aggressive clinical course than does the classical type.

## Clinical Presentation and Behavior

Classical-type ES involves mainly the flexor surface of the fingers, hand, wrist, and forearm, followed by knee, lower leg (pretibial region), proximal extremities (buttocks, thigh, shoulder, and arm), ankle, feet, and toes, but may occur in any location (Fig. 5-1). Most often, at the time of diagnosis small, superficial nodules (3–6 cm) are detected.

Proximal-type ES tends to involve the deep soft tissue of the trunk, genital areas (pubis, vulva, penis), pelvis, perineum, and head and neck region. Larger masses than in C-ES are usually seen (Fig. 5-2).

The classical type of ES tends to occur distally at onset but subsequently it characteristically propagates along fascial planes, tendons, and nerve sheaths. The overall recurrence rate reaches 90%. Most recurrences are generally seen within 1 year of surgery and most likely depend on the adequacy of the first resection. More aggressive surgery performed at expert centers apparently significantly reduces the rate of local recurrences. Metastatic rate ranges in different series between 35 and 40%. Metastases involve lung (50%), regional lymph nodes (35%), scalp (20%), bone, and brain. Classical-type ES often exhibits a protracted clinical course. The 10-year overall survival rates vary from 25 to 50%, with recurrences, metastases, and death being documented up to 20 years following the initial diagnosis. An additional clinical problem is represented by the fact that ES is relatively often diagnosed up to 2 years following onset of clinical symptoms. Proximal-type ES causes earlier tumor-related deaths.

## Morphology and Immunohistochemistry

Morphologically, C-ES shows a characteristic nodular arrangement (Fig. 5-3). The nodules are composed of an admixture of eosinophilic epithelioid and spindle cells (Fig. 5-4) with variable (from mild to overt) nuclear atypia (Figs. 5-5, 5-6, 5-7, and 5-8). Mitotic activity is usually low. The neoplastic nodules may show central necrosis, often generating a

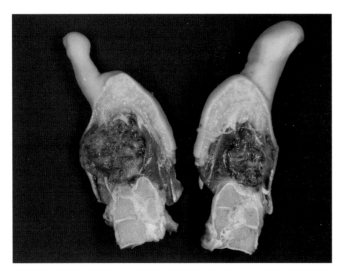

**Fig. 5-1.** Classical-type epithelioid sarcoma. Tumor mass of the foot with extensive infiltration of the soft tissue and bone.

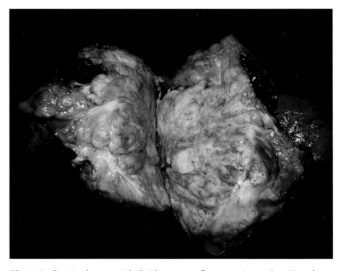

**Fig. 5-2.** Proximal-type epithelioid sarcoma. Gross specimen showing a large, fleshy, deep-seated mass. Multiple foci of necrosis are easily identifiable.

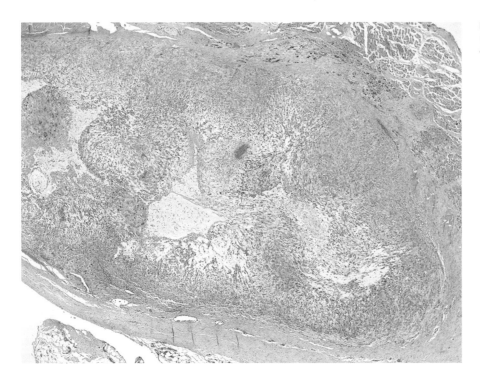

**Fig. 5-3.** Classical-type epithelioid sarcoma. At low magnification, the lesion typically shows a nodular arrangement.

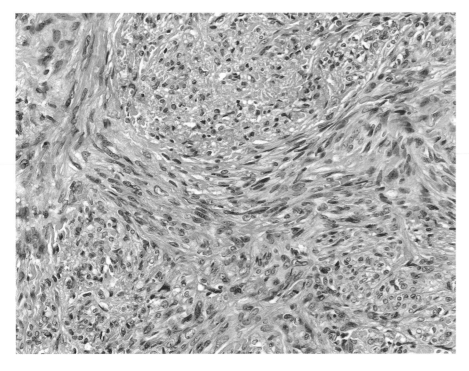

**Fig. 5-4.** Classical-type epithelioid sarcoma. Neoplastic nodules are composed of an admixture of eosinophilic epithelioid and spindle cells. Moderate nuclear atypia and cytologic monomorphism are seen.

pseudogranulomatous appearance, somewhat simulating a rheumatoid nodule or a granuloma annulare (Figs. 5-9 and 5-10). Necrosis tends to be more abundant in larger and/or deep-seated nodules (Fig. 5-11). Perineural and perivascular invasions are commonly seen. Nodules can be well defined or fused into larger masses, forming "geographic" lesions with scalloped margins. Nodules are generally multiple in local recurrences. A pseudoangiomatous pattern due to intratumoral hemorrhage (Fig. 5-12) that can mimic a vascular neoplasm is rarely seen. In some cases, a prominent chronic

inflammatory infiltrate, calcifications, and metaplastic bone formation are described.

A "fibroma-like" variant of ES has been reported by Mirra and coworkers that is mainly composed of fusiform cells, which most likely represent examples of the recently reported entity "pseudomyogenic hemangioendothelioma" and is discussed in detail later in this chapter.

Proximal-type ES also shows a multinodular pattern of growth. The nodules are formed by large, epithelioid, carcinoma-like cells with marked cytologic atypia, vesicular

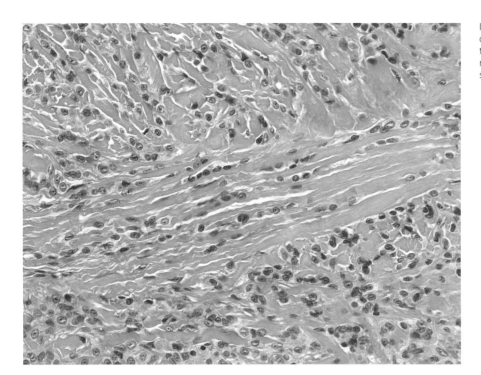

**Fig. 5-5.** Classical-type epithelioid sarcoma. Most often, an epithelioid morphology predominates. In this example, cytologically bland, palely eosinophilic neoplastic cells infiltrating dermal collagen are shown.

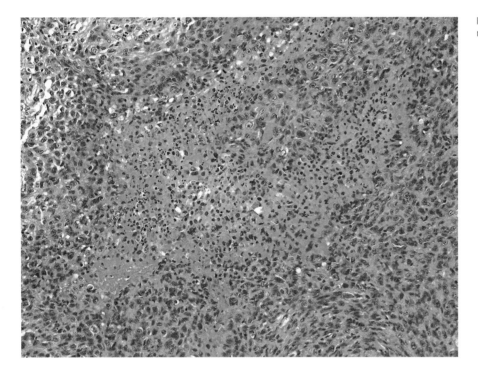

**Fig. 5-6.** Classical-type epithelioid sarcoma. Severe nuclear atypia is shown, associated with necrosis.

nuclei, and prominent nucleoli (Fig. 5-13). The cells are mitotically active and often show a rhabdoid phenotype (Fig. 5-14), characterized by the presence of eosinophilic cytoplasm and eccentric vesicular nuclei with large nucleoli. Interestingly, cases showing hybrid features of both classical-type ES and proximal-type ES have been observed (Fig. 5-15). Similar to C-ES, necrosis tends to be common but not does not feature a granuloma-like morphology (Fig. 5-16). In both C-ES and P-ES, nuclear pleomorphism is relatively rare.

Immunohistochemically, both variants of ES show co-expression of EMA, cytokeratins (both low and high molecular weight) (Fig. 5-17), and vimentin. In contrast to squamous cell carcinoma, cytokeratin 5/6 tends to be negative in ES. CD34 immunopositivity is observed in approximately half of the cases. The vascular marker ERG is expressed in approximately 40% of cases. Importantly, ES characteristically shows loss of nuclear immunoreactivity of INI1 in neoplastic cells (Fig. 5-18). As with any "negative" staining, it is important that positive built-in controls such as normal endothelial cells are always detected.

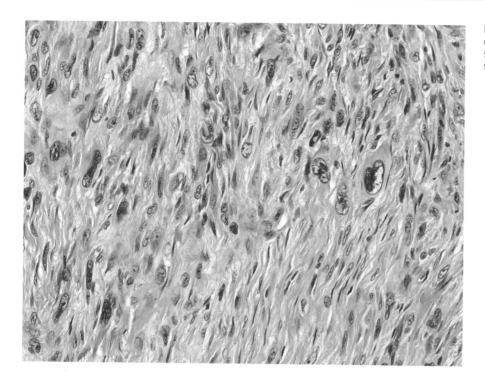

**Fig. 5-7.** Classical-type epithelioid sarcoma. In rare cases of C-ES, significant pleomorphism can be seen, associated with cytologically bland neoplastic spindle cells.

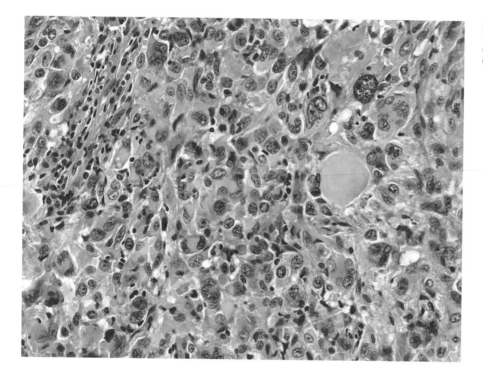

**Fig. 5-8.** Classical-type epithelioid sarcoma. Diffusely severe cytologic atypia (somewhat overlapping that of P-ES) can be rarely observed in C-ES.

## Molecular Genetics

The *SMARCB1/hSNF5/INI1* gene maps at chromosome 22q11.2 and is inactivated in most cases, therefore explaining the loss of INI1 protein expression observed in epithelioid sarcoma. The switch/sucrose nonfermenting (SWI/SNF) complex is an ATPase-dependent multi-subunit complex involved in chromatin remodeling and transcriptional regulation. This complex contributes to the regulation of differentiation and cell proliferation. Growing evidence indicates a key role of SWI/SNF complex subunits in tumor suppression. INI1 is ubiquitously expressed in all normal human tissue types. The mechanism of INI1 inactivation in ES is heterogeneous, including epigenetic silencing and deletions in 20–50% of cases, whereas translocation and point mutations are very rare. Interestingly, INI1 loss appears to be associated with upregulation of EZH2 (the catalytic subunit of the multi-protein histone methyltransferase [HMT] complex known as a polychrome repressive complex [PRC]) that represents a promising molecular therapeutic target.

225

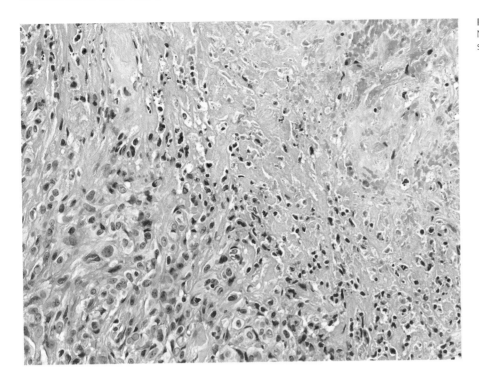

**Fig. 5-9.** Classical-type epithelioid sarcoma. Neoplastic nodules show central necrosis and somewhat mimic a granuloma annulare.

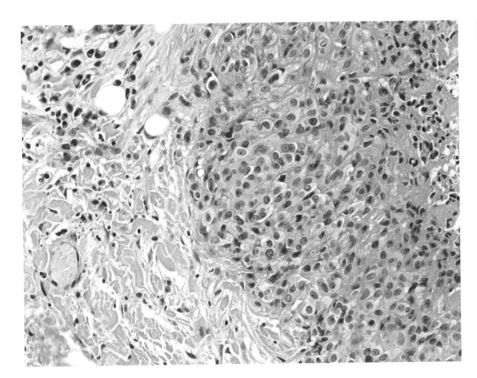

**Fig. 5-10.** Classical-type epithelioid sarcoma. Neoplastic cell surrounding necrotic areas exhibits moderate cytologic atypia: Mitotic figures are easily identified.

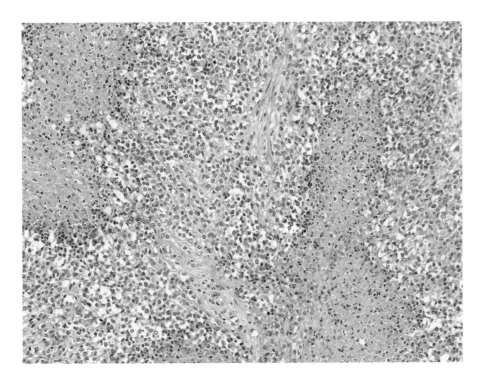

**Fig. 5-11.** Classical-type epithelioid sarcoma. In deep-seated nodules, necrosis tends to be more abundant; however, it keeps the typical "geographic" silhouette.

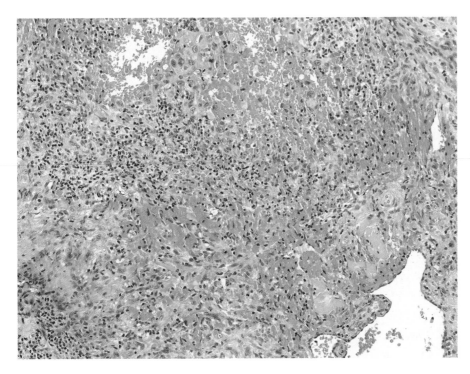

**Fig. 5-12.** Classical-type epithelioid sarcoma. Intratumoral hemorrhage may raise the differential diagnosis with a vascular malignancy. These features have been labeled as "pseudoangiomatous."

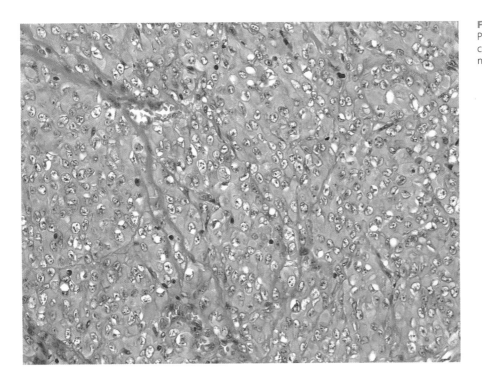

**Fig. 5-13.** Proximal-type epithelioid sarcoma. In P-ES, the cell population assumes an epithelioid carcinoma-like morphology associated with marked nuclear atypia.

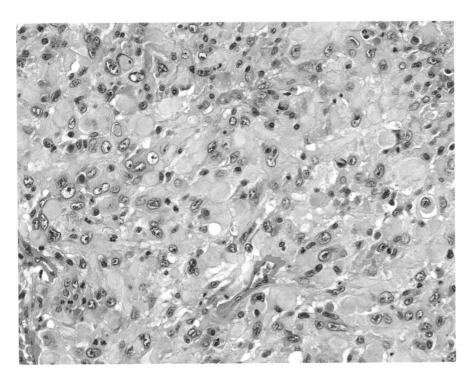

**Fig. 5-14.** Proximal-type epithelioid sarcoma. A rhabdoid (presence of large eosinophilic cytoplasm harboring eccentric macronucleolated nuclei) morphology is often seen in P-ES.

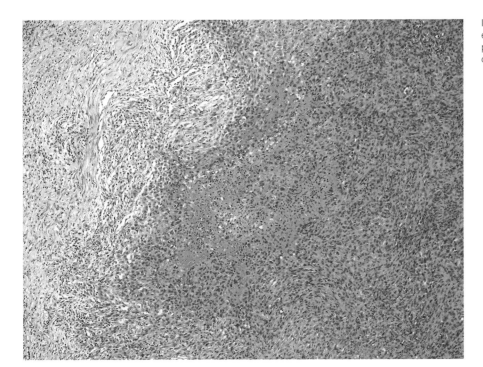

**Fig. 5-15.** Epithelioid sarcoma occasionally may exhibit hybrid features of both classical- and proximal-type ES. Transition of conventional spindle cell areas to high-grade epithelioid is seen.

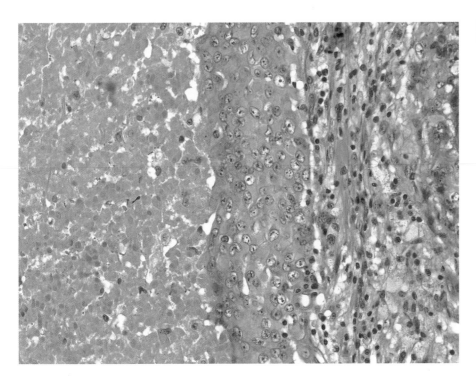

**Fig. 5-16.** Proximal-type epithelioid sarcoma. The tumor shows abundant coagulative necrosis.

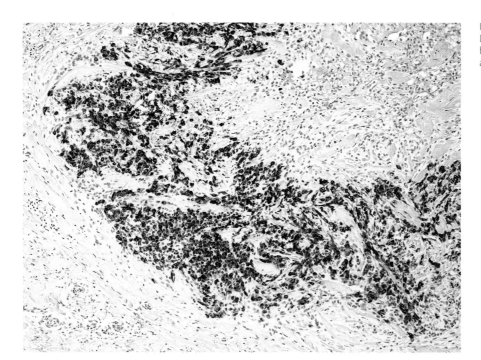

**Fig. 5-17.** Classical-type epithelioid sarcoma. Diffuse expression of cytokeratin is seen, highlighting the distribution of neoplastic cell around large foci of "geographic" necrosis.

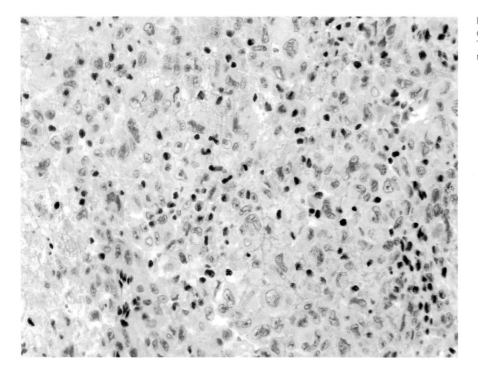

**Fig. 5-18.** Epithelioid sarcoma. Loss of INI1 nuclear expression is very common in both C-ES and P-ES. The presence of INI1-positive endothelial cells represents the positive internal control.

## Differential Diagnosis and Diagnostic Pitfalls

Classical-type ES may exhibit a deceptively bland cytomorphology that represents a major diagnostic challenge as well as a potential source of medical litigation. Granulomatous lesions (rheumatoid nodule, granuloma annulare) certainly enter the differential diagnosis (Figs. 5-19 and 5-20). Absence of expression of epithelial differentiation markers as well as positive immunoreaction for histiocytic markers such as CD68 and CD163 represent extremely valuable diagnostic clues. Sarcomatoid squamous cell carcinoma (SSCC) may also

represent a diagnostic problem, particularly when dealing with elderly patients. However, SSCC is exceptional in young adults and adolescents and is consistently CD34 negative/INI1 positive/cytokeratin 5/6 positive. In addition, p63 immunoreactivity is generally observed in SSCC, whereas it is generally negative in ES.

More important is the differential diagnosis with myoepithelial carcinoma (discussed in detail later in this chapter) that is characterized by a distinctive bimodal pattern of incidence, which in approximately 20% of cases involves the

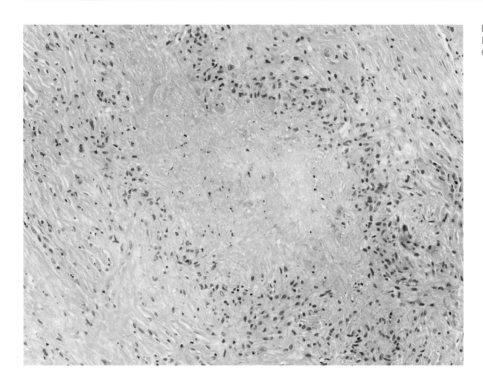

**Fig. 5-19.** Granuloma annulare. Granulomatous lesions such as granuloma annulare may mimic C-ES.

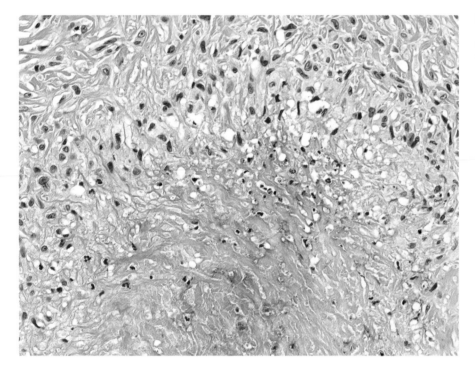

**Fig. 5-20.** Granuloma annulare. This inflammatory lesion generally is cytologically bland; however, C-ES at times may also show unremarkable cytologic atypia.

pediatric age-group. A major pitfall is represented by the fact that myoepithelial carcinoma may also feature loss of INI1 expression (lost in up to 40% in children and in approximately 10% of adult patients). However, myoepithelial carcinoma exhibits a more obvious carcinoma-like appearance and, in addition to the expression of epithelial markers, is generally CD34 negative, and variably expresses S100, glial fibrillary acidic protein (GFAP), and smooth muscle actin. Furthermore, 45% of myoepithelial carcinomas harbor

*EWSR1* rearrangement, which has never been reported in ES. Epithelioid MPNST (discussed later in this chapter) may also show loss of INI1; however, it invariably exhibits diffuse positivity for S100 protein, which is never seen in either C-ES or P-ES.

Epithelioid sarcoma is at risk of being confused with epithelioid vascular malignancies, especially when pseudoangiomatoid features prevail; however, it consistently lacks expression of vascular markers. Nonetheless, it is important to note that the expression of the novel vascular marker ERG has been reported in about 40% of epithelioid sarcoma cases. This finding certainly represents a major diagnostic pitfall, and underlines the concept that the immunohistochemical evaluation of these lesions always requires the use of panels of immunoreagents.

Malignant rhabdoid tumor (MRT) also shows significant morphologic as well as immunophenotypic overlap with P-ES (they both co-express EMA and cytokeratin and exhibit loss of nuclear INI1 immunoreactivity). However, MRT primarily occurs in the deep soft tissues of infants and young children, shows diffuse rhabdoid morphology, and exhibits much higher clinical aggressiveness. Genetically, MRT exhibits *INI1* and *p53* mutations that are much rarer in P-ES.

Unlike ES, epithelioid or rhabdoid melanomas show diffuse expression of S100 sometimes associated with melanocytic markers and retain expression of INI-1. Interestingly, melanoma cells (particularly in metastatic melanoma) may focally express cytokeratins.

**Key Points in Classical-Type Epithelioid Sarcoma Diagnosis**

- Young age
- Acral location
- Admixture of moderately atypical spindle and epithelioid cells
- Expression of epithelial differentiation markers
- Loss of INI1 expression
- Protracted clinical course

**Key Points in Proximal-Type Epithelioid Sarcoma Diagnosis**

- Occurrence in young to middle-aged adults
- Proximal anatomic location
- Predominance of large epithelioid cells with severe atypia
- Aggressive clinical course
- Expression of epithelial differentiation markers
- Loss of INI1 expression

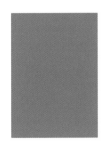

# Malignant Extrarenal Rhabdoid Tumor

## Definition and Epidemiology

Soft tissue malignant rhabdoid tumor (MRT), or extrarenal MRT, is an extremely rare malignant tumor of uncertain differentiation almost exclusively affecting infants and children. Because a rhabdoid phenotype may be present in a broad spectrum of tumors, particularly those occurring in adults, the diagnosis of MRT requires exclusion of an underlining alternative line of differentiation. Extrarenal rhabdoid tumor of soft tissue overlaps morphologically with the pediatric RT of the kidney and central nervous system (so-called atypycal/teratoid rhabdoid tumor). Malignant rhabdoid tumor occurs in children under 3 years of age. Congenital disseminated fatal cases are also reported. Those rare cases occurring in adults most likely represent examples of tumor progression in the context of a variety of malignancies, including carcinoma, mesothelioma, and melanoma.

## Clinical Presentation and Behavior

Malignant rhabdoid tumor of soft tissue occurs in deep, axial locations (neck and paraspinal regions). Malignant rhabdoid tumor can involve skin and visceral locations such as the liver, the heart, and the gastrointestinal system, and represents one of the most aggressive human neoplasms. The outcome is ominous despite multimodal therapies, with overall mortality at 2 years close to 100%.

## Morphology and Immunohistochemistry

Grossly, MRT are non-encapsulated masses, usually less than 5 cm in diameter, soft, gray to tan, with foci of hemorrhage and necrosis.

Histologically, MRT are densely cellular and composed of solid sheets or trabeculae of atypical epithelioid cells. Myxoid stromal change can be observed, often associated with loss of cohesion of neoplastic cells. Large, round to bean-shaped, vesicular nuclei, with prominent, centrally located nucleoli, are harbored within abundant, eosinophilic cytoplasm (Fig. 5-21). Characteristically, a prominent eosinophilic cytoplasmic condensation is seen, which ultrastructurally corresponds to whorls of intermediate filaments (Fig. 5-22). Rarely, MRT may exhibit an organoid, carcinoma-like morphology (Fig. 5-23). High mitotic count and abundant necrosis represent common findings. Malignant rhabdoid tumor shows co-expression of vimentin and cytokeratins (most often in a characteristic dot-like pattern highlighting the cytoplasmic inclusions) and EMA. Immunoreactivity for CD99, synaptophysin, neuron-specific

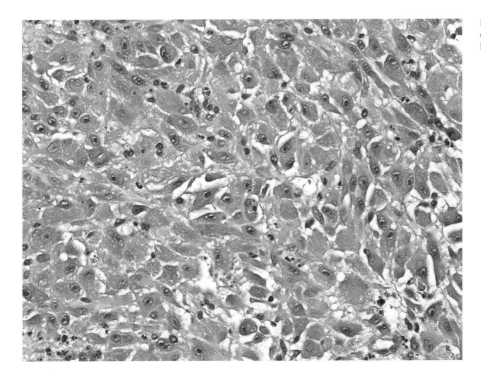

**Fig. 5-21.** Malignant rhabdoid tumor. Neoplastic cells feature abundant eosinophilic cytoplasm harboring vesicular macronucleolated nuclei.

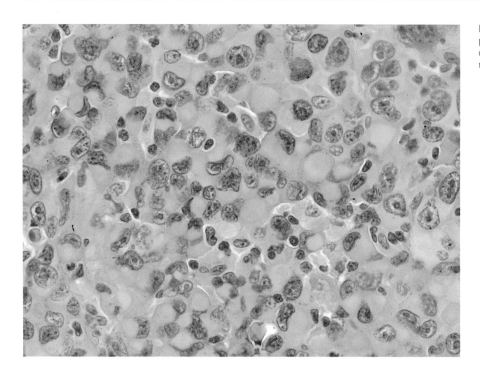

**Fig. 5-22.** Malignant rhabdoid tumor. A prominent eosinophilic hyaline cytoplasmic condensation is often seen. Such inclusions represent whorls of intermediate filaments.

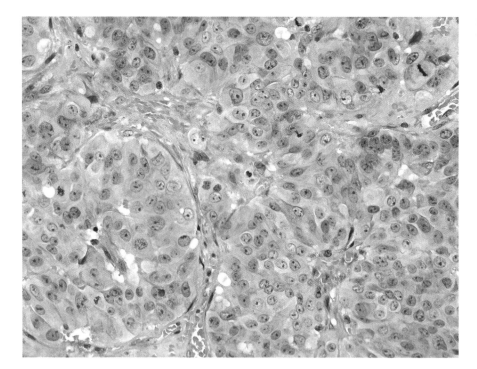

**Fig. 5-23.** Malignant rhabdoid tumor. Sometimes a solid, "carcinoma-like" pattern of growth is seen.

enolase (NSE), actin, and S100 protein is also variably reported; however, in the presence of unusual immunophenotypic features, other neoplasms need to be excluded. An important diagnostic clue is represented by the loss of nuclear expression of INI1, which is observed in almost all cases of MRT (Fig. 5-24). Undifferentiated sarcomas featuring rhabdoid morphology histologically similar to MRT (and equally aggressive) and occurring predominantly in the thoracic region have been recently described. Loss of nuclear expression of SMARCA4 (also belonging with INI1/SMARCB1 to the switch/sucrose

non-fermenting [SWI/SFN] chromatin remodeling complex) has been consistently observed.

## Molecular Genetics

Genetically, soft tissue MRT, when properly defined and provided that other malignancies with rhabdoid features are ruled out, is characterized by aberrations in chromosome region 22q11.2. Gene mutations and/or deletions are involved in approximately 75% of cases of the *SMARCB1/INI1* gene,

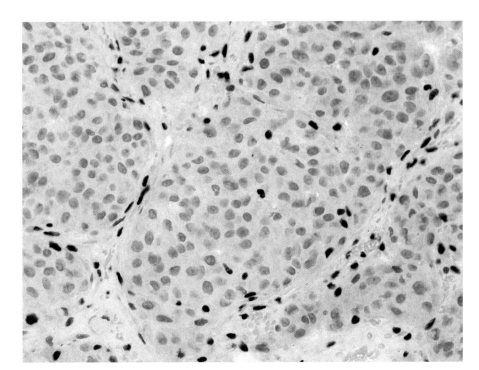

**Fig. 5-24.** Malignant rhabdoid tumor. Loss of nuclear expression of INI1 is characteristically seen in the vast majority of cases. Note the presence of internal positive control represented by endothelial cells.

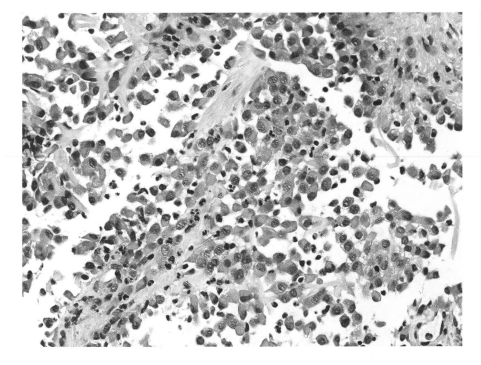

**Fig. 5-25.** Carcinoma with rhabdoid morphology. Undifferentiated carcinoma (and many other malignancies) may overlap morphologically with MRT.

which is also known to be affected in renal as well as central nervous system (CNS) rhabdoid tumors. The remaining 25% of cases show low expression of INI1 secondary to epigenetic mechanisms. These data have greatly contributed to support the concept that, when strictly defined, MRT of soft tissue truly represents a distinctive entity. Germline *INI1* mutations are reported in approximately one-third of patients with sporadic MRT, in which the neoplasm arises at an earlier age (6 months) and appears to be associated with even worse prognosis. As mentioned, SMARCB1/INI1 belongs to the SWI/SFN chromatin remodeling complex that exerts a tumor-supressor function by regulating transcription and promoting cell differentiation. Secondary alterations of the *EWSR1* gene have been reported in SMARCB1-deficient tumors (including MRT) that represent a potential molecular diagnostic pitfall.

## Differential Diagnosis and Diagnostic Pitfalls

Rhabdoid features can be detected in a variety of solid tumors such as carcinoma, meningioma, malignant melanoma, lymphoma, and malignant mesothelioma (also known as "composite rhabdoid tumors") (Fig. 5-25). Application of appropriate differentiation

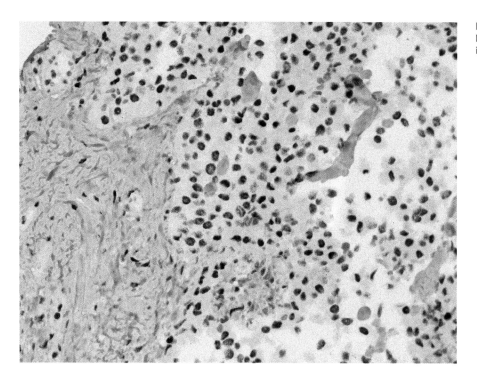

Fig. 5-26. Carcinoma with rhabdoid morphology. Nuclear expression of INI1 is nearly always retained in "rhabdoid" carcinomas.

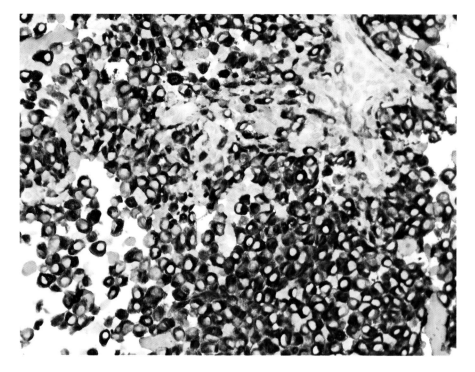

Fig. 5-27. Carcinoma with rhabdoid morphology. Diffuse expression of cytokeratin is seen in this example of rhabdoid undifferentiated carcinoma.

markers permits a correct classification in most cases. INI1 is extremely helpful, as its nuclear expression is most often (but unfortunately not always) retained in all these entities (Figs. 5-26 and 5-27). Rhabdoid features observed in an adult patient should prompt great caution in considering a diagnosis of MRT and prompt a consideration of an alternative diagnosis.

In young patients, the differential diagnosis of a tumor with rhabdoid morphology includes desmoplastic small round cell tumor (DSRCT), epithelioid rhabdomyosarcoma, and proximal-type epithelioid sarcoma (P-ES). Desmoplastic small round cell tumor occurs most often at mesothelium-lined sites in young adults, exhibits a typical polyphenotypic immunophenotype (which most often includes desmin and keratins) associated with retained expression of INI1, and is associated with the rearrangement between the genes *EWSR1* and *WT1*. Rhabdomyosarcoma typically exhibits expression of desmin and myogenin. The most challenging lesion is represented by P-ES, which may exhibit significant morphologic overlap with MRT. However, P-ES in stark contrast with MRT tends to occur in young to middle-aged adults, and approximately 50% of P-ES exhibit CD34 immunoreactivity, something that has never been reported in MRT. A further challenge is represented by the fact that carcinomas arising at various anatomic sites (most often the endometrium, gastrointestinal tract, and lungs) may feature a rhabdoid morphology. Recent data would suggest that expression of claudin represents an important diagnostic clue to separate SMARCA4-deficient carcinomas from SMARCA4-deficient sarcomas.

**Key Points in Malignant Rhabdoid Tumor Diagnosis**

- Predominant in infants and children
- Occurrence in axial deep soft tissues
- High-grade morphology featuring intracytoplasmic eosinophilic inclusions
- Loss of nuclear INI1 expression
- Highly aggressive clinical behavior

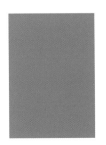

# Malignant Myoepithelioma (Myoepithelial Carcinoma)

## Definition and Epidemiology

Myoepithelial tumors of the soft tissue represent a spectrum of lesions morphologically similar to myoepithelial neoplasms of the salivary gland. Whenever a ductal component is recognized, the term "mixed tumor" is generally adopted, whereas the term "myoepithelioma" is used to designate lesions predominantly composed of myoepithelial cells. Malignant forms are generally identified with the label "myoepithelial carcinoma." Parachordoma is currently considered a variant of myoepithelioma. Myoepithelial tumors are rare and occur equally in males and females, with a peak incidence in the fourth decade. Approximately 20% of cases occur in children wherein myoepithelial carcinoma tends to predominate.

## Clinical Presentation and Behavior

Approximately two-thirds of cases arise in the limbs and limb girdles. The remaining are located in the trunk and the head and neck. Exceptional examples can be seen in the bone or at visceral sites such as the lungs. When located in the soft tissue, approximately 60% tend to be superficially located.

Myoepitheliomas exhibit a local recurrence rate of approximately 20%; however, when followed up for more

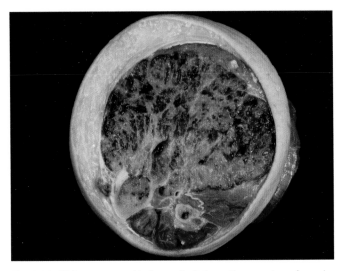

**Fig. 5-28.** Malignant myoepithelioma of soft tissue. Gross specimen from a leg amputation. The tumor mass is well circumscribed with gelatinous/myxoid areas. Infiltration of the bone is seen.

**Fig. 5-29.** Myoepithelioma of soft tissue. Sometimes a spindle cell proliferation featuring eosinophilic cytoplasm is seen.

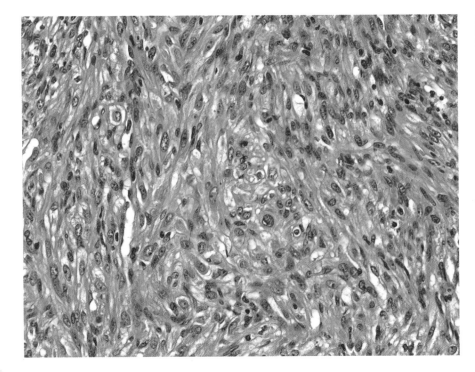

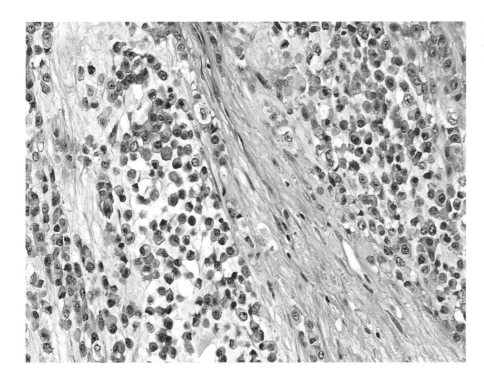

**Fig. 5-30.** Myoepithelioma of soft tissue. An epithelioid morphology is more frequently seen. Tumor cells exhibit abundant eosinophilic cytoplasm.

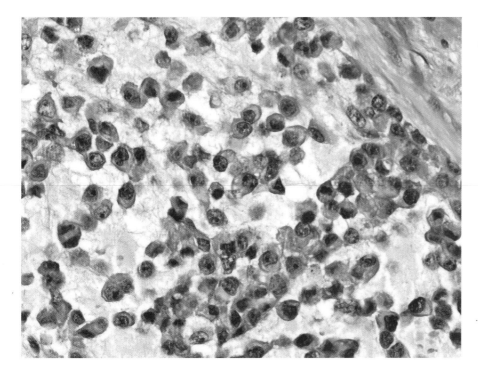

**Fig. 5-31.** Myoepithelioma of soft tissue. At high power, a "plasmocytoid" appearance of neoplastic cells is evident.

than 10 years, a metastatic rate of approximately 10% is observed. Myoepithelial carcinomas (defined as lesions with overt cytologic features of malignancy) most often are aggressive, with local recurrrences and distant metastases observed in half of the cases. The lungs represent the most frequent metastatic site, followed by lymph nodes, bone, and soft tissue.

## Morphology and Immunohistochemistry

Grossly, myoepitheliomas tend to be well circumscribed with a cut surface ranging from gelatinous to firm based on the amount of myxoid matrix. Malignant forms tend to be less well circumscribed (Fig. 5-28).

Microscopically, most cases are composed of a proliferation of spindled (Fig. 5-29) to epithelioid (often

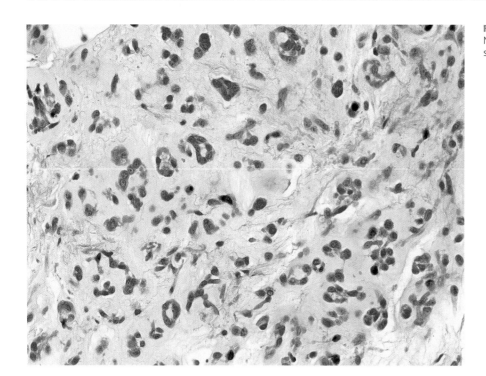

**Fig. 5-32.** Myoepithelioma of soft tissue. Neoplastic cells tend to organize in cords and strands set in a myxochondroid background.

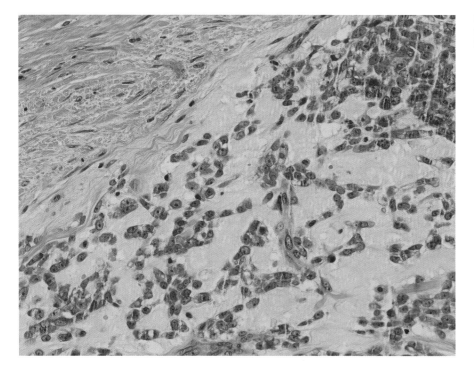

**Fig. 5-33.** Myoepithelioma of soft tissue. Areas of solid growth can be associated with the more typical cord-like pattern of growth.

plasmacytoid) cells (Figs. 5-30 and 5-31), organized in cords, strands, and trabeculae (Figs. 5-32 and 5-33) set in a myxoid or myxochondroid stroma (Fig. 5-34). In one-third of cases, the background is hyalinized (Fig. 5-35). Both myxoid and hyalinized stromata can be seen in the same lesion. A focal ductal component is detectable in approximately 10% of cases (so-called mixed tumors) (Fig. 5-36). Those cases featuring a prominent cytoplasmic vacuolization (somewhat mimicking a chordoma) in the past have been diagnosed as parachordoma (Fig. 5-37). In

about 15% of cases, cartilaginous, bone, or adipocytic metaplasia can be observed. The entity known as ectomesenchymal chondromyxoid tumor most likely represents a variant of myoepithelioma predominatly occurring in the tongue and in the oral cavity.

Myoepithelial carcinoma exhibits overt features of malignancy that include severe nuclear atypia, high mitotic activity, and necrosis (Figs. 5-38 and 5-39). Rarely, a poorly differentiated, round cell morphology can be seen (Fig. 5-40). High-grade cytology remains the best predictor of

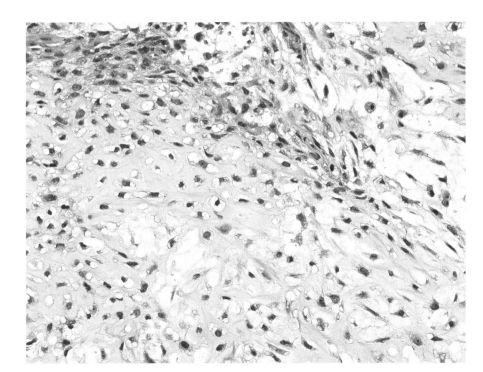

**Fig. 5-34.** Myoepithelioma of soft tissue. Chondroid appearance can at times represent a predominant feature in myoepitheliomas.

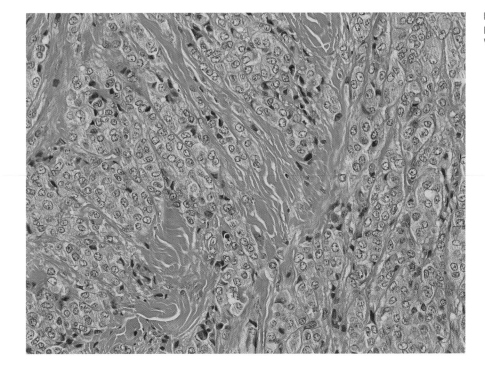

**Fig. 5-35.** Myoepithelioma of soft tissue. The presence of hyaline (instead of or in combination with the more typical myxoid stroma) can be seen.

aggressivenes (Fig. 5-41), whereas the significance of mitotic count as well as of infiltrative pattern of growth is still unclear (Fig. 5-42).

It has to be underlined that myoepitheliomas represent a spectrum of lesions in which, unless obvious high-grade morphology is present, drawing a sharp line between benign and malignant forms is at times difficult.

Immunohistochemically, up to 90% of cases express pan-keratins and S100 protein (Figs. 5-43, 5-44, and 5-45). EMA is also seen in two-thirds of cases, whereas GFAP is detected in

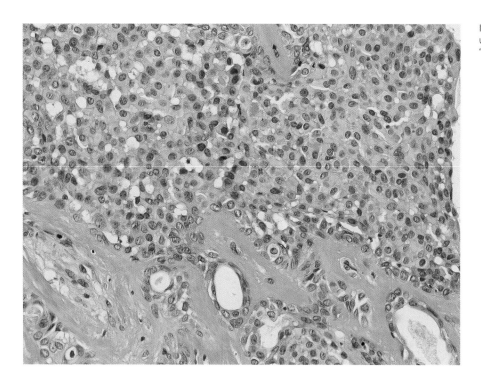

**Fig. 5-36.** Myoepithelioma of soft tissue. When unequivocal ductal differentiation is seen, the label "mixed tumor" is also used.

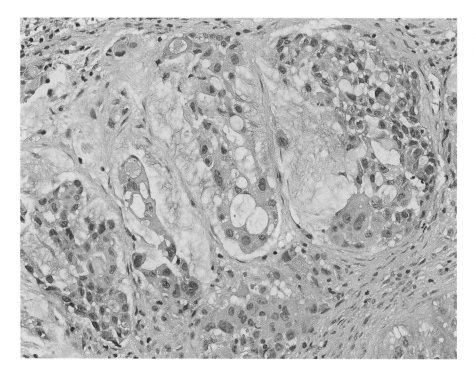

**Fig. 5-37.** Parachordoma. The presence of prominent cytoplasmic vacuolization represents the main feature of those myoepithelial neoplasms that in the past have been labeled as "parachordoma."

about 50% of tumors. Smooth muscle actin is present in one-third of cases, whereas desmin will stain no more than 10% of cases. Interestingly, in contrast to salivary gland lesions, p63 is seen in only about 20% of myoepitheliomas arising in the soft tissues. Loss of INI1/SMARCB1 is observed in approximately one-third of myoepithelial carcinomas.

## Molecular Genetics

*EWSR1* gene rearrangement occurs with an increasing variety of fusion partners (among them *PBX1, PBX3, ZNF444, POU5F1,* and *ATF1*) in approximately 50% of cases. Recently, a small subset of *EWSR1*-negative soft tissue myoepithelial (ME) tumors harboring *FUS* rearrangement was identified, and in

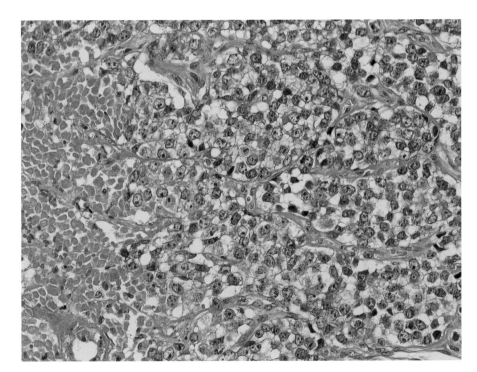

**Fig. 5-38.** Malignant myoepithelioma of soft tissue. Nuclear atypia is clearly evident in this example of malignant myoepithelioma/ myoepithelial carcinoma. In this case, abundant necrosis is seen.

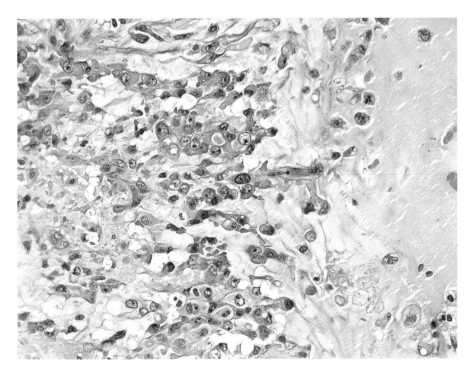

**Fig. 5-39.** Malignant myoepithelioma/ myoepithelial carcinoma of soft tissue. This tumor exhibits a solid pattern of growth.

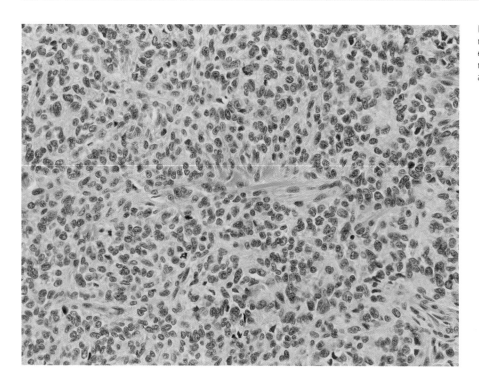

**Fig. 5-40.** Malignant myoepithelioma/ myoepithelial carcinoma of soft tissue. These lesions exhibit a poorly differentiated, round cell morphology. High mitotic activity is easily appreciated.

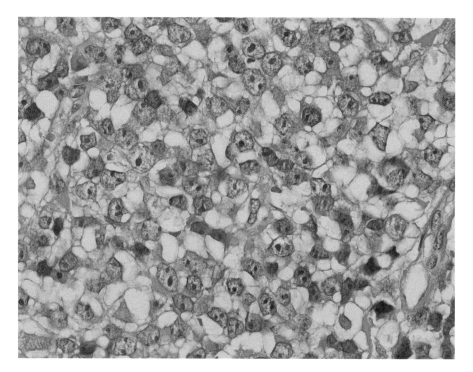

**Fig. 5-41.** Malignant myoepithelioma/ myoepithelial carcinoma of soft tissue. High-grade cytology represents the best predictor of aggressiveness.

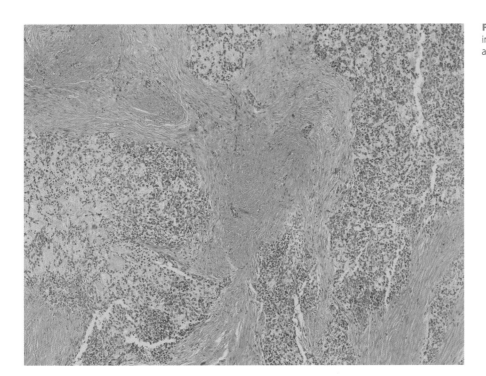

**Fig. 5-42.** Myoepithelioma of soft tissue. An infiltrative pattern of growth does not predict per se aggressive behavior in myoepithelial neoplasms.

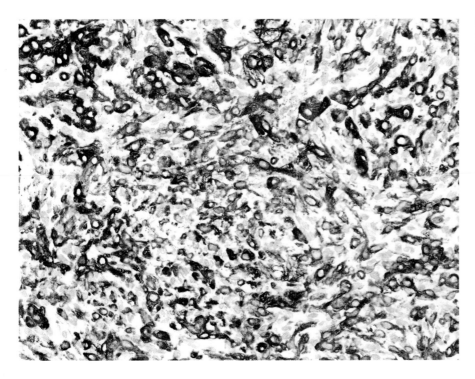

**Fig. 5-43.** Myoepithelioma of soft tissue. Variable expression of cytokeratin is seen in the vast majority of tumors.

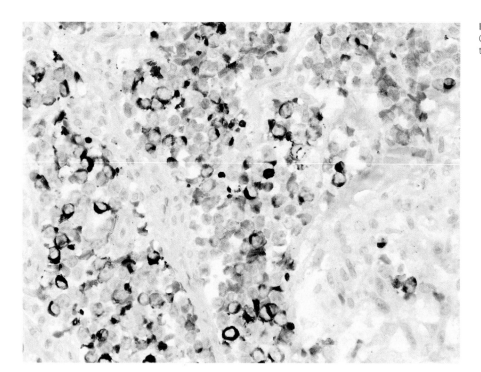

**Fig. 5-44.** Myoepithelioma of soft tissue. Cytokeratin expression at times can be focal and therefore easily overlooked.

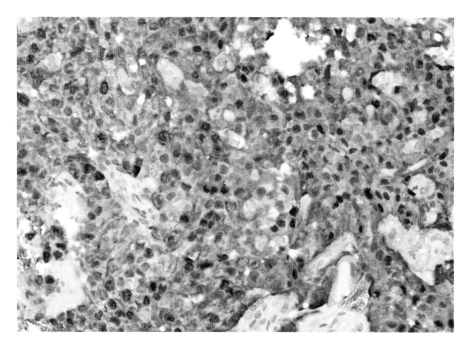

**Fig. 5-45.** Variable expression of S100 protein represents a distinctive immunophenotypical feature of myoepitheliomas.

this subset the most common fusion partner is *KLF17*. Additionally, this last gene is also found as a rare fusion partner of *EWSR1*. *SRF-E2F1* fusion represents a novel genetic aberration among *EWSR1*-negative myoepitheliomas, whereas *PLAG1* gene rearrangement is seen in a subset of myoepitheliomas of the skin and soft tissue featuring ductal differentiation.

## Differential Diagnosis and Diagnostic Pitfalls

The differential diagnosis of myoepithelial neoplasms is primarily with extraskeletal myxoid chondrosarcoma (EMC), metastatic carcinoma, ossifying fibromyxoid tumor (OFMT),

and metastatic and the very rare extra-axial chordomas. Metastatic carcinoma is generally ruled out on the basis of clinical history as well as on the expression of organ-related differentiation markers. Metastatic chordoma may overlap myoepithelial neoplasms both morphologically (epithelioid cell proliferation set in a myxoid background) and immunohistochemically (co-expression of cytokeratins and EMA) (Fig. 5-46). However, aside from pertinent clinical information, chordoma consistently exhibits nuclear expression of brachyury (including those exceptional cases arising primarily in the soft tissue), but which has never been reported in

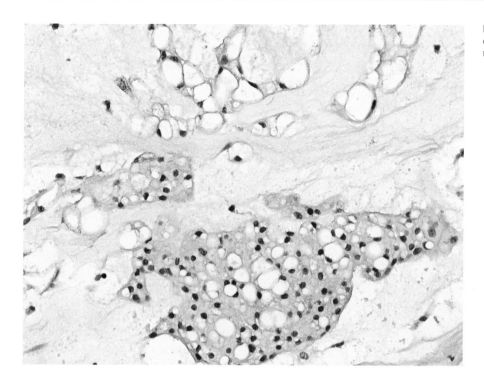

**Fig. 5-46.** Chordoma. The typical cytomorphology composed of an epithelioid cell proliferation set in a myxoid background is shown.

myoepithelial tumors. Ossifying fibromyxoid tumor is a very rare lesion composed of round to oval cell proliferation, frequently co-expressing S100 and desmin and characteristically featuring the presence of a shell of mature bone. Importantly, *PHF1* gene rearrangement is observed in OFMT.

The most challenging differential diagnosis is certainly with EMC, particularly with its high-grade forms. However, EMC tends to be negative for cytokeratins and expresses S100 protein in less than 20% of cases. Nonetheless, there exist cases in which morphologic overlap is significant and only the demonstration of specific gene rearrangements (*EWSR1-NR4A3* being the most frequent genetic aberration in EMC) allows the separation of EMC and myoepithelial tumors. Purely spindle cell myoepitheliomas may be confused with neural neoplasms; however, the expression of epithelial/myoepithelial differentiation markers represent a helpful diagnostic clue. As both myoepithelioma

and EMC share rearrangement of the *EWSR1* gene, fluorescence in situ hybridization (FISH) analysis is not discriminant.

---

**Key Points in Soft Tissue Myoepithelioma/Myoepithelial Carcinoma Diagnosis**

- Spindle/epithelioid proliferation often set in a myxochondroid background
- Benign lesions prevail in adult patients
- Myoepithelial carcinoma shows a peak in the pediatric age-group
- Superficial location most frequent
- Expression of epithelial/myoepithelial differentiation markers and S100 protein
- *EWSR1* and *PLAG1* gene rearrangements mutually exclusive

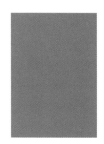

# Pseudomyogenic Hemangioendothelioma

## Definition and Epidemiology

Pseudomyogenic hemangioendothelioma (PMH) is more frequent in males (male-to-female ratio 5:1) with a median age of 30 years, and more than 90% of neoplasms are diagnosed between the second and fifth decade of life. Its first description most likely dates back to 1992, when Mirra and coworkers described four different "histologic pattern subvariants" of epithelioid sarcoma: (1) a granuloma-like variant; (2) an angiosarcoma-like variant; (3) a rhabdoid sarcoma variant; and (4) a rare fibroma-like variant. This last entity was described as a neoplasm composed of a mixture of fibrohistiocytic/myoid cells interspersed among an inflammatory milieu, typically located in the distal extremities of middle-aged men, with a multifocal distribution in the same anatomic region from cutis to bone.

Two subsequent studies have provided a more detailed description of this lesion. In 2003, Billings and colleagues described a series of soft tissue neoplasms with some morphologic and immunophenotypical features in common with ES. Despite the fact that there wasn't clear morphologic evidence of vascular differentiation, the authors demonstrated the expression of some endothelial markers, therefore proposing the term "epithelioid sarcoma–like hemangioendothelioma." More recently, a far larger series was published by Hornick and Fletcher that fully elucidates the clinicopathologic spectrum of this rare lesion, proposing the label "pseudomyogenic hemangioendothelioma" (PMH). This term contains the most relevant morphologic and prognostic features of the neoplasm, highlighting the histopathologic, myogenic-like aspect of the neoplastic cells, the presence of endothelial differentiation, and a rather indolent clinical behavior.

## Clinical Presentation and Behavior

The lower extremities are the most frequently affected anatomic sites, including buttock, thigh, lower leg, ankle, and foot. Less frequently, PMH occurs in the upper extremities, trunk, abdominal wall, and head and neck. Multifocal disease, ranging from 2 to 15 foci, is seen in approximately two-thirds of cases with the involvement of multiple planes of the same anatomic region (dermis, subcutis, skeletal muscle, and underlying bone).

## Morphology and Immunohistochemistry

Macroscopically, tumor nodules are well circumscribed with a tan or white, fibrous to fleshy cut surface (Fig. 5-47).

Microscopically, neoplastic cells are organized in a loose fascicular or sheet-like arrangement, infiltrating the surrounding tissue (Fig. 5-48). Lesional cells exhibit a variable morphology, ranging from plump spindle cells with vesicular nuclei and evident nucleoli (Fig. 5-49) to more epithelioid (Fig. 5-50), rhabdomyoblastic-like elements featuring abundant bright eosinophilic cytoplasm (Fig. 5-51). A myxoid stroma can be noted in some cases (Fig. 5-52). One common feature is the conspicuous inflammatory background, ranging from scattered elements over the neoplastic cells to a dense, prominent infiltrate (Fig. 5-53). Nuclear atypia is generally mild to moderate; however, cases exist in which severe atypia is recognized. Mitotic activity is scant and necrosis rare; however, vascular invasion has been described in a few cases. As Mirra and colleagues had earlier emphasized, the histologic features of the recurrent lesions might be different with a higher degree of atypia and an increased mitotic index with some atypical mitoses.

Despite the pseudomyoid or epithelial-like appearance and the absence of obvious vasoformative morphology, neoplastic cells exhibit immunophenotypic features of endothelial differentiation. Together with the expression of cytokeratin AE1/AE3 (Fig. 5-54), all tumors are positive for FLI1, ERG

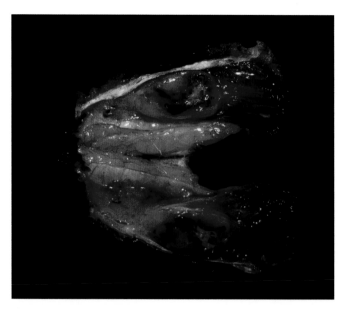

**Fig. 5-47.** Pseudomyogenic hemangioendothelioma. Gross specimen showing a deep-seated, well-circumscribed, fleshy nodule featuring hemorrhagic foci is seen here.

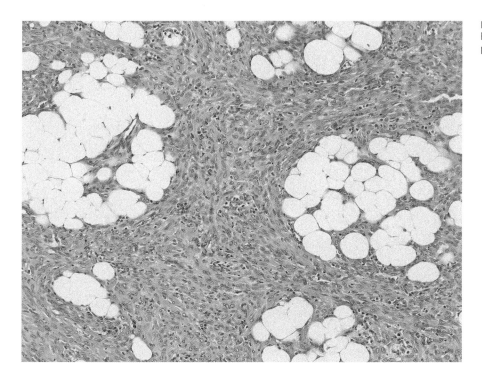

**Fig. 5-48.** Pseudomyogenic hemangioendothelioma. Neoplastic cell proliferation infiltrating the adipose tissue is seen.

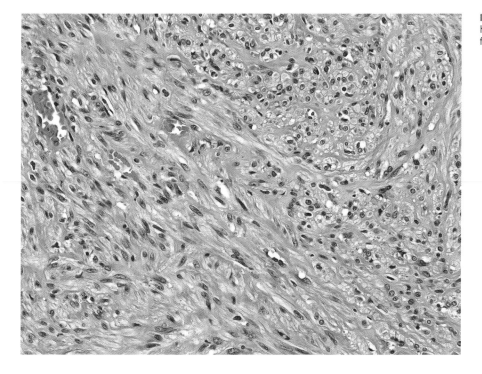

**Fig. 5-49.** Pseudomyogenic hemangioendothelioma. Neoplastic cells range from spindled to an epithelioid shape.

(Fig. 5-55A) and, as a result of the *SERPINE1-FOSB* fusion, strong nuclear expression of FOSB protein is observed (Fig. 5-55B). Multifocal CD31 immunopositivity is seen in approximately 50% of cases. Noteworthy, all tumors tend to be CD34 negative and show preserved nuclear expression of INI1 (SNF5/SMARCB1), further supporting the absence of any relationships with ES.

## Molecular Genetics

Recently, a novel translocation, t(7;19)(q22;q13), has been identified, resulting in the fusion of the *SERPINE1* and *FOSB* genes that further supports the fact that PMH represents a distinctive clinicopathologic entity. This translocation has not been observed thus far in any other bone or soft tissue tumor; therefore, it could be useful for differential diagnostic purposes.

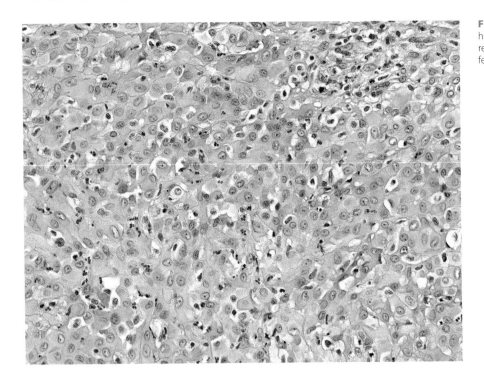

**Fig. 5-50.** Pseudomyogenic hemangioendothelioma. In this example, a relatively monomorphic epithelioid cell population featuring abundant eosinophilic cytoplasm is seen.

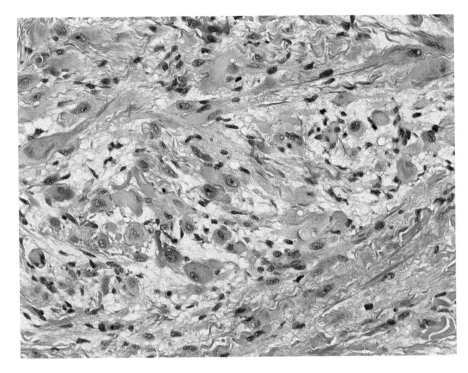

**Fig. 5-51.** Pseudomyogenic hemangioendothelioma. The "myogenic" appearance of tumor cells predominates to the extent that neoplastic cells mimic rhabdomyoblasts.

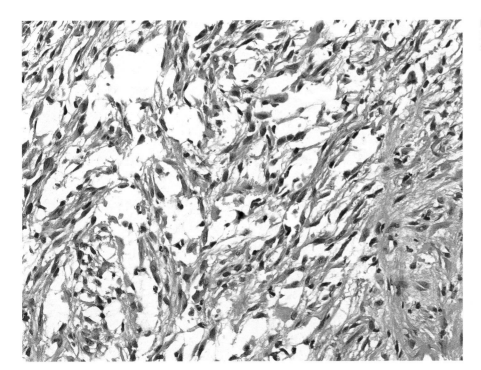

**Fig. 5-52.** Pseudomyogenic hemangioendothelioma. Myxoid change of the stroma is observed relatively often.

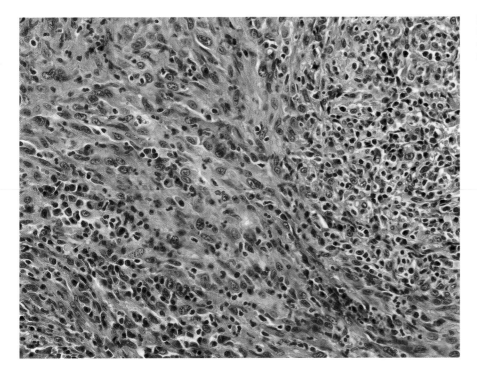

**Fig. 5-53.** Pseudomyogenic hemangioendothelioma. The presence of a conspicuous inflammatory background represents a common feature.

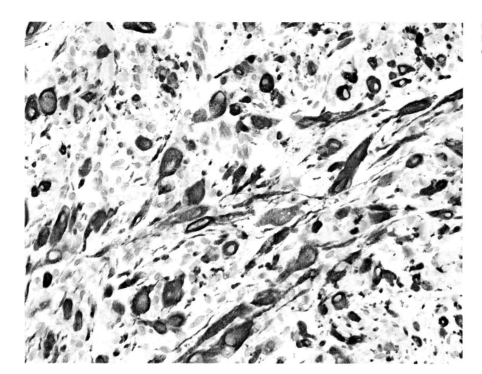

**Fig. 5-54.** Pseudomyogenic hemangioendothelioma. Diffuse expression of cytokeratin AE1/AE3 is typically seen.

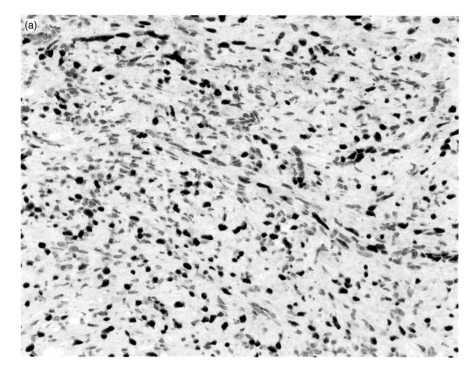

**Fig. 5-55A.** Pseudomyogenic hemangioendothelioma. ERG nuclear immunopositivity is seen in this example. FLI1 would show overlapping results.

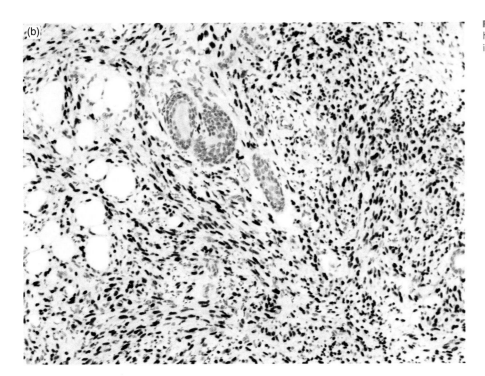

(b)

**Fig. 5-55B.** Pseudomyogenic hemangioendothelioma. FOSB nuclear immunopositivity is seen.

## Differential Diagnosis and Diagnostic Pitfalls

Pseudomyogenic hemangioendothelioma needs to be kept separate from ES. Despite some clinical similarities with ES, PMH exhibits a distinctive myoid appearance, as well as the absence of the "geographic" necrosis so typical of ES. Importantly, ES features loss of nuclear expression of INI1, which, by contrast, is always retained in pseudomyogenic hemangioendothelioma. True myogenic neoplasms are excluded on the basis of the absence of the expression of myogenic markers. As reported in a subsequent section of this chapter, epithelioid hemangioendothelioma expresses keratins only focally, is FOSB negative, and, most important, exhibits nuclear expression of CAMTA1 (or TFE3 in a subset of lesions).

As multiple sites of bone localization can be observed relatively often and in consideration of co-expression of cytokeratin AE1/AE3 and ERG, metastatic prostatic carcinoma needs to be carefully excluded.

**Key Points in Pseudomyogenic Hemangioendothelioma Diagnosis**

- Predominance in male adults
- Often multicentric
- Involvement of multiple anatomic planes
- Spindle/epithelioid cell morphology
- Co-expression of cytokeratin AE1/AE3, endothelial differentiation markers, and FOSB
- *SERPINE1-FOSB* gene fusion
- Indolent clinical course

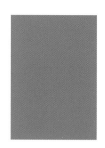

# Epithelioid Hemangioendothelioma

## Definition and Epidemiology

Epithelioid hemangioendothelioma (EHE) is an angiocentric malignant vascular neoplasm featuring striking epithelioid morphology. Soft tissue EHE occurs in almost all age-groups without sex predilection, whereas liver and lung forms predominate in females. In children, it seems to be exceedingly rare.

## Clinical Presentation and Behavior

Epithelioid hemangioendothelioma arises predominantly in the superficial or deep soft tissues of the extremities. Approximately half of the cases show the origin as being the blood vessels. The entity formerly know as intravascular bronchioloalveolar tumor (IVBAT) is currently regarded as a primary pulmonary EHE. Bone and liver can also be involved as primary sites. In general, visceral location is associated with multicentricity, which should not be mistaken for metastatic disease. Epithelioid hemangioendothelioma tends to recur locally in about 20% of cases, and in its classic form, the metastatic rate is less than 20%. The presence of atypical histology (so-called malignant EHE) raises metastatic rates up to 30%. In consideration of this clinical behavior, EHE can no longer be included in the intermediate category and therefore the current WHO classification of soft tissue tumors considers EHE a fully malignant neoplasm. Recent clinical experience would indicate the visceral forms (with the important exception of pleural cases that exhibit significant aggressiveness) may exhibit a rather indolent clinical course when compared with soft tissue EHE.

## Morphology and Immunohistochemistry

Morphologically, EHE is composed of rounded epithelioid eosinophilic cells, organized in strands, cords, or solid nests (Fig. 5-56), often harboring intracytoplasmic vacuoles that may rarely contain red blood cells (Fig. 5-57), set in a myxochondroid background with hemorrhagic foci (Fig. 5-58). In rare cases, neoplastic cells may organize in a cribriform pattern of growth that may mimic invasive carcinoma (Fig. 5-59). Low mitotic activity is generally observed. Approximately 30% of cases feature marked cytologic atypia with prominent nucleoli, focal solid growth pattern, foci of necrosis, and higher mitotic activity (>2 mitoses/10 high-power fields [HPF]), which is associated with more aggressive behavior (Fig. 5-60). As anticipated, these cases are currently termed "malignant EHE."

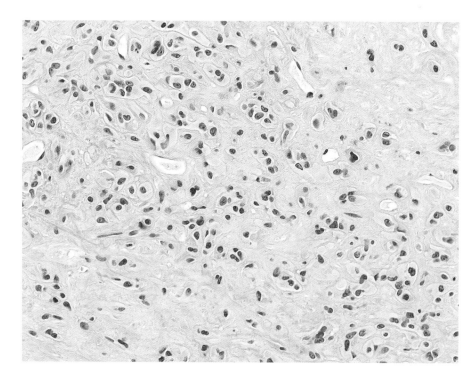

**Fig. 5-56.** Epithelioid hemangioendothelioma. A proliferation of epithelioid eosinophilic cells, organized in strands, cords, or solid nests, is typically seen.

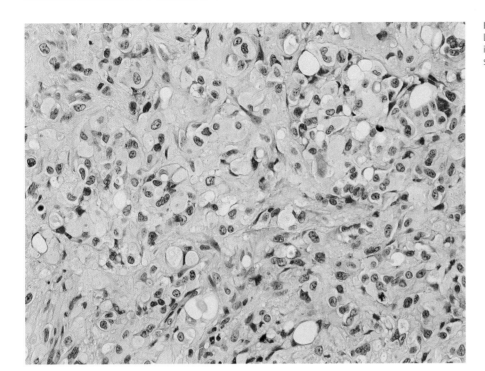

**Fig. 5-57.** Epithelioid hemangioendothelioma. Lesional cells characteristically contain intracytoplasmic vacuoles. Higher nuclear atypia is seen.

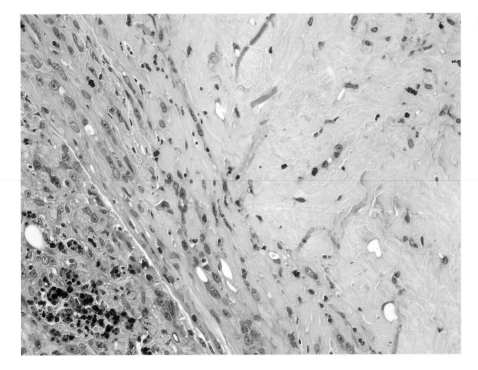

**Fig. 5-58.** Epithelioid hemangioendothelioma. Tumor cells are set in myxochondroid stroma.

When occurring in the lungs, EHE maintains the cytomorphology described above. However, in consideration of its tendency to fill the pulmonary alveoli, it may acquire a distinctive alveolar growth pattern (Fig. 5-61). Liver examples may be challenging, as neoplastic endothelial cells show a tendency to grow in between hepatocytes, somewhat preserving, at first glance, normal liver histology. As most cases are diagnosed on core biopsies, careful examination is mandatory in order to identify the lesion (Figs. 5-62 and 5-63). Immunohistochemically, EHE consistently expresses endothelial differentiation markers such as CD31, CD34, FLI1, and ERG (Fig. 5-64). Focal cytokeratin immunopositivity is observed in less than one-third of cases. Only occasionally can the expression of epithelial differentiation markers be strong and diffuse. Importantly, it has been recently shown that, as a consequence of both *WWTR1-CAMTA1* and *YAP1-TFE3* fusions (see below), nuclear expression of CAMTA1 and TFE3 is consistently observed (Fig. 5-65). TFE3-positive EHE is more vasoformative than is CAMTA1-positive EHE, and it is possible that in the future it will be regarded as a distinctive variant of epithelioid vascular lesions (Fig. 5-66).

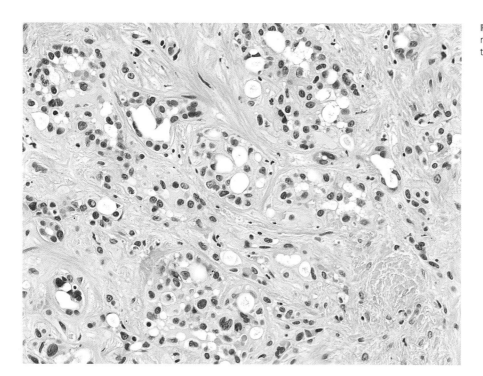

**Fig. 5-59.** Epithelioid hemangioendothelioma. In rare examples, a cribriform pattern of growth is seen that may mimic invasive carcinoma.

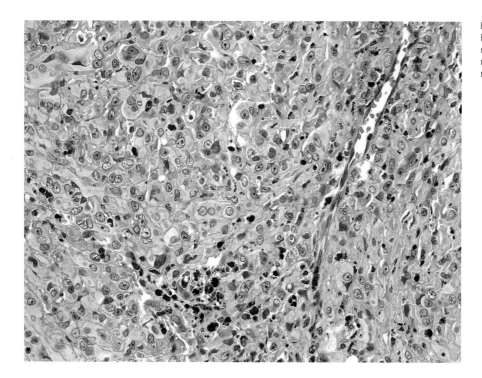

**Fig. 5-60.** Malignant epithelioid hemangioendothelioma. Tumor cells show severe nuclear atypia, focal solid pattern of growth, and mitotic figures. These features are associated with more aggressive clinical behavior.

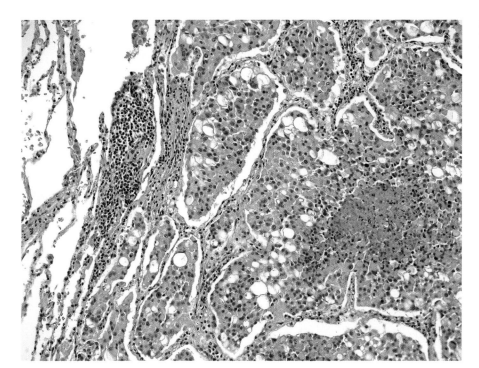

**Fig. 5-61.** Epithelioid hemangioendothelioma of the lungs. Neoplastic cells show a remarkable tendency to fill the pulmonary alveoli.

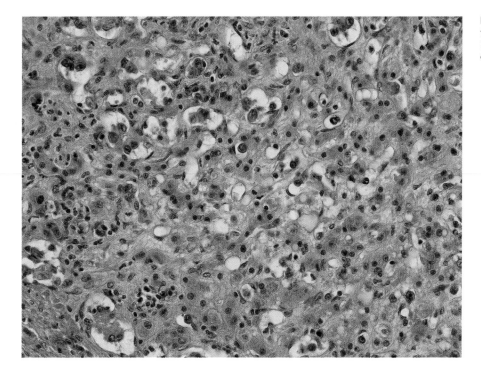

**Fig. 5-62.** Epithelioid hemangioendothelioma of the liver. The infiltrative growth in between residual liver cells can make the identification of neoplastic endothelial cells challenging.

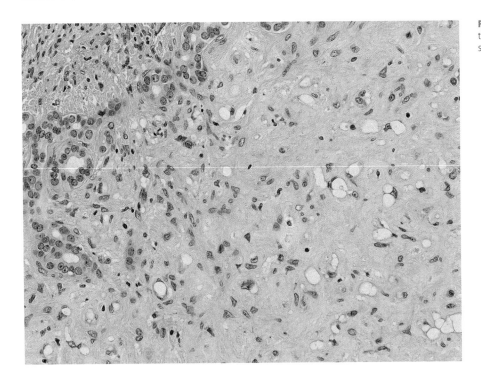

**Fig. 5-63.** Epithelioid hemangioendothelioma of the liver. Residual biliary ducts alongside EHE are seen.

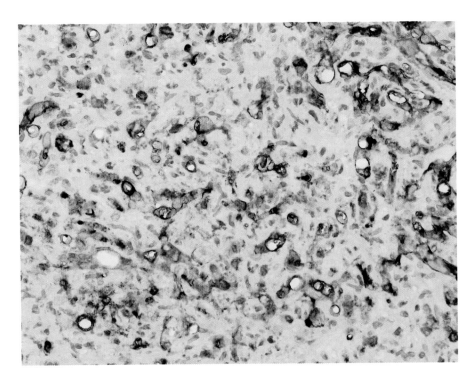

**Fig. 5-64.** Epithelioid hemangioendothelioma. CD31 usefully decorates neoplastic endothelial cells, highlighting the typical cord-like growth pattern.

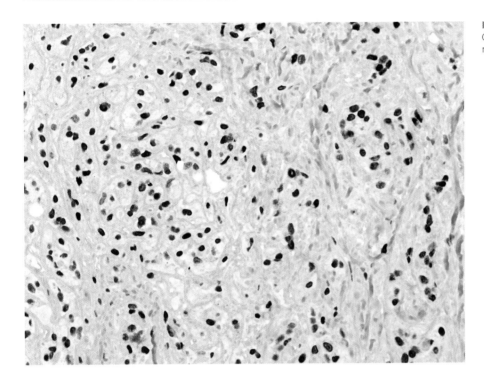

**Fig. 5-65.** Epithelioid hemangioendothelioma. CAMTA1 nuclear expression represents a novel marker, showing high specificity.

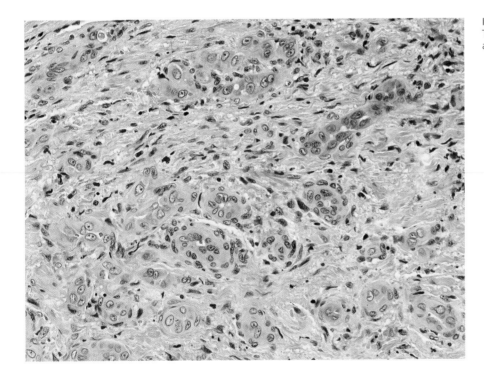

**Fig. 5-66.** Epithelioid hemangioendothelioma. Tumors harboring a *YAP1-TFE3* fusion tend to exhibit a more vasoformative morphology.

## Molecular Genetics

Epithelioid hemangioendothelioma harbors a translocation, t(1;3)(p36.3;q25), that leads to the formation of a *WWTR1-CAMTA1* fusion gene. Very recently, a new genetic aberration, represented by a *YAP1-TFE3* fusion, has been observed in a subset of t(1;3)-negative, morphologically distinct EHEs.

## Differential Diagnosis and Diagnostic Pitfalls

The main differential diagnosis is with primary and metastatic carcinomas (in particular, signet-ring adenocarcinoma metastatic to the pleura); however, consistent expression of endothelial differentiation markers represents a helpful diagnostic clue. As mentioned, the expression of cytokeratin in EHE is generally focal, and those rare cases showing diffuse

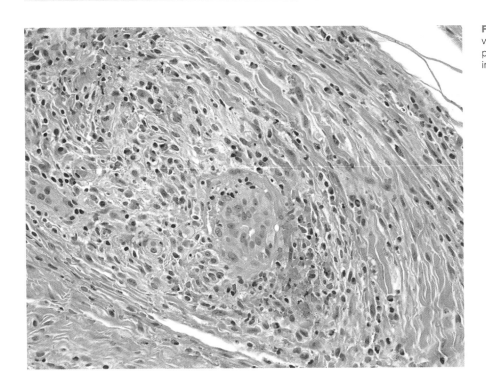

**Fig. 5-67A.** Epithelioid hemangioma. A blood vessel obliterated by an epithelioid endothelial proliferation is seen. Typically, an inflammatory infiltrate rich in eosinophils is present.

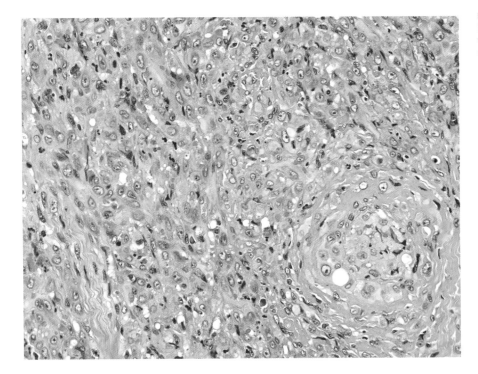

**Fig. 5-67B.** Cellular epithelioid hemangioma. The lesion features higher cellularity when compared with classic epithelioid hemangioma. Some degree of nuclear atypia is also present.

expression may represent a real diagnostic challenge. When dealing with pleural cases, malignant mesothelioma also enters the differential diagnosis. Expression of epithelial differentiation markers, calretinin, and WT1, as well as negativity for endothelial differentiation markers, generally allows accurate diagnosis.

Epithelioid sarcoma may enter the differential diagnosis in consideration of the frequently observed expression of CD34; however, all the true endothelial differentiation markers are consistently negative (with the notable exception of ERG), cytokeratin is invariably and diffusely present in most neoplastic cells, and, as repeatedly mentioned, loss of nuclear INI1 expression is most often observed.

Epithelioid morphology is typically seen in **epithelioid hemangioma** as well as in **epithelioid angiomatous nodules**. However, both lesions are clearly vasoformative, and vascular spaces are accompanied by a smooth muscle, actin-positive pericytic component. Epithelioid hemangioma can be

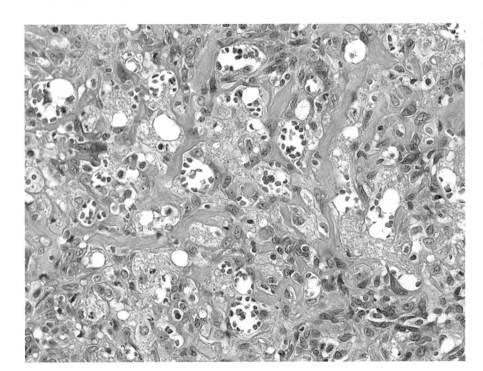

**Fig. 5-68.** Epithelioid angiomatous nodule. This distinctively unilobular intradermal vascular proliferation may feature at times a worrisome cytomorphology.

distinctively cellular; however, nuclear atypia is generally absent. The presence of a mixed inflammatory infiltrate rich in eosinophils is frequently seen (Fig. 5-67A). Recently, a cellular variant of epithelioid hemangioma was reported that featured greater cellularity and multifocal cytologic atypia (Fig. 5-67B). Frequent location on the penis shaft has been recorded, and preliminary data would indicate frequent nuclear expression of FOSB. Epithelioid angiomatous nodules may feature moderate nuclear atypia (and, in fact, most of these lesions in the past were regarded as early examples of epithelioid angiosarcomas); however, their distinctive unilobular silhouette, easily recognizable at low magnification, and the intradermal location allow recognition in most cases (Fig. 5-68).

**Key Points in Epithelioid Hemangioendothelioma Diagnosis**

- Occurrence in the superficial and deep soft tisues of the extremities of adult patients
- Half of the cases are angiocentric
- Lungs, liver, and bone are the most common visceral sites
- Morphology predicts behavior, with cytologic atypia associated with higher metastatic rate
- CAMTA1 expressed in the majority of cases
- Malignant lesion with metastatic rate ranging between 15 and 30%

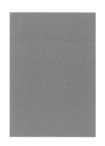

# Epithelioid Angiosarcoma of Soft Tissue

## Definition and Epidemiology

Epithelioid angiosarcoma (EAS) of soft tissue is a high-grade malignancy showing endothelial differentiation that can occur at any age, with a peak incidence in the seventh decade.

## Clinical Presentation and Behavior

Typical presentation is represented by a deep-seated soft tissue mass located in the lower extremities. A significant proportion is observed in the abdominal location or in other visceral sites. Lungs, adrenal glands, heart, and thyroid also represent relatively frequent sites. Multifocality is rarely observed. Soft tissue angiosarcoma has been reported in the context of NF1-associated benign or malignant nerve sheath tumors, and exceptionally it may arise in the context of benign hemangiomas or vascular malformations. Epithelioid angiosarcoma is a very aggressive mesenchymal malignancy to the extent that one-half of patients are expected to die within 1 year after diagnosis. Overall survival at 5 years does not exceed 20%. Distant metastases are most often detected in the lungs, lymph nodes, bone, and soft tissue. Systemic therapy with taxanes or gemcitabine may result in temporary regression of the disease; however, overall prognosis remains dismal.

## Morphology and Immunohistochemistry

Grossly, angiosarcomas of soft tissue most often present as large hemorragic as well as necrotic masses (Fig. 5-69).

The existence of malignant endothelial tumors featuring an epithelioid morphology was first recognized by Rosai in

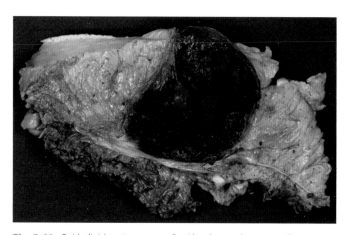

**Fig. 5-69.** Epithelioid angiosarcoma. Grossly, a hemorrhagic as well as necrotic mass is shown.

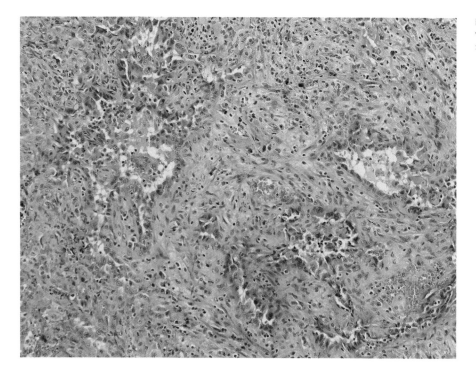

**Fig. 5-70.** Epithelioid angiosarcoma. Irregular vascular spaces lined by epithelioid cells featuring severe cytologic atypia are seen.

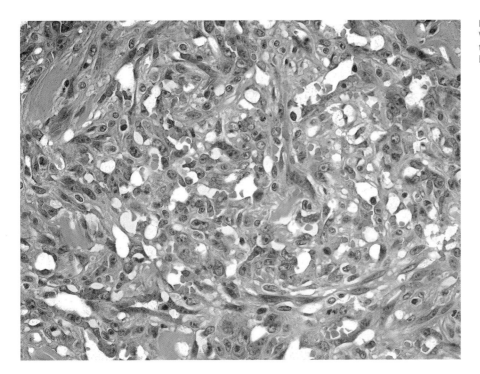

**Fig. 5-71.** Epithelioid angiosarcoma. Vasoformative features in this example are limited to the presence of anastomosing vascular spaces lined by atypical cells.

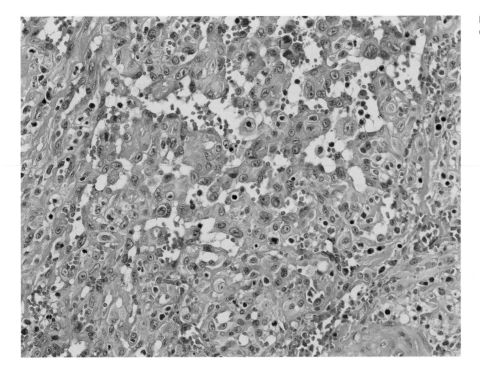

**Fig. 5-72.** Epithelioid angiosarcoma. Tumor cells contain vesicular, macronucleolated nuclei.

cutaneous angiosarcoma and in the thyroid well before it was reported in the soft tissue. Microscopically, EAS is composed of an admixture of spindle and epithelioid cells, with variable (from overt to none) vasoformative morphology (Figs. 5-70, 5-71). In contrast to cutaneous angiosarcoma, epithelioid morphology is more often observed in lesions arising in the deep soft tissues. Typically, neoplastic cells exhibit a large eosinophilic cytoplasm along with distinctive vesicular,

macronucleolated, and often eosinophilic nuclei (Fig. 5-72). Rare cases may feature a predominantly solid growth pattern mimicking a carcinoma (Figs. 5-73 and 5-74).

Immunohistochemically, CD31 (Fig. 5-75), FLI1, and ERG (Fig. 5-76) appear to be the most useful diagnostic markers. It should be remembered that EAS also expresses epithelial differentiation markers such as EMA and cytokeratins in approximately one-third of cases (Fig. 5-77).

263

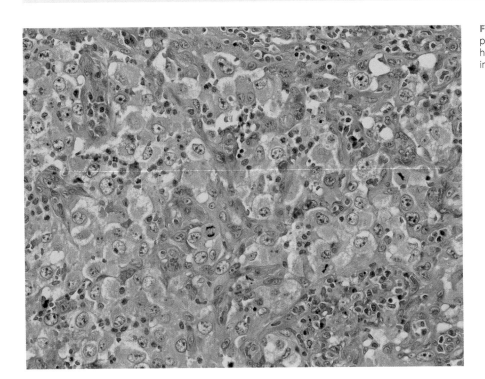

**Fig. 5-73.** Epithelioid angiosarcoma. A solid pattern of growth can be observed associated with high mitotic count. Nuclear features represent an important diagnostic clue.

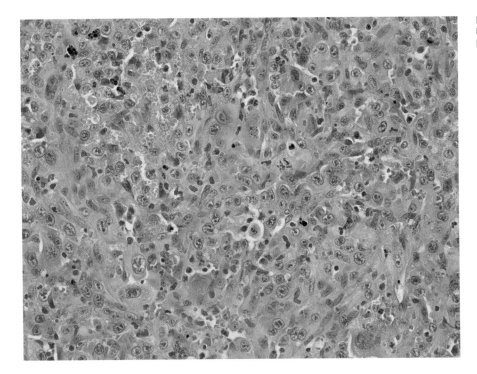

**Fig. 5-74.** Epithelioid angiosarcoma. Undifferentiated EAS can present with a "carcinoma-like"morphology.

## Molecular Genetics

From a genetic standpoint, almost all cases of angiosarcoma tested exhibited complex karyotypic aberrations. As is discussed in Chapter 10, *C-MYC* amplification has been observed in cutaneous angiosarcoma associated with radiotherapy but not in angiosarcoma of deep soft tissues. A recent report has,

however, reported the same alteration in non-RT-associated cutaneous angiosarcomas. *KDR* gene mutations have been reported to occur in approximately 10% of angiosarcomas. Very recently, the presence of recurrent *CIC* gene alterations (including a *CIC-LEUTX* gene fusion in one case) has been reproted in 9% of angiosarcomas featuring solid, epithelioid morphology.

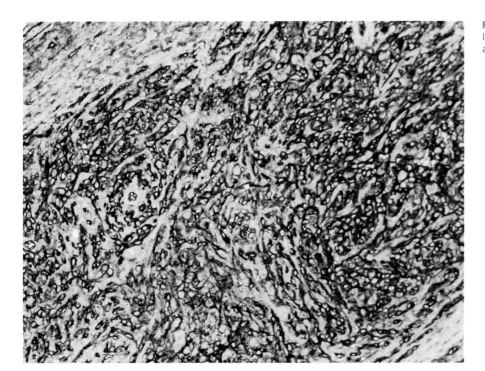

**Fig. 5-75.** Epithelioid angiosarcoma. Immunopositivity for CD31 in tumor cells represents a consistent finding.

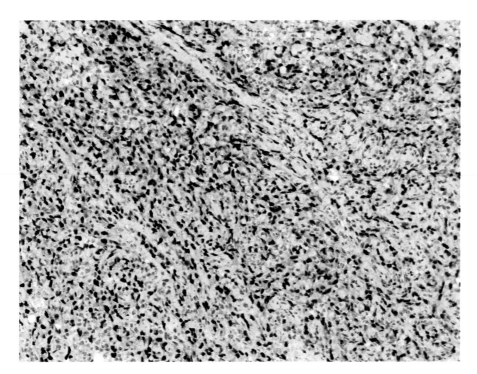

**Fig. 5-76.** Epithelioid angiosarcoma. The novel vascular marker ERG represents a sensitive (but less specific than CD31) marker.

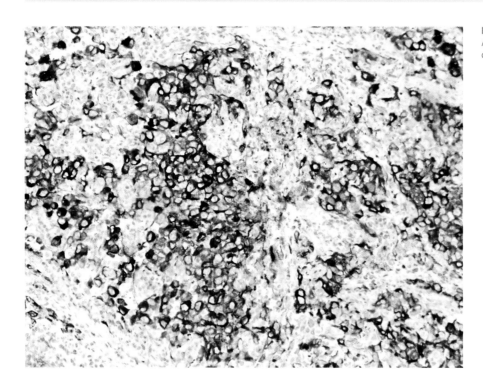

**Fig. 5-77.** Epithelioid angiosarcoma. Approximately one-third of cases express cytokeratin.

## Differential Diagnosis and Diagnostic Pitfalls

Undifferentiated, solid variants of angiosarcoma should be differentiated from metastatic carcinoma as well as from other epithelioid malignancies. Epithelioid angiosarcoma may mimic the angiomatous variant of ES, both in morphology and by the occasional expression of cytokeratin. However, it usually shows more pleomorphism and usually expresses CD31 and ERG. The fact that ES may express CD34 in half of the cases certainly represents a major potential trap.

Differentiating so-called malignant EHE from epithelioid angiosarcoma is sometimes very difficult; however, the presence of extensive solid growth should be generally regarded as a diagnostic clue in favor of EAS. Absence of nuclear expression of CAMTA1/TFE3 also represents a key diagnostic feature of the exclusion of EHE.

A further important diagnostic pitfall is represented by the fact that CD31 also stains intratumoral histiocytes that at times may be abundantly represented. Careful localization of CD31 expression in tumor cells is crucial, also remembering that, in contrast to the more diffuse as well as weaker staining generally observed in histiocytes, neoplastic endothelial cells usually exhibit crisp and intense CD31 membrane staining. Although ERG does not stain histiocyctes, remember that it also decorates prostatic carcinoma.

---

**Key Points in Epithelioid Angiosarcoma Diagnosis**

- Predominance in deep soft tissue of elderly patients
- Striking epithelioid morphology featuring macronucleolated vesicular nuclei
- Vasoformative features may be minimal or absent
- Consistent expression of endothelial differentiation markers
- Highly aggressive malignancy

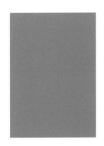

# Epithelioid Malignant Peripheral Nerve Sheath Tumor

## Definition and Epidemiology

Epithelioid malignant peripheral nerve sheath tumor (E-MPNST) represents a distinctive rare variant of MPNST, accounting for approximately 5% of all neural malignancies. Peak incidence is between the third and fourth decade, and generally there is no or only occasional association with neurofibromatosis type 1 (NF1) syndrome. No sex predilection has been observed. Rare cases have been reported arising in the context of benign schwannomas, either sporadic or schwannomatosis related.

## Clinical Presentation and Behavior

Epithelioid MPNST most frequently affects the limbs, the trunk, and the inguinal region. Interestingly, half of the cases arise in the superficial soft tissue or even in the deep dermis. In up to half of the cases, E-MPNST appears to be associated with large nerves or a pre-existing benign neural neoplasm (primarily schwannomas). Clinical behavior for deep-seated tumors is traditionally believed to overlap that of ordinary MPNST, with an overall survival at 5 years approximately 50% in sporadic cases. Metastatic spread to pleura, lungs, and liver is frequently detected. Those 50% of cases arising in the superficial soft tissue pursue a much

better clinical course with prolonged survival. Recent data would actually suggest better outcome (when compared with classic MPNST) also for deep-seated E-MPNST. As for ordinary MPNST, complete surgery represents the therapeutic mainstay.

## Morphology and Immunohistochemistry

Microscopically, E-MPNST usually exhibits a multinodular growth pattern (Fig. 5-78) and is composed of nests and cords of eosinophilic epithelioid cells harboring vesicular, macronucleolated nuclei. Cell clusters are separated by delicate fibrous septa (Fig. 5-79). Sometimes a mucinous background can be observed. Mitotic activity is usually brisk (Fig. 5-80). Perivascular accentuation of cellularity (as in ordinary MPNST) can be observed (Fig. 5-81). At variance with classic MPNST, in which S100 protein stains a minority of cells in no more than half of the cases, epithelioid MPNST usually exhibits strong immunopositivity for S100 in most neoplastic cells (Fig. 5-82). It has also been shown recently that approximately 50% of E-MPNST can exhibit loss of nuclear SMARCB1/INI1 immunoreactivity (Fig. 5-83). Personal experience would indicate that SMARCB1/INI1 loss may be seen even more frequently.

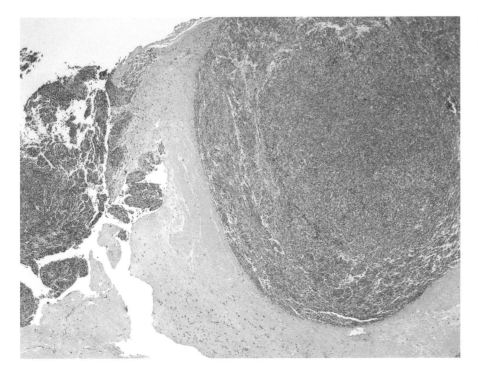

**Fig. 5-78.** Epithelioid MPNST. At low magnification, the tumor often exhibits a multinodular pattern of growth.

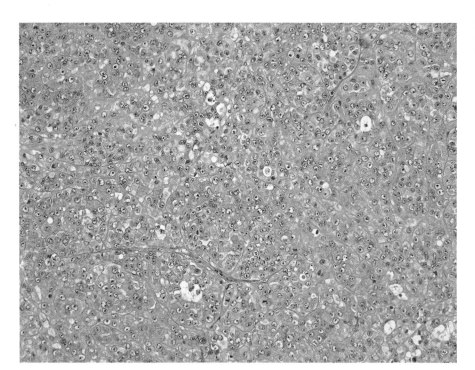

**Fig. 5-79.** Epithelioid MPNST. Clusters of epithelioid neoplastic cells separated by delicate fibrous septa are seen.

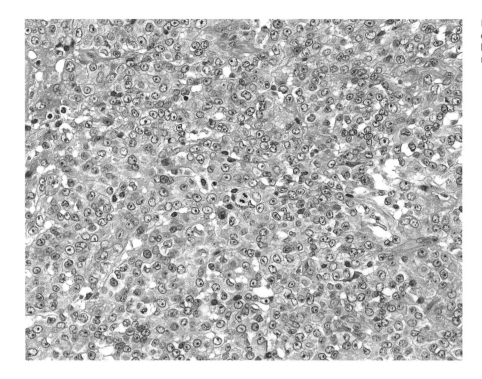

**Fig. 5-80.** Epithelioid MPNST. Neoplastic cells exhibit eosinophilic cytoplasm and vesicular nuclei harboring large, centrally located nucleoli. Brisk mitotic activity is generally seen.

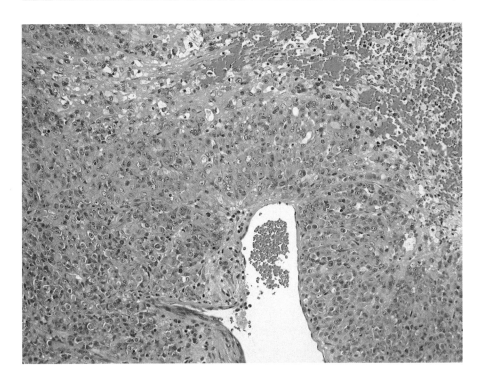

**Fig. 5-81.** Epithelioid MPNST. Perivascular accentuation of celluarity is often seen.

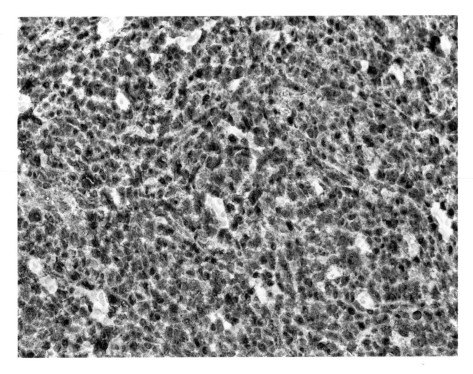

**Fig. 5-82.** Epithelioid MPNST. In contrast to ordinary MPNST, tumor cells feature diffuse S100-positive immunoreactivity.

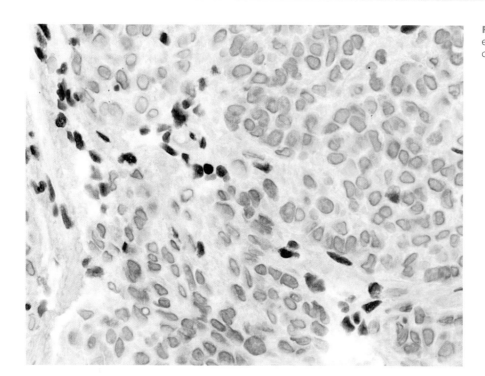

Fig. 5-83. Epithelioid MPNST. Loss of nuclear expression of INI1 is observed in at least half of the cases.

## Molecular Genetics

The relationship between loss of SMARCB1/INI1 and molecular status is poorly understood. Recently, however, a case of E-MPNST developing in a woman with schwannomatosis associated with germline mutation of the *SMARCB1* gene was reported.

## Differential Diagnosis and Diagnostic Pitfalls

The main differential diagnosis is with metastatic amelanotic malignant melanoma. Important differential diagnostic clues are represented by the presence of spindle cell areas (as in ordinary MPNST) and immunonegativity for melanoma markers such as HMB45, MITF-1, or Melan-A.

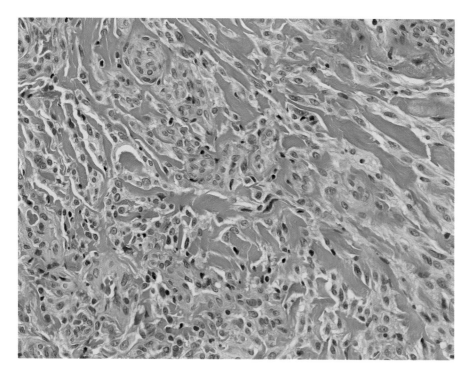

Fig. 5-84. Epithelioid schwannoma. Lesional cells lack cytologic atypia (in particular, macronucleoli are not seen) and mitotic activity is generally absent.

Melanoma does not lose the expression of SMARCB1/INI1. Careful clinical examination by an experienced dermatologist is also strongly advised. Clear cell sarcoma (melanoma of soft parts) also must be differentiated from epithelioid MPNST. In addition to positivity for melanoma markers, clear cell sarcomas most often harbor a rearrangement of the *EWSR1* gene that can be exploited for diagnostic purposes.

Epithelioid benign schwannoma is relatively easily separated from E-MPNST on the basis of the absence of significant atypia as well as mitotic activity (Fig. 5-84). A major pitfall is, however, represented by the fact that immunohistochemical loss of SMARCB1/INI1 nuclear expression can be observed in both entities. The presence of an EMA-positive perineurial component is generally seen at the periphery of the lesion, whereas it is generally absent in E-MPNST.

> **Key Points in Epithelioid Malignant Peripheral Nerve Sheath Tumor Diagnosis**
>
> - Occurrence in the subcutis or deep soft tissue of limbs and groin
> - Striking epithelioid morphology featuring macronucleolated vesicular nuclei
> - Diffuse expression of S100 protein and frequent loss of nuclear expression of SMARCB1/INI1
> - Less aggressive than classic MPNST

# Clear Cell Sarcoma of Soft Parts

## Definition and Epidemiology

Clear cell sarcoma (CCS) of soft parts is a rare soft tissue sarcoma showing features of melanocytic differentiation. Clear cell sarcoma is unrelated to pediatric lesions currently known as clear cell sarcoma of the kidney. First reported in 1965 by Enzinger, CCS usually occurs in adolescents and young adults, with a peak incidence between 20 and 40 years of age. There exists a slight female predominance. Clear cell sarcoma is a slow-growing mass, which presents for months or years. Pain or tenderness is reported in half of the cases. This entity is also referred to as "malignant melanoma of soft parts," a label that has been abandoned because it represents a potential cause of diagnostic confusion.

## Clinical Presentation and Behavior

Clear cell sarcoma mainly involves the extremities (foot and ankle in 40% of cases), followed by knee, thigh, and hand. It is generally deep seated, often attached to tendons and aponeuroses. Cases occurring in the retroperitoneum, bone, penis, and spinal roots are exceptionally reported. Those cases arising in the gastrointestinal (GI) tract (for which the term "malignant gastrointestinal neuroectodermal tumor" has been proposed to differentiate it from ST-CCS) often lack melanocytic differentiation and can be rapidly fatal. It has to be underlined that conventional CCS (identical to those occurring on the soft tissue) may also rarely occur in the GI tract. Clear cell sarcoma is an aggressive neoplasm, with an overall mortality ranging between 35 and 75%. Recurrences and metastases can occur even after 10 years. Nodal metastases are present in about 50% of cases. Lung and bone metastases are also frequent.

Size above 5 cm, necrosis, and local recurrence all represent unfavorable prognostic factors. French Federation of Cancer Centers Sarcoma Group (FNCLCC) grading is not recommended for prognostic stratification.

## Morphology and Immunophenotype

Grossly, ST-CCS is usually of small size (2–6 cm, even if larger tumors are reported), well circumscribed but rarely encapsulated (Fig. 5-85). Cut surface is gray-white and lobulated or multinodular. Pigmented areas can occur. Necrosis, hemorrhage, and cystic degeneration are occasionally seen.

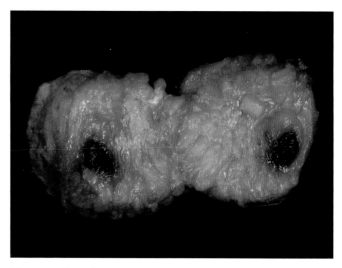

**Fig. 5-85.** Clear cell sarcoma. At gross examination, an unencapsulated, well-circumscribed lobulated mass is seen.

Histologically, CCS is composed of uniform nests and/or fascicles variably composed of epithelioid (Fig. 5-86) and spindle cells (Fig. 5-87) separated by fibrous septa (Fig. 5-88). Abundant clear (Fig. 5-89) or, more frequently (despite the name), eosinophilic cytoplasm is seen (Figs. 5-90 and 5-91) Nuclei are vesicular, round to ovoid, with prominent nucleoli. Multinucleated giant cells are seen in half of the cases (Fig. 5-92), and melanin pigment can be observed (Fig. 5-93). Morphologic variations are represented by the presence of marked pleomorphism (often associated with brisk mitotic activity) (Fig. 5-94), microcystic degeneration, and myxoid change of the stroma (Fig. 5-95). Pleomorphism seems to be more frequent in recurrent lesions as well as in metastases.

Clear cell sarcoma of the GI tract (malignant gastrointestinal neuroectodermal tumor) usually exhibits a monomorphous, round to epithelioid cell morphology (Fig. 5-96), and in up to half of the cases the presence of osteoclast-like giant cells is observed. Neoplastic cells are organized in nests or sheets, and often a pseudopapillary appearance is seen (Fig. 5-97). Spindle cell morphology can be seen in a minority of cases.

Immunohistochemically, CCS exhibits immunoreactivity for S100 protein (Fig. 5-98A), HMB45 (Fig. 5-98B), and other melanoma antigens in almost all cases localized in soft tissue. As mentioned, CCS of the GI tract most often lacks expression of melanocytic markers.

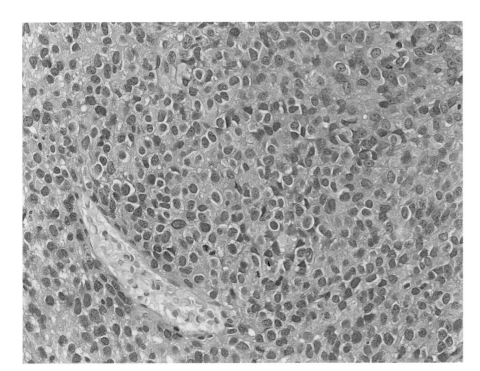

**Fig. 5-86.** Clear cell sarcoma. A monomorphic epithelioid cell proliferation is seen.

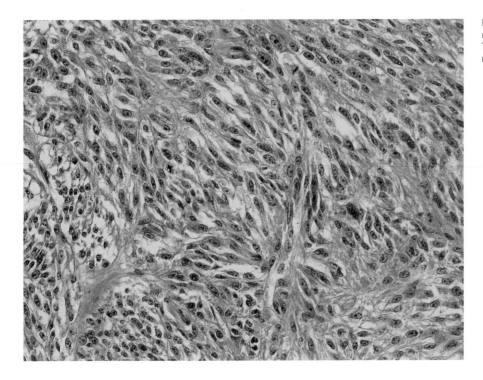

**Fig. 5-87.** Clear cell sarcoma. A uniformly spindled neoplastic cell proliferation is sometimes detected. Tumor cells exhibit vesicular nuclei with large nucleoli.

## Molecular Genetics

Clear cell sarcoma is genetically characterized by the presence of a specific chromosomal translocation, t(12;22)(q13;q12), fusing *EWS* and *ATF1* genes. A variant fusion gene *EWSR1-CREB1* has been recently described in soft part and gastro-intestinal CCS.

273

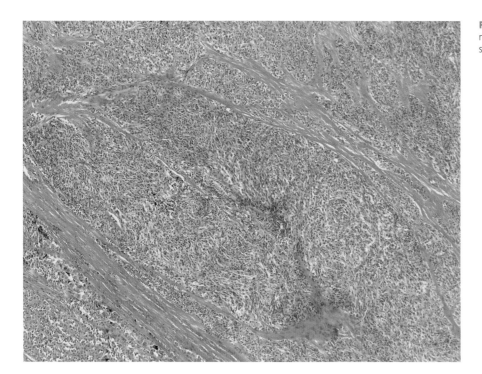

**Fig. 5-88.** Clear cell sarcoma. Most often, neoplastic cells are compartmentalized by fibrous septa.

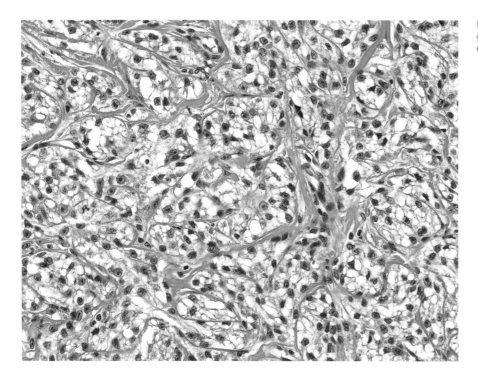

**Fig. 5-89.** Clear cell sarcoma. Less often than generally believed, tumors are entirely composed of cells featuring clear cytoplasm.

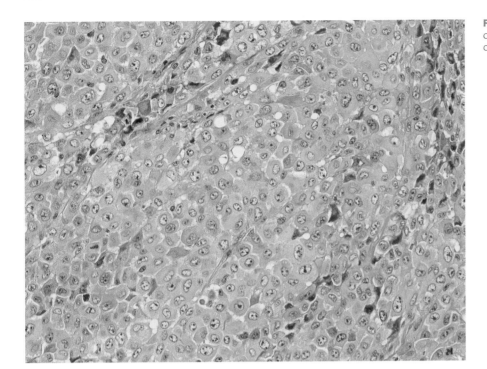

**Fig. 5-90.** Clear cell sarcoma. Most often (in contrast to its label), it is composed of eosinophilic cells. Note the presence of prominent nucleoli.

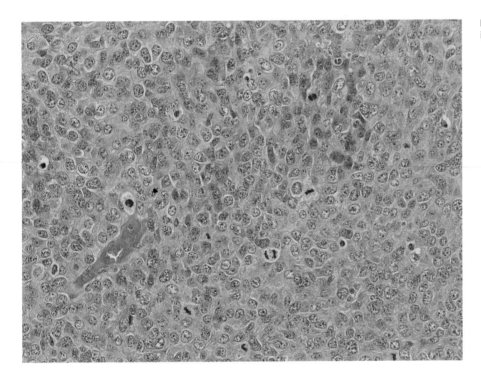

**Fig. 5-91.** Clear cell sarcoma. High mitotic activity is frequently observed.

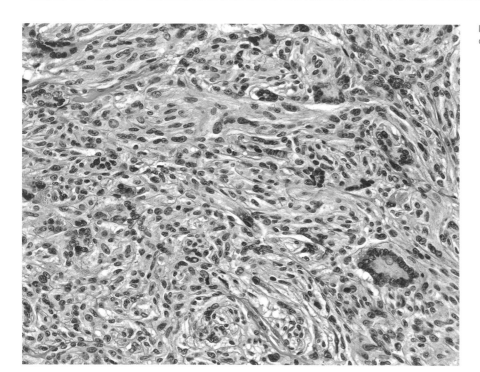

**Fig. 5-92.** Clear cell sarcoma. Multinucleated giant cells are seen in approximately half of the cases.

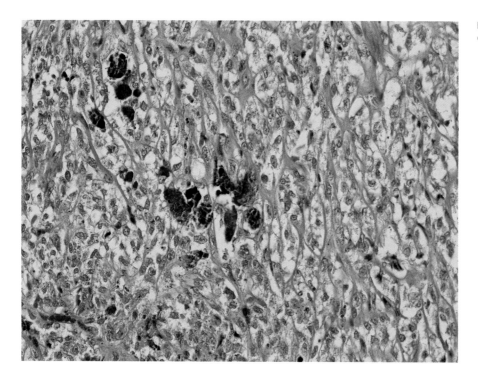

**Fig. 5-93.** Clear cell sarcoma. Melanin pigment is observed in a minority of cases.

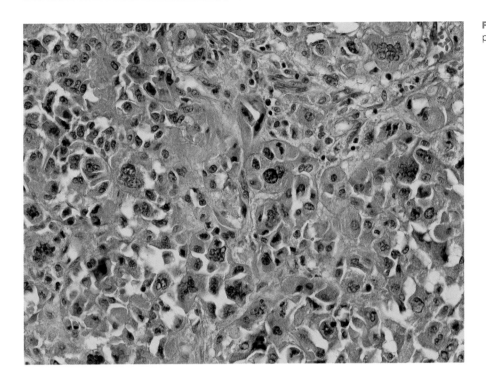

**Fig. 5-94.** Clear cell sarcoma. Rarely, marked pleomorphism can be observed.

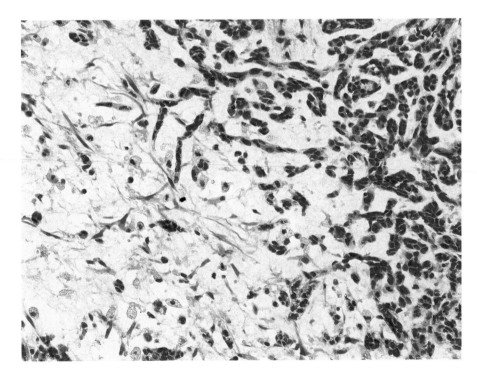

**Fig. 5-95.** Clear cell sarcoma. Prominent myxoid change of the stroma is observed.

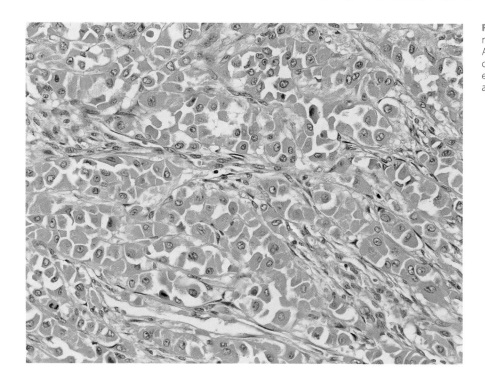

**Fig. 5-96.** Clear cell sarcoma of the GI tract/ malignant gastrointestinal neuroectodermal tumor. A monomorphic epithelioid cell proliferation is most often seen. Dyscohesive tumor cells with eosinophilic cytoplasm and moderate nuclear atypia is seen.

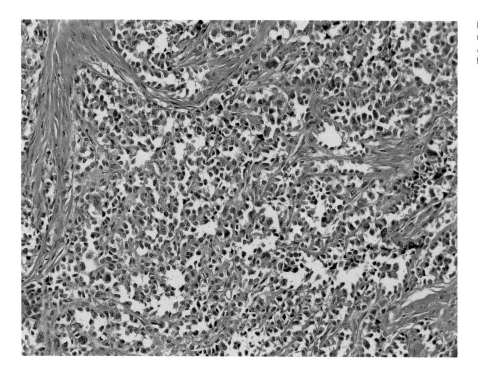

**Fig. 5-97.** Clear cell sarcoma of the GI tract/ malignant gastrointestinal neuroectodermal tumor. A distinctive pseudopapillary architecture is frequently seen.

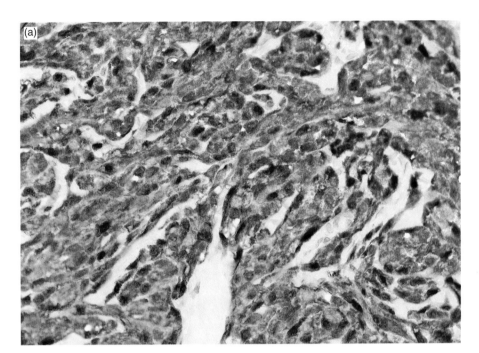

**Fig. 5-98A.** Clear cell sarcoma. S100 immunopositivity is seen in all cases.

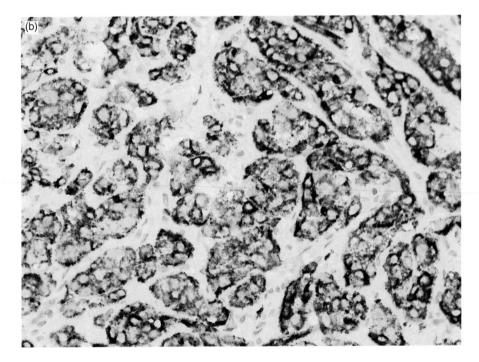

**Fig. 5-98B.** Clear cell sarcoma. HMB45 immunopositivity is seen, featuring the distinctive granular cytoplasmic localization.

## Differential Diagnosis and Diagnostic Pitfalls

The main differential diagnosis is obviously with malignant melanoma. Melanoma can be ruled out on the basis of clinical history (and careful clinical examination by an expert dermatologist) and in the absence of a junctional component (however, epidermis can be ulcerated, thus not allowing evaluation). The presence of fibrous septa as well as of multinucleated cells tends to favor CCS. Unfortunately, metastatic melanoma can at times exhibit complete morphologic overlap with CCS, making genetic analysis such as demonstration of *EWSR1* gene rearrangement the only way to separate them. HMB45 immunopositivity tends to be more diffuse in ST-CCS than in malignant melanoma, but again it is itself not sufficient to allow a diagnosis of certainty. When dealing with CCS (or CCS-like tumors) of the GI tract, the differential diagnosis also includes GIST, in particular considering that rarely GIST may express S100. Immunopositivity for KIT and DOG1 in GIST permits differentiation in most cases.

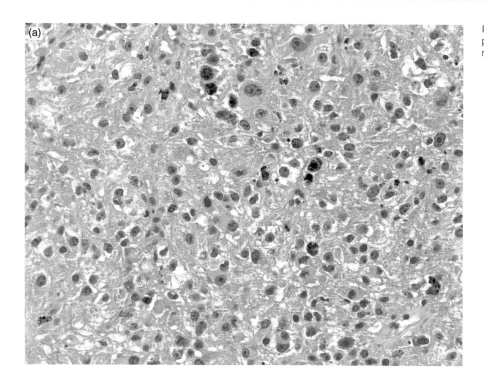

**Fig. 5-99A.** Melanotic schwannoma. The cell population is predominantly epithelioid, featuring round nuclei and macronucleoli.

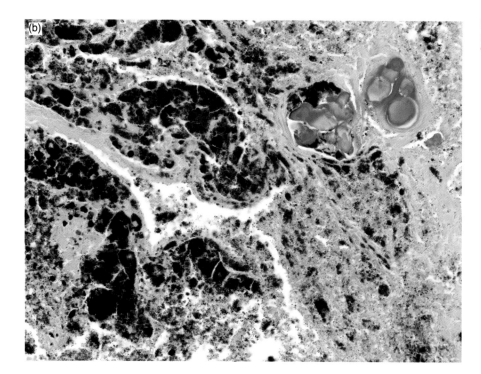

**Fig. 5-99B.** Melanotic schwannoma, psammomatous variant. Laminated calcified corpuscles are easily identified.

Even if clinical presentation is distinct, another lesion, in consideration of extensive melanogenic differentiation, enters the differential diagnosis and is represented by **melanotic schwannoma** (MS). Melanotic schwannoma is a rare neural neoplasm showing hybrid features of nerve sheath and melanocytic differentiation. Peak incidence is in the fourth decade and the most frequently affected anatomic locations are the spinal nerves and spinal ganglia. A psammomatous variant exists that is associated with the Carney complex (myxomas,

spotty pigmentation, and endocrine abnormalities) in 50% of cases.

Microscopically, MS is usually composed of solid sheets of epithelioid cells harboring round, macronucleolated nuclei and associated with abundant melanin pigment (Fig. 5-99A). The psammomatous variant features the presence of a variable number of concentric calcifications (psammoma bodies) (Fig. 5-99B). The neoplastic cell population may also focally assume a spindled morphology

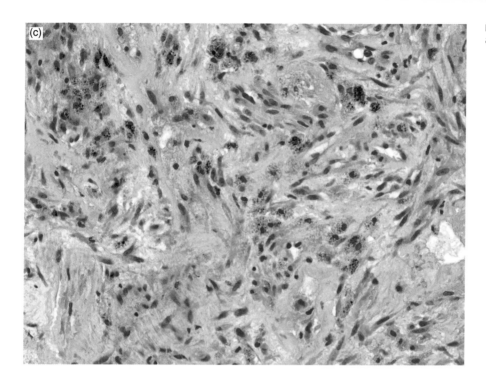

**Fig. 5-99C.** Melanotic schwannoma. A variably abundant spindle cell component can be observed.

(Fig. 5-99C). Melanotic schwannoma exhibits immunopositivity for S100 in most neoplastic cells. As a consequence of the abundant number of melanosomes, common melanoma markers are also all positive. Main differential diagnosis is with malignant melanoma, and in many cases the differential diagnosis is primarily based upon clinical presentation rather than on morphologic findings. Malignant behavior associated with metastatic spread is observed in 10 to 15% of cases and is associated with nuclear atypia and mitotic activity; however, it may be unrelated to morphologic features of malignancy.

---

**Key Points in Clear Cell Sarcoma Diagnosis**

- Predominance in extremities of adolescents and young adults.
- Melanoma-like cytomorphology
- Multinodular pattern of growth with presence of fibrous septa
- Consistent expression of melanocytic differentiation markers (much less so in GI tract examples)
- *EWSR1* rearranged in most cases
- Clinically aggressive malignancy

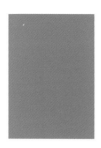

# Sclerosing Epithelioid Fibrosarcoma

## Definition and Epidemiology

Sclerosing epithelioid fibrosarcoma (SEF) represents an exceedingly rare mesenchymal fibroblastic malignancy that can easily be confused with metastatic carcinoma. First reported by Enzinger and coworkers in 1995, it tends to occur in middle-aged and elderly patients (median age 45 years), with no sex predilection.

## Clinical Presentation and Behavior

Most cases arise in the deep soft tissue of the limbs and limb girdles, followed by the trunk and the head and neck region. Exceptionally rare visceral cases have also been reported. Sclerosing epithelioid fibrosarcoma is characterized by aggressive clinical behavior, with 10 to 20% of patients presenting with metastatic disease at diagnosis. In approximately 50% of cases, there is local recurrence, with metastatic spread being reported in up to 80% of cases, most often affecting the pleuropulmonary region, bone, and central nervous system. Interestingly, distant metastases may occur several years after diagnosis. Surgery still represents the therapeutic mainstay, whereas conventional systemic therapies seem to play a limited role.

## Morphology and Immunophenotype

Macroscopically, SEF is usually well demarcated, often showing a lobular or multinodular pattern of growth. Those exceptional cases arising at visceral sites may exhibit a more infiltrative pattern of growth. Microscopically, SEF is composed of an infiltrative proliferation of epithelioid cells, often featuring a clear cytoplasm, organized in cords, strands, and nests, and set in a distinctively prominent sclerotic collagen background (Figs. 5-100 and 5-101). Most cases are cytologically uniform with scanty mitoses; however, foci of pleomorphism (Fig. 5-102), hypercellularity (Fig. 5-103), and high mitotic activity are rarely encountered, particularly in recurrent lesions. Some cases may exibit areas indistinguishable from low-grade fibromyxoid sarcoma (LGFMS), an entity morphologically as well as genetically closely related to SEF. Immunophenotypically, SEF exhibits EMA positivity in approximately 50% of cases. Most important, two-thirds of cases show strong cytoplasmic immunoreactivity for MUC4

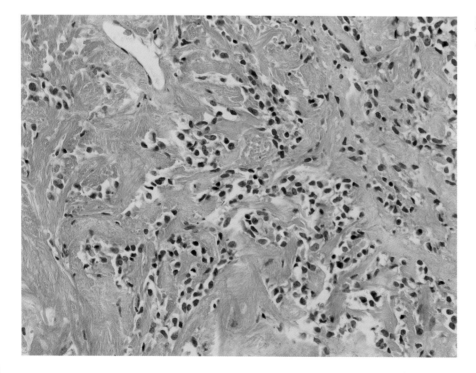

**Fig. 5-100.** Sclerosing epithelioid fibrosarcoma. The presence of a cytologically bland cell set in a densely sclerotic collagen stroma is shown.

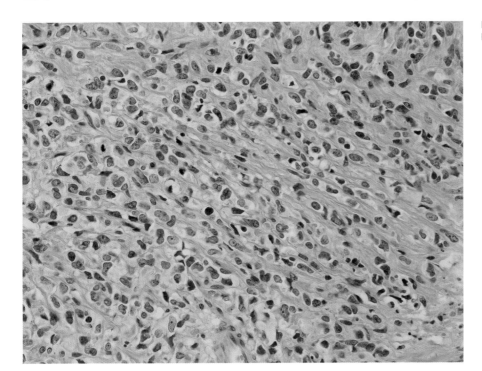

**Fig. 5-101.** Sclerosing epithelioid fibrosarcoma. Neoplastic cells most often feature clear cytoplasm.

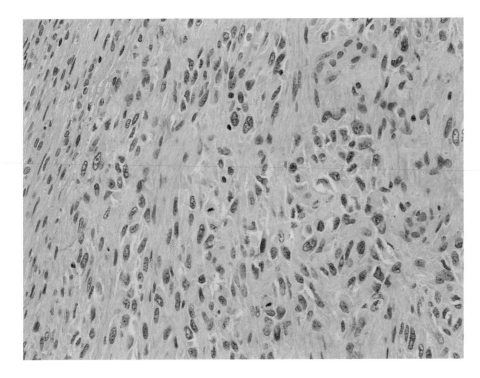

**Fig. 5-102.** Sclerosing epithelioid fibrosarcoma. Foci of pleomorphism are rarely seen (most often in recurrences).

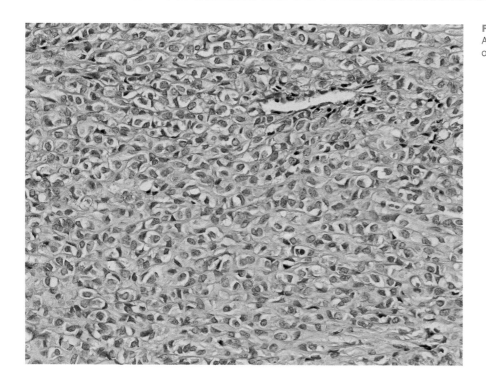

**Fig. 5-103.** Sclerosing epithelioid fibrosarcoma. Areas of hypercellularity can be observed (most often in recurrences).

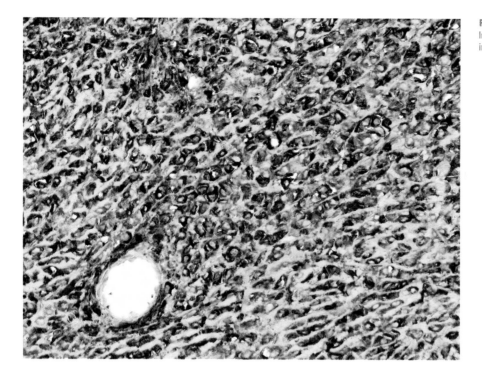

**Fig. 5-104.** Sclerosing epithelioid fibrosarcoma. Immunopositivity for MUC4 represents an important diagnostic clue.

(Fig. 5-104), a finding that further supports the relationship between LGFMS and SEF.

## Molecular Genetics

In contrast to the marked predominance of *FUS-CREB3L2* t (7;16)(q33;p11) in LGFMS, the genetics of SEF is more heterogeneous, more often exhibiting *FUS-CREB3L1* t(11;16) and *EWSR1-CREB3L1* t(11;22) gene fusions.

## Differential Diagnosis and Diagnostic Pitfalls

The main challenge is represented by the differential diagnosis with metastatic carcinoma. As SEF expresses EMA in half of the cases, the morphologic overlap with epithelial malignancies can represent a potential source of misclassification. MUC4 immunopositivity may be expressed in epithelial malignancies; however, cytokeratins tend to be consistently negative in SEF. Epithelioid vascular neoplasms are easily ruled out on the basis

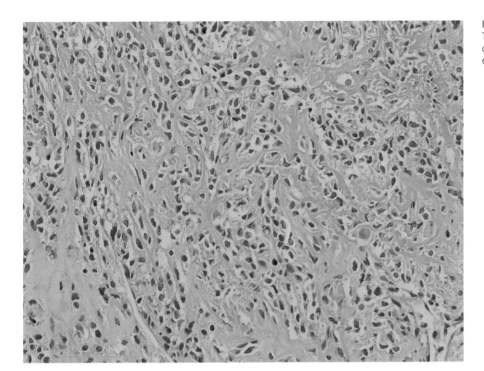

**Fig. 5-105.** Sclerosing epithelioid fibrosarcoma. The sclerotic collagen may mimic malignant osteoid, raising the differential diagnosis with extraskeletal osteosarcoma.

of the absence of vasoformative features as well as lack of expression of all vascular differentiation markers. Extraskeletal osteosarcoma may enter the differential diagnosis, as the distinctive sclerotic collagen of SEF may mimic neoplastic osteoid (Fig. 5-105). However, extraskeletal osteosarcoma is MUC4 negative, whereas it exhibits intense SATB2 nuclear immunopositivity. Sclerosing rhabdomyosarcoma may also be the source of diagnostic confusion but is easily recognized on the basis of the presence of desmin and myogenin immunopositivity.

**Key Points in Sclerosing Epithelioid Fibrosarcoma Diagnosis**

- Predominance in limbs and limb girdles of adults and elderly patients
- Striking epithelioid morphology associated with sclerotic collagen
- Expression of MUC4 in most cases
- Aggressive clinical behavior with delayed systemic spread

# Alveolar Soft Part Sarcoma

## Definition and Epidemiology

Alveolar soft part sarcoma (ASPS), first reported in 1952 by Christopherson and coworkers, is an extremely rare mesenchymal malignancy of uncertain lineage, representing less than 1% of all soft tissue sarcomas. It is most common in adolescents and young adults between 15 and 35 years of age. Females predominate before 30 years of age.

## Clinical Presentation and Behavior

Alveolar soft part sarcoma usually presents as a slow-growing, painless mass. As the presence of the primary soft tissue mass is frequently missed, metastases (most frequently to lungs and brain) at times represent the first clinical sign. Alveolar soft part sarcoma occurs most frequently in the lower extremities, especially in the deep soft tissue of the anterior aspect of the thigh, and in the buttock of adults. In the pediatric age-group, it involves primarily the head and neck region (orbit and tongue). Alveolar soft part sarcoma has also been occasionally described in a number of other sites, such as female genital tract, mediastinum, lung, stomach, and bone. Metastases can occur early, even before the discovery of the primary tumor, or late, even decades after detection of the primary tumor, the most common sites being the lungs, bone, and brain. Brain metastases are more common with ASPS than with any other soft tissue sarcoma. Overall survival for localized disease is about 60% at 5 years, dropping to 50% at 10 years, and then to less than 10% at 20 years. Prognosis seems to be related to age at presentation (risk of metastases increases with age) and tumor size (larger tumors are more frequently associated with metastases at diagnosis). FNCLCC grading is not recommended for assessing prognosis. Alveolar soft part sarcoma is generally regarded as chemoresistant; however, recently some clinical responses have been shown using Met inhibitors or the multitarget agent sunitinib. Removal of lung metastasis is generally undertaken in the attempt to prolong survival.

## Morphology and Immunophenotype

Grossly, ASPS tends to be poorly circumscribed, yellow-white to gray-red, friable, and soft (Fig. 5-106). Necrosis and hemorrhage can be present. Frequently, it is surrounded by large-caliber blood vessels. Histologically, dense, fibrous trabeculae of varying thickness divide the tumor mass into compartments. These compartments are formed by cells arranged in nests set in a thin, connective tissue network containing a sinusoidal

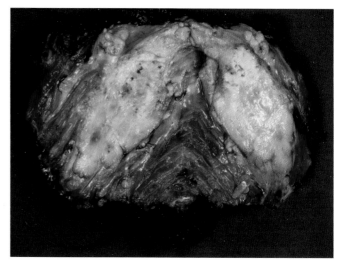

**Fig. 5-106.** Alveolar soft part sarcoma. Grossly, the tumor most often presents as a poorly circumscribed, deep-seated mass.

vasculature (Fig. 5-107). Centrally to the nests are foci of necrosis and/or cellular loss of cohesion (so-called alveolar pattern because of its vague resemblance to normal lung alveoli) (Fig. 5-108). This pattern of growth can be absent in pediatric cases wherein a more solid morphology is often seen (Fig. 5-109). The neoplastic cells are typically large, rounded or, more often, polygonal, with vesicular, often multiple nuclei with prominent nucleoli, and abundant granular eosinophilic cytoplasm (Fig. 5-110). Cellular borders are sharp and mitoses uncommon. Necrosis and hemorrhage may be found, especially in larger tumors. Rhomboid or rod-shaped crystalline PAS+ inclusions are evident in the cytoplasm of some neoplastic cells. Vascular invasion is frequently observed.

Immunohistochemically, ASPS may show immunoreactivity for muscle specific actin and rarely for desmin. Reported cytoplasmic MyoD1 immunoreactivity most likely represents unspecific staining. Strong and diffuse nuclear immunopositivity of the nuclear transcription factor TFE3 is typically present (Fig. 5-111).

## Molecular Genetics

Genetically, ASPS is characterized by the presence of a specific translocation, t(X;17)(p11;q25), leading to the fusion transcript between ASPL and TFE3.

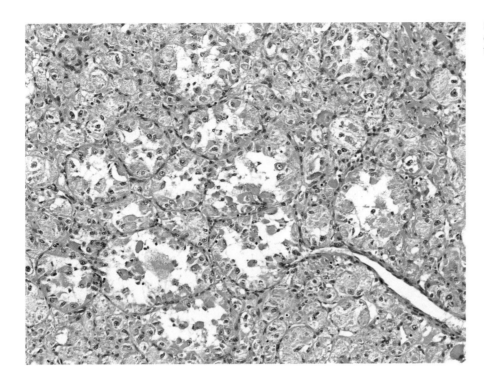

**Fig. 5-107.** Alveolar soft part sarcoma. Neoplastic cells are organized in nests separated by thin, fibrovascular septa.

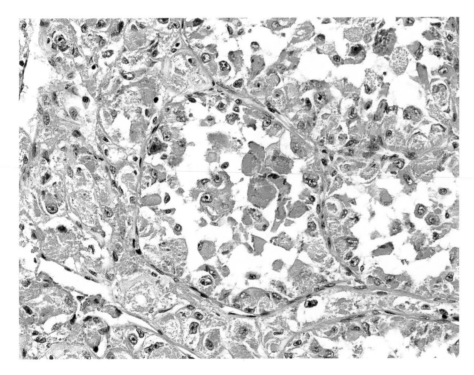

**Fig. 5-108.** Alveolar soft part sarcoma. Loss of cell cohesion determines the characteristic pseudoalveolar architecture.

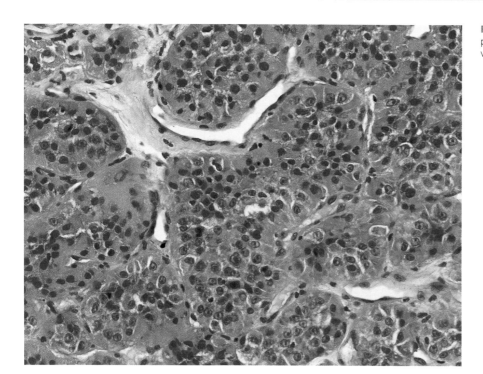

**Fig. 5-109.** Alveolar soft part sarcoma. A solid pattern of growth is most often seen in the pediatric variant.

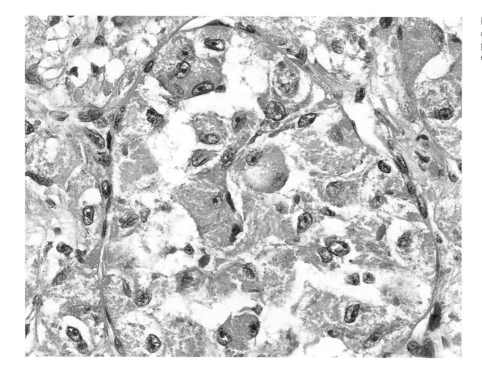

**Fig. 5-110.** Alveolar soft part sarcoma. Lesional cells are often polygonal, with vesicular nuclei, prominent nucleoli, and abundant granular eosinophilic cytoplasm.

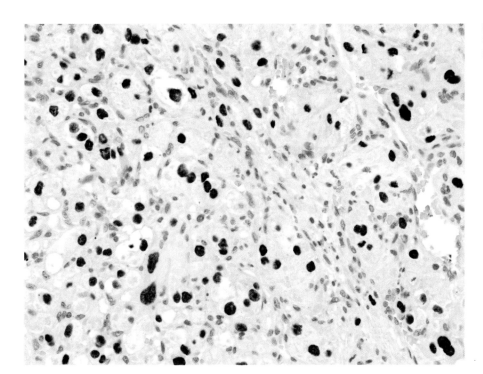

**Fig. 5-111.** Alveolar soft part sarcoma. TFE3 nuclear immunopositivity is characteristically present.

## Differential Diagnosis and Diagnostic Pitfalls

Alveolar soft part sarcoma can be confused with paraganglioma, a neoplasm characterized by a nesting growth pattern, expression of endocrine markers (synaptophysin and chromogranin), and the presence of S100-positive sustentacular cells, easily identifiable at the periphery of nests. Metastatic chromophobe renal cell carcinoma can be distinguished on the basis of the expression of keratins, CD10 and PAX8 immunopositivity. Another potential pitfall is represented by the fact that a subset of pediatric renal cell carcinomas shares with ASPS the t(X;17) translocation and consequently also exhibits TFE3 immunoreactivity. Malignant PEComa rarely exhibits TFE3 immunopositivity, which may result in misclassification; however, it more strikingly shows nuclear atypia and distinctive cytoplasmic granularity and features immunopositivity for melanoma as well as myogenic markers.

| Key Points in Alveolar Soft Part Sarcoma Diagnosis |
| --- |
| • Predominance in the lower extremities of adolescents and young adults |
| • Striking epithelioid morphology |
| • Nesting pattern of growth |
| • Nuclear expression of TFE3 |
| • Prolonged clinical course with high tendency to metastatic spread to the lungs |

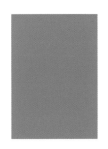

# Pecoma of Soft Tissue (PEComa)

## Definition and Epidemiology

The concept of perivascular epithelioid cell (PEC) and neoplasm thereof (PEComas) was pioneered by Bonetti and colleagues in 1992. They described lesions composed of neoplastic cells apparently originating from the walls of blood vessels. These cells exhibited a peculiar biphenotypic immunophenotype, featuring both myogenic and melanocytic differentiation. Currently, the term "PEComa" has gained broad acceptance and this label includes (actually generating some potential confusion) renal and extrarenal angiomyolipoma (AML), lymphangioleiomyomatosis (LAM), clear cell "sugar" tumor, and clear cell myomelanocytic tumor of the falciform ligament/ligamentum teres. PEComas (with the exclusion of angiomyolipoma) are very rare. Lymphangioleiomyomatosis is not included in this section because of its distinctive clinical and morphologic (being predominatly composed of spindle cells) features. Conventional angiomyolipomas of the kidney are not addressed in depth (with the exception of the monotypic epithelioid variant), as they are most often benign and in fact almost always detected as an incidental radiologic finding.

## Clinical Presentation and Behavior

PEComas seem to occur at almost any age, with a peak incidence in the fourth decade, and exhibit a striking predilection for females. PEComas may occur anywhere, including the skin; however, they most often arise in the retroperitoneum, the abdominopelvic region, uterus, and gastrointestinal tract. Malignant PEComas are exceedingly rare, and the most common metastatic sites are represented by the liver, lymph nodes, lungs, and bone. In consideration of the activation of the mTOR pathway, anti-mTOR inhibitors have been used with some success. Renal AML shows predominance in females, with the exception of those 50% of cases arising in the context of tuberous sclerosis complex (TSC).

## Morphology and Immunophenotype

PEComas usually exhibit a nested pattern of growth (Fig. 5-112). Neoplastic cells are epithelioid, featuring an abundant granular eosinophilic or clear cytoplasm (Figs. 5-113 and 5-114). An extremely variable combination of epithelioid and spindle cells is seen (Fig. 5-115). The proportion of eosinophilic and clear cells is also

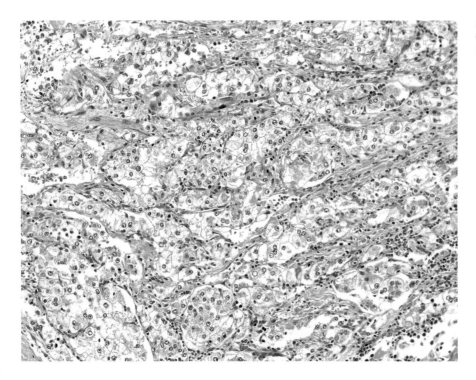

**Fig. 5-112.** PEComa. Neoplastic cells are most often organized in nests. Tumor cells have large polygonal cytoplasm.

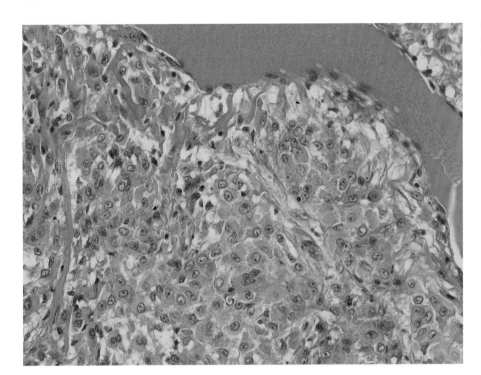

**Fig. 5-113.** PEComa. A predominantly eosinophilic epithelioid cell proliferation can be seen.

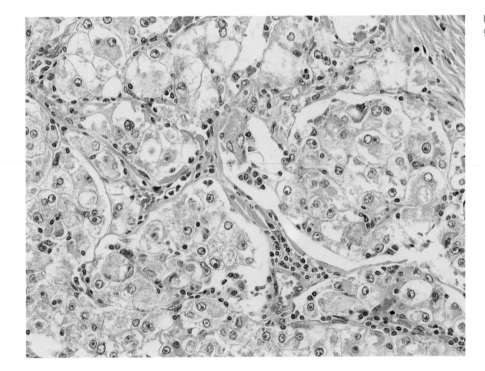

**Fig. 5-114.** PEComa. The presence of clear, granular cytoplasm is frequently observed.

extremely variable (Fig. 5-116). An intimate connection with the walls of blood vessels represents a relatively common finding (Fig. 5-117). A recently reported variant of PEComa features the presence of a dense sclerotic collagenous stroma, and it has been consequently named "sclerosing PEComa" (Figs. 5-118 and 5-119). Very occasionally, melanocytic pigment can be observed (Fig. 5-120). Cytologic atypia not associated with significant mitotic activity is sometimes seen but does not necessarily imply aggressive behavior (Fig. 5-121).

As mentioned, malignant PEComa is extremely rare, and criteria of malignancy are not well established. However, aggressive clinical behavior is primarily seen in those cases featuring a combination of the following criteria of malignancy: i.e., tumor size greater than 5 cm, presence of severe nuclear atypia, hypercellularity, presence of necrosis (Fig. 5-122), and high mitotic activity (greater than 1 mitosis/50HPF) (Fig. 5-123). Mitotic activity appears to be the strongest predictor, followed by necrosis; however, further validation is certainly needed.

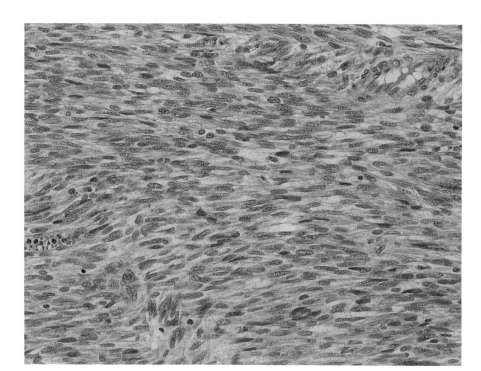

**Fig. 5-115.** PEComa. More rarely, tumors may be entirely composed of a spindle cell population.

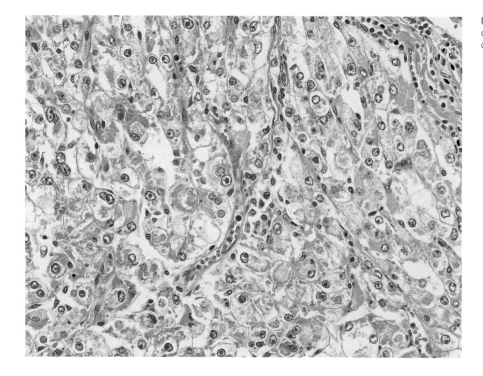

**Fig. 5-116.** PEComa. A variable combination of clear cell and eosinophilic epithelioid cells is most often seen.

Conventional AML, as mentioned, is generally benign and typically exhibits a variable combination of mature fat, thick-walled blood vessels and smooth muscle (Fig. 5-124). An epithelioid component can be seen that can become predominant. Purely epithelioid AML (Fig. 5-125) is currently also called PEComa, and in these cases (among which aggressive behavior can be observed) the same criteria of malignancy previously discussed are applied.

Immunohistochemically, HMB45 represents the most sensitive marker (Fig. 5-126). PEComas also variably exhibit Melan-A, MITF-1, and muscle markers such as smooth muscle actin (seen in approximately 80% of cases), desmin (Fig. 5-127), h-caldesmon, and calponin. Approximately 5–10% of cases may exhibit TFE3 nuclear immunoreactivity, which may be associated with TFE3 gene rearrangement. TFE3 nuclear expression seems to be seen more frequently in lesions featuring an epithelioid morphology that is also associated with a predominantly melanogenic (rather than myogenic) immunophenotype. In AML, myogenic differentition markers are more robustly expressed than melanocytic markers.

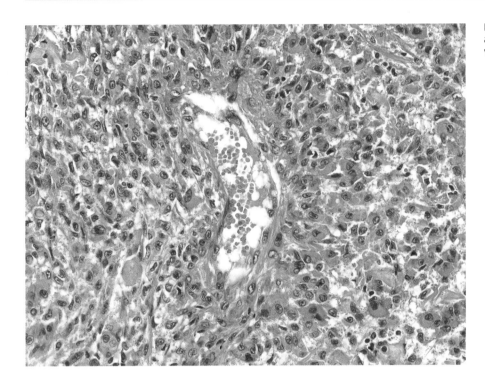

**Fig. 5-117.** PEComa. Neoplastic cells often exhibit an intimate connection with the wall of blood vessels.

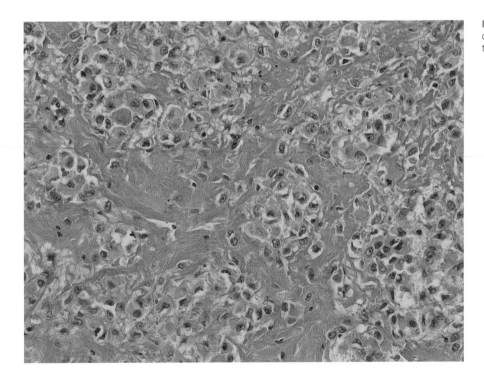

**Fig. 5-118.** Sclerosing PEComa. Epithelioid tumor cells set in abundant sclerotic collagen represent the diagnostic hallmark.

## Molecular Genetics

Frequent deletion of the 16p region wherein the *TSC2* gene maps is seen. The genetic aberration underlies the potential link with TSC2-associated neoplasms such as angiomyolipomas. Clinical signs of TSC are much less frequent in non-LAM/non-AML PEComas (approximately 8–10%). However, sporadic PEComas are also associated with 16p aberrations that lead to the activation of the mTOR pathway. *TFE3* gene rearrangement has been reported in a subset of PEComas.

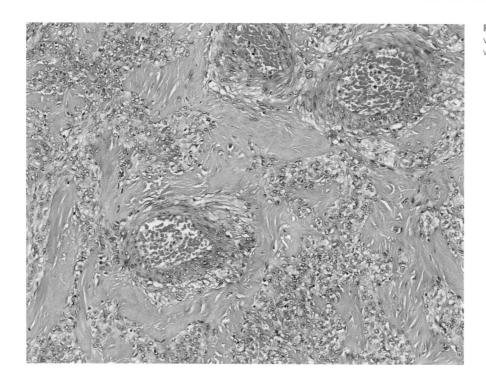

**Fig. 5-119.** Sclerosing PEComa. Similar to classic variants, the close relationship of neoplastic cells with blood vessels is also seen.

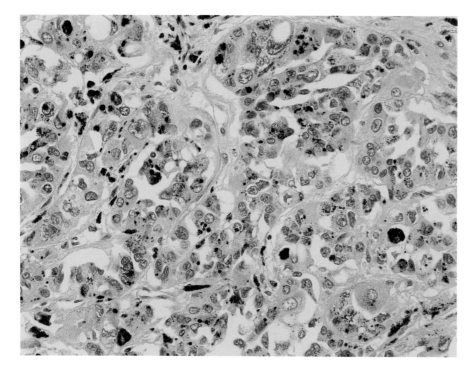

**Fig. 5-120.** PEComa. Rarely, tumor cells may contain melanin pigment.

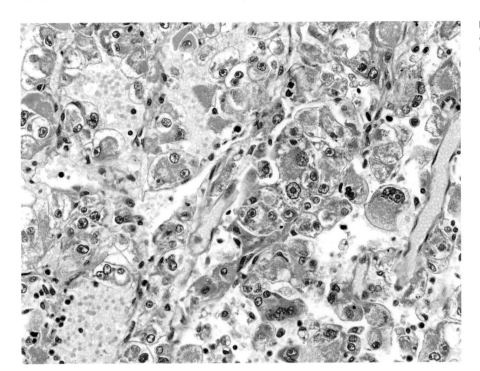

**Fig. 5-121.** PEComa. Tumor cells show cytologic atypia not associated with mitotic activity (symplastic type).

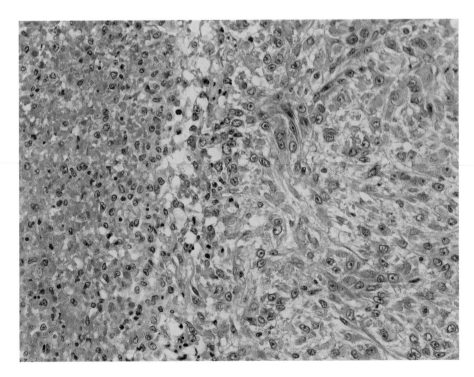

**Fig. 5-122.** Malignant PEComa. Tumor cells exhibit severe cytologic atypia associated with abundant coagulative necrosis.

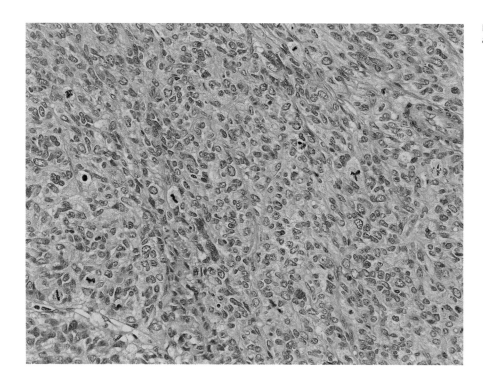

**Fig. 5-123.** Malignant PEComa. High mitotic activity and atypical mitoses are seen.

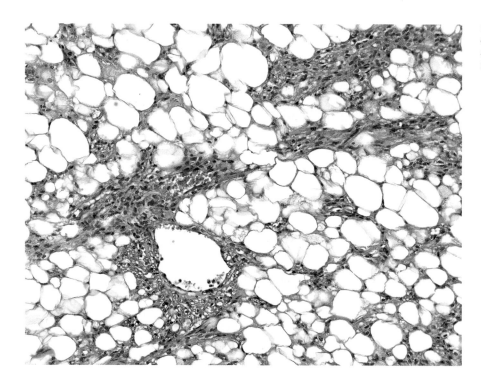

**Fig. 5-124.** Angiomyolipoma. The tumor is composed of a combination of blood vessels, adipose tissue, and a spindle/epithelioid cell population.

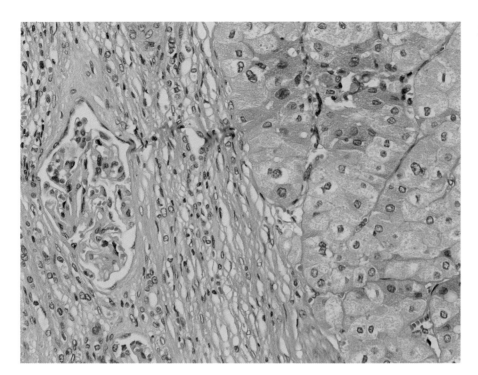

**Fig. 5-125.** Epithelioid angiomyolipoma. Renal tumors purely composed of epithelioid cells (currently grouped under the label "PEComa") may express clinically aggressive behavior.

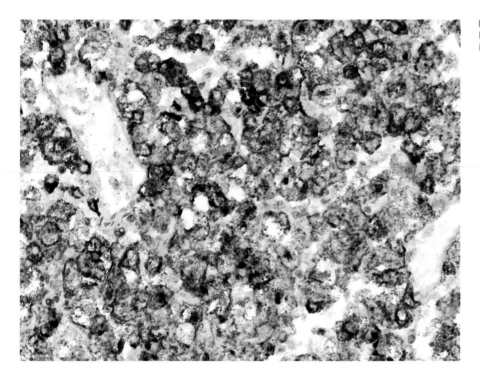

**Fig. 5-126.** PEComa. Neoplastic cells express HMB45, which represents the most sensitive immunophenotypic marker.

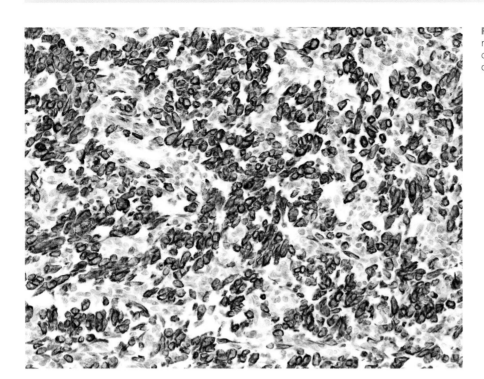

**Fig. 5-127.** PEComa. The co-expression of melanocytic and myogenic markers (desmin, in this case) represents a key diagnostic clue to the diagnosis.

## Differential Diagnosis and Diagnostic Pitfalls

Differential diagnosis primarily includes malignant melanoma and clear cell sarcoma. Both entities exhibit strong S100 immunopositivity, which is never seen in PEComa. Clear cell sarcoma features the rearrangement of the *EWSR1* gene that is absent on both PEComa and malignant melanoma. In consideration of the visceral location, epithelioid GIST enters the differential diagnosis; however, it can be ruled out rather easily on the basis of identification of KIT and/or DOG1 immunoreactivity. Clear cell carcinoma is easily recognized on the basis of the expression of cyokeratin. Alveolar soft part sarcomas can be challenging, as these may rarely share with PEComa expression of TFE3; however, ASPS never exhibits the distinctive myomelanocytic phenotype of PEComa. Epithelioid leiomyosarcoma can also be confused with PEComa; however, it always lacks expression of melanocytic markers, and cytoplasm most often lack the distinctive granularity of PEComas. Having said that, it has to be underlined that epithelioid leiomyosarcoma is exceedingly rare, which means that when dealing with an epithelioid tumor featuring expression of myogenic markers, PEComa should represent the first diagnostic option and menocytic markers checked carefully. Another possible differential is represented by the extremely rare **malignant variant of granular cell tumor** (GCT). Malignant GCT accounts for no more than 2% of all GCT. In addition to the typical cell population featuring eosinophilic granular cytoplasm, malignant forms exhibit a combination of the following histologic features: cytologic atypia, spindling, more than 2 mitoses/10HPF, and tumor necrosis (Fig. 5-128). The presence of fewer than three criteria would qualify a GCT as "atypical."

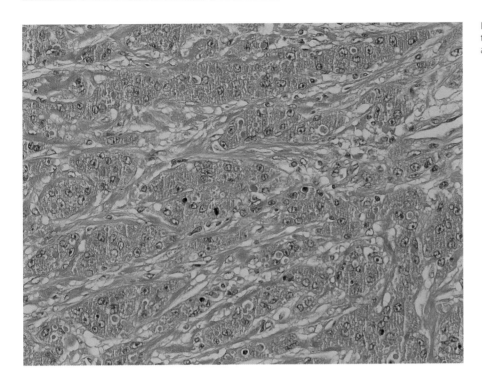

**Fig. 5-128.** Malignant granular cell tumor. Nest of tumor cells exhibits nuclear atypia and mitotic activity.

**Key Points in Pecoma of Soft Tissue (PEComa) Diagnosis**

- Predominance in female patients
- Variable combination of spindled and epithelioid morphology
- Granular clear cell or eosinophilic cytoplasm
- Biphenotypic myogenic and melanogenic phenotype
- TFE3 expression observed in a minority of cases
- Aggressiveness associated with high-grade morphology

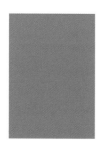

# Variants of Soft Tissue Sarcomas Featuring Epithelioid Morphology

## Epithelioid Pleomorphic Liposarcoma

Pleomorphic liposarcoma is a high-grade pleomorphic sarcoma, most often occurring in deep soft tissue of the limbs (or, rarely, in the trunk) of elderly patients, showing variable amounts (from focal to massive) of adipocytic differentiation. Pleomorphic liposarcoma is extensively discussed in Chapter 7. Microscopically, four main histologic presentations can be encountered: (1) an "MFH-like" pleomorphic/spindle cell sarcoma featuring scattered lipoblasts or sheets of lipoblasts; (2) rare cases overlap morphologically with intermediate to high-grade myxofibrosarcoma, except for the presence of lipoblasts; (3) lesions entirely composed of pleomorphic, multivacuolated lipoblasts; and (4) importantly, up to one-third of cases exhibit a very distinctive epithelioid morphology and pose significant diagnostic problems (Figs. 5-129 and 5-130). Interestingly, epithelioid pleomorphic liposarcoma relatively often arises at visceral locations. The presence of pleomorphic multivacuolated lipoblasts (which can be very few and therefore easily overlooked) set in a monomorphic epithelioid cell proliferation represent the most valuable diagnostic clue. Immunohistochemically, focal expression of EMA and cytokeratin is relatively often observed.

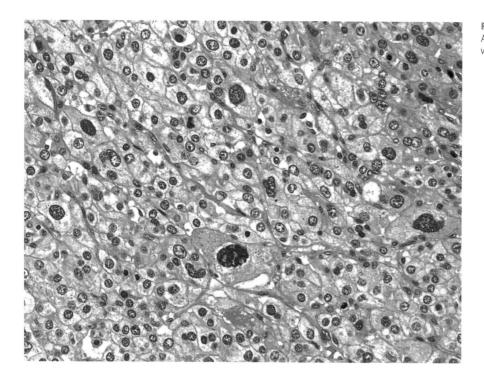

**Fig. 5-129.** Epithelioid pleomorphic liposarcoma. An epithelioid cell proliferation is seen associated with multifocal nuclear pleomorphism.

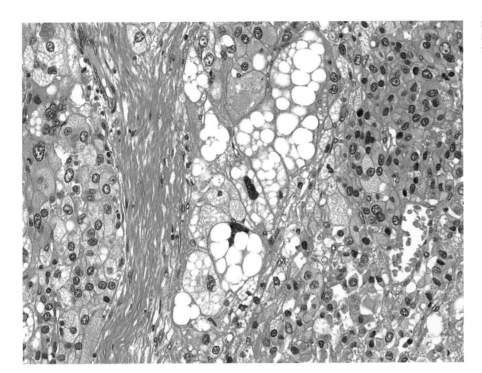

**Fig. 5-130.** Epithelioid pleomorphic liposarcoma. Pleomorphic multivacuolated lipoblasts are seen scattered in epithelioid cell proliferation.

## Differential Diagnosis and Diagnostic Pitfalls

The main differential diagnosis of epithelioid pleomorphic liposarcoma (E-PLPS) is with epithelial malignancies such as metastatic renal cell carcinoma and adrenal cortical carcinoma. The most important diagnostic clue is represented by the detection of multivacuolated pleomorphic lipoblasts, along with negativity for epithelial markers. As lipoblasts can be scanty and therefore easily overlooked, extensive sampling is mandatory. At visceral locations (which are relatively

frequent), epithelioid GIST also enters the differential diagnosis (see below). Most cases, however, will stain for CD117 and/or DOG1, which are consistently negative in E-PLPS.

## Epithelioid GIST

Gastrointestinal stromal tumors (GISTs) are covered in detail in Chapter 4. However, it is important to remember that approximately 20% of GISTs feature a distinctive epithelioid morphology (Fig. 5-131). Epithelioid-cell GISTs are more common in the

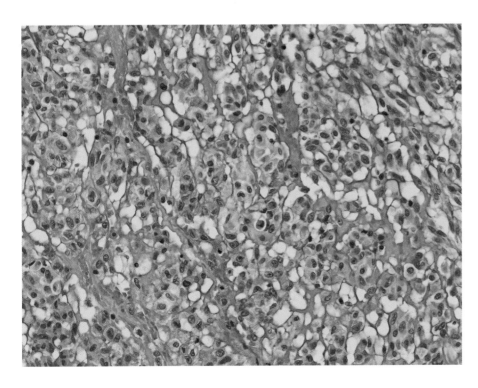

**Fig. 5-131.** Epithelioid GIST. The tumor is composed of a monomorphic epithelioid cell proliferation exhibiting plasmacytoid features.

stomach and include those that are PDGFRA-mutated. An important potential diagnostic pitfall is represented by the fact that up to 30% of gastric epithelioid cells may be CD117 (kit) negative. Positive staining for DOG1 usually helps in confirming the diagnosis in most cases. The recently recognized group of so-called succinate dehydrogenase (SDH)-deficient GIST also shows a tendency to exhibit an epithelioid morphology, which is also associated with a distinctive multinodular pattern of growth. SDH-deficient GISTs tend to predominate in young patients (but not exclusively), and in stark contrast with KIT-associated GISTs exhibit a tendency to spread to regional lymph nodes. Both PDGFRA-associated GISTs and SDH-deficient GISTs tend to share a rather indolent clinical course. Immunohistochemically, the loss of expression of SDHB can be used diagnostically as evidence of mutation of one of the genes encoding for the different SDH subunits.

## Differential Diagnosis and Diagnostic Pitfalls

Main differential diagnosis (which is extremely important in consideration of the specific targeted treatments currently available that are linked to GIST diagnosis) is with epithelioid smooth muscle tumors, to the extent that epithelioid GIST has been in the past also termed "leiomyoblastomas." GIST and smooth muscle tumor may share expression of smooth muscle markers; however, KIT and DOG1 expression is strictly restricted to GIST. A very rare entity that can exceptionally arise in the GI tract (primarily in the stomach) is represented by glomus tumor. Glomus tumor, in its most common form, occurs in the distal extremities of middle-aged adults. It typically features a monomorphic epithelioid cell proliferation with sharply defined cytoplasmic borders, often organized in a perivascular pattern of growth (Fig. 5-132). Immunohistochemically, smooth muscle actin is most often expressed, along with focal CD34 immunopositivity, in approximately half of the cases. Glomus tumor is generally benign; however, malignant forms do exist. These are usually deep seated, greater than 2 cm in size, and associated wth severe cytologic atypia and miotic count exceeding 5 mitoses/50HPF (Fig. 5-133). However, these criteria have not been validated for visceral location.

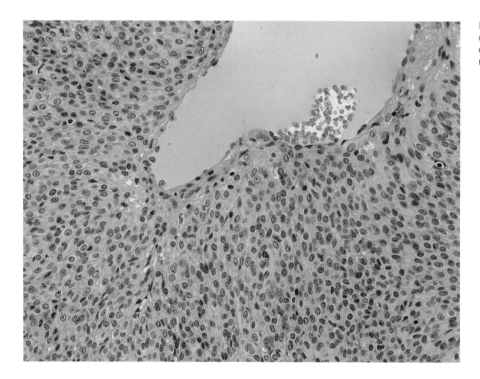

**Fig. 5-132.** Glomus tumor. Tumor cells are organized in a perivascular pattern of growth and exhibit a monomorphic epithelioid cell morphology.

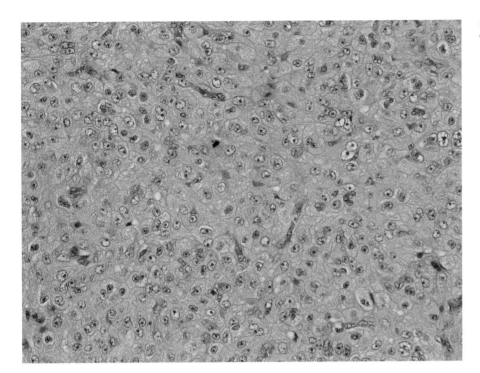

**Fig. 5-133.** Malignant glomus tumor. Significant cytologic atypia and mitotic activity are seen.

## Epithelioid Myxofibrosarcoma

Myxofibrosarcoma is discussed in Chapter 8. Myxofibrosarcoma may rarely feature an epithelioid morphology to the extent that it may simulate metastatic mucinous adenocarcinoma (Fig. 5-134). However, it retains the typical multinodular architecture as well as the presence of distinctive, thin-walled archiform blood vessels (Fig. 5-135). Epithelioid myxofibrosarcoma is always high grade and exhibits higher clinical aggressiveness than do ordinary myxofibrosarcomas. Immunohistochemically, multifocal expression of epithelial differentiation markers (primarily EMA) can be seen. Most relevant, differential diagnosis is with metastatic carcinoma wherein diffuse expression of cytokeratins represents a helpful diagnostic clue.

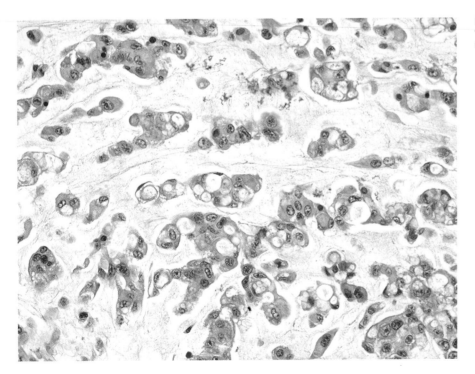

**Fig. 5-134.** Epithelioid myxofibrosarcoma. A "carcinoma-like" morphologic mimicking of a mucinous adenocarcinoma is seen.

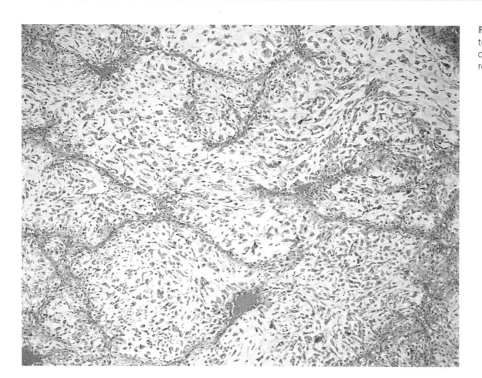

**Fig. 5-135.** Epithelioid myxofibrosarcoma. Similar to conventional myxofibrosarcoma, the presence of distinctive archiform, thin-walled blood vessels represents a helpful diagnostic clue.

## Epithelioid Leiomyosarcoma

Leiomyosarcoma is discussed in the chapter dedicated to spindle cell sarcoma, as most often it exhibits a spindle cell and/or pleomorphic morphology. However, there exist extremely rare cases that are almost entirely composed of epithelioid neoplastic cells (Fig. 5-136). Most examples of epithelioid leiomyosarcomas (E-LMS) actually occur in the uterus; however, examples can also be seen in the somatic soft tissues.

Epithelioid leiomyosarcoma retains variable expression of smooth muscle actin, desmin, and h-caldesmon. As already discussed in this chapter, main differential diagnosis is with PEComa, in which the demonstration of the expression of melanocytic markers (HMB45 and/or Melan-A) represents a most helpful diagnostic clue. As mentioned, epithelioid GIST expresses KIT and/or DOG1, which are always negative in true smooth muscle tumors.

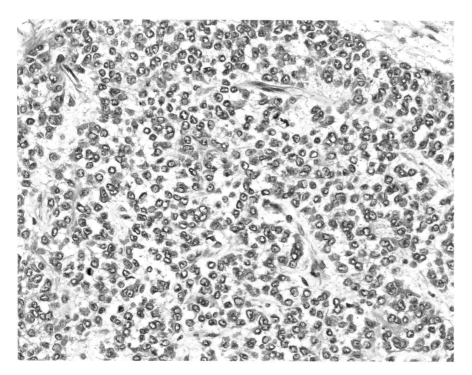

**Fig. 5-136.** Epithelioid leiomyosarcoma. Tumor cells exhibit an epithelioid cell morphology and feature eosinophilic cytoplasm.

# Epithelioid Rhabdomyosarcoma

Very recently, an epithelioid variant of rhabdomyosarcoma (RMS), reminiscent of poorly differentiated carcinoma or melanoma, was reported.

Epithelioid RMS tends to occur in the extremities of adult patients (peak incidence in the seventh decade), with a predilection for men. Visceral location is also observed.

Histologically, epithelioid RMS is composed of diffuse sheets of tumor cells featuring high-grade epithelioid morphology and lacking the morphologic features of either embryonal or alveolar RMS.

The tumor cells are characterized by abundant amphophilic to eosinophilic cytoplasm and large vesicular nuclei with irregular nuclear contours (Fig. 5-137). Nucleoli tend to be large and prominent, similar to those seen in melanoma, and are occasionally multiple. Rarely, multinucleate cells are found; however, in contrast to usual pleomorphic RMS, E-RMS shows less nuclear atypia or very focal cytologic pleomorphism (Fig. 5-138). Mitotic activity is generally high, with frequent atypical forms.

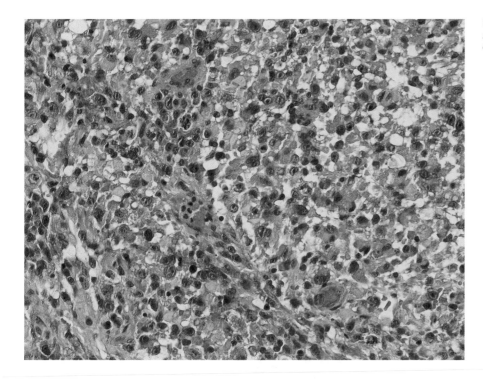

**Fig. 5-137.** Epithelioid rhabdomyosarcoma. Atypical epithelioid tumor cells feature deeply eosinophilic cytoplasm.

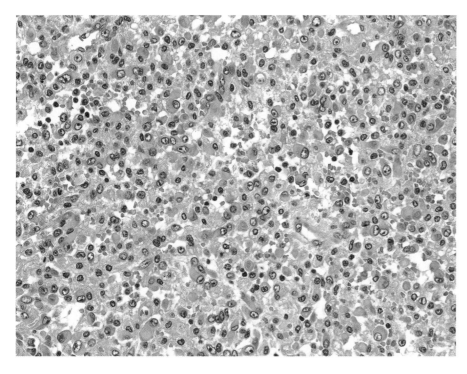

**Fig. 5-138.** Epithelioid rhabdomyosarcoma. In this example, a monomorphic "rhabdoid" cell proliferation is seen.

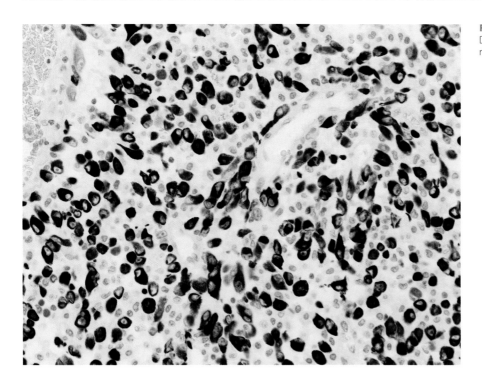

**Fig. 5-139.** Epithelioid rhabdomyosarcoma. Desmin is the most sensitive marker for rhabdomyosarcoma.

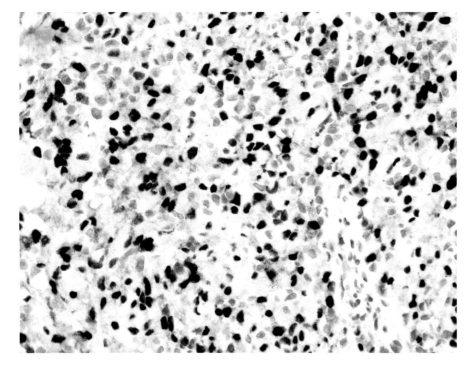

**Fig. 5-140.** Epithelioid rhabdomyosarcoma. Myogenin is the most specific marker for rhabdomyosarcoma.

Immunohistochemically, the neoplasm is desmin (Fig. 5-139) and myogenin (Fig. 5-140) positive, with variable expression from diffuse to multifocal. Focal positivity for cytokeratin and S100 can be observed.

## Differential Diagnosis and Diagnostic Pitfalls

The differential diagnosis of E-RMS includes metastatic carcinoma, melanoma, angiosarcoma, epithelioid leiomyosarcoma, and malignant PEComa. Importantly, all these entities lack

expression of myogenin, which still represents a very specific as well as extremely helpful diagnostic marker.

## Epithelioid Inflammatory Myofibroblastic Sarcoma

A distinctive, aggressive intra-abdominal variant of inflammatory myofibroblastic tumor (IMT) with epithelioid morphology has been recently reported. In consideration of aggressive behavior, the designation "epithelioid inflammatory myofibroblastic

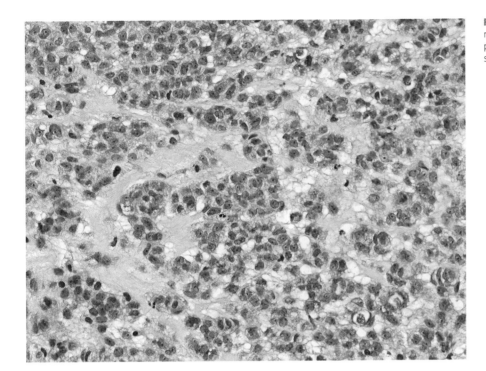

**Fig. 5-141.** Epithelioid inflammatory myofibroblastic tumor. The tumor shows a proliferation of atypical epithelioid cells organized in sheets.

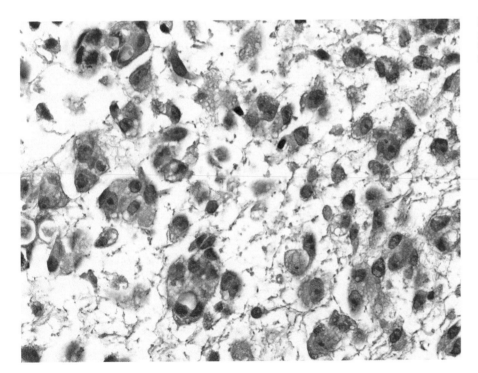

**Fig. 5-142.** Epithelioid inflammatory myofibroblastic tumor. Tumor cells exhibit macronucleolated vesicular nuclei and eosinophilic cytoplasm.

sarcoma" (E-IMT) has been proposed. This variant more often affects males of any age, ranging from 7 months to 63 years (peak incidence in the third decade) and tends to occur intraabdominally.

Histologically, tumor cells exhibit an epithelioid to round shape and grow in solid sheets (Fig. 5-141). A variably prominent inflammatory (predominantly neutrophils and small lymphocytes) infiltrate is most often observed. Neoplastic cells are embedded in a variable myxoid, collagenous, or mixed stroma (Fig. 5-142). The tumor cells have vesicular nuclei with large

nucleoli and variable amounts of amphophilic or eosinophilic cytoplasm. Focal necrosis can be present. Mitotic activity is very variable, ranging from 1 to 18 per high-power field.

Immunohistochemically, E-IMT exhibits a distinctive perinuclear membrane pattern of ALK staining, which correlates with the presence of a *RANBP2-ALK* gene fusion. Recently, a novel *RRBP1-ALK* fusion was reported. Tumor cells also variably express desmin, smooth muscle actin, and CD30 (Fig. 5-143), whereas they are cytokeratin and S100 negative.

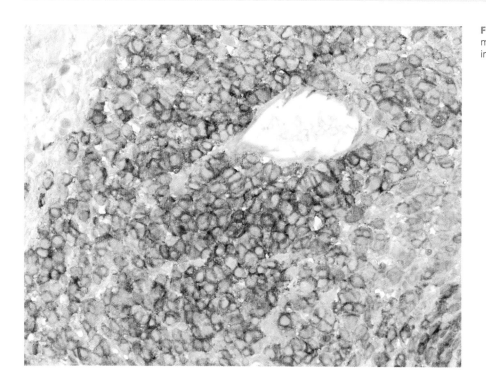

**Fig. 5-143.** Epithelioid inflammatory myofibroblastic tumor. CD30 (in addition to ALK1) immunopositivity is often seen.

## Differential Diagnosis and Diagnostic Pitfalls

The unusual epithelioid-to-round-cell morphology, along with the markedly atypical nuclear features, may lead to a rather broad differential diagnosis including anaplastic large cell lymphoma (ALCL) and epithelioid variants of leiomyosarcoma, rhabdomyosarcoma, myxofibrosarcoma, and undifferentiated sarcoma. The recognition of this distinctive tumor type is especially relevant, given the recent development of ALK-targeted therapy, which may provide effective treatment for these aggressive tumors.

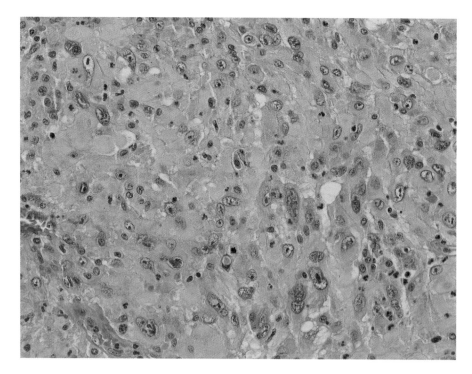

**Fig. 5-144.** Undifferentiated epithelioid sarcoma. An epithelioid cell neoplastic proliferation is seen, featuring multifocal marked nuclear pleomorphism.

# Undifferentiated Epithelioid Sarcoma

Undifferentiated epithelioid sarcoma (UES) has been recognized recently within the 2013 WHO classification of bone and soft tissue sarcomas. Shared views among experts indicate that a group of aggressive epithelioid mesenchymal malignancies lacking a specific line of differentiation exist.

Most often, these lesions exhibit epithelioid morphology associated with high-grade nuclear atypia (Fig. 5-144). At the moment, UES as a group is still poorly defined and the differential diagnosis is very broad, also including metastatic carcinoma and melanoma. Close clinicopathologic correlation is mandatory in order to avoid misclassification.

## Chapter 5 Selected Key References

### Epithelioid Sarcoma

- Agaimy A. The expanding family of SMARCB1(INI1)-deficient neoplasia: implications of phenotypic, biological, and molecular heterogeneity. *Adv Anat Pathol.* 2014;21:394–410.

- Arber DA, Kandalaft PL, Mehta P, Battifora H. Vimentin-negative epithelioid sarcoma. The value of an immunohistochemical panel that includes CD34. *Am J Surg Pathol.* 1993;17:302–7.

- Bos GD, Pritchard DJ, Reiman HM, et al. Epithelioid sarcoma. An analysis of fifty-one cases. *J Bone Joint Surg Am.* 1988;70:862–70.

- Chase DR, Enzinger FM. Epithelioid sarcoma. Diagnosis, prognostic indicators and treatment. *Am J Surg Pathol.* 1985;9:241–63.

- Chase DR, Enzinger FM, Weiss SW, Langloss JM. Keratin in epithelioid sarcoma. An immunohistochemical study. *Am J Surg Pathol.* 1984;8:435–41.

- Enzinger FM. Epithelioid sarcoma. A sarcoma simulating a granuloma or a carcinoma. *Cancer.* 1970;26:1029–41.

- Evans HL, Baer SC. Epithelioid sarcoma: a clinicopathologic and prognostic study of 26 cases. *Semin Diagn Pathol.* 1993;10:286–91.

- Guillou L, Wadden C, Coindre JM, Krausz T, Fletcher CD. "Proximal-type" epithelioid sarcoma, a distinctive aggressive neoplasm showing rhabdoid features. Clinicopathologic, immunohistochemical, and ultrastructural study of a series. *Am J Surg Pathol.* 1997;21:130–46.

- Halling AC, Wollan PC, Pritchard DJ, Vlasak R, Nascimento AG. Epithelioid sarcoma: a clinicopathologic review of 55 cases. *Mayo Clin Proc.* 1996;71:636–42.

- Hollmann TJ, Hornick JL. INI1-deficient tumors: diagnostic features and molecular genetics. *Am J Surg Pathol.* 2011;35:47–63.

- Hornick JL, Dal Cin P, Fletcher CD. Loss of INI1 expression is characteristic of both conventional and proximal-type epithelioid sarcoma. *Am J Surg Pathol.* 2009;33:542–50.

- Italiano A. Role of the EZH2 histone methyltransferase as a therapeutic target in cancer. *Pharmacol Ther.* 2016;165:26–31.

- Kodet R, Smelhaus V, Newton WA, et al. Epithelioid sarcoma in childhood: an immunohistochemical, electron microscopic, and clinicopathologic study of 11 cases under 15 years of age and review of the literature. *Pediatr Pathol.* 1994;14:433–51.

- Kohashi K, Izumi T, Oda Y, et al. Infrequent SMARCB1/ INI1 gene alteration in epithelioid sarcoma: a useful tool in distinguishing epithelioid sarcoma from malignant rhabdoid tumor. *Hum Pathol.* 2009;40:349–55.

- Modena P, Luaki E, Facchinetti F, et al. SMARCB1/INI1 tumor suppressor gene is frequently inactivated in epithelioid sarcomas. *Cancer Res.* 2005;65:4012–19.

- Miettinen M, Fanburg-Smith JC, Virolainen M, Shmookler BM, Fetsch JF. Epithelioid sarcoma: an immunohistochemical analysis of 112 classical and variant cases and a discussion of the differential diagnosis. *Hum Pathol.* 1999;30:934–42.

- Miettinen M, Wang Z, Sarlomo-Rikala M, et al. ERG expression in epithelioid sarcoma: a diagnostic pitfall. *Am J Surg Pathol.* 2013;37:1580–5.

- Wick MR, Manivel JC. Epithelioid sarcoma and isolated necrobiotic granuloma: a comparative immunocytochemical study. *J Cutan Pathol.* 1986;13:253–60.

### Malignant Extrarenal Rhabdoid Tumor or MRT of Soft Tissue

- Biegel JA, Tan L, Zhang F, et al. Alterations of the hSNF5/INI1 gene in central nervous system atypical teratoid/ rhabdoid tumors and renal and extrarenal rhabdoid tumors. *Clin Cancer Res.* 2002;8:3461–7.

- Bittesini L, Dei Tos AP, Fletcher CDM. Malignant melanoma showing rhabdoid differentiation. Further evidence of a non- specific histologic pattern. *Histopathology.* 1992;20:167–70.

- Fanburg-Smith JC, Hengge M, Hengge UR, Smith JS Jr, Miettinen M. Extrarenal rhabdoid tumors of soft tissue: a clinicopathologic and immunohistochemical study of 18 cases. *Ann Diagn Pathol.* 1998;2:351–62.

- Huang SC, Zhang L, Sung YS, et al. Secondary EWSR1 gene abnormalities in SMARCB1-deficient tumors with 22q11-12 regional deletions: potential pitfalls in interpreting EWSR1 FISH results. *Genes Chromosomes Cancer.* 2016;55:767–76.

- Judkins AR. Immunohistochemistry of INI1 expression: a new tool for old challenges in CNS and soft tissue pathology. *Adv Anat Pathol.* 2007;14:335–9.

- Le Loarer F, Watson S, Pierron G, et al. SMARCA4 inactivation defines a group of undifferentiated thoracic malignancies transcriptionally related to BAF-deficient sarcomas. *Nat Genet.* 2015;47:1200–5.

- Margol AS, Judkins AR. Pathology and diagnosis of SMARCB1-deficient tumors. *Cancer Genetics.* 2014;207:358–64.

- Oda Y, Tsuneyoshi M. Extrarenal rhabdoid tumors of soft tissue: clinicopathological and molecular genetic review and distinction from other soft-tissue sarcomas with rhabdoid features. *Pathol Int.* 2006;56:287–95.

- Parham DM, Weeks DA, Beckwith JB. The clinicopathologic spectrum of putative extrarenal rhabdoid tumors. An analysis of 42 cases studied with immunohistochemistry or electron microscopy. *Am J Surg Pathol.* 1994;18:1010–29.

- Sauter JL, Graham RP, Larsen BT, et al. SMARCA4-deficient thoracic sarcoma: a distinctive clinicopathological entity with undifferentiated rhabdoid morphology and aggressive behavior. *Mod Pathol.* 2017;30:1422–32.

- Schaefer IM, Agaimy A, Fletcher CD, Hornick JL. Claudin-4 expression distinguishes SWI/SNF complex-deficient undifferentiated carcinomas from sarcomas. *Mod Pathol.* 2017;30:539–48.

- Sigauke E, Rakheja D, Maddox DL, et al. Absence of expression of SMARCB1/INI1 in malignant rhabdoid tumors of the central nervous system, kidneys and soft tissue: an immunohistochemical study with implications for diagnosis. *Mod Pathol*. 2006;**19**:717–25.
- Sotelo-Avila C, Gonzalez-Crussi F, DeMello D, et al. Renal and extrarenal rhabdoid tumors in children: a clinicopathologic study of 14 patients. *Semin Diagn Pathol*. 1986;**3**:151–63.
- Wick MR, Ritter JH, Dehner LP. Malignant rhabdoid tumors: a clinicopathologic review and conceptual discussion. *Semin Diagnostic Pathol*. 1995;**12**:233–48.

## Myoepithelioma/Myoepithelial Carcinoma

- Agaram NP, Chen HW, Zhang L, et al. EWSR1-PBX3: a novel gene fusion in myoepithelial tumors. *Genes Chromosomes Cancer*. 2015;**54**:63–71.
- Antonescu CR, Zhang L, Chang NE, et al. EWSR1-POU5F1 fusion in soft tissue myoepithelial tumors. A molecular analysis of sixty-six cases, including soft tissue, bone, and visceral lesions, showing common involvement of the EWSR1 gene. *Genes Chromosomes Cancer*. 2010;**49**: 1114–24.
- Antonescu CR, Zhang L, Shao SY, et al. Frequent PLAG1 gene rearrangements in skin and soft tissue myoepithelioma with ductal differentiation. *Genes Chromosomes Cancer*. 2013;**52**:675–82.
- Attwooll C, Tariq M, Harris M, et al. Identification of a novel fusion gene involving hTAFII68 and CHN from a t(9;17)(q22;q11.2) translocation in an extraskeletal myxoid chondrosarcoma. *Oncogene*. 1999;**18**:7599–601.
- Fisher C. Parachordoma exists–but what is it? *Adv Anat Pathol*. 2000;**7**:141–8.
- Gleason BC, Fletcher CD. Myoepithelial carcinoma of soft tissue in children: an aggressive neoplasm analyzed in a series of 29 cases. *Am J Surg Pathol*. 2007;**31**:1813–24.
- Hallor KH, Teixeira MR, Fletcher CD, et al. Heterogeneous genetic profiles in soft tissue myoepitheliomas. *Mod Pathol*. 2008;**21**:1311–19.
- Hornick JL, Fletcher CD. Myoepithelial tumors of soft tissue: a clinicopathologic and immunohistochemical study of 101 cases with evaluation of prognostic parameters. *Am J Surg Pathol*. 2003;**27**:1183–96.
- Huang SC, Chen HW, Zhang L, et al. Novel FUS-KLF17 and EWSR1-KLF17 fusions in myoepithelial tumors. *Genes Chromosomes Cancer*. 2015;**54**:267–75.
- Kilpatrick SE, Hitchcock MG, Kraus MD, Calonje E, Fletcher CD. Mixed tumors and myoepitheliomas of soft tissue: a clinicopathologic study of 19 cases with a unifying concept. *Am J Surg Pathol*. 1997;**21**:13–22.
- Leduc C, Zhang L, Öz B, et al. Thoracic myoepithelial tumors: a pathologic and molecular study of 8 cases with review of the literature. *Am J Surg Pathol*. 2016;**40**:212–23.
- Le Loarer F, Zhang L, Fletcher CD, et al. Consistent SMARCB1 homozygous deletions in epithelioid sarcoma and in a subset of myoepithelial carcinomas can be reliably detected by FISH in archival material. *Genes Chromosomes Cancer*. 2014;**53**:475–86.
- Puls F, Arbajian E Magnusson L, et al. Myoepithelioma of bone with a novel FUS-POU5F1 fusion gene. *Histopathology*. 2014;**65**:917–22.
- Sciot R, Dal Cin P, Fletcher C, et al. t(9;22)(q22-31;q11-12) is a consistent marker of extraskeletal myxoid chondrosarcoma: evaluation of three cases. *Mod Pathol*. 1995;**8**:765–8.
- Thway K, Fisher C. Myoepithelial tumor of soft tissue: histology and genetics of an evolving entity. *Adv Anat Pathol*. 2014;**21**:411–19.
- Tirabosco R, Mangham DC, Rosenberg AE, et al. Brachyury expression in extra-axial skeletal and soft tissue chordomas: a marker that distinguishes chordoma from mixed tumor/myoepithelioma/parachordoma in soft tissue. *Am J Surg Pathol*. 2008;**32**:572–80.
- Urbini M, Astolfi A, Indio V, et al. Identification of SRF-E2F1 fusion transcript in EWSR-negative myoepithelioma of the soft tissue. *Oncotarget*. 2017;**8**:60036–45.

## Pseudomyogenic Hemangioendothelioma

- Billings SD, Folpe AL, Weiss SW. Epithelioid sarcoma-like hemangioendothelioma. *Am J Surg Pathol*. 2003;**27**:48–57.
- Hornick JL, Fletcher CD. Pseudomyogenic hemangioendothelioma: a distinctive, often multicentric tumor with indolent behavior. *Am J Surg Pathol*. 2011;**35**:190–201.
- Hung YP, Fletcher CD, Hornick JL. FOSB is a useful diagnostic marker for pseudomyogenic hemangioendothelioma. *Am J Surg Pathol*. 2017;**41**:596–606.
- Inyang A, Mertens F, Puls F, et al. Primary pseudomyogenic hemangioendothelioma of bone. *Am J Surg Pathol*. 2016;**40**:587–98.
- Mirra JM, Kessler S, Bhuta S, Eckardt J. The fibroma-like variant of epithelioid sarcoma. A fibrohistiocytic/myoid cell lesion often confused with benign and malignant spindle cell tumors. *Cancer*. 1992;**69**:1382–95.
- Righi A, Gambarotti M, Picci P, Dei Tos AP, Vanel D. Primary pseudomyogenic haemangioendothelioma of bone: report of two cases. *Skel Radiol*. 2015;**44**:727–31.
- Trombetta D, Magnusson L, von Steyern FV, et al. Translocation t(7;19)(q22;q13): a recurrent chromosome aberration in pseudomyogenic hemangioendothelioma? *Cancer Genetics*. 2011;**204**:211–15.
- Walther C, Tayebwa J, Lilljebjorn H, et al. A novel SERPINE1-FOSB fusion gene results in transcriptional up-regulation of FOSB in pseudomyogenic haemangioendothelioma. *J Pathol*. 2014;**23**:534–40.

## Epithelioid Hemangioendothelioma and Its Differential Diagnosis

- Anderson T, Zhang L, Hameed M, et al. Thoracic epithelioid malignant vascular tumors: a clinicopathologic study of 52 cases with emphasis on pathologic grading and molecular studies of WWTR1-CAMTA1 fusions. *Am J Surg Pathol*. 2015;**39**:132–9.
- Antonescu CR, Chen HW, Zhang L, et al. ZFP36-FOSB fusion defines a subset of epithelioid hemangioma with atypical features. *Genes Chromosomes Cancer*. 2014;**53**:951–9.
- Antonescu CR, Le Loarer F, Mosquera JM, et al. Novel YAP1-TFE3 fusion defines a distinct subset of epithelioid hemangioendothelioma. *Genes Chromosomes Cancer*. 2013;**52**:775–84.
- Bhagavan BS, Dorfman HD, Murthy MS, Eggleston JC. Intravascular bronchiolo-alveolar tumor (IVBAT): A low-grade sclerosing epithelioid angiosarcoma of lung. *Am J Surg Pathol*. 1982;**6**:41–52.
- Dietze O, Davies SE, Williams R, Portmann B. Malignant epithelioid haemangioendothelioma of the liver: a clinicopathological and histochemical

study of 12 cases. *Histopathology.* 1989;**15**:225–37.

- Doyle LA, Fletcher CD, Hornick JL. Nuclear expression of CAMTA1 distinguishes epithelioid hemangioendothelioma from histologic mimics. *Am J Surg Pathol.* 2016;**40**:94–102

- Errani C, Zhang L, Sung YS, et al. A novel WWTR1-CAMTA1 gene fusion is a consistent abnormality in epithelioid hemangioendothelioma of different anatomic sites. *Genes Chromosomes Cancer.* 2011;**50**:644–53.

- Gomez-Arellano LI, Ferrari-Carballo T, Dominguez-Malagon HR. Multicentric epithelioid hemangioendothelioma of bone. Report of a case with radiologic-pathologic correlation. *Ann Diagn Pathol.* 2012;**16**:43–7.

- Huang SC, Zhang L, Sung YS, et al. Frequent FOS gene rearrangements in epithelioid hemangioma: a molecular study of 58 cases with morphologic reappraisal. *Am J Surg Pathol.* 2015;**39**:1313–21.

- Mendlick MR, Nelson M, Pickering D, et al. Translocation t(1;3)(p36.3;q25) is a nonrandom aberration in epithelioid hemangioendothelioma. *Am J Surg Pathol.* 2001;**25**: 684–7.

- Mentzel T, Beham A, Calonje E, Katenkamp D, Fletcher CD. Epithelioid hemangioendothelioma of skin and soft tissues: clinicopathologic and immunohistochemical study of 30 cases. *Am J Surg Pathol.* 1997;**21**:363–74.

- Miettinen M, Wang ZF, Paetau A, et al. ERG transcription factor as an immunohistochemical marker for vascular endothelial tumors and prostatic carcinoma. *Am J Surg Pathol.* 2011;**35**:432–41.

- Rossi S, Orvieto E, Furlanetto A, et al. Utility of the immunohistochemical detection of FLI-1 expression in round cell and vascular neoplasm using a monoclonal antibody. *Mod Pathol.* 2004;**17**:547–52.

- Weiss SW, Enzinger FM. Epithelioid hemangioendothelioma: a vascular tumor often mistaken for a carcinoma. *Cancer.* 1982;**50**:970–81.

- Weiss SW, Ishak KG, Dail DH, Sweet DE, Enzinger FM. Epithelioid hemangioendothelioma and related lesions. *Semin Diagn Pathol.* 1986;**3**:259–87.

## Epithelioid Angiosarcoma

- Eusebi V, Carcangiu ML, Dina R, Rosai J. Keratin-positive epithelioid angiosarcoma of thyroid. A report of four cases. *Am J Surg Pathol.* 1990;**14**:737–47.

- Fletcher CD, Beham A, Bekir S, Clarke AM, Marley NJ. Epithelioid angiosarcoma of deep soft tissue: a distinctive tumor readily mistaken for an epithelial neoplasm. *Am J Surg Pathol.* 1991;**15**:915–24.

- Meis-Kindblom JM, Kindblom LG. Angiosarcoma of soft tissue: a study of 80 cases. *Am J Surg Pathol.* 1998;**22**:683–97.

- Rosai J, Sumner HW, Kostianovsky M, Perez-Mesa C. Angiosarcoma of the skin. A clinicopathologic and fine structural study. *Hum Pathol.* 1976;**7**:83–109.

- Rossi S, Fletcher CD. Angiosarcoma arising in hemangioma/vascular malformation: report of four cases and review of the literature. *Am J Surg Pathol.* 2002;**26**:1319–29.

- Shon W, Sukov WR, Jenkins SM, Folpe AL. MYC amplification and overexpression in primary cutaneous angiosarcoma: a fluorescence in-situ hybridization and immunohistochemical study. *Mod Pathol.* 2014;**27**:509–15.

- Stacchiotti S, Palassini E, Sanfilippo R, et al. Gemcitabine in advanced angiosarcoma: a retrospective case series analysis from the Italian Rare Cancer Network. *Ann Oncol.* 2012;**23**:501–8.

## Epithelioid MPNST and Its Differential Diagnosis

- Allison KH, Patel RM, Goldblum JR, Rubin BP. Superficial malignant peripheral nerve sheath tumor: a rare and challenging diagnosis. *Am J Clin Pathol.* 2005;**124**:685–92.

- Carter JM, O'Hara C, Dundas G, et al. Epithelioid malignant peripheral nerve sheath tumor arising in a schwannoma, in a patient with "neuroblastoma-like" schwannomatosis and a novel germline SMARCB1 mutation. *Am J Surg Pathol.* 2012;**36**:154–60.

- DiCarlo EF, Woodruff JM, Bansal M, Erlandson RA. The purely epithelioid malignant peripheral nerve sheath tumor. *Am J Surg Pathol.* 1986;**10**:478–90.

- Jo VY, Fletcher CD. Epithelioid malignant peripheral nerve sheath tumor: clinicopathologic analysis of 63 cases. *Am J Surg Pathol.* 2015;**39**:673–82.

- Jo VY, Fletcher CDM. SMARCB1/INI1 loss in epithelioid schwannoma: a clinicopathologic and immunohistochemical study of 65 cases. *Am J Surg Pathol.* 2017;**41**:1013–22.

- Laskin WB, Weiss SW, Bratthauer GL. Epithelioid variant of malignant peripheral nerve sheath tumor (malignant epithelioid schwannoma). *Am J Surg Pathol.* 1991;**15**:1136–45.

- Lodding P, Kindblom LG, Angervall L. Epithelioid malignant schwannoma. A study of 14 cases. *Virchows Archiv.* 1986;**409**:433–51.

- McCormack LJ, Hazard JB, Dickson JA. Malignant epithelioid neurilemoma (schwannoma). *Cancer.* 1954;**7**:725–8.

- McMenamin ME, Fletcher CD. Expanding the spectrum of malignant change in schwannomas: epithelioid malignant change, epithelioid malignant peripheral nerve sheath tumor, and epithelioid angiosarcoma: a study of 17 cases. *Am J Surg Pathol.* 2001;**25**:13–25.

- Yamamoto T. Epithelioid malignant schwannoma of the superficial soft tissues vs. metastatic amelanotic melanoma. *J Cutan Pathol.* 2002;**29**:569.

- Yousem SA, Colby TV, Urich H. Malignant epithelioid schwannoma arising in a benign schwannoma. A case report. *Cancer.* 1985;**55**:2799–803.

## Clear Cell Sarcoma and Its Differential Diagnosis

- Alexiev BA, Chou PM, Jennings LJ. Pathology of melanotic schwannoma. *Arch Pathol Lab Med.* 2018 Jan 26. [Epub ahead of print]

- Antonescu CR, Nafa K, Segal NH, Dal Cin P, Ladanyi M. EWS-CREB1: a recurrent variant fusion in clear cell sarcoma – association with gastrointestinal location and absence of melanocytic differentiation. *Clin Cancer Res.* 2006;**15**:5356–62.

- Antonescu CR, Tschernyavsky SJ, Woodruff JM, et al. Molecular diagnosis of clear cell sarcoma: detection of EWS-ATF1 and MITF-M transcripts and histopathological and ultrastructural analysis of 12 cases. *J Mol Diagn.* 2002;**4**:44–52.

- Carney JA. Psammomatous melanotic schwannoma. A distinctive, heritable tumor with special associations, including cardiac myxoma and the

Cushing syndrome. *Am J Surg Pathol.* 1990;**14**:206–22.

- Chung EB, Enzinger FM. Malignant melanoma of soft parts. A reassessment of clear cell sarcoma. *Am J Surg Pathol.* 1983;**7**:405–13.

- Dim DC, Cooley LD, Miranda RN. Clear cell sarcoma of tendons and aponeuroses: a review. *Arch Pathol Lab Med.* 2007;**131**:152–6.

- Enzinger FM. Clear-cell sarcoma of tendons and aponeuroses. An analysis of 21 cases. *Cancer.* 1965;**18**: 1163–74.

- Graadt van Roggen JF, Mooi WJ, Hogendoorn PC. Clear cell sarcoma of tendons and aponeuroses (malignant melanoma of soft parts) and cutaneous melanoma: exploring the histogenetic relationship between these two clinicopathological entities. *J Pathol.* 1998;**186**:3–7.

- Granter SR, Weilbaecher KN, Quigley C, Fletcher CD, Fisher DE. Clear cell sarcoma shows immunoreactivity for microphthalmia transcription factor: further evidence for melanocytic differentiation. *Mod Pathol.* 2001;**14**:6–9.

- Kawai A, Hosono A, Nakayama R, et al. Japanese Musculoskeletal Oncology G: clear cell sarcoma of tendons and aponeuroses: a study of 75 patients. *Cancer.* 2007;**109**:109–16.

- Kosemehmetoglu K, Folpe AL. Clear cell sarcoma of tendons and aponeuroses, and osteoclast-rich tumour of the gastrointestinal tract with features resembling clear cell sarcoma of soft parts: a review and update. *J Clin Pathol.* 2010;**63**:416–23.

- Panagopoulos I, Mertens F, Isaksson M, Mandahl N. Absence of mutations of the BRAF gene in malignant melanoma of soft parts (clear cell sarcoma of tendons and aponeuroses). *Cancer Genet Cytogenet.* 2005;**156**:74–6.

- Sara AS, Evans HL, Benjamin RS. Malignant melanoma of soft parts (clear cell sarcoma). A study of 17 cases, with emphasis on prognostic factors. *Cancer.* 1990;**65**: 367–74.

- Stockman DL, Miettinen M, Suster S, et al. Malignant gastrointestinal neuroectodermal tumor: clinicopathologic, immunohistochemical, ultrastructural, and molecular analysis of 16 cases with a reappraisal of clear cell sarcoma-like tumors of the gastrointestinal tract. *Am J Surg Pathol.* 2012;**36**:857–68.

- Torres-Mora J, Dry S, Li X, et al. Malignant melanotic schwannian tumor: a clinicopathologic,
immunohistochemical, and gene expression profiling study of 40 cases, with a proposal for the reclassification of "melanotic schwannoma." *Am J Surg Pathol.* 2014;**38**:94–105.

- Wang J, Thway K. Clear cell sarcoma-like tumor of the gastrointestinal tract: an evolving entity. *Arch Pathol Lab Med.* 2015;**139**:407–12.

- Zambrano E, Reyes-Mugica M, Franchi A, Rosai J. An osteoclast-rich tumor of the gastrointestinal tract with features resembling clear cell sarcoma of soft parts: reports of 6 cases of a GIST simulator. *Int J Surg Pathol.* 2003;**11**:75–81.

## Sclerosing Epithelioid Fibrosarcoma

- Antonescu CR, Rosenblum MK, Pereira P, Nascimento AG, Woodruff JM. Sclerosing epithelioid fibrosarcoma: a study of 16 cases and confirmation of a clinicopathologically distinct tumor. *Am J Surg Pathol.* 2001;**25**:699–709.

- Arbajian E, Puls F, Magnusson L, et al. Recurrent EWSR1-CREB3L1 gene fusions in sclerosing epithelioid fibrosarcoma. *Am J Surg Pathol.* 2014;**38**:801–8.

- Argani P, Lewin JR, Edmonds P, et al. Primary renal sclerosing epithelioid fibrosarcoma: report of 2 cases with EWSR1-CREB3L1 gene fusion. *Am J Surg Pathol.* 2015;**39**:365–73.

- Doyle LA, Hornick JL. EWSR1 rearrangements in sclerosing epithelioid fibrosarcoma. *Am J Surg Pathol.* 2013;**37**:1630–1.

- Doyle LA, Wang WL, Dal Cin P, et al. MUC4 is a sensitive and extremely useful marker for sclerosing epithelioid fibrosarcoma: association with FUS gene rearrangement. *Am J Surg Pathol.* 2012;**36**:1444–51.

- Guillou L, Benhattar J, Gengler C, et al. Translocation-positive low-grade fibromyxoid sarcoma: clinicopathologic and molecular analysis of a series expanding the morphologic spectrum and suggesting potential relationship to sclerosing epithelioid fibrosarcoma: a study from the French Sarcoma Group. *Am J Surg Pathol.* 2007;**31**:1387–402.

- Meis-Kindblom JM, Kindblom LG, Enzinger FM. Sclerosing epithelioid fibrosarcoma. A variant of fibrosarcoma simulating carcinoma. *Am J Surg Pathol.* 1995;**19**:979–93.

- Stockman DL, Ali SM, He J, Ross JS, Meis JM. Sclerosing epithelioid fibrosarcoma presenting as intraabdominal
sarcomatosis with a novel EWSR1-CREB3L1 gene fusion. *Hum Pathol.* 2014;**45**:2173–8.

- Wang WL, Evans HL, Meis JM, et al. FUS rearrangements are rare in 'pure' sclerosing epithelioid fibrosarcoma. *Mod Pathol.* 2012;**25**:846–53.

## Alveolar Soft Part Sarcoma

- Argani P, Antonescu CR, Illei PB, et al. Primary renal neoplasms with the ASPL-TFE3 gene fusion of alveolar soft part sarcoma: a distinctive tumor entity previously included among renal cell carcinomas of children and adolescents. *Am J Surg Pathol.* 2001;**159**:179–92.

- Argani P, Lal P, Hutchinson B, et al. Aberrant nuclear immunoreactivity for TFE3 in neoplasms with TFE3 gene fusions: a sensitive and specific immunohistochemical assay. *Am J Surg Pathol.* 2003;**27**:750–61.

- Aulmann S, Longerich T, Schirmacher P, Mechtersheimer G, Penzel R. Detection of the ASPSCR1-TFE3 gene fusion in paraffin-embedded alveolar soft part sarcomas. *Histopathology.* 2007;**50**:881–6.

- Christopherson WM, Foote FW Jr, Stewart FW. Alveolar soft-part sarcomas: structurally characteristic tumors of uncertain histogenesis. *Cancer.* 1952;**5**:100–11.

- Fanburg-Smith JC, Miettinen M, Folpe AL, Weiss SW, Childers EL. Lingual alveolar soft part sarcoma; 14 cases: novel clinical and morphological observations. *Histopathology.* 2004;**45**:526–37.

- Folpe AL, Deyrup AT. Alveolar soft-part sarcoma: a review and update. *J Clin Pathol.* 2006;**59**:1127–32.

- Kayton ML, Meyers P, Wexler LH, Gerald WL, LaQuaglia MP. Clinical presentation, treatment, and outcome of alveolar soft part sarcoma in children, adolescents, and young adults. *J Ped Surg.* 2006;**41**:187–93.

- Ladanyi M, Lui MY, Antonescu CR, et al. The der(17)t(X;17)(p11;q25) of human alveolar soft part sarcoma fuses the TFE3 transcription factor gene to ASPL, a novel gene at 17q25. *Oncogene.* 2001;**20**:48–57.

- Lieberman PH, Brennan MF, Kimmel M, et al. Alveolar soft-part sarcoma. A clinico-pathologic study of half a century. *Cancer.* 1989;**63**:1–13.

- Orbach D, Brennan B, Casanova M, et al. Paediatric and adolescent alveolar soft part sarcoma: A joint series from European cooperative groups. *Pediatr Blood Cancer.* 2013;**60**:1826–32.

- Portera CA Jr, Ho V, Patel SR, et al. Alveolar soft part sarcoma: clinical course and patterns of metastasis in 70 patients treated at a single institution. *Cancer.* 2001;**91**:585–91.
- Tsuda M, Davis IJ, Argani P, et al. TFE3 fusions activate MET signaling by transcriptional up-regulation, defining another class of tumors as candidates for therapeutic MET inhibition. *Cancer Res.* 2007;**67**:919–29.

## Pecoma of Soft Tissue (PEComa)

- Argani P, Aulmann S, Illei PB, et al. A distinctive subset of PEComas harbors TFE3 gene fusions. *Am J Surg Pathol.* 2010;**34**:1395–406.
- Bleeker JS, Quevedo JF, Folpe AL. "Malignant" perivascular epithelioid cell neoplasm: risk stratification and treatment strategies. *Sarcoma.* **2012**;54:1626.
- Bonetti F, Pea M, Martignoni G, Zamboni G. PEC and sugar. *Am J Surg Pathol.* 1992;**16**:307–8.
- Doyle LA, Hornick JL, Fletcher CD. PEComa of the gastrointestinal tract: clinicopathologic study of 35 cases with evaluation of prognostic parameters. *Am J Surg Pathol.* 2013;**37**:1769–82.
- Folpe AL, Goodman ZD, Ishak KG, et al. Clear cell myomelanocytic tumor of the falciform ligament/ligamentum teres: a novel member of the perivascular epithelioid clear cell family of tumors with a predilection for children and young adults. *Am J Surg Pathol.* 2000;**24**:1239–46.
- Folpe AL, Kwiatkowski DJ. Perivascular epithelioid cell neoplasms: pathology and pathogenesis. *Hum Pathol.* 2010;**41**:1–15.
- Hornick JL, Fletcher CD. PEComa: what do we know so far? *Histopathology.* 2006;**48**:75–82.
- Hornick JL, Fletcher CD. Sclerosing PEComa: clinicopathologic analysis of a distinctive variant with a predilection for the retroperitoneum. *Am J Surg Pathol.* 2008;**32**:493–501.
- Martignoni G, Pea M, Reghellin D, Zamboni G, Bonetti F. PEComas: the past, the present and the future. *Virchows Arch.* 2008;**452**:119–32.
- Nese N, Martignoni G, Fletcher CD, et al. Pure epithelioid PEComas (so-called epithelioid angiomyolipoma) of the kidney: a clinicopathologic study of 41 cases: detailed assessment of morphology and risk stratification. *Am J Surg Pathol.* 2011;**35**:161–76.

- Pan CC, Chung MY, Ng KF, et al. Constant allelic alteration on chromosome 16p (TSC2 gene) in perivascular epithelioid cell tumour (PEComa): genetic evidence for the relationship of PEComa with angiomyolipoma. *J Pathol.* 2008;**214**:387–93.
- Schoolmeester JK, Dao LN, Sukov WR, et al. TFE3 Translocation-associated perivascular epithelioid cell neoplasm (pecoma) of the gynecologic tract: morphology, immunophenotype, differential diagnosis. *Am J Surg Pathol.* 2015;**39**:394–404.
- Schoolmeester JK, Howitt BE, Hirsch MS, et al. Perivascular epithelioid cell neoplasm (PEComa) of the gynecologic tract: clinicopathologic and immunohistochemical characterization of 16 cases. *Am J Surg Pathol.* 2014;**38**:176–88.
- Shen Q, Rao Q, Xia QY, et al. Perivascular epithelioid cell tumor (PEComa) with TFE3 gene rearrangement: clinicopathological, immunohistochemical, and molecular features. *Virchows Arch.* 2014;**465**:607–13.
- Stacchiotti S, Marrari A, Dei Tos AP, Casali PG. Targeted therapies in rare sarcomas: IMT, ASPS, SFT, PEComa, and CCS. *Hematol Oncol Clin North Am.* 2013;**27**:1049–61.
- Wagner AJ, Malinowska-Kolodziej I, Morgan JA, et al. Clinical activity of mTOR inhibition with sirolimus in malignant perivascular epithelioid cell tumors: targeting the pathogenic activation of mTORC1 in tumors. *J Clin Oncol.* 2010;**28**:835–40.

## Variants of Soft Tissue Sarcomas Featuring Epithelioid Morphology

## Epithelioid Pleomorphic Liposarcoma

- Dei Tos AP, Mentzel T, Fletcher CD. Primary liposarcoma of the skin: a rare neoplasm with unusual high grade features. *Am J Dermatopathol.* 1998;**20**:332–8.
- Gebhard S, Coindre JM, Michels JJ, et al. Pleomorphic liposarcoma: clinicopathologic, immunohistochemical, and follow-up analysis of 63 cases: a study from the French Federation of Cancer Centers Sarcoma Group. *Am J Surg Pathol.* 2002;**26**:601–16.
- Ghadimi MP, Liu P, Peng T, et al. Pleomorphic liposarcoma: clinical observations and molecular variables. *Cancer.* 2011;**117**:5359–69.
- Hornick JL, Bosenberg MW, Mentzel T, et al. Pleomorphic liposarcoma: clinicopathologic analysis of 57 cases. *Am J Surg Pathol.* 2004;**28**:1257–67.
- Huang HY, Antonescu CR. Epithelioid variant of pleomorphic liposarcoma: a comparative immunohistochemical and ultrastructural analysis of six cases with emphasis on overlapping features with epithelial malignancies. *Ultrastruct Pathol.* 2002;**26**:299–308.
- Miettinen M, Enzinger FM. Epithelioid variant of pleomorphic liposarcoma: a study of 12 cases of a distinctive variant of high-grade liposarcoma. *Mod Pathol.* 1999;**12**:722–8.

## Epithelioid GIST

- Agaimy A, Otto C, Braun A, et al. Value of epithelioid morphology and PDGFRA immunostaining pattern for prediction of PDGFRA mutated genotype in gastrointestinal stromal tumors (GISTs). *Int J Clin Exp Pathol.* 2013;**6**:1839–46.
- Agaimy A, Wang LM, Eck M, Haller F, Chetty R. Loss of DOG-1 expression associated with shift from spindled to epithelioid morphology in gastric gastrointestinal stromal tumors with KIT and platelet-derived growth factor receptor alpha mutations. *Ann Diagn Pathol.* 2013;**17**:187–91.
- Folpe AL, Fanburg-Smith JC, Miettinen M, Weiss SW. Atypical and malignant glomus tumors: analysis of 52 cases, with a proposal for the reclassification of glomus tumors. *Am J Surg Pathol.* 2001;**25**:1–12.
- Gaal J, Stratakis CA, Carney JA, et al. SDHB immunohistochemistry: a useful tool in the diagnosis of Carney-Stratakis and Carney triad gastrointestinal stromal tumors. *Mod Pathol.* 2011;**24**:147–51.
- Miettinen M, Wang ZF, Sarlomo-Rikala M, et al. Succinate dehydrogenase-deficient GISTs: a clinicopathologic, immunohistochemical, and molecular genetic study of 66 gastric GISTs with predilection to young age. *Am J Surg Pathol.* 2011;**35**:1712–21.
- Schaefer IM, Strobel P, Cameron S, et al. Rhabdoid morphology in gastrointestinal

stromal tumours (GISTs) is associated with PDGFRA mutations but does not imply aggressive behaviour. *Histopathology*. 2014;**64**:421–30.

## Epithelioid Myxofibrosarcoma

- Nascimento AF, Bertoni F, Fletcher CD. Epithelioid variant of myxofibrosarcoma: expanding the clinicomorphologic spectrum of myxofibrosarcoma in a series of 17 cases. *Am J Surg Pathol*. 2007;**31**:99–105.

## Epithelioid Leiomyosarcoma

- Eyden B. Epithelioid leiomyosarcoma of the external deep soft tissue. *Arch Pathol Lab Med*. 2003;**127**:402–4.
- Suster S. Epithelioid leiomyosarcoma of the skin and subcutaneous tissue. Clinicopathologic, immunohistochemical, and ultrastructural study of five cases. *Am J Surg Pathol*. 1994;**18**:232–40.
- Yamamoto T, Minami R, Ohbayashi C, Inaba M. Epithelioid leiomyosarcoma of the external deep soft tissue. *Arch Pathol Lab Med*. 2002;**126**:468–70.

## Epithelioid Rhabdomyosarcoma

- Bowe SN, Ozer E, Bridge JA, Brooks JS, Iwenofu OH. Primary intranodal epithelioid rhabdomyosarcoma. *Am J Clin Pathol*. 2011;**136**:587–92.
- Jo VY, Marino-Enriquez A, Fletcher CD. Epithelioid rhabdomyosarcoma: clinicopathologic analysis of 16 cases of a morphologically distinct variant of rhabdomyosarcoma. *Am J Surg Pathol*. 2011;**35**:1523–30.
- Seidal T, Kindblom LG, Angervall L. Rhabdomyosarcoma in middle-aged and elderly individuals. *APMIS*. 1989;**97**:236–48.
- Suarez-Vilela D, Izquierdo-Garcia FM, Alonso-Orcajo N. Epithelioid and rhabdoid rhabdomyosarcoma in an adult patient: a diagnostic pitfall. *Virchows Arch*. 2004;**445**:323–5.
- Zin A, Bertorelle R, Dall'Igna P, et al. Epithelioid rhabdomyosarcoma: a clinicopathologic and molecular study. *Am J Surg Pathol*. 2014;**38**:273–8.

## Epithelioid Inflammatory Myofibroblastic Sarcoma

- Butrynski JE, D'Adamo DR, Hornick JL, et al. Crizotinib in ALK-rearranged inflammatory myofibroblastic tumor. *N Engl J Med*. 2010;**28**;363:1727–33.
- Lee JC, Li CF, Huang HY, et al. ALK oncoproteins in atypical inflammatory myofibroblastic tumours: novel RRBP1-ALK fusions in epithelioid inflammatory myofibroblastic sarcoma. *J Pathol*. 2017;**241**:316–323.
- Marino-Enriquez A, Wang WL, Roy A, et al. Epithelioid inflammatory myofibroblastic sarcoma: An aggressive intra-abdominal variant of inflammatory myofibroblastic tumor with nuclear membrane or perinuclear ALK. *Am J Surg Pathol*. 2011;**35**:135–44.

# Round Cell Sarcomas

## Alberto Righi MD, Marco Gambarotti MD, and Angelo Paolo Dei Tos MD

## Introduction

Round cell sarcomas (also called small round blue cell tumors) represent a heterogeneous group of poorly differentiated, diagnostically challenging mesenchymal malignancies, most often occurring in the pediatric and young adult population. Careful recognition of the different disease entities is extremely important in consideration of the availability of specific systemic treatments. In addition, the round cell tumors category also includes a variety of non-mesenchymal neoplasms (i.e., lymphoma and leukemia, neuroendocrine tumors, malignant melanoma, and neuroblastoma) that for several reasons may represent a source of diagnostic error. Diagnostic accuracy strictly depends upon the integration of morphologic, immunohistochemical (Table 6.1), and molecular features (Tables 6.2, 6.3, and 6.4). Interestingly, all round cell sarcomas

feature specific genetic aberrations that play a key role in the diagnostic workup. The *EWSR1* gene is by far the most frequently involved gene; however, it is rearranged with different partners in distinct round cell sarcoma subtypes such as Ewing sarcoma, desmoplastic small round cell sarcoma, and round cell liposarcoma (Table 6.5). Paradoxically, in inexperienced hands fluorescence in situ hybridization (FISH) analysis of *EWSR1* often becomes itself a cause of diagnostic confusion. In our experience, molecular diagnosis needs to be mandatorily interpreted in context with morphology and with the results of immunophenotypic analysis. The latest WHO classification recognizes the existence of undifferentiated round cell sarcomas. However, since the publication of that classification, the concept that most of these lesions could be actually classified on the basis of the driving genetic abnormality is gaining broad acceptance.

**Table 6.1** Immunophenotypic features of round cell sarcomas

| Sarcoma type | CD99 | Cytokeratin | Desmin | Myogenin | S100 | SOX9 | EMA | WT1*** |
|---|---|---|---|---|---|---|---|---|
| Alveolar rhabdomyosarcoma | – | 50% | >90% | 100% | 30% | – | – | – |
| Desmoplastic small round cell tumor | 60%* | >90% | >90% | – | 10% | – | >90% | 70% |
| Ewing sarcoma | 100% | 30% | 5% | – | 10% | – | – | – |
| Mesenchymal chondrosarcoma | >90%* | – | – | – | 100%** | >80% | – | – |
| Round cell synovial sarcoma | >80%* | 40% | – | – | 30% | – | >90% | – |
| Round cell liposarcoma | – | – | – | – | 70% | – | – | – |

\*    CD99 in non-Ewing sarcomas never features thick membrane immunostaining
\*\*   Only in the cartilaginous component
\*\*\* C-terminus WT1

**Table 6.2** Genetics of round cell sarcomas (not including Ewing sarcoma)

| Sarcoma type | Cytogenetic alterations | Molecular alterations |
|---|---|---|
| Alveolar rhabdomyosarcoma | t(2;13)(q35;q14)<br>t(1;13)(p36;q14)<br>t(2;22)(q35;p23)<br>t(2;8)(q35;q13)<br>t(x;2)(q35;q13) | PAX3-FOXO1A<br>PAX7-FOXO1A<br>PAX3-NCOA1<br>PAX3-NCOA2<br>PAX3-AFX |
| Desmoplastic small round cell tumor | t(11;22)(p13;q12) | EWSR1-WT1 |
| Mesenchymal chondrosarcoma | t(8;8)(q13;q21) | HEY1-NCOA2 |
| Round cell liposarcoma | t(12;16)(q13;p11)<br>t(12;22)(q13;q12) | FUS-DDIT3<br>EWSR1-DDIT3 |
| Synovial sarcoma | t/X;18)(p11;q11) | SYT-SSX, SSX2, SSX4 |

**Table. 6.3** Molecular genetics of Ewing sarcoma

| EWSR1-ETS fusion partners | | |
|---|---|---|
| Cytogenetic alterations | Gene fusion | Percentage of cases (%) |
| t(11;22)(q24;q12) | FLI1 | 90–95 |
| t(21;22)(q22;q12) | ERG | <10 |
| t(7;22)(p22;q12) | ETV1 | <1 |
| t(2;22)(q33;q12) | FEV | <1 |
| t(17;22)(q21;q12) | E1A-F | <1 |
| **EWSR1-non-ETS fusion partners** | | |
| Cytogenetic alterations | Gene fusion | Percentage of cases (%) |
| inv(22)(q12;q12) | PATZ1 | <1 |
| t(2;22)(q13;q12) | SP3 | <1 |
| t(20;22)(q13;q12)* | NFATc2 | <1 |
| t(4;22)(q31;q12) | SMARCA5 | <1 |
| t(6;22)(q21;q12) | POU5F1 | <1 |
| **FUS-ETS fusion partners** | | |
| Cytogenetic alterations | Gene fusion | Percentage of cases (%) |
| t(16;21)(p11;q22) | ERG | <1 |
| t(2;16)(q35;p11) | FEV | <1 |

\*  Amplification of the fusion transcript by FISH.

**Table 6.4** Molecular alteration in undifferentiated round cell sarcoma (EWS-like sarcomas)

| *CIC* rearrangement | |
|---|---|
| Cytogenetic alterations | Gene fusion |
| t(4;19)(q35;q13) | *DUX4* |
| t(10;19)(q26;q13) | *DUX4L* |
| t(x;19)(q13;q13) | *FOXO4* |

| *BCOR* rearrangement | |
|---|---|
| Cytogenetic alterations | Gene fusion |
| inv(x)(p11.4;11.22) | *CCNB3* |
| t(x;14)(p11;q31) | *MAML3* |
| t(x;22)(p11;q13) | *ZC3H7B* |
| t(x; 12)(p11;q13)) | *KMT2D* |

| Other | |
|---|---|
| Cytogenetic alterations | Gene fusion |
| t(16;20)(q13;p11) | *FUS-NFATc2* |
| t(12;15)(p13;q25.3) | *ETV6-NTRK3* |

**Table 6.5** Histotypes featuring rearrangement of the *EWSR1* gene

| Histotype | Cytogenetic alterations | Molecular alterations |
|---|---|---|
| Angiomatoid fibrous histiocytoma | t(12;22)(q13;q12)<br>t(2;22)(q33;q12) | *EWSR1-ATF1*<br>*EWSR1-CREB1* |
| Clear cell sarcoma | t(12;22)(q13;q12)<br>t(2;22)(q33;q12) | *EWSR1-ATF1*<br>*EWSR1-CREB1* |
| Low-grade fibromyxoid sarcoma/Sclerosing epithelioid fibrosarcoma | t(11;22)(p11;q12) | *EWSR1-CREB3L1* |
| Angiosarcoma | t(12;22)(q13;q12) | *EWSR1-ATF1* |
| Hemangioma of bone | t(18;22)(q23;q12) | *EWSR1-NFATC1* |
| Desmoplastic small round cell tumor | t(11;22)(p13;q12) | *EWSR1-WT1* |
| Extraskeletal myxoid chondrosarcoma | t(9;22)(q22;q12) | *EWSR1-NR4A3* |
| Myoepithelial tumor of soft tissue | t(6;22)(p21;q12)<br>t(19;22)(q13;q12)<br>t(1;22)(q23;q12)<br>t(9;22)(q33.2;q12)<br>t(1;22)(p34.1;q12) | *EWSR1-POU5F1*<br>*EWSR1-ZNF444*<br>*EWSR1-PBX1*<br>*EWSR1–PBX3*<br>*EWSR1-KLF17* |
| Myxoid/round cell liposarcoma | t(12;22)(q13;q12) | *EWSR1-DDIT3* |

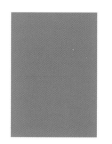

# Ewing Sarcoma

## Definition and Epidemiology

Ewing sarcoma (EWS) represents a poorly differentiated, round cell sarcoma of bone and soft tissue, showing variable neuroectodermal differentiation and sharing rearrangements of the *EWSR1* gene that, in most cases, fuses with a member of the ETS family of transcription factors. The first description dates back to 1918 when Arthur Purdy Stout reported a round cell neoplasm featuring rosettes in the ulnar nerve of a 42-year-old. James Ewing later described a similar lesion in 1921, occurring in the radius of a 14-year-old female.

Ewing sarcoma is rare, accounting for less than 1% of all soft tissue sarcomas. Overall, the peak incidence is between the first and second decade (approximately 80% of cases); however, it can present at any age, particularly when arising in the soft tissue. Interestingly, EWS predominates in the Caucasian population. In the past, the term "primitive neuroectodermal tumor" (PNET) was adopted to identify better-differentiated forms of EWS (those showing well-formed rosettes or pseudorosettes). This label has been abandoned, as it simply reflects a morphologic variation within the same tumor entity and is clinically irrelevant.

## Clinical Presentation and Outcome

The most frequent anatomic location of EWS is actually the metaphysis of long bones. However, we will focus mainly on EWS arising primarily in the soft tissue that represents approximately 20% of all EWS. Extraskeletal Ewing sarcoma occurs in the deep soft tissues of the paravertebral region and proximal portions of the lower and upper extremities. Visceral locations such as kidney, pancreas, and meninges have been documented. Primary cutaneous Ewing sarcoma represents a well-known (albeit rare) possible clinical presentation. When dealing with axial tumors, because of osseous involvement it is frequently difficult to determine whether the origin was in bone or soft tissue. This is also true for so-called Askin tumor (examples of Ewing sarcoma involving the thoracopulmonary region and labeled eponymically after Dr. Fred Askin) in which point of origin at a rib at times cannot be excluded. The involvement of a major nerve that leads to neurologic symptomatology is reported in up to one-third of cases, as with the very first example of this entity, described by Stout in 1918. The prognosis of extraskeletal EWS is poor; however, using multimodal therapy (which includes surgical resection and/or radiation therapy and chemotherapy), long-term survival has increased from less than 10% to approximately 30 to 40%. Histopathologic assessment of the percentage of tumor necrosis following induction chemotherapy represents a key prognostic parameter in bone; however, its value in soft tissue is less clear. Several studies had claimed that the presence of a type 1 *EWS-FLI1* fusion (EWS exon 7 is linked in frame with exon 6 of FLI1) represents an independent, positive prognostic factor; however, a recent large series has not confirmed this assumption. The analysis of cell cycle regulators has also provided potentially valuable information regarding the prognosis of this important family of round cell sarcomas: p53 expression seems to delineate a small subset of EWS with a remarkably poor clinical outcome, and the same effect appears to be determined by deletion of the *INK4A* gene. Yet unpublished data would also suggest that primary cutaneous EWS, in contrast to deep-seated lesions, pursues a rather indolent clinical course.

## Morphology and Immunohistochemistry

The gross appearance of these neoplasms reflects their rapid growth and is usually represented by a large, multilobulated soft tissue mass, featuring extensive necrosis and/or hemorrhage (Fig. 6-1). Microscopically, the morphologic findings mirror the degree of neuroectodermal differentiation. Most examples of EWS share a predominantly lobular architecture (Fig. 6-2). Most often, neoplastic cells exhibit round or ovoid vesicular nuclei with fine chromatin, distinct nuclear membrane, and poorly defined, scanty cytoplasm. Extravasated erythrocytes are often seen (Fig. 6-3). Cytoplasmic clearing represents a relatively frequent microscopic finding (Fig. 6-4). At times, neoplastic cells feature more abundant cytoplasm with discernible nucleoli (Fig. 6-5). A variable number of rosettes (from scarce to numerous) can be detected and are traditionally interpreted as evidence of neuroectodermal differentiation. Most frequently, the rosettes are of the Homer-Wright type, similar to those seen in neuroblastoma (Fig. 6-6), but occasionally Flexner-Wintersteiner rosettes (Fig. 6-7) or perivascular pseudorosettes (Fig. 6-8) are found. As mentioned, those cases exhibiting numerous rosettes in the past were termed peripheral PNETs. Intracytoplasmic glycogen, highlighted by PAS stains, is present in the majority of undifferentiated cases but only in less than half of EWS containing rosettes. Mitotic activity tends to be remarkably high, and interestingly, mitotic figures are always typical (Fig. 6-9). Necrosis is almost always present (Fig. 6-10) and can be extensive, sometimes leaving collars of viable tumor cells around the richly ramified capillary network. Rarely, EWS may feature cytoplasmic eosinophilia that, when associated with formation of microcystic change of the stroma, may represent a source of diagnostic confusion with alveolar rhabdomyosarcoma (Fig. 6-11). Occasionally, EWS shows atypical cytologic features represented by the presence of spindling or of large anaplastic tumor cells. However, these features are currently associated with *CIC-DUX4-* or with *BCOR*-associated round cell sarcomas (to be discussed separately).

Immunohistochemically, CD99 (the product of the MIC2 antigen) certainly represents the most useful marker. Strong CD99 membrane immunopositivity is seen in practically all examples of EWS, independently from the degree of

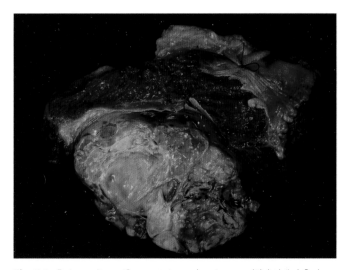

**Fig. 6-1.** Ewing sarcoma. Gross specimen showing a multilobulated, fleshy, deep-seated mass with large areas of necrosis.

differentiation (Fig. 6-12). The presence of neuroectodermal differentiation in EWS can be demonstrated by occasional immunopositivity for S100 protein, CD57, neurofilaments. Occasional expression of desmin can be observed. However, all these markers exhibit high variability, eventually proving to be of scant diagnostic utility. Expression of cytokeratin is observed in approximately 30% of cases. FLI1 and ERG immunopositivity can be seen in those EWSs harboring a *EWSR1-FLI1* and a *EWSR1-ERG* gene fusion, respectively. Recently, it has been shown that consistent expression of PAX7 represents a further promising diagnostic tool. Interestingly, PAX7 expression seems to be restricted to those EWSs demonstrating a fusion between *EWSR1* and *FLI1*, *ERG*, and *NFATc2*.

## Genetics

The central karyotypic anomaly is a t(11;22), with other variants found in about 15% of cases (see Table 6.3). The so-called Ewing sarcoma translocation is the best-known example of sarcoma translocation, as it was the first one to be identified as well as the first from which the involved genes were cloned. Molecularly, the result of the t(11;22) is a fusion of the *EWSR1* gene that contains an RNA-binding domain with the *FLI1* (Friend Leukemia virus Integration site 1) gene on 11q24 belonging to the ETS (avian Erythroblastosis virus Transforming Sequence) family of transcription factor. The replacement of the RNA-binding domain of the *EWSR1* gene with the DNA-binding domain of the *FLI1* gene (or related genes) leads to the formation of a novel transcription factor. *EWSR1* can fuse with other members of the ETS family (*ERG* being the second-most prevalent, followed by *ETV1* and *FEV*) and can also be replaced in the fusion with *ERG* and *FEV* by the *FUS* gene. *FUS* encodes a protein belonging to the TET family, the aminoacidic sequence

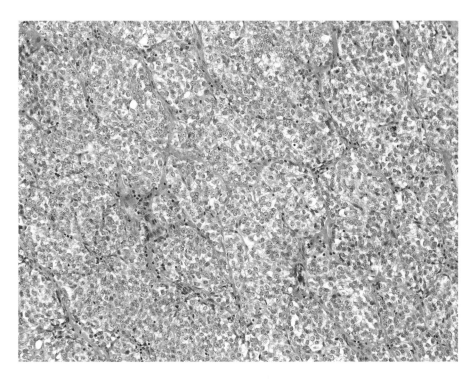

**Fig. 6-2.** Ewing sarcoma. At low power, a lobular pattern of growth is usually seen.

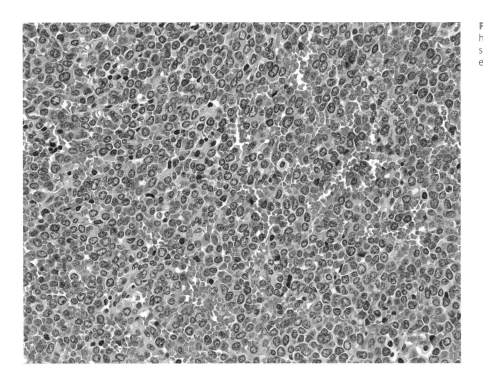

**Fig. 6-3.** Ewing sarcoma. The neoplastic cells often have round vesicular nuclei and poorly defined, scanty cytoplasm. The presence of extravasated erythrocytes represents a relatively frequent finding.

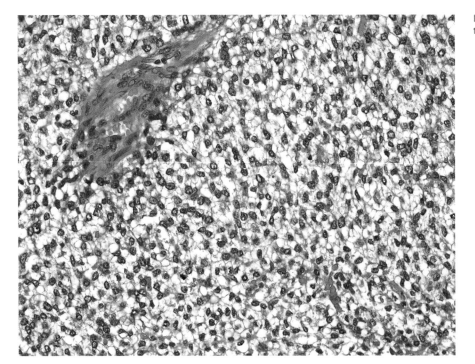

**Fig. 6-4.** Ewing sarcoma. Cytoplasmic clearing due to high glycogen content is frequently observed.

of which significantly overlaps with that generated by *EWSR1.* The possibility of detecting these karyotypic abnormalities by means of molecular genetics on a routine basis has greatly increased diagnostic accuracy.

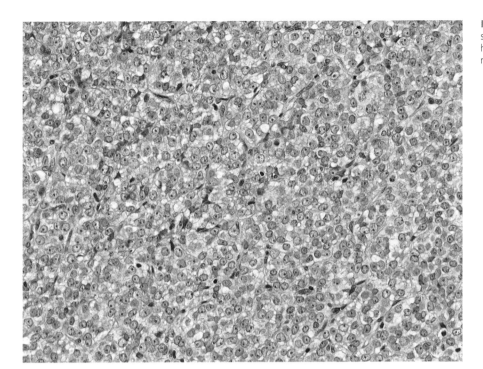

**Fig. 6-5.** Ewing sarcoma. Cytoplasm can sometimes be more abundant. The neoplastic cells have a distinct nuclear membrane with prominent nucleoli.

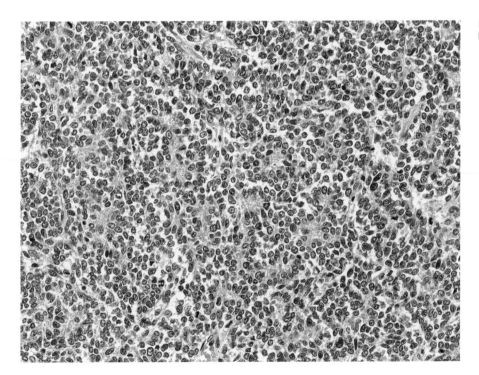

**Fig. 6-6.** Ewing sarcoma. At times, numerous Homer-Wright rosettes are seen.

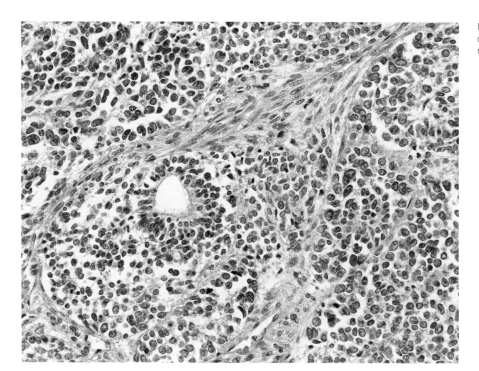

**Fig. 6-7.** Ewing sarcoma. The tumor is composed of large cells, and occasionally Flexner-Wintersteiner rosette formation is shown.

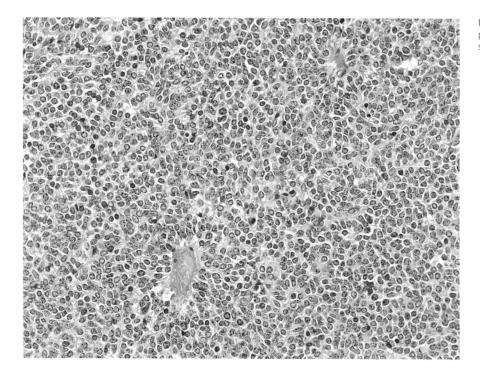

**Fig. 6-8.** Ewing sarcoma. Perivascular pseudorosettes in a classical background of Ewing sarcoma.

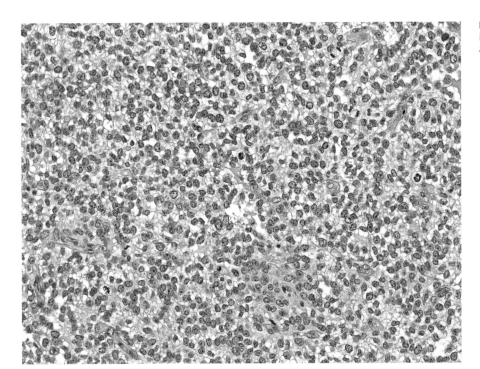

**Fig. 6-9.** Ewing sarcoma. Mitotic activity is typically brisk and almost always mitotic figures are non-atypical.

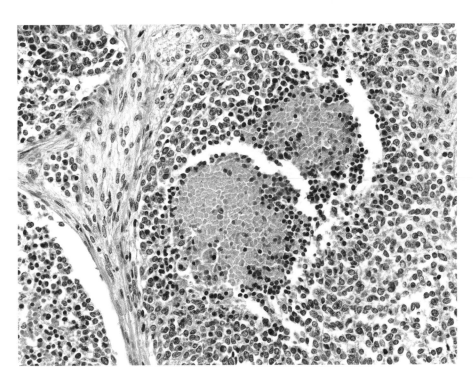

**Fig. 6-10.** Ewing sarcoma. The presence of necrotic foci represents a relatively common histologic finding.

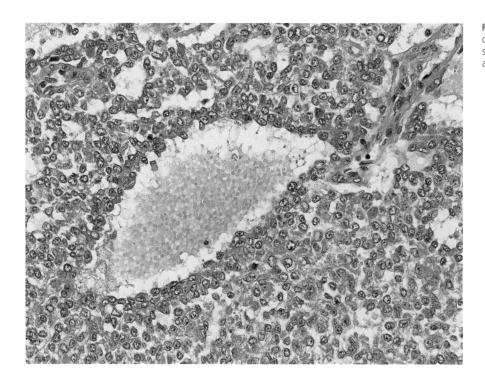

**Fig. 6-11.** Ewing sarcoma. The tumor is composed of round cells with eosinophilic cytoplasm. In the stroma, a prominent microcystic change is appreciable.

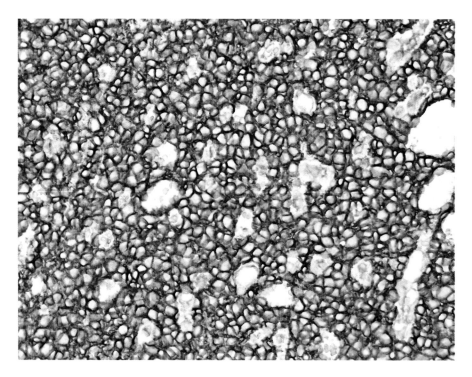

**Fig. 6-12.** Ewing sarcoma. The presence of strong membranous CD99 immunostaining is seen in virtually all examples of Ewing sarcoma.

## Differential Diagnosis and Diagnostic Pitfalls

The differential diagnosis of EWS is rather broad and includes the solid variant of alveolar rhabdomyosarcoma (ARMS), desmoplastic small round cell tumor (DSRCT), poorly differentiated round cell synovial sarcoma (PDSS), small cell osteosarcoma, malignant lymphoma, neuroblastoma in children, mesenchymal chondrosarcoma, and, when dealing with cutaneous EWS, Merkel cell carcinoma (MCC). CD99 immunopositivity is certainly important; however, it can be variably expressed in a broad variety of neoplasms including lymphoblastic lymphoma, DSRCT, and PDSS. In most non-EWS cases, CD99 tends to decorate the cytoplasm diffusely, very rarely featuring the crisp, intense membranous pattern of staining typically seen in EWS. Conversely, absence of CD99 immunoreactivity in a round cell sarcoma virtually excludes EWS from the differential diagnosis.

As mentioned, EWS may sometimes mimic the pseudoalveolar pattern of growth of ARMS, therefore creating some morphologic overlap. However, myogenin expression is never

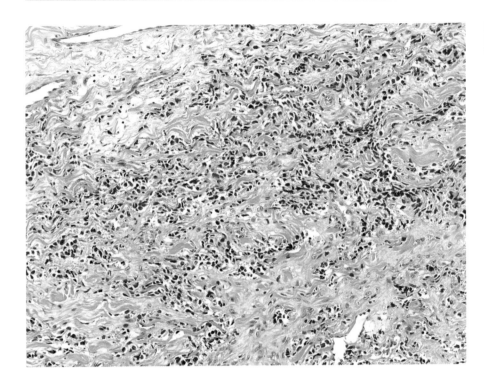

**Fig. 6-13.** Ewing sarcoma. The presence of dense sclerotic stroma is frequently seen when Ewing sarcoma occurs in the paraspinal soft tissues.

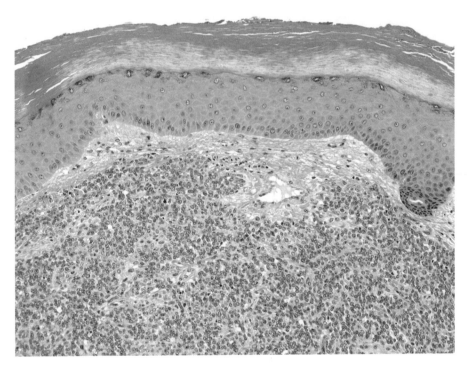

**Fig. 6-14.** Ewing sarcoma. Ewing sarcoma may occur primarily as a cutaneous neoplasm.

seen in EWS and, in contrast to ARMS, it typically features rearrangement of the *EWSR1* gene instead of the *FOXO1* gene. Ewing sarcoma may be confused with DSRCT when occurring in the soft tissues of the paraspinal region wherein it is often associated with heavily collagenized stroma (Fig. 6-13). The differential diagnosis relies upon the very distinctive clinical DSRCT presentation (the vast majority occurs in mesothelium-lined sites of young males) as well as on its distinctive polyphenotypic immunoprofile represented by variable co-expression of epithelial, myogenic, and

neuroectodermal differentiation markers. Importantly, as EWS (which may express cytokeratin in up to 30% of cases) shares with DSRCT the presence of *EWSR1* gene rearrangement, a break-apart FISH approach is not sufficient to differentiate it. As is discussed later in this chapter, poorly differentiated round cell synovial sarcoma can be separated from EWS on the basis of the expression of EMA and TLE1 and, most of all, by the demonstration of the rearrangement of the *SYT* gene. Mesenchymal chondrosarcoma is also discussed in detail later on; however, in brief, it is typically biphasic and

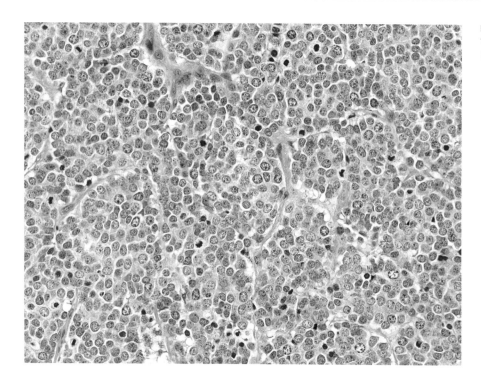

**Fig. 6-15.** Merkel cell carcinoma. Tumor cells feature round nuclei with characteristic "salt and pepper" chromatin.

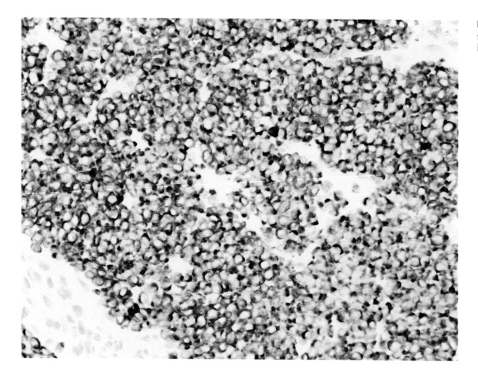

**Fig. 6-16.** Merkel cell carcinoma. Neoplastic cells show a distinctive "dot-like" cytoplasmic immunopositivity for cytokeratin 20.

features islands of mature cartilage. Extraosseous extension of round cell osteosarcoma may at times represent a major challenge; however, the combination of CD99 negativity (or weak positivity), presence of malignant osteoid, SATB2 immunopositivity, and absence of *EWSR1* gene rearrangements all contribute to arrival at the correct diagnosis. Metastatic neuroblastoma tends to occur in children younger than 2 years, is CD99 negative, expresses the recently described marker PHOXI2B, and again lacks involvement of the *EWRS1* gene.

The availability of *EWSR1* break-apart probes coupled with morphologic observation certainly represents an important diagnostic adjunct; however, it may also lead to potential diagnostic confusion. In fact, as shown in Table 6.5, the *EWSR1* gene exhibits a high degree of molecular promiscuity and its rearrangement can be detected in a variety of unrelated soft tissue neoplasm. Evaluation of genetic analysis in context with morphology is therefore mandatory.

As mentioned, EWS can occur as a primarily cutaneous neoplasm, raising the problem of making the distinction between it and Merkel cell carcinoma (MCC) (Fig. 6-14) and round cell examples of myoepithelial carcinomas. Merkel cell carcinoma represents a clinically aggressive, primarily cutaneous high-grade neuroendocrine carcinoma most often related to polyoma virus and, in approximately 20% of cases, to ultraviolet (UV) exposure. Most often, MCC exhibits a very distinctive cytomorphology characterized by round nuclei featuring the typical "salt and pepper" chromatin (Fig. 6-15). However, it is important to remember that about 30% of EWS do express cytokeratins and that, on the other hand, MCC can express CD99 in approximately 30% of cases. As neuroendocrine markers can be detected in both lesions (of course, much more consistently in MCC), dot-like CK20 immunopositivity in MMC appears to be extremely helpful, as it has been consistently negative in all cases of EWS tested so far (Fig. 6-16). Myoepithelial carcinoma is discussed in detail in Chapter 5. It most often exhibits variable co-expression of EMA, cytokeratin, smooth muscle actin, and S100. One major potential pitfall is represented by the fact that the *EWSR1* gene may also be rearranged in myoepithelial carcinoma (approximately 40% of cases in the adult population). Again, FISH analysis is therefore not adequate to sort out this specific differential diagnosis.

Ewing sarcoma has been increasingly reported to occur at visceral sites. When occurring in the kidney, the main differential diagnosis is with the so-called adult variant of Wilms' tumor, particularly when undifferentiated blastemal areas predominate. It has to be stressed that CD99 is usually negative in Wilms' tumor, making immunohistochemistry extremely important in the differential diagnosis. As a consequence, most adult-type Wilms' tumors have now been reclassified as EWS, following either immunohistochemical or molecular genetics analysis.

The existence of atypical forms of Ewing sarcomas also deserves a brief comment. It is in fact now our impression that most cases actually represent examples of other tumor entities, in particular malignant myoepitheliomas and most important other recently described distinctive Ewing-like sarcomas such as *CIC-DUX4-* and *BCOR-CCNB3*-associated round cell sarcomas.

### Key Points in Ewing Sarcoma Diagnosis

- Occurrence in the bone and soft tissue of young adults
- Presence of lobular growth pattern, geographic necrosis, cellular monomorphism, high mitotic count
- CD99 strongly positive with a thick membrane staining pattern
- Rearrangement of the *EWSR1* gene with various partners
- Aggressive clinical course

# CIC-DUX4-Associated Round Cell Sarcoma

## Definition and Epidemiology

So-called CIC-DUX4-associated sarcoma represents an extremely rare, undifferentiated round cell malignancy characterized by high prevalence of *CIC* gene rearrangements. *CIC* generally fuses with one of the *DUX4* retrogenes, located on either 4q35 or 10q26.3. CIC-DUX4 fusion-positive round cell sarcomas were first reported in 2006 by Kawamura-Saito, although the description of the translocation t(4;19) dates back to 1996.

In the 2013 WHO classification, CIC-DUX4 fusion-positive round cell sarcomas were temporarily assigned to the category of undifferentiated round cell sarcomas but were also regarded as a possible variant of Ewing sarcoma. However, there exist now sufficient clinical, morphologic, and genetic features to consider them as a distinct entity. Age range is rather broad, with peak incidence in the third decade. Occurrence in the pediatric age-group is observed in approximately 20% of cases. Male-to-female ratio is 1:1.3.

## Clinical Presentation and Behavior

CIC-DUX4 fusion-positive round cell sarcomas occur in deep or superficial soft tissue of the trunk, limbs, or head and neck region, sometimes with secondary bone involvement; rarely, they arise from viscera. Occurrence primarily in bone seems to be comparatively very rare. These tumors generally have a dismal prognosis, with lung metastasis at presentation. Poor histologic response to standard chemotherapeutic protocols for Ewing sarcomas is reported; however, experience is still rather limited.

## Morphology and Immunohistochemistry

Morphologically, CIC-DUX4 fusion-positive round cell sarcoma shows a lobular growth pattern, with lobules of various sizes separated by thin fibrous septa. Confluent geographic areas of necrosis represent a relatively frequent finding (Fig. 6-17). Most often, CIC-DUX4 fusion-positive round cell sarcoma exhibits infiltrative margins with invasion of adjacent anatomic structures. Cytologically, mild to moderate pleomorphism is seen that contrasts with the monotonous appearance of Ewing sarcoma (Figs. 6-18 and 6-19). In particular, areas with vesicular nuclei, often with readily identifiable nucleoli, are present, and abundant cytoplasm is present, often with clear cell change (somewhat reminiscent of renal cell carcinoma) (Fig. 6-20). Myxoid change of the stroma also represents a relatively frequent finding (Fig. 6-21). In rare cases, neoplastic cells acquire an epithelioid morphology featuring eosinophilic, rhabdoid-like cytoplasm (Fig. 6-22). Rarely, focal cell spindling can be observed. Mitotic count is generally high (often exceeding 40 mitoses/10 high-power fields [HPF]).

Immunohistochemically, these tumors are only focally positive or negative for CD99, whereas cytoplasmic and/or nuclear immunoreactivity for WT1 (n-terminus) has been reported. Recently, it has been shown that the nuclear expression of ETV4 and of DUX4 is observed in the majority of cases.

## Molecular Genetics

CIC-DUX4-associated round cell sarcomas fail to demonstrate the cytogenetic abnormality of Ewing sarcoma, lacking rearrangement of *EWSR1* or of other members of the TET family. However, upregulation of the PEA3 subclass of the ETS family of genes has been shown, therefore providing some link with Ewing sarcoma. The *CIC-DUX4* fusion results from either a t(4;19)(q35;q13) or a t(10;19)(q26;q13) translocation, and harbors the majority of the *CIC* gene, whereas it does not contain the homeodomains of *DUX4*. The *CIC-DUX4* fusion product seems to act as an aberrant transcription factor with transforming capacity.

The *CIC* gene is the human homolog of the *Drosophila* gene *capicua*. It encodes a high-mobility group box transcription factor and is involved in the development of the central nervous system. The *DUX4* gene encodes for a double homeobox transcription factor, two genomic copies of which are, as already mentioned, located within polymorphic macrosatellite repeats on 4q35 and 10q26. Its normal function is poorly understood and its expression is normally suppressed in differentiated cells. *DUX4* has been involved in the pathogenesis of facioscapulohumeral muscular dystrophy. At present, the demonstration of *CIC* gene rearrangement is mandatory for the diagnosis (see Table 6.4). As a consequence of the genomic aberration, upregulation of the *ETV4* gene is observed, leading to nuclear overexpression of the protein thereof. Rare cases of undifferentiated round cell sarcoma featuring a *CIC-FOXO4* gene fusion have been reported.

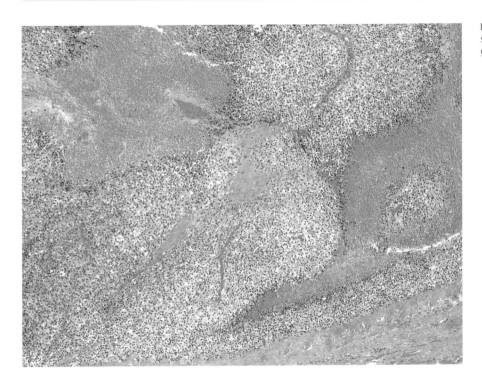

**Fig. 6-17.** CIC-DUX4-associated round cell sarcoma. At low power, large areas of confluent geographic necrosis are most often seen.

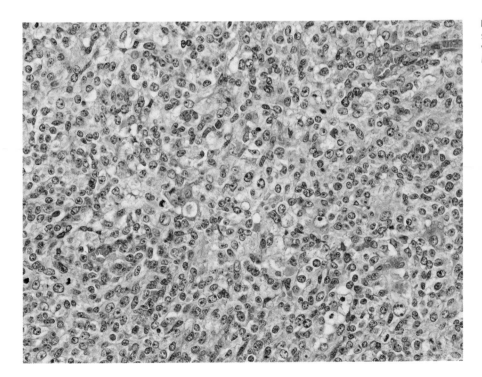

**Fig. 6-18.** CIC-DUX4-associated round cell sarcoma. The tumor cells exhibit vesicular nuclei with prominent nucleoli and scant, pale cytoplasm. Mitotic figures are numerous.

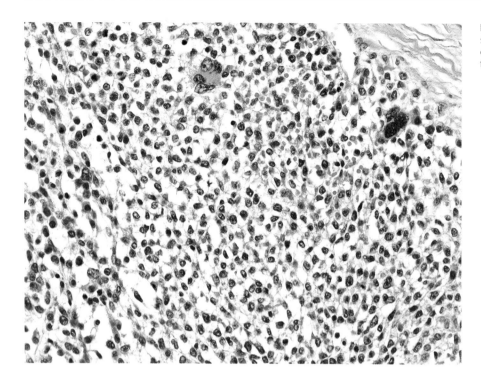

**Fig. 6-19.** CIC-DUX4-associated round cell sarcoma. The presence of scattered pleomorphic cells represents a relatively common morphologic finding.

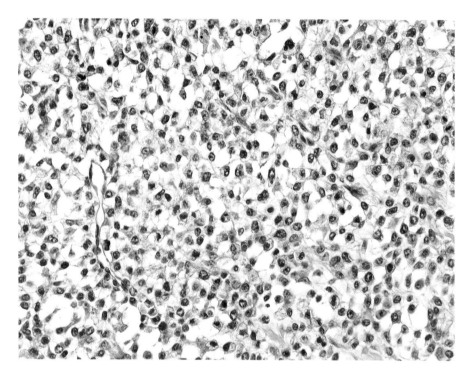

**Fig. 6-20.** CIC-DUX4-associated round cell sarcoma. Tumor cells relatively often feature abundant clear cytoplasm, somewhat mimicking renal cell carcinoma.

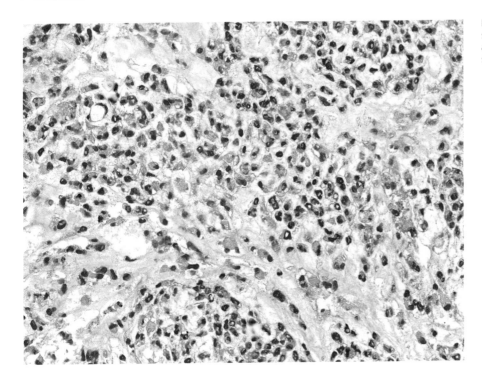

**Fig. 6-21.** CIC-DUX4-associated round cell sarcoma. Myxoid change of the stroma represents another common finding of this subset of round cell sarcomas.

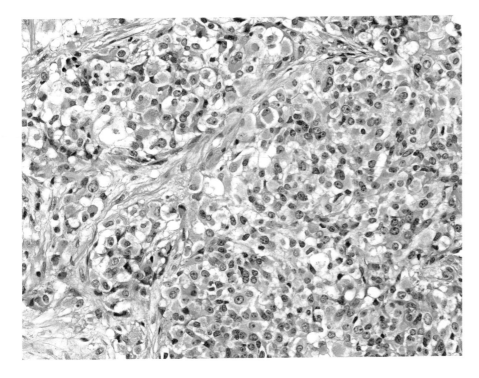

**Fig. 6-22.** CIC-DUX4-associated round cell sarcoma. The presence of epithelioid morphology is sometimes seen. Rhabdoid-like morphology can be also observed.

## Differential Diagnosis and Diagnostic Pitfalls

The main differential diagnosis of CIC-DUX4-associated round cell sarcomas is EWS and other round cell sarcomas of soft tissues.

In contrast to EWS, CIC-DUX4-associated round cell sarcomas occur predominantly in soft tissues or, rarely, in viscera, whereas Ewing sarcoma is more frequently found in bone. Morphologically, the presence of cytoplasmic clearing, multifocal pleomorphism, and geographic necrosis, as well as of myxoid degeneration of the stroma in a round cell sarcoma, allows us to

suspect CIC-DUX4-associated round cell sarcoma. Importantly, the absence of diffuse membrane-type immunopositivity for CD99 generally does not support the diagnosis of Ewing sarcoma.

All of the other soft tissue tumors that enter in the differential diagnosis (high-grade "round cell" liposarcoma, poorly differentiated "round cell" synovial sarcoma, and other small round cell sarcomas) are generally characterized by specific translocations, and all of them lack *CIC* gene rearrangements. Therefore, molecular analysis showing *CIC* rearrangement is currently regarded as mandatory for the diagnosis.

## Key Points in CIC-DUX4 Fusion-Positive Round Cell Sarcomas Diagnosis

- Occurrence in the soft tissue (rarely viscera) of young adults
- Lobular growth pattern, geographic necrosis, mild to moderate pleomorphism, high mitotic count, presence of myxoid stroma
- CD99 focally positive or negative; cytoplasmic and/or nuclear immunoreactivity for WT1 (n-terminus); nuclear expression of ETV4 and DUX4
- *CIC* rearrangement, generally with *DUX4*
- Dismal prognoses, with poor histologic response to standard chemotherapeutic protocols for Ewing sarcoma

# BCOR-CCNB3 (EWING-LIKE) SARCOMA

## Definition and Epidemiology

Recently described by Pierron and coworkers, BCOR-CCNB3 fusion-positive sarcoma is a new member of the "Ewing-like" family of tumors. It arises in bone and soft tissue, and harbors a novel gene fusion involving an intra-chromosomal X paracentric inversion. Since the first description in 2012, fewer than 50 cases have been published in the literature. This *BCOR-CCNB3* fusion gene was identified in 4% (24/594) of undifferentiated "Ewing-like" round cell sarcomas lacking *EWSR1* gene rearrangements. In a large, mono-institutional series reporting on 250 small round cell sarcomas, the ratio of BCOR-CCNB3 sarcomas to classical Ewing sarcomas was 1:27. A male predominance is reported, with a peak incidence in the second decade. Children and adolescents can also be affected.

## Clinical Presentation and Behavior

BCOR-CCNB3 sarcomas appear to occur in either bone or soft tissue, with slight bone predominance. BCOR-CCNB3 sarcomas more frequently involve the pelvis or lower limbs with an equal distribution between axial (paraspinal, chest wall, and pelvis) and extra-axial (ankle, calcaneus, and thigh) locations. Visceral sites (i.e., kidney) can be exceptionally observed. The clinical outcome for patients with BCOR-CCNB3 is currently unclear, in consideration of the small number of reported patients as well as of the heterogeneity of the administered treatment regimens. The vast majority of BCOR-CCNB3 sarcomas present as a localized disease, with only 15% of patients showing lung or bone metastases at diagnosis. Overall recurrence and metastatic rate (primarily to the lungs) are approximately 30% and 35%, respectively. Overall survival somewhat overlaps with that of Ewing sarcoma (most data refer to primary bone lesions) with 5-year and 10-year survival rates of 78% and 56%, respectively; however, as more cases are identified, a slightly more indolent clinical behavior seems to emerge with 10-year survival rates reaching 70%. A longer overall survival is significantly linked to location of the primary tumor in the extremities versus axial skeleton and soft tissues. In contrast to Ewing sarcoma, no association between survival and metastatic disease at diagnosis is reported.

## Morphology and Immunohistochemistry

The morphologic spectrum of BCOR-CCNB3 sarcoma is broad, with tumors predominately composed of a diffuse proliferation of round tumor cells featuring a small amount of ill-defined pale to eosinophilic cytoplasm (Fig. 6-23) and/or short spindle tumor cells arranged in short fascicles or whorls (Fig. 6-24). Nuclei are angulated and hyperchromatic with finely dispersed chromatin. In the majority of cases, nucleoli are not readily discernible. Significant variation in cellularity is sometimes seen, with hypocellular areas often being associated with myxoid change of the stroma, and occasionally containing angulated, thin-walled vessels. Small areas of tumor cell necrosis are seen in almost all cases. Mitotic count is often brisk, with a median of 20 mitoses per 10 high-power fields; however, there exist cases featuring lower proliferative activity. When compared with the primary tumor, recurrent and metastatic lesions show an increased cellularity and a higher degree of pleomorphism, occasionally simulating undifferentiated pleomorphic sarcoma.

Immunohistochemically, almost all tested tumors exhibit strong and diffuse BCOR as well as cyclin B3 (CCNB3) nuclear positivity (Fig. 6-25), with only a few cases showing patchy staining associated with some background cytoplasmic staining. In an extensive screening of approximately 1,000 tumor samples, including a spectrum of pediatric tumors, adult sarcomas, and brain tumors, only the BCOR-CCNB3-associated sarcomas showed very high nuclear expression levels of CCNB3.

Apart from CCNB3 positivity, the immunohistochemical profile shows broad overlap with that seen in classic Ewing sarcoma, although CD99 staining is generally weaker or totally absent. Despite molecular evidence of activation of the Wnt pathway generated by expression profiling of BCOR-CCNB3 sarcoma, no nuclear staining for beta-catenin is observed. Positivity for TLE1, SATB2, and cyclin-D1 has been recently reported.

## Molecular Genetics

BCOR-CCNB3 mRNA originates from a paracentric inversion on the X-chromosome and splicing of the end of the *BCOR* coding sequence to the *CCNB3* exon 5 splice acceptor site. The resultant fusion protein is composed of full-length *BCOR*, a transcriptional repressor encoding the Bcl-6 co-repressor, and the C-terminus of *CCNB3*, a cyclin normally expressed in leptotene and zygotene of meiosis. More recently, BCOR was found to be a core component of a variant PRC1.1 complex associated with chromatin remodeling and histone modifications. In vitro studies suggest that the fusion BCOR-CCNB3 protein is oncogenic and drives proliferation in this sarcoma. Recently, novel fusion partners have been identified (see Table 6.4).

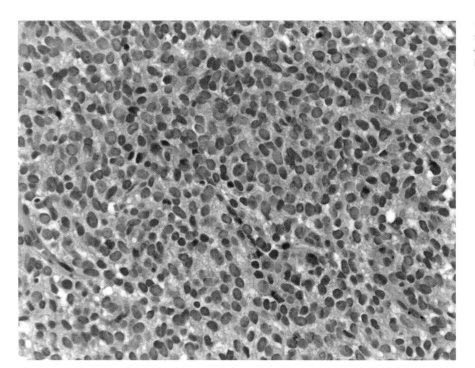

**Fig. 6-23.** BCOR-CCNB3-associated round cell sarcoma. This example is composed of a monotonous, undifferentiated round cell proliferation.

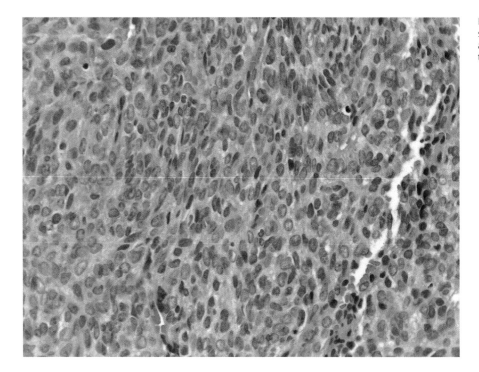

**Fig. 6-24.** BCOR-CCNB3-associated round cell sarcoma. The presence of cell spindling represents a relatively distinctive morphologic feature of this tumor entity.

Despite remarkable clinical and occasionally pathologic similarities with Ewing sarcoma, gene profiling and single-nucleotide polymorphic (SNP) allele array analyses indicate that this new group of tumors is biologically distinct from Ewing sarcoma.

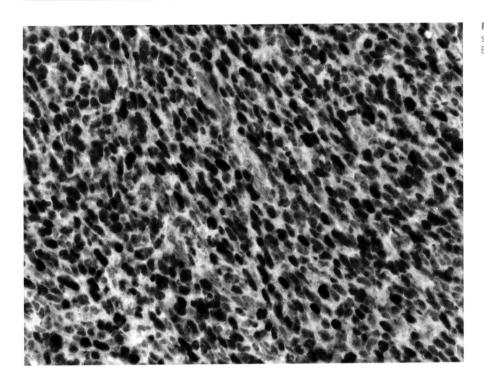

**Fig. 6-25.** BCOR-CCNB3-associated round cell sarcoma. Strong nuclear immunoreactivity for cyclin B3 is typically seen.

## Differential Diagnosis and Diagnostic Pitfalls

BCOR-CCNB3 sarcoma needs to be distinguished from all other round cell as well as spindle sarcomas, in particular Ewing sarcoma, poorly differentiated synovial sarcoma, CIC-DUX4 sarcoma, and, when dealing with primary bone tumor, small cell osteosarcoma. Presence of diffuse CCNB3 nuclear immunopositivity in a round cell neoplasm should prompt consideration of a diagnosis of BCOR-CCNB3 sarcoma. However, a major diagnostic pitfall is represented by the fact that weak to moderate cytoplasmic staining of CCNB3 is also identified in some cases of classic Ewing sarcoma, alveolar rhabdomyosarcoma, and very focally in some synovial sarcomas. In order to accept CCBN3 immunostains as valid, nuclear localization needs to be mandatorily present and, in any case, evaluated in context with morphology and with the results of molecular genetic findings. Regarding synovial sarcoma, a further potential pitfall is represented by the fact that it seems to share the expression of TLE1 with BCOR sarcoma. In the case of the differential diagnosis with small cell osteosarcoma, the presence of malignant osteoid matrix represents

a key diagnostic finding. In this context, SATB2 immunopositivity is unhelpful, as it is observed in both entities. The relationships between BCOR-CCNB3 sarcoma and a group of pediatric lesions sharing BCOR involvement (namely, undifferentiated round cell tumor of soft tissue, clear cell sarcoma of the kidney, and primitive myxoid mesenchymal tumor) need to be further elucidated, but it is possible that they are part of a morphologic/genetic spectrum.

**Key Points in BCOR-CCNB3 Sarcoma Diagnosis**

- Occurrence in adolescents and young adults
- Male prevalence
- Bone origin predominance
- Pelvis or lower limb anatomic location
- Small round to plump and/or short spindle tumor cells
- Immunohistochemical expression of CCNB3, a highly sensible and specific marker
- *BCOR-CCNB3* fusion transcript
- More indolent clinical course compared to *CIC*-rearranged sarcoma

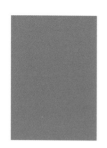

# Extraskeletal Mesenchymal Chondrosarcoma

## Definition and Epidemiology

Mesenchymal chondrosarcoma (MCHS) is a rare subtype of high-grade sarcoma of bone and soft tissue, characterized by a biphasic pattern, composed of undifferentiated neoplastic cells associated with areas of mature cartilage. It accounts for approximately 3% of all chondrosarcomas and may affect any age-group, with a peak incidence in the second and third decades. No sex predilection is observed. Primary bone MCHS is three time as frequent as soft tissue MCHS.

## Clinical Presentation and Outcome

Mesenchymal chondrosarcoma most often occurs in the craniofacial bones, ribs, pelvic bones, and spine. Up to one-third of cases arise primarily in the soft tissues. The most common extraskeletal site is represented by the meninges. Among the somatic soft tissue locations, the lower leg is more frequently involved. Exceptional visceral cases have been also reported. Mesenchymal chondrosarcoma is an aggressive tumor with a high frequency of distant metastasis, primarily to the lungs, even several years after diagnosis. The overall survival rate is about 50% at 5 years and 25% at 10 years. There is no evidence of prognostic value of any histologic feature. The treatment of choice is surgical resection.

## Morphology and Immunophenotype

Macroscopically, MCHS is usually a large, white to tan soft mass with areas of calcification (Fig. 6-26). Microscopically, MCHS has a typical biphasic pattern, with richly cellular, undifferentiated, small mesenchymal cells intermixed with islands of well-differentiated cartilage (Fig. 6-27). In the round cell component, neoplastic cells are variably arranged in sheet-like structures (closely mimicking Ewing sarcoma) (Fig. 6-28); however, they frequently organize around branching, thin-walled vascular spaces featuring a hemangiopericytoma-like pattern (Fig. 6-29). More rarely, a spindle cell neoplastic population predominates (Fig. 6-30). The transition from cellular foci to matrix-producing areas is usually abrupt, but less frequently can be gradual. The extension of the cartilaginous component is variable, from small foci (Fig. 6-31) to large, well-defined masses (Fig. 6-32). Metaplastic bone can be rarely observed (Fig. 6-33). Immunohistochemically, the undifferentiated component may be CD99 positive, making the distinction from Ewing sarcoma difficult, while the cartilaginous component is S100 protein positive. Recently, positive nuclear staining for SOX-9, a master regulator protein of the differentiation of mesenchymal cells into chondrocytes, has been detected both in the cartilaginous component of the tumor and in the undifferentiated neoplastic cells.

## Genetics

Mesenchymal chondrosarcoma is characterized genetically by a recurrent *HEY1-NCOA2* fusion. As both genes are found on chromosome 8 (8q21.1 and 8q13.3, respectively), the fusion may be determined by interstitial deletions, which would be difficult to recognize using classic cytogenetic tools. A molecular diagnostic approach is therefore recommended.

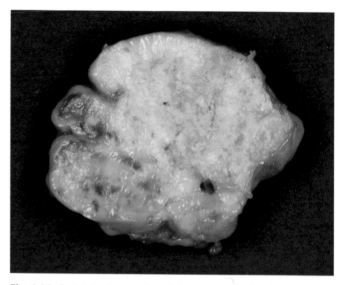

**Fig. 6-26.** Extraskeletal mesenchymal chondrosarcoma. Grossly, the tumor often features a white to yellow, glistening cut surface. Whitish spots of calcification are seen.

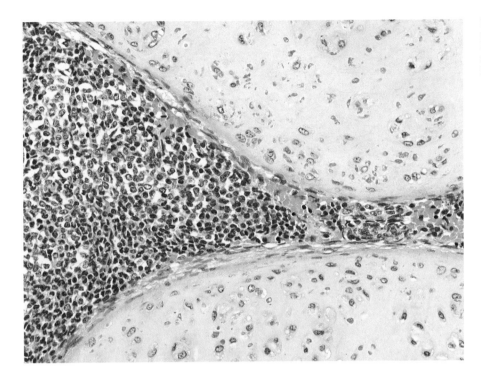

**Fig. 6-27.** Extraskeletal mesenchymal chondrosarcoma. The tumor features a distinctive biphasic pattern showing areas composed of undifferentiated round cells, side by side with islands of well-differentiated cartilage.

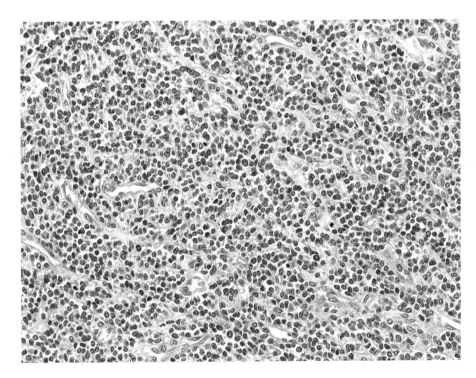

**Fig. 6-28.** Extraskeletal mesenchymal chondrosarcoma. Undifferentiated round cell areas may mimic Ewing sarcoma.

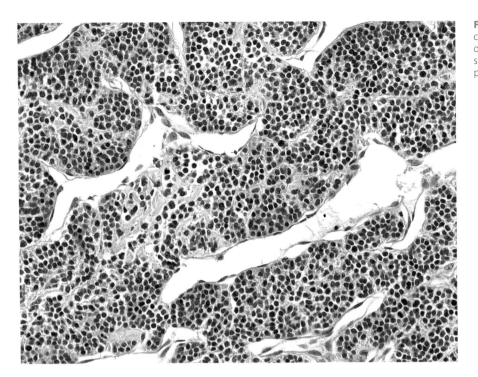

**Fig. 6-29.** Extraskeletal mesenchymal chondrosarcoma. The tumor cells are often organized around branching, thin-walled vascular spaces, also called "hemangiopericytoma-like pattern."

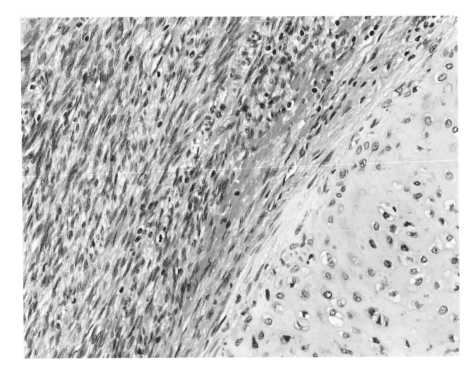

**Fig. 6-30.** Extraskeletal mesenchymal chondrosarcoma. Rarely, the undifferentiated component features a spindle cell morphology.

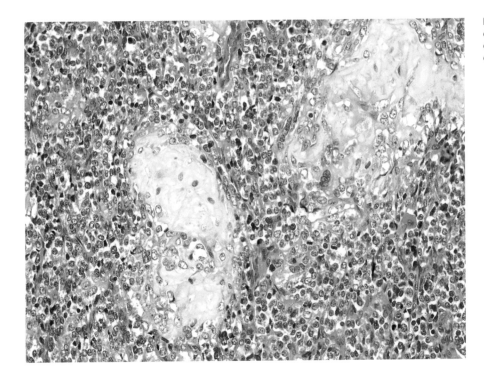

**Fig. 6-31.** Extraskeletal mesenchymal chondrosarcoma. Some cases have small cartilaginous foci through the round cell component.

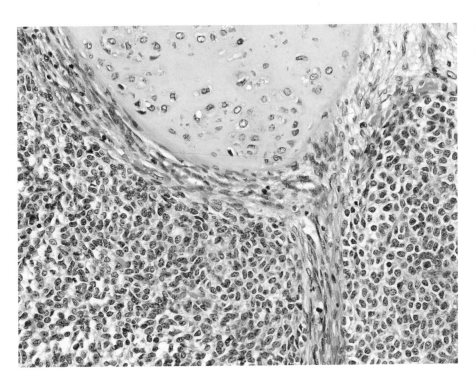

**Fig. 6-32.** Extraskeletal mesenchymal chondrosarcoma. Note the large island of cartilaginous tissue.

**339**

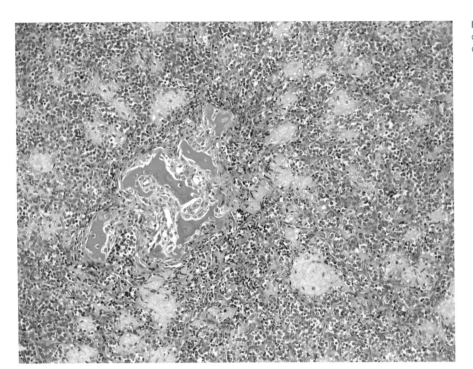

**Fig. 6-33.** Extraskeletal mesenchymal chondrosarcoma. The presence of metaplastic bone can be rarely observed.

## Differential Diagnosis and Diagnostic Pitfalls

The main differential diagnosis of MCHS is primarily with other small round cell sarcomas, principally with Ewing sarcoma and poorly differentiated round cell synovial sarcoma, and it is particularly challenging when the amount of differentiated cartilaginous areas is limited. Round cell poorly differentiated synovial sarcoma is particularly challenging, as it tends to share with MCHS the presence of a prominent hemangiopericytoma-like vascular pattern. Furthermore, both lesions may feature areas of calcification and bone metaplasia. Cytokeratin and EMA positivity, along with nuclear expression of TLE1, support the diagnosis of synovial sarcoma, which is also characterized genetically by a specific t(X;18) translocation.

A major potential diagnostic pitfall is represented by the fact that MCHS may share with Ewing sarcoma diffuse expression of CD99. However, positivity is usually more limited than in Ewing sarcoma and almost never features the distinctive, thick membrane pattern of staining. The demonstration of *EWSR1* and *NCOA2* gene rearrangement in Ewing sarcoma and in MCHS, respectively, represents an extremely helpful diagnostic finding.

In those rare examples of MCHS featuring spindle cell morphology, main differential diagnosis is with malignant peripheral nerve sheath tumor with chondrogenic heterologous differentiation. Clinical presentation, SOX-9 immunopositivity, and *NCOA2* gene rearrangement all represent important clues to the correct diagnosis.

---

**Key Points in Extraskeletal Mesenchymal Chondrosarcoma Diagnosis**

- Occurrence in bone and soft tissue
- Biphasic histologic pattern (undifferentiated round cell and mature cartilage)
- Hemangiopericytoma-like vascular network
- Expression of SOX-9
- Presence of *HEY1-NCOA2* fusion transcript
- Clinically aggressive neoplasm

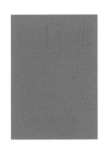

# Desmoplastic Small Round Cell Tumor

## Definition and Epidemiology

Desmoplastic small round cell tumor (DSRCT) is a highly malignant, polyphenotypic mesenchymal neoplasm associated with a prominent fibrous stroma. First reported by Gerald and Rosai in 1991 (the first case was actually presented at a United States and Canadian Academy of Pathology [USCAP] meeting in 1988 and published in 1989), DSRCT mainly affects young adults, with a peak incidence in the second decade. Male patients outnumber females 4:1.

## Clinical Presentation and Outcome

Desmoplastic small round cell tumor most often arises in mesothelium-lined surfaces. In its most frequent intra-abdominal presentation, DSRCT usually causes abdominal pain associated with ascites, abdominal distension, and/or intestinal obstruction. At surgery, the lesion usually presents as a large intra-abdominal mass associated with multiple peritoneal smaller implants. Metastases to locoregional lymph nodes are also observed.

Originally described as a predominantly intra-abdominal malignancy, a broader distribution has gradually emerged that includes the pleura and the tunica vaginalis. Extraserous locations have been occasionally reported, including primary renal cases occurring in children and rare examples observed in the head and neck region. Desmoplastic small round cell tumor is extremely aggressive, with a dismal prognosis. Even if improved survival seems to be achieved by high-dose chemotherapy regimens associated with extensive surgery, most patients die either of advanced uncontrolled local disease or of distant metastases within 48 months after diagnosis.

## Morphology and Immunophenotype

Grossly, the neoplastic masses tend to be solid, firm, and multilobulated with a gray-white, occasionally cystic cut surface. Necrosis represents a relatively common gross finding (Fig. 6-34). Histologically, at low power DSRCT is characterized by the presence of sharply demarcated clusters of small rounded cells, separated by a hypocellular spindle cell desmoplastic stroma (Fig. 6-35). The shape of cellular clusters may vary, ranging from centrally necrotic large islands to cord-like structures (Figs. 6-36 and 6-37). Rarely, neoplastic cells arrange in "Indian files," somewhat mimicking lobular carcinoma of the breast (Fig. 6-38). In up to one-third of cases, DSRCT exhibits variable growth patterns that include tubular arrangement, an insular pattern simulating carcinoid tumors

(Fig. 6-39), multicystic patterns, and adenoid cystic-like patterns.

In typical cases, tumor cells are usually uniform in size and shape and are characterized by small to medium size and round to oval shape, featuring hyperchromatic nuclei, inconspicuous nucleoli, and variable (from scanty to abundant) cytoplasm (Figs. 6-40 and 6-41). Mitotic figures are usually numerous (Fig. 6-42), and prominent necrosis is frequently observed (Fig. 6-43). More rarely, rhabdoid, spindle cell, or even signet-ring cell morphology has been observed; however, marked pleomorphism is not a typical feature of DSRCT. Rare cases of DSRCT exhibit a striking epithelioid morphology that makes the differential diagnosis with true epithelial malignancies very challenging (Fig. 6-44). It is also important to mention that pseudorosettes can occasionally be observed, making the differential diagnosis in Ewing sarcoma even more challenging (Fig. 6-45).

Desmoplastic small round cell tumor exhibits a remarkably distinctive polyphenotypic immunohistochemical profile, which consists of immunopositivity for epithelial (cytokeratins, EMA), myogenic (desmin), and neural/neuronal (neuron-specific enolase, S100 protein, CD57) differentiation markers. Cytokeratin immunoreactivity is observed in the vast majority of cases (Fig. 6-46). It is worth noting that all DSRCTs tested so

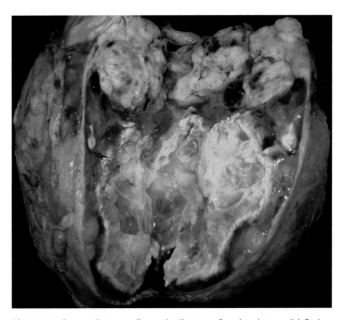

**Fig. 6-34.** Desmoplastic small round cell tumor. Grossly, a large solid, fleshy mass with cystic changes and areas of necrosis is seen.

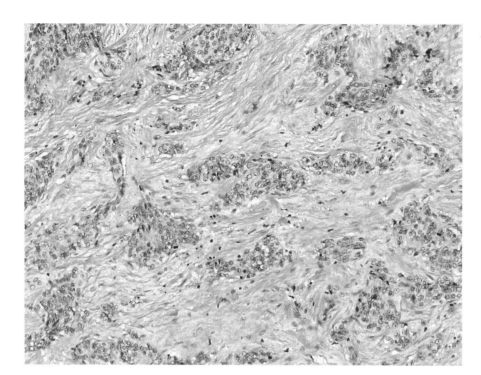

**Fig. 6-35.** Desmoplastic small round cell tumor. The tumor is composed of well-demarcated nests of round neoplastic cells, separated by a desmoplastic stroma.

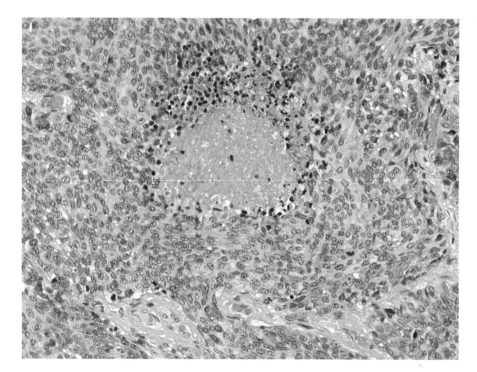

**Fig. 6-36.** Desmoplastic small round cell tumor. Central areas of necrosis are often seen with neoplastic cell clusters.

far appear to be negative for both cytokeratin 20 and cytokeratin 5/6 (usually expressed in normal mesothelium and mesotheliomas). EMA immunopositivity is also present in most examples of DSRCTs and appears to be slightly more sensitive than cytokeratins in detecting epithelial differentiation.

One of the most characteristic immunohistochemical features of DSRCT is represented by the expression of desmin. A distinctive dot-like pattern of staining represented by tiny paranuclear globules is observed (Fig. 6-47). DSRCT also tends to exhibit immunohistochemical features of neural differentiation. The expression of neural differentiation markers is very variable, but both neuron-specific enolase (NSE) and CD57 have tested positive in about two-thirds of cases. Unfortunately, considering the poor specificity of both markers, the presence of either NSE or CD57 immunopositivity cannot be regarded as unequivocal evidence of neural

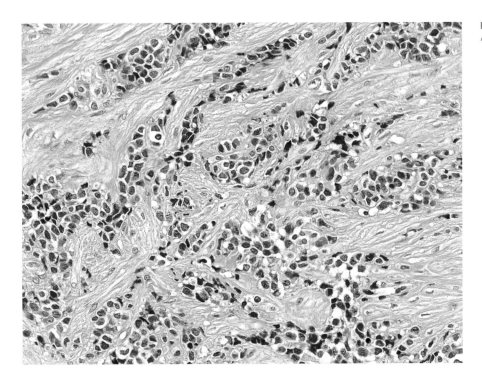

**Fig. 6-37.** Desmoplastic small round cell tumor. A cord-like pattern of growth is often seen.

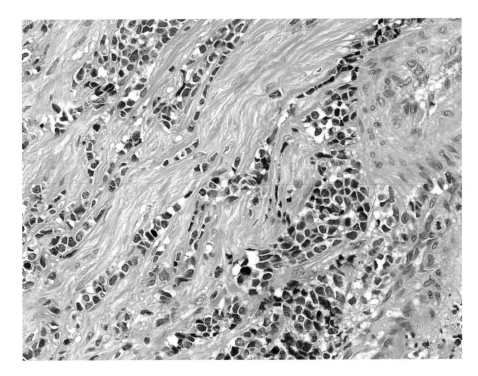

**Fig. 6-38.** Desmoplastic small round cell tumor. In some cases, the neoplastic cells are arranged in "Indian file" pattern, somewhat mimicking lobular carcinoma of the breast.

differentiation. Other, more specific markers of neural/neuronal differentiation, such as synaptophysin and chromogranin, have been reported in approximately 20% of cases; however, in our experience they seem to be negative. An additional immunophenotypic marker is represented by nuclear expression of C-terminus WT1.

## Genetics

Cytogenetically, DSRCT is characterized by a reciprocal translocation, t(11;22)(p13;q12), that was first reported by Sawyer in 1992. In 1994, Ladanyi first demonstrated that the Wilms' tumor gene (*WT1*) fuses with the *EWSR1* gene, resulting in its oncogenic activation. The fusion protein functions as a novel transcription factor that possesses the ability to transactivate genes overlapping with those normally regulated by *WT1*. One of the most interesting targets is represented by the platelet-derived growth factor alpha (*PDGFA*), a powerful fibroblast growth factor whose function may play a key role in the development of the desmoplastic fibroblastic stroma that is typically seen in DSRCT.

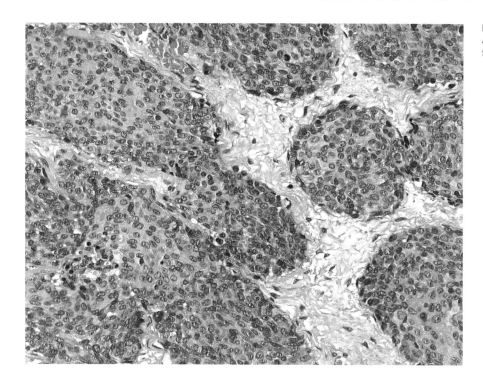

**Fig. 6-39.** Desmoplastic small round cell tumor. An "organoid" insular pattern of growth is sometimes seen.

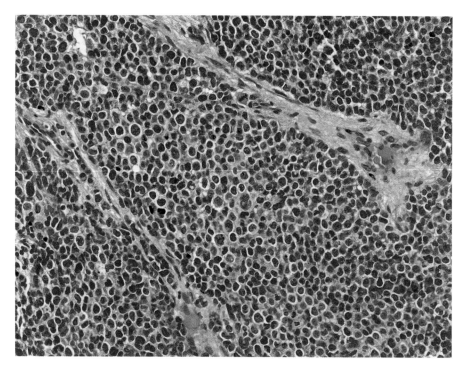

**Fig. 6-40.** Desmoplastic small round cell tumor. Tumor cells tend to be uniformly round, featuring hyperchromatic nuclei and scanty cytoplasm.

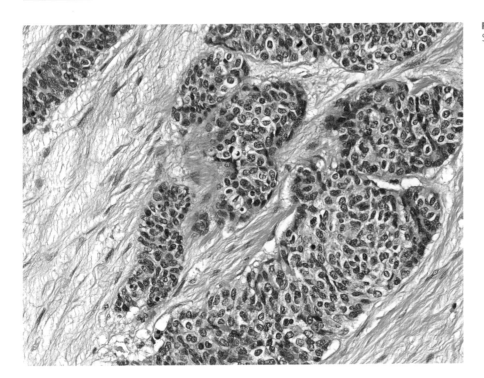

**Fig. 6-41.** Desmoplastic small round cell tumor. Sometimes cytoplasm tend to be abundant.

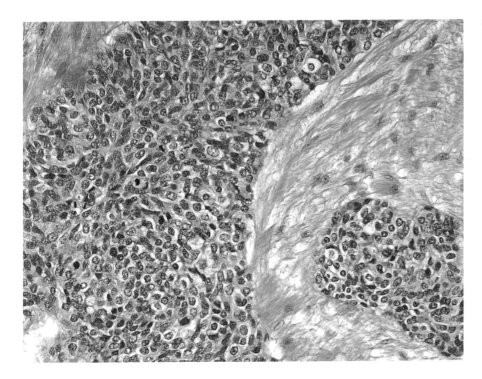

**Fig. 6-42.** Desmoplastic small round cell tumor. A high mitotic activity is often seen.

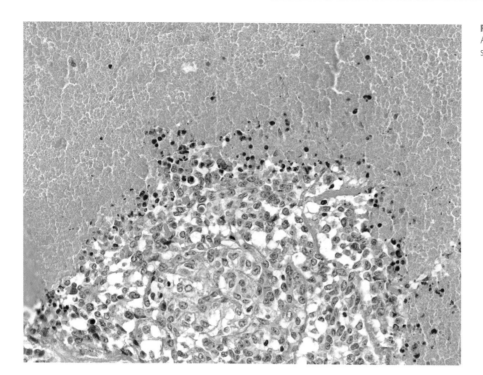

**Fig. 6-43.** Desmoplastic small round cell tumor. A large area of confluent coagulative necrosis is shown in this case.

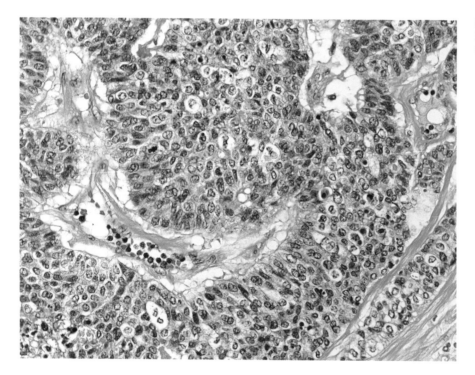

**Fig. 6-44.** Desmoplastic small round cell tumor. Pseudoglandular, epithelial-like features are rarely seen.

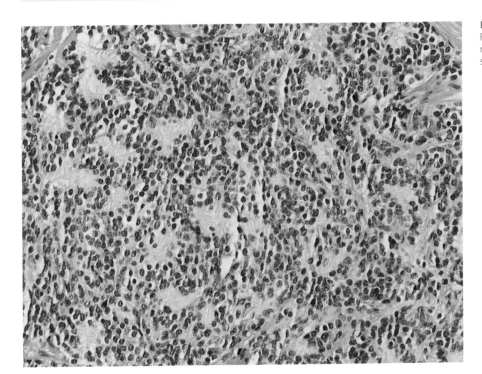

**Fig. 6-45.** Desmoplastic small round cell tumor. Rarely, the presence of numerous pseudorosettes may generate diagnostic confusion with Ewing sarcoma.

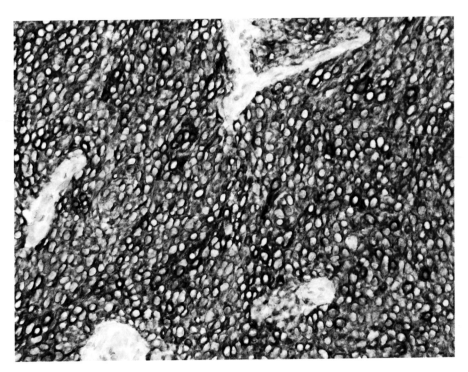

**Fig. 6-46.** Desmoplastic small round cell tumor. Strong immunopositivity for cytokeratin is shown in the vast majority of cases.

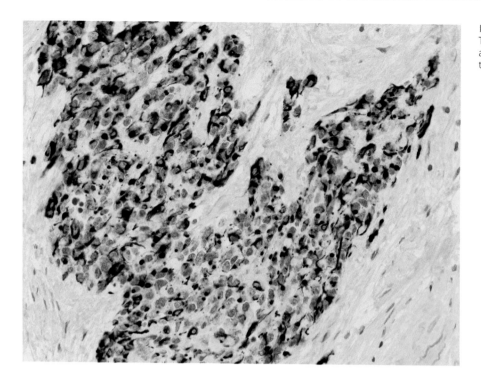

**Fig. 6-47.** Desmoplastic small round cell tumor. The presence of desmin immunostaining with a dot-like pattern represents a distinctive feature of the tumor.

## Differential Diagnosis and Diagnostic Pitfalls

The existence of polyphenotypic neoplasms morphologically similar to DSRCT but containing chimeric transcripts associated with the EWS category (EWS-FLI1 and EWS-ERG) underlines the importance of strict correlation between conventional morphology and genetic analysis. As the differential diagnosis includes Ewing sarcoma, it has to be stressed that CD99 immunopositivity is observed in less that 20% of DSRCT. However, in contrast to the thick membrane pattern observed in ES/PNET, CD99 tends to decorate diffusely the cytoplasm of the DSRCT neoplastic cells. Of course, the expression of myogenic markers raises the problem of some immunomorphologic overlap with the solid variant of alveolar rhabdomyosarcoma. However, both myogenin and MyoD1 (both members of the family of myogenic regulatory factors and sensitive as well as specific markers of skeletal muscle differentiation) have proved negative in all DSRCT tested so far. In consideration of the occurrence in serous-lined anatomic sites, malignant mesothelioma and metastatic carcinoma also need to be ruled out, as they can both be associated with desmoplastic reaction of the stroma. In this context, the demonstration of *EWSR1* gene rearrangement represents an extremely valuable finding. A final potential pitfall is represented by the fact that desmoplasia at times can be minimal, making the diagnosis extremely challenging.

### Key Points in Desmoplastic Small Round Cell Tumor Diagnosis

- Occurrence in mesothelium-lined anatomic sites of young males
- Round cell proliferation associated with desmoplastic stroma
- Polyphenotypic immunophenotype
- Presence of EWSR1/WT1 chimeric transcript
- Dismal prognosis despite multimodal therapy

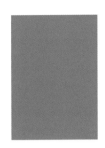

# Alveolar Rhabdomyosarcoma

## Definition and Epidemiology

Alveolar rhabdomyosarcoma (ARMS) is a malignant, round cell neoplasm showing skeletal muscle differentiation and is most often associated with *FOXO1* gene rearrangement. Two main variants of ARMS are currently recognized: classic ARMS and solid ARMS. Mixed embryonal/alveolar rhabdomyosarcomas usually lacks *FOXO1* gene aberrations and are currently considered closer to embryonal rhabdomyosarcoma (ERMS). Alveolar rhabdomyosarcoma accounts for approximately 20% of all rhabdomyosarcoma, and even if most often occur in adolescents and young adults, ARMS can actually be seen at any age.

## Clinical Presentation and Outcome

Alveolar rhabdomyosarcoma commonly involves the extremities (about 40%), including acral sites, followed by the paraspinal and perineal regions and paranasal sinuses. In further support of a close link between mixed forms and ERMS, these are more frequent in sites such as the urogenital tract and the orbit, wherein ERMS is more frequent. Alveolar rhabdomyosarcoma tends to be high stage at presentation, with distant metastases involving lymph nodes and bone marrow. An extremely rare, aggressive clinical presentation is that which mimics an acute leukemia with widespread bone marrow dissemination.

Alveolar rhabdomyosarcoma is a high-grade neoplasm, with a 3-year, disease-free survival of approximately 50% and it is more aggressive than ERMS. Treatment variably combines chemotherapy, surgery, and radiotherapy. Stage and post-surgical evaluation are predictive of outcome. A solid morphology seems not to have an impact on survival. The presence of PAX3/FOXO1 fusion transcript in metastatic cases at presentation has been associated with worse outcome (4-year overall survival rate of 75% for PAX7/FOXO1 vs. 8% for PAX3/FOXO1); however, other studies have not confirmed this finding. The sites of metastases are the same as those for embryonal rhabdomyosarcoma: lungs (60%), lymph node (50%), bone (40%), liver (25%), and brain (25%), but they are twice as frequent.

## Morphology and Immunophenotype

Grossly, ARMS forms an expansive, rapidly growing mass with a fleshy, pale yellow to white cut surface, with variable amounts of fibrous tissue, hemorrhage, and necrosis (Fig. 6-48). Microscopically, undifferentiated round cells organized in sheets, subdivided into nests by fibrovascular septa, compose classic forms of ARMS (Fig. 6-49). A scant eosinophilic (or, more rarely, clear) cytoplasm harbors hyperchromatic round nuclei (Fig. 6-50). Typically, loss of cohesion of neoplastic cells at the center of the nests occurs, somewhat resembling lung alveoli (Fig. 6-51). Multinucleated neoplastic giant cells are relatively often seen (Fig. 6-52).

The same cell population as in the classic form composes the solid variant of ARMS. However, a solid, diffuse pattern of growth predominates to the extent that the alveolar pattern is no longer recognizable (Fig. 6-53). Immunohistochemically, diffuse immunoreactivity for desmin (Fig. 6-54) and myogenin (Fig. 6-55) is typically seen. Importantly, in contrast to both ERMS and pleomorphic RMS, myogenin and/or MyoD1 decorate the vast majority of neoplastic cells. Up to 50% of cases may express cytokeratins that can be associated with expression of neuroendocrine markers (chromogranin and synaptophysin).

## Genetics

Alveolar rhabdomyosarcoma is characterized by two mutually exclusive PAX-FOXO1 rearrangements: a *PAX3-FOXO1* fusion (80%) and a *PAX7/FOXO1* fusion (20%). A third group is characterized by *PAX/FOXO1* fusion negativity (20%), but as discussed most of them are currently placed within the ERMS group. Gene expression arrays of ARMS show that fusion-positive cases form a distinct, tightly coherent molecular signature entity with impressive homogeneity, whereas fusion-negative cases tend to be molecularly dissimilar and overlap with the more heterogeneous ERMS. This correlates with aggressive behavior. Alternative translocations

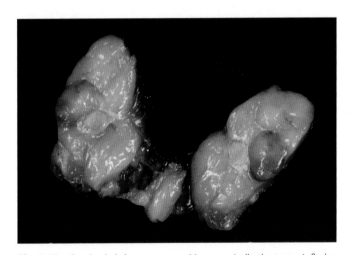

**Fig. 6-48.** Alveolar rhabdomyosarcoma. Macroscopically, the tumor is fleshy, featuring a pale, glistening cut surface with a central necrotic area.

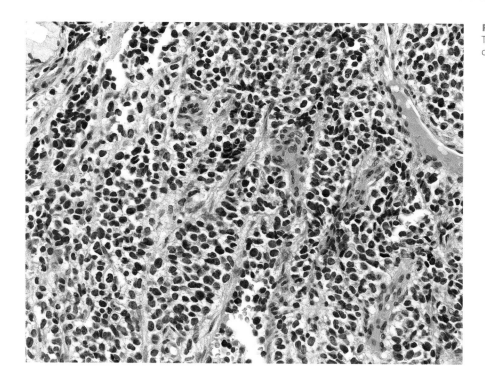

**Fig. 6-49.** Alveolar rhabdomyosarcoma. The tumor is composed of a round cell proliferation organized in nests separated by fibrovascular septa.

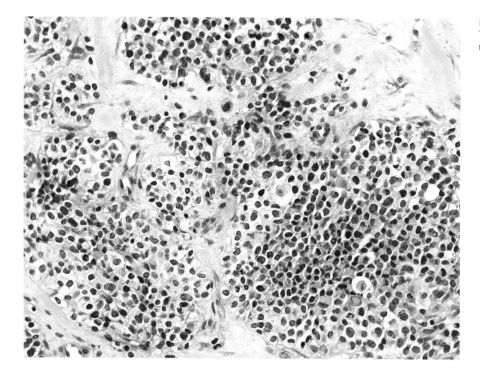

**Fig. 6-50.** Alveolar rhabdomyosarcoma. The neoplastic cells feature hyperchromatic round nuclei and scant eosinophilic cytoplasm.

producing PAX3-NCOA1 and PAX3-NCOA2 chimeric transcripts have been reported in some cases of ARMS (see Table 6.2). Fusion proteins are potent transcriptional activators with proven oncogenic activity.

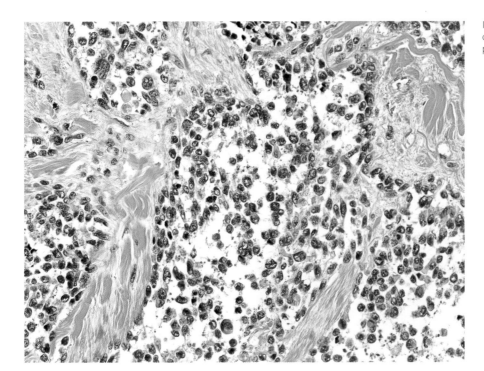

**Fig. 6-51.** Alveolar rhabdomyosarcoma. Loss of cohesion of neoplastic cells at the center of the nest produces the distinctive "alveolar" morphology.

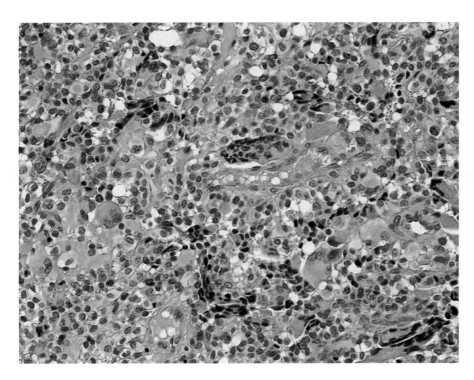

**Fig. 6-52.** Alveolar rhabdomyosarcoma. Giant cell with rhabdomyoblastic differentiation scattered through round neoplastic cells is seen.

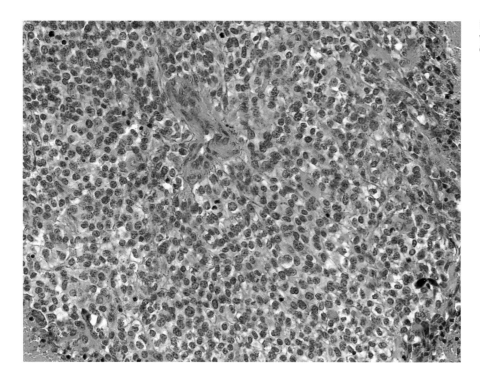

**Fig. 6-53.** Alveolar rhabdomyosarcoma (solid variant). The tumor cells show a solid, diffuse pattern of growth.

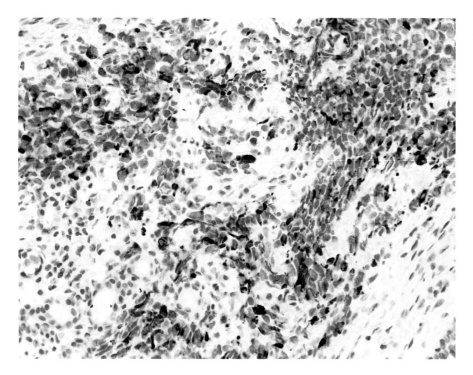

**Fig. 6-54.** Alveolar rhabdomyosarcoma. Diffuse expression of desmin is typically seen.

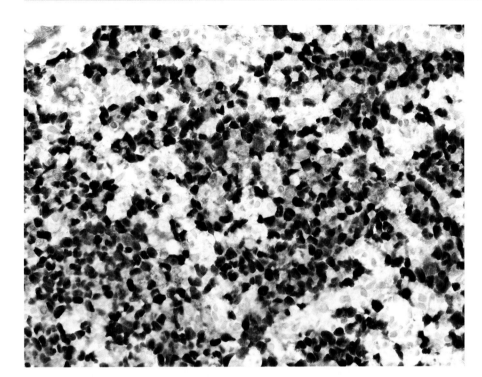

**Fig. 6-55.** Alveolar rhabdomyosarcoma. Nuclear immunostaining for myogenin is seen in the majority of neoplastic cells.

## Differential Diagnosis and Diagnostic Pitfalls

The differential diagnosis includes all small round cell neoplasms, including Ewing sarcoma/PNET, poorly differentiated synovial sarcoma, desmoplastic small round cell tumor, and mesenchymal chondrosarcoma. With the exception of desmoplastic small round cell tumor (which expresses desmin in a distinctive dot-like pattern but is myogenin/MyoD1 negative), all the others fail to express myogenic markers consistently. Embryonal rhabdomyosarcoma is discussed in detail in Chapter 4; however, it often features a heterogeneous cell population containing a variable number of rhabdomyoblasts set in a myxoid stroma. In contrast to the diffuse immunoreactivity observed in ARMS, myogenin usually decorates not more than 30–40% of ERMS neoplastic cells, which, in addition, never harbor *FOXO1* gene rearrangements. The distinction between ARMS and ERMS is extremely important in consideration of the differences in terms of clinical outcome. As mentioned, ARMS can express epithelial and neuroendocrine markers, raising the differential diagnosis with neuroendocrine carcinoma and olfactory neuroblastoma. Again, expression of skeletal differentiation markers and genetic findings represent helpful confirmatory tools.

| Key Points in Alveolar Rhabdomyosarcoma Diagnosis |
| --- |
| • Occurrence in the distal extremities and the head and neck region of adolescents and young adults |
| • Round cell morphology, often featuring an alveolar (rarely solid) pattern of growth |
| • Expression of desmin, myogenin, and MyoD1 |
| • Presence of rearrangement of the *FOXO1* gene |
| • Aggressive clinical behavior |

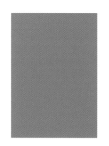

# Variants of Soft Tissue Sarcomas Featuring a Round Cell Morphology

## Poorly Differentiated Round Cell Synovial Sarcoma

Synovial sarcoma is discussed in detail in Chapter 4. Synovial sarcoma is a mesenchymal spindle cell tumor displaying variable epithelial differentiation. It can occur at any age, with a peak incidence between the first and the third decade. The most common clinical presentation is a mass in the soft tissues of the lower extremities, especially around the knee and the ankle. Trunk, head and neck, and mediastinum are also among the most common sites. Even if typical of somatic soft tissues, synovial sarcoma is also described at visceral sites, such as the lungs (wherein it represents by far the most common mesenchymal malignancy), the mediastinum, and the gastrointestinal tract. Less than 20% of cases feature an undifferentiated round cell morphology that is associated with higher clinical aggressiveness.

Grossly, poorly differentiated round cell synovial sarcoma exhibits a fleshy appearance often associated with hemorrhagic and pseudocystic changes (Fig. 6-56). Microscopically, it is composed of an undifferentiated round cell population most often organized as a solid pattern of growth (Fig. 6-57). Hemangiopericytoma-like blood vessels can be observed, but

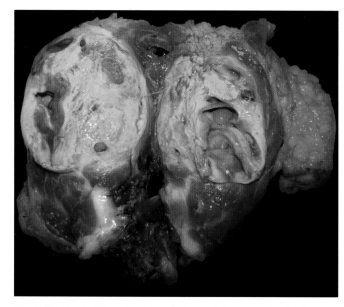

**Fig. 6-56.** Poorly differentiated round cell synovial sarcoma. Grossly, the tumor is a well-demarcated fleshy mass with cystic changes and areas of necrosis.

**Fig. 6-57.** Poorly differentiated round cell synovial sarcoma. The neoplastic cells feature round nuclei with prominent nucleoli and poorly defined cytoplasm.

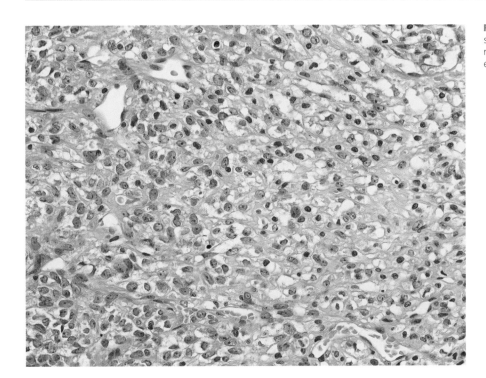

**Fig. 6-58.** Poorly differentiated round cell synovial sarcoma. An extremely helpful diagnostic clue is represented by the presence of pericellular eosinophilic collagen.

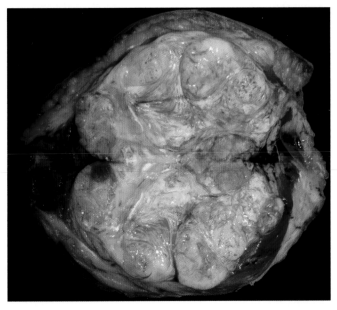

**Fig. 6-59.** Round cell myxoid liposarcoma. Grossly, the neoplastic mass is most often well circumscribed. The cut surface is gelatinous to fleshy with areas of necrosis.

## Differential Diagnosis and Diagnostic Pitfalls

Poorly differentiated round cell synovial sarcoma exhibits significant morphologic overlap with Ewing sarcoma and mesenchymal chondrosarcoma, including CD99 immunopositivity. Expression of EMA and TLE1 and the presence of *SYT* gene rearrangement represent extremely helpful diagnostic findings. As mentioned, cytokeratins may be entirely negative, therefore representing a potential diagnostic pitfall. FISH analysis appears to be a valuable tool, as *SYT* gene rearrangements have so far proved extremely specific for synovial sarcoma.

## High-Grade "Round Cell" Myxoid Liposarcoma

Myxoid liposarcoma is discussed in detail in Chapter 8. It represents the second-most common group of adipocytic malignancies (after well-differentiated liposarcoma), accounting for about one-third of all liposarcomas. The peak incidence of myxoid liposarcoma is between the third and fifth decade, and occurs predominantly in the limbs (particularly the thigh).

The presence of hypercellularity or round cell differentiation is associated with worsening prognosis. Different cut-off values, ranging between 5 and 25%, have been set by independent studies. Myxoid liposarcoma tends to recur repeatedly and to metastasize to both bone and soft issue locations, including the retroperitoneum. Standard treatment is represented by wide surgical resection. In high-grade lesions, adjuvant therapy (radiotherapy and/or chemotherapy) may be associated. The drug trabectedin appears to be a highly promising treatment for metastatic myxoid liposarcoma.

Grossly, high-grade myxoid liposarcoma is most often well circumscribed and features a fleshy appearance with multiple foci of necrosis (Fig. 6-59). Myxoid/round cell liposarcoma is

less often than in classic examples of synovial sarcoma. The presence of pericellular collagen represents an extremely helpful diagnostic clue (Fig. 6-58). Immunohistochemically, EMA represents the most sensitive markers, whereas cytokeratin can be frequently negative. TLE1 immunopositivity is also seen. Molecularly, poorly differentiated round cell synovial sarcoma shares with all synovial sarcoma variants the presence of the specific chromosomal translocation t(X;18) (p11;q11), which fuses the gene *SYT* with *SSX1, SSX2,* and, rarely, *SSX4.*

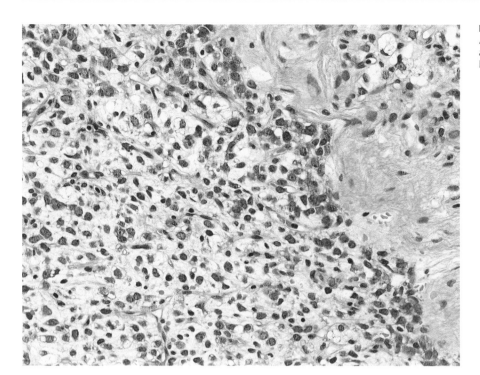

**Fig. 6-60.** Round cell myxoid liposarcoma. A round cell population often organized in a perivascular pattern of growth, with scattered lipoblasts, is frequently observed.

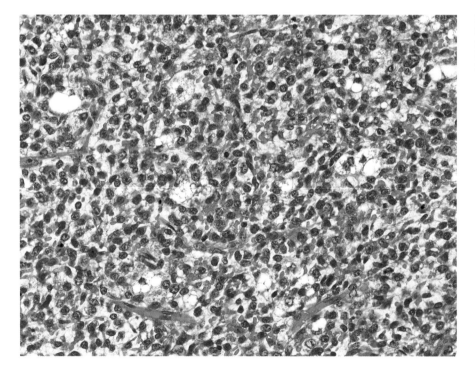

**Fig. 6-61.** Round cell myxoid liposarcoma (pure form). A highly cellular round cell population with numerous small, branching blood vessels is seen. Mitotic activity may be low despite high-grade morphology.

defined by the presence of hypercellular areas (which most frequently begin to form in a perivascular distribution) featuring (but not always) undifferentiated round cell morphology and ranging in extent between 5 and 80% (Fig. 6-60). Pure round cell liposarcoma is a rare neoplasm in which hypercellularity or round cell differentiation accounts for more than 80% of tumor tissue (Fig. 6-61). Adipocytic differentiation in pure round cell liposarcoma is often barely appreciable. Myxoid liposarcoma usually exhibits S100 immunopositivity,

which tends to be retained in the hypercellular/round cell areas. As mentioned, hypercellularity in myxoid liposarcoma is not always associated with the presence of round cell morphology, and rather often neoplastic cells retain a spindled shape (Fig. 6-62). Myxoid liposarcoma, independently of grade of differentiation, is characterized by two main karyotypic aberrations: a t(12;16) that fuses the *DDIT3* (formerly *CHOP*) gene on 12q13 with the *FUS* (or *TLS*) gene on 16p11, and t(12;22) that fuses *DDIT3* with *EWSR1* on 22q12.

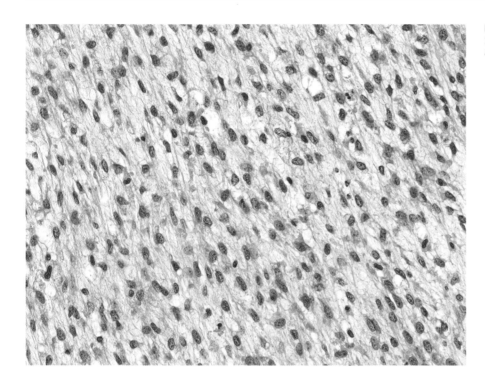

**Fig. 6-62.** Round cell myxoid liposarcoma. Sometimes, the cellular areas, despite the name, are actually composed of spindle cells.

## Differential Diagnosis and Diagnostic Pitfalls

Poorly differentiated round cell liposarcoma in its pure form enters the differential diagnosis with all other round cell sarcomas. As adipocytic differentiation represented by the presence of monovacuolated lipoblasts can be minimal and therefore easily overlooked, demonstration of *DDIT3* gene rearrangements represents the most effective confirmatory diagnostic technique. However, it has to be remembered that pure round cell morphology in myxoid liposarcoma is extremely rare, and most often differentiated areas are recognizable. An important diagnostic clue is represented by the presence of a thin-walled, plexiform vascular network that tends to be retained in high-grade areas.

## Chapter 6 Selected Key References

### Ewing Sarcoma and Its Differential Diagnosis

- Ambros IM, Ambros PF, Strehl S, et al. MIC2 is a specific marker for Ewing's sarcoma and peripheral primitive neuroectodermal tumors. Evidence for a common histogenesis of Ewing's sarcoma and peripheral primitive neuroectodermal tumors from MIC2 expression and specific chromosome aberration. *Cancer.* 1991;**67**:1886–93.

- Askin FB, Rosai J, Sibley RK, Dehner LP, McAlister WH. Malignant small cell tumor of the thoracopulmonary region in childhood: a distinctive clinicopathologic entity of uncertain histogenesis. *Cancer.* 1979;**43**:2438–51.

- Aurias A, Rimbaut C, Buffe D, Zucker JM, Mazabraud A. Translocation involving chromosome 22 in Ewing's sarcoma. A cytogenetic study of four fresh tumors. *Cancer Genet Cytogenet.* 1984;**12**:21–5.

- Charville GW, Wang WL, Ingram DR, et al. EWSR1 fusion proteins mediate PAX7 expression in Ewing sarcoma. *Mod Pathol.* 2017;**30**:1312–20.

- Chen S, Deniz K, Sung YS, et al. Ewing sarcoma with ERG gene rearrangements: A molecular study focusing on the prevalence of FUS-ERG and common pitfalls in detecting EWSR1-ERG fusions by FISH. *Genes Chromosomes Cancer.* 2016;**55**:340–9.

- de Alava E, Antonescu CR, Panizo A, et al. Prognostic impact of P53 status in Ewing sarcoma. *Cancer.* 2000;**15**;89:783–92.

- de Alava E, Kawai A, Healey JH, et al. EWS-FLI1 fusion transcript structure is an independent determinant of prognosis in Ewing's sarcoma. *J Clin Oncol.* 1998;**16**:1248–55.

- Dedeurwaerdere F, Giannini C, Sciot R, et al. Primary peripheral PNET/Ewing's sarcoma of the dura: a clinicopathologic entity distinct from central PNET. *Mod Pathol.* **200**;15:673–8.

- Dehner LP. Primitive neuroectodermal tumor and Ewing's sarcoma. *Am J Surg Pathol.* 1993;**17**:1–13.

- Delattre O, Zucman J, Melot T, et al. The Ewing family of tumors – a subgroup of small-round-cell tumors defined by specific chimeric transcripts. *N Engl J Med.* 1994;**331**:294–9.

- Delattre O, Zucman J, Plougastel B, et al. Gene fusion with an ETS DNA-binding domain caused by chromosome translocation in human tumours. *Nature.* 1992;**10**(359):162–5.

- Folpe AL, Goldblum JR, Rubin BP, et al. Morphologic and immunophenotypic diversity in Ewing family tumors: a study of 66 genetically confirmed cases. *Am J Surg Pathol.* 2005;**29**:1025–33.

- Folpe AL, Hill CE, Parham DM, O'Shea PA, Weiss SW. Immunohistochemical detection of FLI-1 protein expression: a study of 132 round cell tumors with emphasis on CD99-positive mimics of Ewing's sarcoma/primitive neuroectodermal tumor. *Am J Surg Pathol.* 2000;**24**:1657–62.

- Hasegawa SL, Davison JM, Rutten A, Fletcher JA, Fletcher CD. Primary cutaneous Ewing's sarcoma: immunophenotypic and molecular cytogenetic evaluation of five cases. *Am J Surg Pathol.* 1998;**22**:310–18.

- Hung YP, Lee JP, Bellizzi AM, Hornick JL. PHOX2B reliably distinguishes neuroblastoma among small round blue cell tumours. *Histopathology.* 2017;**71**:786–94.

- Jeon IS, Davis JN, Braun BS, et al. A variant Ewing's sarcoma translocation (7;22) fuses the EWS gene to the ETS gene ETV1. *Oncogene.* 1995;**10**:1229–34.

- Jimenez RE, Folpe AL, Lapham RL, et al. Primary Ewing's sarcoma/primitive neuroectodermal tumor of the kidney: a clinicopathologic and immunohistochemical analysis of 11 cases. *Am J Surg Pathol.* 2002;**26**:320–7.

- Kawamura-Saito M, Yamazaki Y, Kaneko K, et al. Fusion between CIC and DUX4 up-regulates PEA3 family genes in Ewing-like sarcomas with t(4;19)(q35; q13) translocation. *Hum Mol Genet.* 2006;**15**:2125–37.

- Le Deley MC, Delattre O, Schaefer KL, et al. Impact of EWS-ETS fusion type on disease progression in Ewing's sarcoma/peripheral primitive neuroectodermal tumor: prospective results from the cooperative Euro-E.W.I.N.G. 99 trial. *J Clin Oncol.* 2010;**20**:1982–8.

- Le Loarer F, Pissaloux D, Coindre JM, Tirode F, Vince DR. Update on families of round cell sarcomas other than classical Ewing sarcomas. *Surg Pathol Clin.* 2017;**10**:587–620.

- Lessnick SL, Dei Tos AP, Sorensen PH, et al. Small round cell sarcomas. *Semin Oncol.* 2009;**36**:338–46.

- Miettinen M. Keratin 20: immunohistochemical marker for gastrointestinal, urothelial, and Merkel cell carcinomas. *Mod Pathol.* 1995;**8**:384–8.

- Moll R, Löwe A, Laufer J, Franke WW. Cytokeratin 20 in human carcinomas. A new histodiagnostic marker detected by monoclonal antibodies. *Am J Pathol.* 1992;**140**:427–47.

- Nicholson SA, McDermott MB, Swanson PE, Wick MR. CD99 and cytokeratin-20 in small-cell and basaloid tumors of the skin. *Appl Immunohistochem Mol Morphol.* 2000;**8**:37–41.

- Parham DM, Hijazi Y, Steinberg SM, et al. Neuroectodermal differentiation in Ewing's sarcoma family of tumors does not predict tumor behavior. *Hum Pathol.* 1999;**30**:911–18.

- Peter M, Couturier J, Pacquement H, et al. A new member of the ETS family fused to EWS in Ewing tumors. *Oncogene.* 1997;**13**(14):1159–64.

- Righi A, Gambarotti M, Longo S, et al. Small cell osteosarcoma: clinicopathologic, immunohistochemical, and molecular analysis of 36 cases. *Am J Surg Pathol.* 2015;**39**:691–9.

- Romeo S, Dei Tos AP. Soft tissue tumors associated with EWSR1 translocation. *Virchows Arch.* 2010;**456**:219–34.

- Rossi S, Orvieto E, Furlanetto A, et al. Utility of the immunohistochemical detection of FLI-1 expression in round cell and vascular neoplasm using a monoclonal antibody. *Mod Pathol.* 2004;**17**:547–52.

- Schmidt D, Herrmann C, Jürgens H, Harms D. Malignant peripheral neuroectodermal tumor and its necessary distinction from Ewing's sarcoma. A report from the Kiel Pediatric Tumor Registry. *Cancer.* 1991;**15**(68):2251–9.

- Sorensen PH, Lessnick SL, Lopez-Terrada D, et al. A second Ewing's sarcoma translocation, t(21;22), fuses the EWS gene to another ETS-family transcription factor, ERG. *Nat Genet.* 1994;**6**:146–51.

- Stout AP. A tumor of the ulnar nerve. *Proc N Y Pathol Soc.* 1918;**18**:2–12.

- Szuhai K, IJszenga M, Tanke HJ, et al. Detection and molecular cytogenetic characterization of a novel ring chromosome in a histological variant of Ewing sarcoma. *Cancer Genet Cytogenet.* 2007;**172**:12–22.

- Terrier P, Henry-Amar M, Triche TJ, et al. Is neuro-ectodermal differentiation of Ewing's sarcoma of bone associated with an unfavourable prognosis? *Eur J Cancer.* 1995;**31A**:307–14.

- Thorner P, Squire J, Chilton-MacNeil S, et al. Is the EWS/FLI-1 fusion transcript specific for Ewing sarcoma and peripheral primitive neuroectodermal tumor? A report of four cases showing this transcript in a wider range of tumor types. *Am J Pathol.* 1996;**148**:1125–38.

- Urano F, Umezawa A, Hong W, Kikuchi H, Hata J. A novel chimera gene between EWS and E1A-F, encoding the adenovirus E1A enhancer-binding protein, in extraosseous Ewing's sarcoma. *Biochem Biophys Res Commun.* 1996;**15**(219):608–12.

- Wei G, Antonescu CR, de Alava E, et al. Prognostic impact of INK4A deletion in Ewing sarcoma. *Cancer.* 2000;**15**(89):793–9.

- Zogopoulos G, Teskey L, Sung L, et al. Ewing sarcoma: favourable results with combined modality therapy and conservative use of radiotherapy. *Pediatr Blood Cancer.* 2004;**43**:35–9.

## CIC-DUX4-Associated Round Cell Sarcoma

- Antonescu CR, Owosho AA, Zhang L, et al. Sarcomas with CIC-rearrangements are a distinct pathologic entity with aggressive outcome: a clinicopathologic and molecular study of 115 cases. *Am J Surg Pathol.* 2017;**41**:941–9.

- Choi EY, Thomas DG, McHugh JB, et al. Undifferentiated small round cell sarcoma with t(4;19)(q35;q13.1) CIC-DUX4 fusion: a novel highly aggressive soft tissue tumor with distinctive histopathology. *Am J Surg Pathol.* 2013;**37**:1379–86.

- Graham C, Chilton-MacNeill S, Zielenska M, Somers GR. The CIC-DUX4 fusion transcript is present in a subgroup of pediatric primitive round cell sarcomas. *Hum Pathol.* 2012;**43**:180–9.

- Hung YP, Fletcher CD, Hornick JL. Evaluation of ETV4 and WT1 expression in CIC-rearranged sarcomas and histologic mimics. *Mod Pathol.* 2016;**29**:1324–34.

- Italiano A, Sung YS, Zhang L, et al. High prevalence of CIC fusion with double-homeobox (DUX4) transcription factors in EWSR1-negative undifferentiated small blue round cell sarcomas. *Genes Chromosomes Cancer.* 2012;**51**:207–18.

- Kawamura-Saito M, Yamazaki Y, Kaneko K, et al. Fusion between CIC and DUX4 up-regulates PEA3 family genes in Ewing-like sarcomas with t(4;19)(q35; q13) translocation. *Hum Mol Genet.* 2006 **15**:2125–37.

- Le Guellec S, Velasco V, Pérot G, et al. ETV4 is a useful marker for the diagnosis of CIC-rearranged undifferentiated round-cell sarcomas: a study of 127 cases including mimicking lesions. *Mod Pathol.* 2016;**29**:1523–31.

- Le Loarer F, Pissaloux D, Coindre JM, Tirode F, Vince DR. Update on families of round cell sarcomas other than classical Ewing sarcomas. *Surg Pathol Clin.* 2017;**10**:587–620.

- Richkind KE, Romansky SG, Finklestein JZ. t(4;19)(q35;q13.1): a recurrent change in primitive mesenchymal tumors? *Cancer Genet Cytogenet.* 1996;**87**:71–4.

- Siegele B, Roberts J, Black JO, et al. DUX4 immunohistochemistry is a highly sensitive and specific marker for CIC-DUX4 fusion-positive round cell tumor. *Am J Surg Pathol.* 2017;**41**:423–9.

- Smith SC, Buehler D, Choi EY, et al. CIC-DUX sarcomas demonstrate frequent MYC amplification and ETS-family transcription factor expression. *Mod Pathol.* 2015;**28**:57–68.

- Specht K, Sung YS, Zhang L, et al. Distinct transcriptional signature and immunoprofile of CIC-DUX4 fusion-positive round cell tumors compared to EWSR1-rearranged Ewing sarcomas: further evidence toward distinct pathologic entities. *Genes Chromosomes Cancer.* 2014;**53**:622–33.

- Sugita S, Arai Y, Aoyama T, et al. NUTM2A-CIC fusion small round cell sarcoma: a genetically distinct variant of CIC-rearranged sarcoma. *Hum Pathol.* 2017;**65**:225–30.

- Sugita S, Arai Y, Tonooka A, Hama N, et al. A novel CIC-FOXO4 gene fusion in undifferentiated small round cell sarcoma: a genetically distinct variant of Ewing-like sarcoma. *Am J Surg Pathol.* 2014;**38**:1571–6.

- Yoshida A, Arai Y, Kobayashi E, et al. CIC break-apart fluorescence in-situ hybridization misses a subset of CIC-DUX4 sarcomas: a clinicopathological and molecular study. *Histopathology.* 2017;**71**:461–9.

- Yoshimoto T, Tanaka M, Homme M, et al. CIC-DUX4 induces small round cell sarcomas distinct from Ewing sarcoma. *Cancer Res.* 2017;**77**:2927–37.

## BCOR-CCNB3 (Ewing-Like) Sarcoma

- Argani P, Kao YC, Zhang L, et al. Primary renal sarcomas with BCOR-CCNB3 gene fusion: a report of 2 cases showing histologic overlap with clear cell sarcoma of kidney, suggesting further link between BCOR-related sarcomas of the kidney and soft tissues. *Am J Surg Pathol.* 2017;**41**:1702–12.

- Chiang S, Lee CH, Stewart CJR, et al. BCOR is a robust diagnostic immunohistochemical marker of genetically diverse high-grade endometrial stromal sarcoma, including tumors exhibiting variant morphology. *Mod Pathol.* 2017;**30**:1251–61.

- Cohen-Gogo S, Cellier C, Coindre JM, et al. Ewing-like sarcomas with BCOR-CCNB3 fusion transcript: a clinical, radiological and pathological retrospective study from the Société Française des Cancers de L'Enfant. *Pediatr Blood Cancer.* 2014;**61**:2191–8.

- Creytens D. SATB2 and TLE1 Expression in BCOR-CCNB3 (Ewing-like) sarcoma, mimicking small cell osteosarcoma and poorly differentiated synovial sarcoma. *Appl Immunohistochem Mol Morphol.* 2017 Oct 27. [Epub ahead of print]

- Kao YC, Owosho AA, Sung YS, et al. BCOR-CCNB3 fusion positive sarcomas: a clinicopathologic and molecular analysis of 36 cases with comparison to morphologic spectrum and clinical behavior of other round cell sarcomas. *Am J Surg Pathol.* 2017 Oct 25. [Epub ahead of print]

- Kao YC, Sung YS, Zhang L, et al. BCOR Overexpression is a highly sensitive marker in round cell sarcomas with BCOR genetic abnormalities. *Am J Surg Pathol.* 2016a;**40**:1670–8.

- Kao YC, Sung YS, Zhang L, et al. Recurrent BCOR internal tandem duplication and YWHAE-NUTM2B fusions in soft tissue undifferentiated round cell sarcoma of infancy: overlapping genetic features with clear cell sarcoma of kidney. *Am J Surg Pathol.* 2016b;**40**:1009–20.

- Lewis N, Soslow RA, Delair DF, et al. ZC3H7B-BCOR high-grade endometrial stromal sarcomas: a report of 17 cases of a newly defined entity. *Mod Pathol.* 2017 Dec 1. [Epub ahead of print]

- Ludwig K, Alaggio R, Zin A, et al. BCOR-CCNB3 Undifferentiated sarcoma-does immunohistochemistry help in the identification? *Pediatr Dev Pathol.* 2017;**20**:321–9.

- Mariño-Enriquez A, Lauria A, Przybyl J, et al. BCOR internal tandem duplication in high-grade uterine sarcomas. *Am J Surg Pathol.* 2017 Dec 1. [Epub ahead of print]

- Matsuyama A, Shiba E, Umekita Y, et al. Clinicopathologic diversity of undifferentiated sarcoma with BCOR-CCNB3 fusion: analysis of 11 cases with a reappraisal of the utility of immunohistochemistry for BCOR and CCNB3. *Am J Surg Pathol.* 2017;**41**:1713–21.

- Peters TL, Kumar V, Polikepahad S, et al. BCOR-CCNB3 fusions are frequent in undifferentiated sarcomas of male children. *Mod Pathol.* 2015;**28**:575–86.

- Pierron G, Tirode F, Lucchesi C, et al. A new subtype of bone sarcoma defined by BCOR-CCNB3 gene fusion. *Nat Genet.* 2012;**44**:461–6.

- Puls F, Niblett A, Marland G, et al. BCOR-CCNB3 (Ewing-like) sarcoma: a clinicopathologic analysis of 10 cases, in comparison with conventional Ewing sarcoma. *Am J Surg Pathol.* 2014;**38**:1307–18.

- Specht K, Zhang L, Sung YS, et al. Novel BCOR-MAML3 and ZC3H7B-BCOR gene fusions in undifferentiated small blue round cell sarcomas. *Am J Surg Pathol.* 2016 Apr;**40**(4):433–42.

- Wong MK, Ng CCY, Kuick CH, et al. Clear cell sarcomas of the kidney are characterised by BCOR gene abnormalities, including exon 15 internal tandem duplications and BCOR-CCNB3 gene fusion. *Histopathology.* 2018;**72**:320–9.

## Extraskeletal Mesenchymal Chondrosarcoma

- Bertoni F, Picci P, Bacchini P, et al. Mesenchymal chondrosarcoma of bone and soft tissues. *Cancer.* 1983;**52**:533–41.

- Frezza AM, Cesari M, Baumhoer D, et al. Mesenchymal chondrosarcoma: prognostic factors and outcome in 113 patients. A European Musculoskeletal Oncology Society study. *Eur J Cancer.* 2015;**51**:374–81.

- Guccion JG, Font RL, Enzinger FM, Zimmerman LE. Extraskeletal mesenchymal chondrosarcoma. *Arch Pathol.* 1973;**95**:336–40.

- Hoang MP, Suarez PA, Donner LR, et al. Mesenchymal chondrosarcoma: a small cell neoplasm with polyphenotypic differentiation. *Int J Surg Pathol.* 2000;**8**:291–301.

- Jacobs JL, Merriam JC, Chadburn A, et al. Mesenchymal chondrosarcoma of the orbit. Report of three new cases and review of the literature. *Cancer.* 1994;**73**:399–405.

- Knott PD, Gannon FH, Thompson LD. Mesenchymal chondrosarcoma of the sinonasal tract: a clinicopathological study of 13 cases with a review of the literature. *Laryngoscope.* 2003;**113**:783–90.

- Nakashima Y, Unni KK, Shives TC, Swee RG, Dahlin DC. Mesenchymal chondrosarcoma of bone and soft tissue. A review of 111 cases. *Cancer.* 1986;**57**:2444–53.

- Naumann S, Krallman PA, Unni KK, et al. Translocation der(13;21)(q10;q10) in skeletal and extraskeletal mesenchymal chondrosarcoma. *Mod Pathol.* 2002;**15**:572–6.

- Nussbeck W, Neureiter D, Söder S, Inwards C, Aigner T. Mesenchymal chondrosarcoma: an immunohistochemical study of 10 cases examining prognostic significance of proliferative activity and cellular differentiation. *Pathology.* 2004;**36**:230–3.

- Suster S, Moran CA. Malignant cartilaginous tumors of the mediastinum: clinicopathological study of six cases presenting as extraskeletal soft tissue masses. *Hum Pathol.* 1997;**28**:588–94.
- Tsuda Y, Ogura K, Hakozaki M, et al. Mesenchymal chondrosarcoma: a Japanese Musculoskeletal Oncology Group (JMOG) study on 57 patients. *J Surg Oncol.* 2017;**115**:760–7.
- Wang L, Motoi T, Khanin R, et al. Identification of a novel, recurrent HEY1-NCOA2 fusion in mesenchymal chondrosarcoma based on a genome-wide screen of exon-level expression data. *Genes Chromosomes Cancer.* 2012;**51**:127–39.
- Wehrli BM, Huang W, De Crombrugghe B, Ayala AG, Czerniak B. Sox9, a master regulator of chondrogenesis, distinguishes mesenchymal chondrosarcoma from other small blue round cell tumors. *Hum Pathol.* 2003;**34**:263–9.

## Desmoplastic Small Round Cell Tumor

- Antonescu CR, Gerald WL, Magid MS, Ladanyi M. Molecular variants of the EWS-WT1 gene fusion in desmoplastic small round cell tumor. *Diagn Mol Pathol.* 1998;**7**:24–8.
- Barnoud R, Sabourin JC, Pasquier D, et al. Immunohistochemical expression of WT1 by desmoplastic small round cell tumor: a comparative study with other small round cell tumors. *Am J Surg Pathol.* 2000;**24**:830–6.
- Cummings OW, Ulbright TM, Young RH, et al. Desmoplastic small round cell tumors of the paratesticular region. A report of six cases. *Am J Surg Pathol.* 1997;**21**:219–25.
- de Alava E, Ladanyi M, Rosai J, Gerald WL. Detection of chimeric transcripts in desmoplastic small round cell tumor and related developmental tumors by reverse transcriptase polymerase chain reaction. A specific diagnostic assay. *Am J Pathol.* 1995;**147**:1584–91.
- Froberg K, Brown RE, Gaylord H, Manivel C. Intra-abdominal desmoplastic small round cell tumor: immunohistochemical evidence for up-regulation of autocrine and paracrine growth factors. *Ann Clin Lab Sci.* 1999;**29**:78–85.
- Gerald WL, Ladanyi M, de Alava E, et al. Clinical, pathologic, and molecular spectrum of tumors associated with t(11;22)(p13;q12): desmoplastic small round-cell tumor and its variants. *J Clin Oncol.* 1998;**16**:3028–36.
- Gerald WL, Miller HK, Battifora H, et al. Intra-abdominal desmoplastic small round-cell tumor. Report of 19 cases of a distinctive type of high-grade polyphenotypic malignancy affecting young individuals. *Am J Surg Pathol.* 1991;**15**:499–513.
- Gerald WL, Rosai J. Case 2. Desmoplastic small cell tumor with divergent differentiation. *Pediatr Pathol.* 1989;**9**:177–83.
- Gerald WL, Rosai J, Ladanyi M. Characterization of the genomic breakpoint and chimeric transcripts in the EWS-WT1 gene fusion of desmoplastic small round cell tumor. *Proc Natl Acad Sci U S A.* 1995;**92**:1028–32.
- Gonzalez-Crussi F, Crawford SE, Sun CC. Intraabdominal desmoplastic small-cell tumors with divergent differentiation. Observations on three cases of childhood. *Am J Surg Pathol.* 1990;**14**:633–42.
- Hill DA, Pfeifer JD, Marley EF, et al. WT1 staining reliably differentiates desmoplastic small round cell tumor from Ewing sarcoma/primitive neuroectodermal tumor. An immunohistochemical and molecular diagnostic study. *Am J Clin Pathol.* 2000;**114**:345–53.
- Kushner BH, LaQuaglia MP, Wollner N, et al. Desmoplastic small round-cell tumor: prolonged progression-free survival with aggressive multimodality therapy. *J Clin Oncol.* 1996;**14**:1526–31.
- Ladanyi M, Gerald W. Fusion of the EWS and WT1 genes in the desmoplastic small round cell tumor. *Cancer Res.* 1994;**54**:2837–40.
- Lae ME, Roche PC, Jin L, Lloyd RV, Nascimento AG. Desmoplastic small round cell tumor: a clinicopathologic, immunohistochemical, and molecular study of 32 tumors. *Am J Surg Pathol.* 2002;**26**:823–35.
- Lee SB, Kolquist KA, Nichols K, et al. The EWS-WT1 translocation product induces PDGFA in desmoplastic small round-cell tumour. *Nat Genet.* 1997;**17**:309–13.
- Mohamed M, Gonzalez D, Fritchie KJ, et al. Desmoplastic small round cell tumor: evaluation of reverse transcription-polymerase chain reaction and fluorescence in situ hybridization as ancillary molecular diagnostic techniques. *Virchows Arch.* 2017;**471**:631–40.
- Mora J, Modak S, Cheung NK, et al. Desmoplastic small round cell tumor 20 years after its discovery. *Future Oncol.* 2015;**11**:1071–81.
- Ordi J, de Alava E, Torné A, et al. Intraabdominal desmoplastic small round cell tumor with EWS/ERG fusion transcript. *Am J Surg Pathol.* 1998;**22**:1026–32.
- Ordóñez NG. Desmoplastic small round cell tumor: I: a histopathologic study of 39 cases with emphasis on unusual histological patterns. *Am J Surg Pathol.* 1998a;**22**:1303–13.
- Ordóñez NG. Desmoplastic small round cell tumor: II: an ultrastructural and immunohistochemical study with emphasis on new immunohistochemical markers. *Am J Surg Pathol.* 1998b;**22**:1314–27.
- Ordóñez NG, Zirkin R, Bloom RE. Malignant small-cell epithelial tumor of the peritoneum coexpressing mesenchymal-type intermediate filaments. *Am J Surg Pathol.* 1989;**3**:413–21.
- Parkash V, Gerald WL, Parma A, Miettinen M, Rosai J. Desmoplastic small round cell tumor of the pleura. *Am J Surg Pathol.* 1995;**19**:659–65.
- Rachfal AW, Luquette MH, Brigstock DR. Expression of connective tissue growth factor (CCN2) in desmoplastic small round cell tumour. *J Clin Pathol.* 2004;**57**:422–5.
- Sawyer JR, Tryka AF, Lewis JM. A novel reciprocal chromosome translocation t(11;22)(p13;q12) in an intraabdominal desmoplastic small round-cell tumor. *Am J Surg Pathol.* 1992;**16**:411–16.
- Tison V, Cerasoli S, Morigi F, et al. Intracranial desmoplastic small-cell tumor. Report of a case. *Am J Surg Pathol.* 1996;**20**:112–17.
- Trupiano JK, Machen SK, Barr FG, Goldblum JR. Cytokeratin-negative desmoplastic small round cell tumor: a report of two cases emphasizing the utility of reverse transcriptase-polymerase chain reaction. *Mod Pathol.* 1999;**12**:849–53.
- Variend S, Gerrard M, Norris PD, Goepel JR. Intra-abdominal neuroectodermal tumour of childhood with divergent differentiation. *Histopathology.* 1991;**18**:45–51.
- Wang LL, Perlman EJ, Vujanic GM, et al. Desmoplastic small round cell tumor of the kidney in childhood. *Am J Surg Pathol.* 2007;**31**:576–84.

## Alveolar Rhabdomyosarcoma

- Arnold MA, Anderson JR, Gastier-Foster JM, et al. Histology, fusion status, and outcome in alveolar rhabdomyosarcoma with low-risk clinical features: a report from the Children's Oncology Group. *Pediatr Blood Cancer.* 2016;**63**:634–9.

- Bahrami A, Gown AM, Baird GS, Hicks MJ, Folpe AL. Aberrant expression of epithelial and neuroendocrine markers in alveolar rhabdomyosarcoma: a potentially serious diagnostic pitfall. *Mod Pathol.* 2008;**21**:795–806.

- Barr FG, Galili N, Holick J, et al. Rearrangement of the PAX3 paired box gene in the paediatric solid tumour alveolar rhabdomyosarcoma. *Nat Genet.* 1993;**3**:113–17.

- Callender TA, Weber RS, Janjan N, et al. Rhabdomyosarcoma of the nose and paranasal sinuses in adults and children. *Otolaryngol Head Neck Surg.* 1995;**112**: 252–7.

- Davicioni E, Anderson MJ, Finckenstein FG, et al. Molecular classification of rhabdomyosarcoma– genotypic and phenotypic determinants of diagnosis: a report from the Children's Oncology Group. *Am J Pathol.* 2009;**174**:550–64.

- Douglass EC, Shapiro DN, Valentine M, et al. Alveolar rhabdomyosarcoma with the t(2;13): cytogenetic findings and clinicopathologic correlations. *Med Pediatr Oncol.* 1993;**21**:83–7.

- Enterline HT, Horn RC Jr. Alveolar rhabdomyosarcoma; a distinctive tumor type. *Am J Clin Pathol.* 1958;**29**:356–66.

- Enzinger FM, Shiraki M. Alveolar rhabdomyosarcoma. An analysis of 110 cases. *Cancer.* 1969;**24**:18–31.

- Harms D. Alveolar rhabdomyosarcoma: a prognostically unfavorable rhabdomyosarcoma type and its necessary distinction from embryonal rhabdomyosarcoma. *Curr Top Pathol.* 1995;**89**:273–96.

- Kubo T, Shimose S, Fujimori J, Furuta T, Ochi M. Prognostic value of PAX3/7-FOXO1 fusion status in alveolar rhabdomyosarcoma: systematic review and meta-analysis. *Crit Rev Oncol Hematol.* 2015;**96**:46–53.

- Leroy X, Petit ML, Fayoux P, Aubert S, Escande F. Aberrant diffuse expression of synaptophysin in a sinonasal alveolar rhabdomyosarcoma. *Pathology.* 2007;**39**: 275–6.

- Newton WA Jr, Gehan EA, Webber BL, et al. Classification of rhabdomyosarcomas and related sarcomas. Pathologic aspects and proposal for a new classification – an Intergroup Rhabdomyosarcoma Study. *Cancer.* 1995;**76**:1073–85.

- Parham DM, Qualman SJ, Teot L, et al; Soft Tissue Sarcoma Committee of the Children's Oncology Group. Correlation between histology and PAX/FKHR fusion status in alveolar rhabdomyosarcoma: a report from the Children's Oncology Group. *Am J Surg Pathol.* 2007;**31**:895–901.

- Perel Y, Ansoborlo S, Bernard P, Rivel J, Micheau M. Alveolar rhabdomyosarcoma presenting as leukemia. *J Pediatr Hematol Oncol.* 1998;**20**:94.

- Reid MM, Saunders PW, Bown N, et al. Alveolar rhabdomyosarcoma infiltrating bone marrow at presentation: the value to diagnosis of bone marrow trephine biopsy specimens. *J Clin Pathol.* 1992;**45**: 759–62.

- Rudzinski ER, Anderson JR, Chi YY, et al. Histology, fusion status, and outcome in metastatic rhabdomyosarcoma: A report from the Children's Oncology Group. *Pediatr Blood Cancer.* 2017 **64**(12).

- Rudzinski ER, Anderson JR, Hawkins DS, et al. The World Health Organization Classification of Skeletal Muscle Tumors in Pediatric Rhabdomyosarcoma: a report from the Children's Oncology Group. *Arch Pathol Lab Med.* 2015;**139**:1281–7.

- Rudzinski ER, Teot LA, Anderson JR, et al. Dense pattern of embryonal rhabdomyosarcoma, a lesion easily confused with alveolar rhabdomyosarcoma: a report from the Soft Tissue Sarcoma Committee of the Children's Oncology Group. *Am J Clin Pathol.* 2013;**140**:82–90.

- Sorensen PH, Lynch JC, Qualman SJ, et al. PAX3-FKHR and PAX7-FKHR gene fusions are prognostic indicators in alveolar rhabdomyosarcoma: a report from the children's oncology group. *J Clin Oncol.* 2002;**20**:2672–9.

- Stegmaier S, Poremba C, Schaefer KL, et al. Prognostic value of PAX-FKHR fusion status in alveolar rhabdomyosarcoma: a report from the cooperative soft tissue sarcoma study group (CWS). *Pediatr Blood Cancer.* 2011;**57**:406–14.

- Thompson LDR, Jo VY, Agaimy A, et al. Sinonasal tract alveolar rhabdomyosarcoma in adults: a clinicopathologic and immunophenotypic study of fifty-two cases with emphasis on epithelial immunoreactivity. *Head Neck Pathol.* 2017;1–12. [Epub ahead of print]

- Turc-Carel C, Lizard-Nacol S, Justrabo E, et al. Consistent chromosomal translocation in alveolar rhabdomyosarcoma. *Cancer Genet Cytogenet.* 1986;**19**:361–2.

- Yasuda T, Perry KD, Nelson M, et al. Alveolar rhabdomyosarcoma of the head and neck region in older adults: genetic characterization and a review of the literature. *Hum Pathol.* 2009;**40**:341–8.

## Poorly Differentiated Round Cell Synovial Sarcoma

- de Silva MV, McMahon AD, Paterson L, Reid R. Identification of poorly differentiated synovial sarcoma: a comparison of clinicopathological and cytogenetic features with those of typical synovial sarcoma. *Histopathology.* 2003;**43**:220–30.

- Fisher C. Synovial sarcoma. *Ann Diagn Pathol.* 1998;**2**:401–21.

- Fligman I, Lonardo F, Jhanwar SC, et al. Molecular diagnosis of synovial sarcoma and characterization of a variant SYT-SSX2 fusion transcript. *Am J Pathol.* 1995;**147**:1592–9.

- Folpe AL, Schmidt RA, Chapman D, Gown AM. Poorly differentiated synovial sarcoma: immunohistochemical distinction from primitive neuroectodermal tumors and high-grade malignant peripheral nerve sheath tumors. *Am J Surg Pathol.* 1998;**22**: 673–82.

- Guillou L, Benhattar J, Bonichon F, et al. Histologic grade, but not SYT-SSX fusion type, is an important prognostic factor in patients with synovial sarcoma: a multicenter, retrospective analysis. *J Clin Oncol.* 2004;**22**:4040–50.

- Machen SK, Easley KA, Goldblum JR. Synovial sarcoma of the extremities: a clinicopathologic study of 34 cases, including semi-quantitative analysis of spindled, epithelial, and poorly differentiated areas. *Am J Surg Pathol.* 1999;**23**:268–75.

- Pelmus M, Guillou L, Hostein I, et al. Monophasic fibrous and poorly differentiated synovial sarcoma: immunohistochemical reassessment of 60 t(X;18)(SYT-SSX)-positive cases. *Am J Surg Pathol.* 2002;**26**:1434–40.

- van de Rijn M, Barr FG, Xiong QB, et al. Poorly differentiated synovial sarcoma: an analysis of clinical, pathologic, and molecular genetic features. *Am J Surg Pathol.* 1999;**23**:106–12.

## High-Grade "Round Cell" Myxoid Liposarcoma

- Antonescu CR, Tschernyavsky SJ, Decuseara R, et al. Prognostic impact of P53 status, TLS-CHOP fusion transcript structure, and histological grade in myxoid liposarcoma: a molecular and clinicopathologic study of 82 cases. *Clin Cancer Res*. 2001;7:3977–87.

- Dei Tos AP, Wadden C, Fletcher CDM. S-100 protein staining in liposarcoma. Its diagnostic utility in the high grade myxoid (round cell) variant. *Appl Immunohistochem*. 1996;4:95–101.
- de Vreeze RS, de Jong D, Tielen IH, et al. Primary retroperitoneal myxoid/round cell liposarcoma is a nonexisting disease: an immunohistochemical and molecular biological analysis. *Mod Pathol*. 2009;22: 223–31.
- Hoffman A, Ghadimi MP, Demicco EG, et al. Localized and metastatic myxoid/round cell liposarcoma: clinical and molecular observations. *Cancer*. 2013;119:1868–77.
- Kilpatrick SE, Doyon J, Choong PF, Sim FH, Nascimento AG. The clinicopathologic spectrum of myxoid and round cell liposarcoma. A study of 95 cases. *Cancer*. 1996;77: 1450–8.
- Knight JC, Renwick PJ, Dal Cin P, Van den Berghe H, Fletcher CD. Translocation t(12;16)(q13;p11) in myxoid liposarcoma and round cell liposarcoma: molecular and cytogenetic analysis. *Cancer Res*. 1995;55:24–7.
- Orvieto E, Furlanetto A, Laurino L, Dei Tos AP. Myxoid and round cell liposarcoma: a spectrum of myxoid adipocytic neoplasia. *Semin Diagn Pathol*. 2001;18:267–73.
- Smith TA, Easley KA, Goldblum JR. Myxoid/round cell liposarcoma of the extremities. A clinicopathologic study of 29 cases with particular attention to extent of round cell liposarcoma. *Am J Surg Pathol*. 1996;20:171–80.
- Tallini G, Akerman M, Dal Cin P, et al. Combined morphologic and karyotypic study of 28 myxoid liposarcomas. Implications for a revised morphologic typing, (a report from the CHAMP Group). *Am J Surg Pathol*. 1996;20: 1047–55.

# Pleomorphic Sarcomas

Angelo Paolo Dei Tos MD

## Introduction

During the past two decades, the classification of pleomorphic sarcomas has evolved significantly. In fact, from 1980 until early 2000, so-called pleomorphic and storiform malignant fibrous histiocytoma (MFH) represented the most frequently diagnosed sarcoma, accounting for approximately 40% of adult mesenchymal malignancies. The 2002 WHO classification of soft tissue tumors clearly indicated that MFH, at best, represented a synonym for undifferentiated pleomorphic sarcomas, denying the status of distinct clinicopathologic entity. In 2013, the latest WHO classification formally declared the extinction of MFH. However, the consensus achieved in the context of the new WHO classification of soft tissue tumors represents only the final step in a long conceptual evolution.

Historically, Ozzello, O'Brien, and Stout introduced the term malignant fibrous histiocytoma in the medical literature in the early 1960s. These authors, who are among the founders of modern surgical pathology, were impressed by the acquisition of phagocytic properties observed in cultured fibroblasts. Therefore, based on the combination of morphology and tissue culture analysis, they suggested that this group of soft tissue sarcomas, showing a pleomorphic phenotype and a storiform or cartwheel-like growth pattern, would be derived from histiocytes. As a result, the findings generated by an "ancillary technique" overcame the observations of conventional morphology, leading to the creation of a novel nosologic category. The existence of MFH as a well-defined clinicopathologic entity rapidly became very popular and, by the mid 1980s, pleomorphic and storiform MFH represented the most common sarcoma in adults. However, in the same way that an ancillary technique somewhat created MFH, ancillary techniques significantly contributed to its demolition. In fact, with the advent of electron microscopy, immunohistochemistry, and molecular genetics, it became clear that the so-called facultative fibroblast theory had no scientific grounds. In 1992, a milestone paper written by Christopher Fletcher eventually brought attention to the concept that MFH merely represented a morphologic pattern shared by a wide variety of poorly differentiated malignant neoplasms. This careful analysis of a series of 159 "MFHs" retrieved from the files of St. Thomas Hospital in London demonstrated that 63% of the cases could be reclassified (with the support of immunohistochemistry and/or electron microscopy) as specific types of pleomorphic sarcoma and 12.6% as non-mesenchymal malignancies (primarily melanomas, sarcomatoid carcinomas, and lymphomas). Of the 42 cases (approximately half of which consisted of small biopsies) with no demonstrable line of differentiation, only a small fraction (13%

of the total) was morphologically compatible with the MFH "category." Over 25 years after its creation, pleomorphic MFH appears to be a heterogeneous group of unrelated lesions. Such a reappraisal generated a sharp debate. However, even the most recent gene-profiling studies have further confirmed the validity of this conceptual shift, since MFHs do not form a discrete cluster.

The main discussion today, over 20 years since that publication, focuses on whether accurate subclassification of pleomorphic sarcomas is worthwhile or not from the prognostic and therapeutic points of view. First, separation of true sarcomas from carcinomas, melanomas, and lymphomas showing sarcomatoid, pleomorphic morphology is of paramount importance if the difference in prognosis and, more important, in therapy is considered. At present, such differential diagnoses are based mainly on an accurate and careful histopathologic examination, accompanied by an immunohistochemical workup that includes a panel of differentiation markers. Second, it has also become evident that the presence of myogenic differentiation among high-grade pleomorphic sarcomas identifies a group of tumors characterized by particularly poor prognosis. This finding has been further confirmed by other studies, underlining beyond any doubt the clinical relevance of pleomorphic sarcoma histotyping. During the past decade, primarily as a consequence of more accurate phenotyping, the percentage of pleomorphic, unclassifiable sarcomas that would fit in the former category of MFH has dropped dramatically. And in fact, with the disappearing of the prototypical storiform-pleomorphic form of MFH, its progeny has also undergone a profound nosologic reappraisal. Myxoid MFH has now been renamed "myxofibrosarcoma" to underline the fibroblastic line of differentiation of this neoplasm. Inflammatory MFH is now regarded as an inflammatory variant of well-differentiated /dedifferentiated liposarcoma. As anticipated in 1971 by Salm and Sissons, giant cell MFH represents a wastebasket category, which includes specific sarcoma types, such as leiomyosarcoma with osteoclastic giant cells, giant cell tumor of soft tissue, and examples of extraskeletal osteosarcoma. Angiomatoid MFH (the most recently coined variant) is no longer considered a malignant neoplasm, it harbors a specific genetic anomaly, and, as the ultimate line of differentiation remains to be elucidated, it is currently listed among the neoplasms of uncertain differentiation.

This chapter focuses on high-grade sarcomas featuring constitutively pleomorphic morphology and on pleomorphic variants of sarcomas. The integration of morphologic, immunohistochemical (Table 7.1), and molecular features will be discussed. We also consider those lesions that, despite showing significant pleomorphism, tend to exhibit a distinctively indolent clinical behavior.

**Table 7.1** Immunohistochemical features of pleomorphic sarcomas

| | Smooth muscle actin | Desmin | h-Caldesmon | Myogenin | MDM2 | S100 | CD34 | Pankeratin | SATB2 |
|---|---|---|---|---|---|---|---|---|---|
| Pleomorphic rhabdomyosarcoma | <5% focal | > 95% | – | 100% focal | – | <10% | – | – | – |
| Pleomorphic leiomyosarcoma | 70% | 70% | 90% | – | – | – | – | 10% | – |
| Pleomorphic liposarcoma | – | – | – | – | – | 30% | – | – | – |
| Dedifferentiated liposarcoma | 50% focal | 10% | 15% | 2% | 100% | – | – | – | – |
| Extraskeletal osteosarcoma | – | – | – | – | – | focally + if chondroblastic | – | – | 95% |
| Pleomorphic myxofibrosarcoma | 40% focal | – | – | – | – | – | 30% focal | – | – |
| Pleomorphic MPNST | – | – focally + in MTT | – | – focally + in MTT | – | 30% focal | – | – | – |
| PHAT | – | – | – | – | – | – | 50% | – | – |
| AFX | 40% focal | – | – | – | – | – | – | – | – |
| UPS | Focal | – | – | – | – | – | – | – | – |

**Legends:**

AFX: Atypical fibroxanthoma

MPNST: Malignant peripheral nerve sheath tumor

MTT: Malignant triton tumor

PHAT: Pleomorphic hyalinizing angiectatic tumor

UPS: Undifferentiated pleomorphic sarcoma

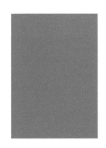

# Pleomorphic Rhabdomyosarcoma

## Definition and Epidemiology

Pleomorphic rhabdomyosarcoma (P-RMS) is a high-grade sarcoma showing evidence of skeletal muscle differentiation. No embryonal or alveolar component should be identified. Pleomorphic rhabdomyosarcoma is very rare, accounting for less than 5% of all RMS. Peak incidence of P-RMS is in the sixth decade, whereas it is extremely rare in childhood; the vast majority of sarcomas displaying features of pleomorphic RMS in children actually represents examples of embryonal RMS with anaplastic features, and true P-RMS should be regarded as exceptional.

## Clinical Presentation and Outcome

Pleomorphic rhabdomyosarcoma occurs almost exclusively in the deep soft tissue of the lower limbs; however, it has also been reported in other locations, such as the chest wall, upper extremites, pelvis, and retroperitoneum. Treatment is a combination of chemotherapy, surgery, and radiotherapy. Metastases are most commonly observed in the lungs. Prognosis is poor for both localized and metastatic disease, with an overall survival at 5 years of approximately 30%. A high relapse rate and a poor and short-lived response to standard chemotherapy is most often observed.

## Morphology and Immunophenotype

Grossly, P-RMS represents a well-circumscribed, often large (usually ranging between 10 and 30 cm) mass. The cut surface is red-gray and firm, with variable areas of hemorrhage and necrosis (Fig. 7-1).

Microscopically, pleomorphic RMS is composed of an admixture of round to spindle cells and polygonal cells organized in a very variable growth pattern that is most often solid (Fig. 7-2), but can be fascicular (Fig. 7-3), rarely storiform, and hemangiopericytoma-like. Necrosis is generally abundant (Fig. 7-4), and inflammatory infiltrates are frequently observed. In some cases, myxoid change of the

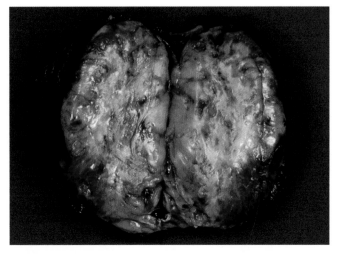

**Fig. 7-1.** Pleomorphic rhabdomyosarcoma. Gross specimen exhibits well-circumscribed borders, abundant necrosis, and hemorrhagic foci.

stroma can be detected (Fig. 7-5). The presence of large polygonal, spindle, tadpole, and racquet-like cells featuring abundant, deeply eosinophilic cytoplasm represents one of the most useful diagnostic clues (Figs. 7-6 and 7-7). Contrary to common belief, cross striations represent an extremely rare finding. Immunohistochemically, the majority of tumor cells express desmin (Fig. 7-8), whereas myogenin expression is most often limited to a few neoplastic cells (Fig. 7-9). As myogenin represents a nuclear transcription factor, only nuclear staining need be considered, and cytoplasmic positivity should be disregarded. Interestingly, most cases tend to be negative for both smooth muscle actin (overall, less than 5% RMS are smooth muscle actin positive) and h-caldesmon.

## Genetics

Pleomorphic rhabdomyosarcoma shows highly complex karyotypes with numerical and unbalanced structural changes.

365

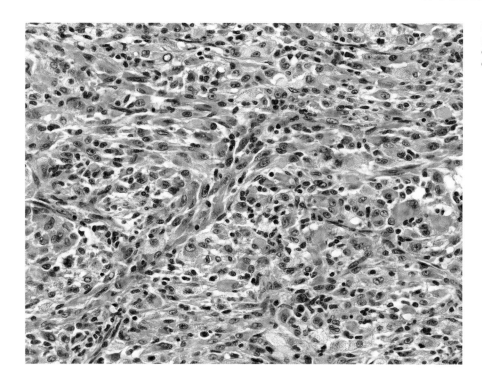

**Fig. 7-2.** Pleomorphic rhabdomyosarcoma. A solid proliferation of spindle, polygonal, and pleomorphic cells is seen. Neoplastic cells feature abundant eosinophilic cytoplasm.

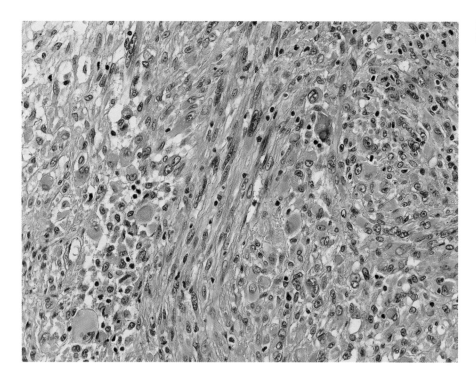

**Fig. 7-3.** Pleomorphic rhabdomyosarcoma. Neoplastic cells can focally arrange in fascicles.

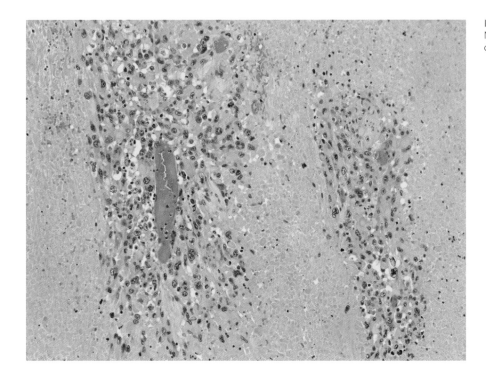

**Fig. 7-4.** Pleomorphic rhabdomyosarcoma. Necrosis tends to be abundant. Viable neoplastic cells are seen around blood vessels.

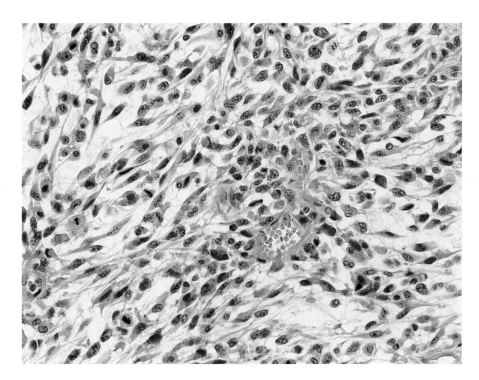

**Fig. 7-5.** Pleomorphic rhabdomyosarcoma. Myxoid change of the stroma can be observed. Neoplastic cells maintain the typical nuclear pleomorphism and cytoplasmic eosinophilia.

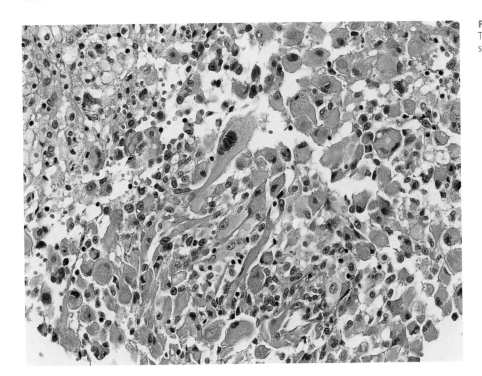

**Fig. 7-6.** Pleomorphic rhabdomyosarcoma. The tumor is composed of eosinophilic polygonal, spindle, tadpole, and racquet-like neoplastic cells.

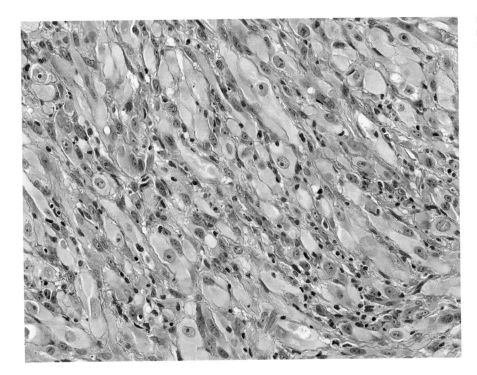

**Fig. 7-7.** Pleomorphic rhabdomyosarcoma. Rarely, neoplastic cells somewhat mimic normal striated muscle cells.

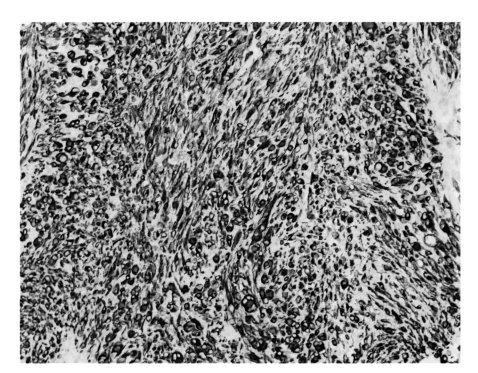

**Fig. 7-8.** Pleomorphic rhabdomyosarcoma. Diffuse desmin immunopositivity is most often seen.

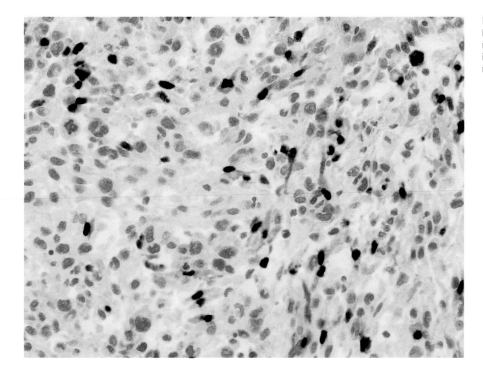

**Fig. 7-9.** Pleomorphic rhabdomyosarcoma. In contrast to what is observed in alveolar rhabdomyosarcoma, myogenin nuclear immunoreactivity is generally seen in a minority of neoplastic cells.

## Differential Diagnosis and Diagnostic Pitfalls

Differential diagnosis includes all other pleomorphic sarcoma subtypes. Distinction from pleomorphic leiomyosarcoma (LMS) is particularly challenging, even if clinically not that relevant. Morphologically, neoplastic cells in pleomorphic RMS tend to exhibit more striking cytoplasmic eosinophilia and more extreme variation in cell size than pleomorphic LMS. Conversely, the presence of better-differentiated areas composed of fascicles of spindle cells featuring fibrillary

eosinophilic cytoplasm represent a useful diagnostic clue in favor of LMS. As mentioned, there exists a trend for pleomorphic RMS to display a desmin +/SMA– phenotype, but occasional exceptions can be detected. Immunoreactivity for h-caldesmon is preferentially seen in LMS. The demonstration of nuclear positivity for myogenin is currently accepted as an unquestionable demonstration of rhabdomyoblastic differentiation. It has to be underlined that, in contrast to what is usually observed in alveolar RMS (and to a lesser extent in embryonal rhabdomyosarcoma), myogenin positivity is most

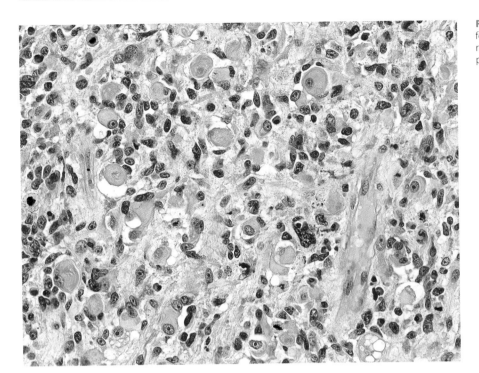

**Fig. 7-10.** Carcinosarcoma. Polygonal cells featuring abundant eosinophilic cytoplasm represent rhabdomyoblastic differentiation in this pelvic recurrence of uterine carcinosarcoma.

often (but not always) limited to a small fraction of neoplastic cells. Importantly, when interpreting myogenin immunostains, a major diagnostic pitfall is represented by the presence of residual non-neoplastic striated muscle cells.

It has to be remembered that heterologous striated muscle differentiation is rarely observed in other high-grade neoplasms, in particular malignant peripheral nerve sheath tumors (so-called malignant triton tumor), and in a small fraction of dedifferentiated liposarcomas. Malignant peripheral nerve sheath tumor (MPNST) is discussed in detail in Chapter 4; however, as emphasized later, MPNST very rarely features a pleomorphic morphology. Importantly, diffuse MDM2-positive immunoreactivity and/or *MDM2* gene amplification is never seen on pleomorphic RMS, whereas it represents a consistent finding in dedifferentiated liposarcoma.

When dealing with abdominal masses arising in female patients, it is important to remember that a rhabdomyoblastic component is frequently observed in both adenosarcoma and carcinosarcoma (malignant mixed mullerian tumor) of both uterus and ovary. In carcinosarcomas, often the carcinomatous component can be minimal and therefore easily overlooked, leading to an erroneous diagnosis of rhabdomyosarcoma (Fig. 7-10). Before making a diagnosis of primary rhabdomyosarcoma of the uterus, careful examination of the clinical history as well as use of epithelial differentiation markers on different blocks are strongly advised. Extrarenal rhabdoid tumor (ERT) also enters the differential diagnosis; however, ERT arises exclusively in the pediatric age-group, and immunophenotypically it is myogenin negative and typically exhibits loss of nuclear expression of INI1.

**Key Points in Pleomorphic Rhabdomyosarcoma Diagnosis**

- Occurrence in the limbs of adults and elderly patients
- Presence of intense cytoplasmic eosinophilia
- Expression of desmin and myogenin
- Expression of myogenin always multifocal
- Aggressive clinical behavior

# Pleomorphic Liposarcoma

## Definition and Epidemiology

Pleomorphic liposarcoma (P-LPS) is a high-grade pleomorphic sarcoma showing histologic evidence of adipocytic differentiation represented by the presence of a variable number of pleomorphic lipoblasts. It represents the most rare variant of liposarcoma, accounting for no more than 5% of all lipogenic malignancies. Pleomorphic liposarcoma occurs in patients usually in or after the sixth decade of life, with slight male predominance.

## Clinical Presentation and Behavior

Pleomorphic liposarcoma occurs predominantly in the lower limbs, particularly the thigh, followed by the upper extremities and the retroperitoneum. It is a high-grade sarcoma associated with relatively poor survival rates. The metastatic rate is between 30 and 50% (occurring most often in the lungs), and overall mortality ranges between 40 and 50%. Interestingly, tumor grade according to the French Federation of Cancer Centers Sarcoma Group (FNCLCC) system (grade 2 versus grade 3) does not seem to affect prognosis. Rare cases of P-LPS have also been reported in the skin; however, in these rare cases the clinical outcome appears largely benign, complete removal being usually curative.

## Morphology and Immunohistochemistry

Grossly, pleomorphic liposarcoma most often presents as a large, fleshy mass featuring necrotic areas (Fig. 7-11).

The main diagnostic clue to defining adipocytic differentiation in a pleomorphic sarcoma is the presence of pleomorphic lipoblasts, and their identification often requires careful histopathologic examination of an optimally sampled neoplasm. Lipoblasts show irregular, hyperchromatic, scalloped nuclei, and prominent nucleoli set in a multivacuolated, abundant cytoplasm (Fig. 7-12). Most cases tend to fit into one of four main morphologic subsets: (1) Approximately two-thirds are represented by a non-distinctive, high-grade pleomorphic/spindle cell sarcoma with scattered lipoblasts or sheets of lipoblasts (Fig. 7-13). (2) As discussed in more detail in Chapter 5, in less than one-third of cases a high-grade pleomorphic sarcoma with predominantly epithelioid cell population and scattered lipoblasts is seen (Fig. 7-14). (3) A smaller group of cases overlaps morphologically with intermediate to high-grade myxofibrosarcoma, except for the presence of

lipoblasts (Figs. 7-15 and 7-16). (4) Even more rarely, pleomorphic liposarcoma is composed entirely of pleomorphic, multivacuolated lipoblasts (Fig. 7-17). These neoplasms are usually rich in mitotic figures, primarily atypical, and necrosis can be extensive (Fig. 7-18).

An extremely important diagnostic clue (particularly useful when lipoblasts are scanty) is represented by the presence of extreme nuclear atypia. In this context, nuclear pseudoinclusions and multinucleation represent relatively frequent findings (Fig. 7-19). These morphologic features should always prompt a careful search of lipogenic features that may require extensive sampling of the tumor.

As mentioned, the diagnosis of pleomorphic liposarcoma primarily relies upon the identification of lipoblasts; as a consequence, immunohistochemistry plays a minor role. However, in those cases in which few lipoblasts are present, S100 protein may at times prove helpful in highlighting their presence.

## Molecular Genetics

Pleomorphic liposarcoma always exhibits complex karyotypes. Loss of the *RB1* gene, as well as mutations of *TP53* and *NF1* genes, has been reported. Importantly (in contrast to well-differentiated/dedifferentiated liposarcoma), amplification of *MDM2/CDK4* genes is generally not observed.

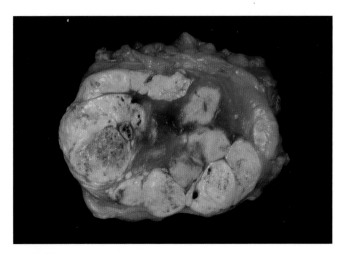

**Fig. 7-11.** Pleomorphic liposarcoma. Gross specimen showing fleshy areas, abundant necrosis, and areas of myxoid degeneration.

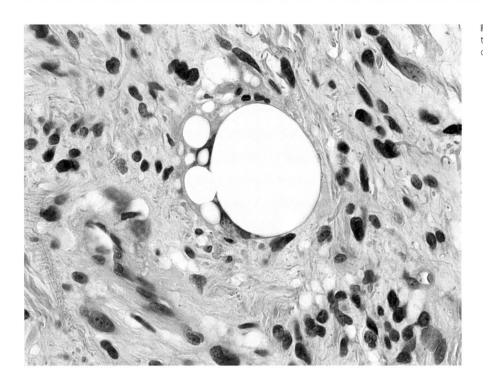

**Fig. 7-12.** Pleomorphic liposarcoma. Lipoblasts typically feature hyperchromatic nuclei indented by cytoplasmic vacuoles.

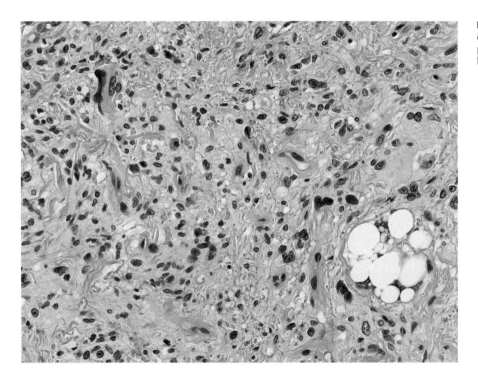

**Fig. 7-13.** Pleomorphic liposarcoma. The tumor is composed of a high-grade pleomorphic cell proliferation containing scattered pleomorphic lipoblasts.

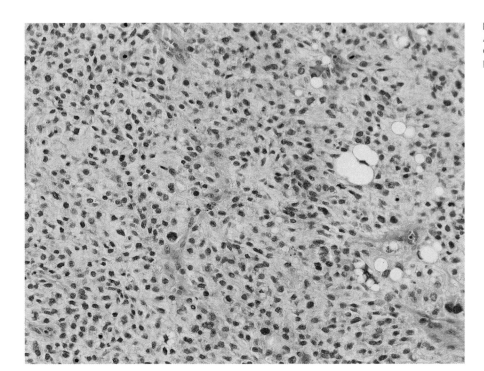

**Fig. 7-14.** Pleomorphic liposarcoma. Approximately one-third of cases exhibit an epithelioid cell population associated with pleomorphic lipoblasts.

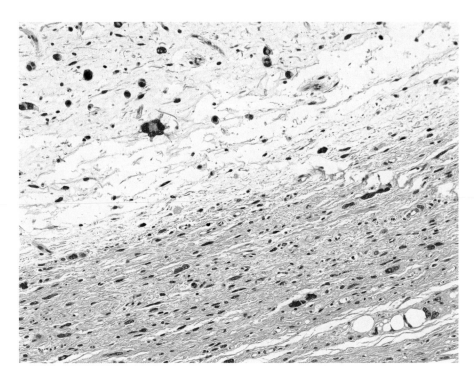

**Fig. 7-15.** Pleomorphic liposarcoma. Myxofibrosarcoma-like areas can predominate. The detection of lipoblasts represents the key diagnostic clue.

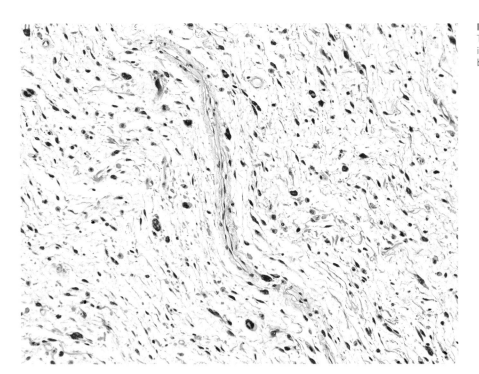

**Fig. 7-16.** Pleomorphic liposarcoma. The morphologic overlap with myxofibrosarcoma includes the presence of capillary-sized, archiform blood vessels.

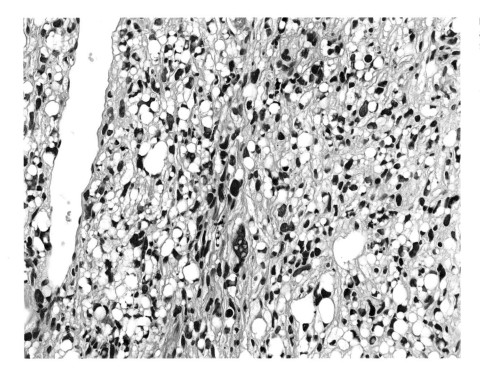

**Fig. 7-17.** Pleomorphic liposarcoma. Rarely, a diffuse proliferation of pleomorphic lipoblasts is seen.

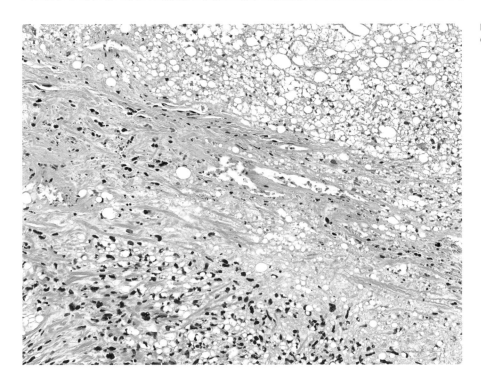

**Fig. 7-18.** Pleomorphic liposarcoma. The presence of necrosis represents a relatively common finding.

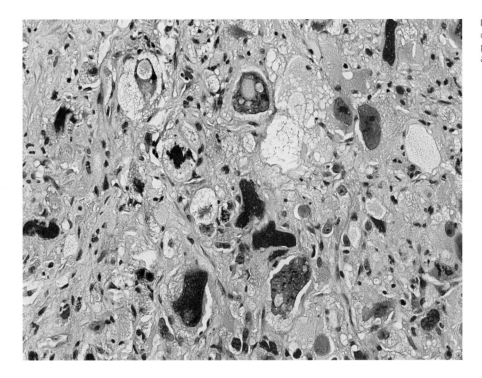

**Fig. 7-19.** Pleomorphic liposarcoma. The presence of extreme cytologic atypia is very typical of pleomorphic liposarcoma and should prompt a search for lipoblasts.

## Differential Diagnosis and Diagnostic Pitfalls

When pleomorphic liposarcoma occurs in the retroperitoneum, the most relevant differential diagnosis is with dedifferentiated liposarcoma, particularly with the so-called homologous lipogenic variant. The absence in pleomorphic liposarcoma of MDM2 expression and/or amplification represents the key diagnostic clue.

Extensive myxoid change can be observed in P-LPS, causing potential diagnostic confusion with both myxofibrosarcoma and myxoid liposarcoma. Myxofibrosarcoma is most often superficial and multinodular and never features the presence of lipoblasts. A potential pitfall is represented by pseudolipoblasts (mucin-laden neoplastic cells) that, however, most often lack the typical punched-out nuclear morphology of true lipoblasts. Myxoid liposarcoma never exhibits nuclear pleomorphism (a feature that should always lead to reconsidering such a diagnosis), lipoblasts are most often mononucleated, and a distinctive rearrangement of the *DDIT3* gene that fuses with

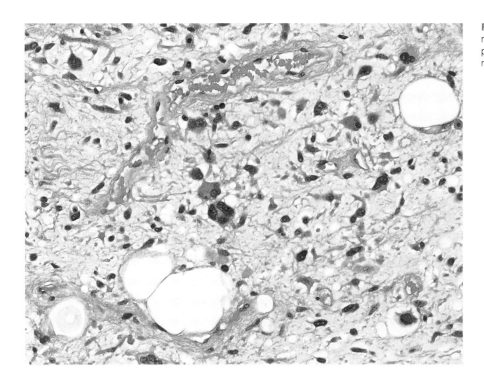

Fig. 7-20. Pleomorphic lipoma. Florette-like multinucleated cells are seen, featuring significant pleomorphism. Lipoblasts can be seen and should not lead to a diagnosis of malignancy.

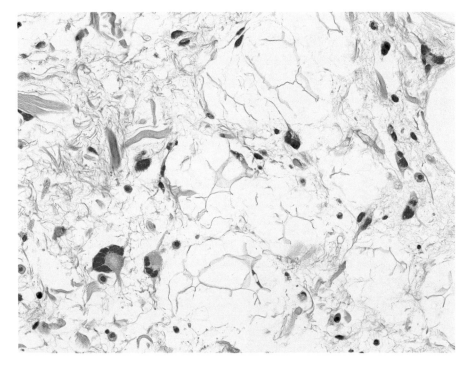

Fig. 7-21. Pleomorphic lipoma. The presence of coarse eosinophilic collagen fibers represents an important diagnostic clue.

the *FUS* gene or, more rarely, with the *EWSR1* gene is detected molecularly.

Another major diagnostic pitfall is represented by **pleomorphic lipoma**. Pleomorphic lipoma is a benign lipogenic lesion that represents a morphologic and genetic continuum with spindle cell lipoma. Pleomorphic lipoma (as spindle cell lipoma) primarily occurs in the head and neck of middle-aged patients. Microscopically, it is characterized by a spindle-cell proliferation admixed with a mature adipocytic component that may include lipoblasts, and associated with the

presence of distinctive multinucleated (florette-like) neoplastic cells (Fig. 7-20). Significant nuclear pleomorphism is only occasionally observed. Helpful diagnostic clues are represented by the presence of thick eosinophilic collagen bundles (Fig. 7-21) and the absence of significant mitotic activity. Immunohistochemically, pleomorphic lipoma exhibits CD34 immunopositivity and often shows loss of RB1 nuclear expression. Of course, both immunohistochemical findings need to be interpreted in context with morphology, as loss of RB1 can also be observed in pleomorphic liposarcoma. It has very recently

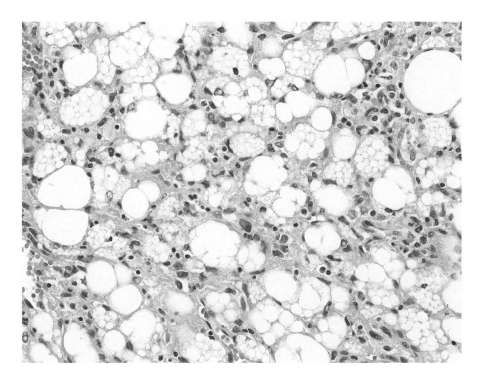

**Fig. 7-22.** Silicone granuloma. The presence of silicone-laden macrophages may mimic pleomorphic liposarcoma. The absence of nuclear pleomorphism should be noted.

been suggested that rarely pleomorphic lipoma exhibits greater cytologic atypia that can be associated with the presence of scattered mitotic figures. These lesions have been labeled as atypical pleomorphic lipomatous tumors and seem to be associated with a rather indolent clinical behavior.

A relatively well-known pseudosarcomatous simulator of pleomorphic liposarcoma is represented by granulomatous reactions to silicone implants (Fig. 7-22). Silicone-laden macrophages may closely mimic a "lipoblastic" proliferation and lead to an erroneous diagnosis of liposarcoma. An extremely helpful morphologic clue is represented by the absence of nuclear atypia that, by contrast, is invariably seen in pleomorphic liposarcoma.

It is our experience that pleomorphic liposarcoma is at times under-recognized and often placed within the "undifferentiated pleomorphic sarcoma ex-MFH" category. One reason is that pleomorphic lipoblasts may often be present only in minimal amounts and therefore are overlooked. Careful (and sometimes extensive) sampling is therefore mandatory.

| Key Points in Pleomorphic Liposarcoma Diagnosis |
| --- |
| • Occurrence in the limbs of adult patients |
| • High-grade pleomorphic sarcoma featuring variable amounts of pleomorphic lipoblasts |
| • Striking nuclear atypia |
| • Clinically aggressive neoplasm |

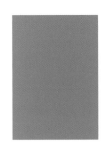

# Dedifferentiated Liposarcoma

## Definition and Epidemiology

Dedifferentiated liposarcoma (DDLPS) represents both a morphologically and biologically fascinating lesion, in which transition from well-differentiated (WD) liposarcoma to non-lipogenic (most often high-grade) sarcoma is observed. Evans first described dedifferentiated liposarcoma in 1979, co-opting this term from David Dahlin's description of tumor progression in chondrosarcoma. Since then, it has become clear that transition sometimes is not abrupt, that dedifferentiation can rarely feature a "low-grade" appearance and even be lipogenic in nature.

Dedifferentiation in WD liposarcoma tends to occur more frequently in the primary tumor (90%) but can also be observed in recurrences (10%). Peak incidence is in the sixth and seventh decades of life, and males are more frequently affected than females.

## Clinical Presentation and Outcome

The vast majority of DDLPS occurs in the retroperitoneum (including the paratesticular region) of adult patients. Approximately 10% of cases are seen in the limbs, in the mediastinum, the head and neck region, and (exceptionally) in the skin. When dealing with the retroperitoneal location, diagnosis tends to be delayed. Recent molecular data focusing on the genomic profile of pleomorphic sarcoma of the limbs would suggest the dedifferentiated liposarcoma at this location might be under-recognized.

The biologic behavior of DDLPS represents one of the most fascinating enigmas of tumor biology: (1) Despite high-grade morphology, and with the exception of cases showing rhabdomyoblastic differentiation, it tends to be less aggressive than other types of high-grade pleomorphic sarcomas occurring at the same location. (2) Dedifferentiated liposarcoma can recur as an entirely WD liposarcoma. (3) In contrast to WD liposarcoma, dedifferentiation is associated with a 15–20% metastatic rate. Long-term survival rates for retroperitoneal DDLPS certainly indicate a more accelerated course; however, mortality is related more to uncontrolled local recurrences than to metastatic spread. Contrary to common belief, recently published studies have shown that the application of the FNCLCC grading system may help to stratify DDLPS prognostically. Furthermore, the presence of myogenic differentiation (particularly when rhabdomyoblastic in type) appears to be associated with remarkably poorer prognosis. It has recently been suggested that high amplification levels of both MDM2 and CDK4 correlate with decreased disease-free survival.

Standard treatment of DDLPS is represented by wide surgical resection that, in its most common location represented by the retroperitoneum, should include adjacent viscera. This strategy is aimed at delaying the time to the first local recurrence and, it is hoped, prolonging overall survival. As multivisceral resection is associated with higher morbidity (an unnecessary risk when dealing with other pleomorphic sarcomas occurring in the retroperitoneum), accurate recognition of DDLPS represents a key step in clinical decision making.

## Morphology and Immunohistochemistry

Grossly, dedifferentiated liposarcoma usually presents as a multinodular mass with yellow cut surface, containing firm tan-gray areas. Sometimes a distinct firm nodule is seen in the context of adipose tissue (Fig. 7-23). Microscopically, the transition from well-differentiated liposarcoma to high-grade sarcoma tends to be abrupt (Fig. 7-24); however, cases exist in which this can be more gradual, and exceptionally low-grade and high-grade areas appear to be co-mingled (Figs. 7-25 and 7-26). Morphologically, dedifferentiated areas exhibit a remarkable histologic variability. Most often, morphologic

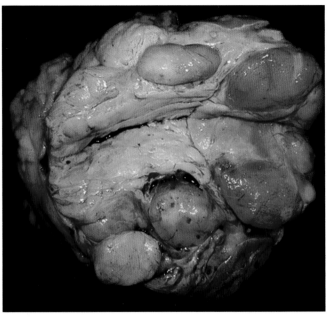

**Fig. 7-23.** Dedifferentiated liposarcoma. Most often, surgical specimens attain large size and feature a combination of adipocytic and fleshy features.

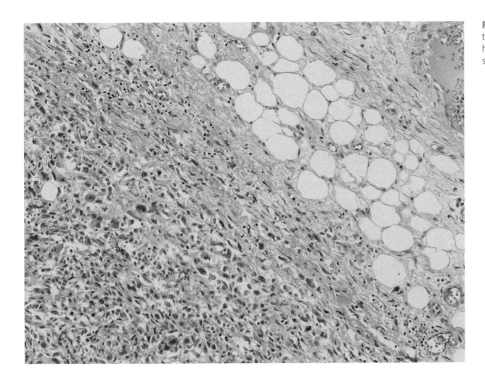

**Fig. 7-24.** Dedifferentiated liposarcoma. Abrupt transition from well-differentiated liposarcoma to high-grade, non-lipogenic sarcoma is most often seen.

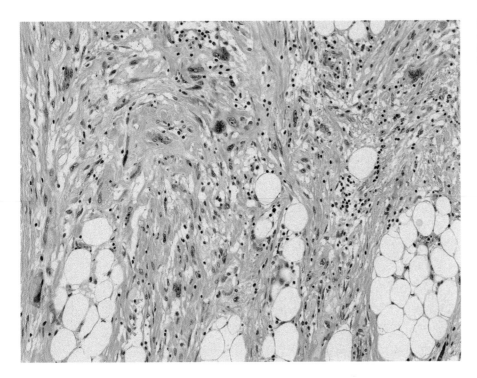

**Fig. 7-25.** Dedifferentiated liposarcoma. A spindle cell and pleomorphic component is intimately admixed with a well-differentiated lipogenic component.

overlap with undifferentiated pleomorphic sarcoma (Fig. 7-27) is seen, and less frequently high-grade, myxofibrosarcoma-like features are observed (Fig. 7-28). Often, the dedifferentiated component is composed of a hypercellular spindle cell proliferation lacking significant pleomorphism and exhibiting a distinctive storiform pattern of growth (Fig. 7-29). A relatively rare morphologic variation is represented by a dedifferentiated component featuring a primitive, undifferentiated, round cell (Fig. 7-30) or spindle cell (Fig. 7-31) appearance. Interestingly, DDLPS may exhibit the presence

of fascicles of bland spindle cells with a cellularity somewhat intermediate between WD sclerosing liposarcoma and the usual high-grade areas. "Low-grade dedifferentiation" is the term proposed to describe these areas and in part overlaps with the "cellular" variants of well-differentiated liposarcoma described by Evans (Fig. 7-32). Low-grade dedifferentiated areas can feature variable morphologies somewhat mimicking desmoid fibromatosis or solitary fibrous tumors (Fig. 7-33). Inflammatory myofibroblastic, tumor-like features have also been reported, and rarely morphologic overlap with

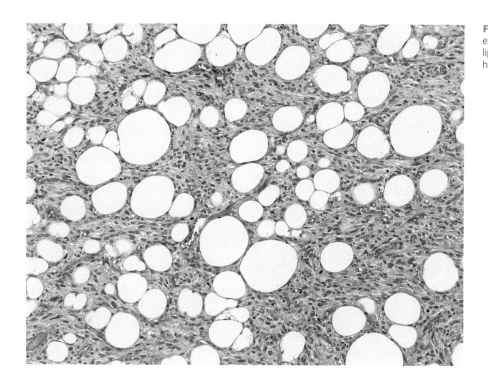

**Fig. 7-26.** Dedifferentiated liposarcoma. In this example of co-mingled dedifferentiated liposarcoma, the high-grade component is hypercellular but lacks significant pleomorphism.

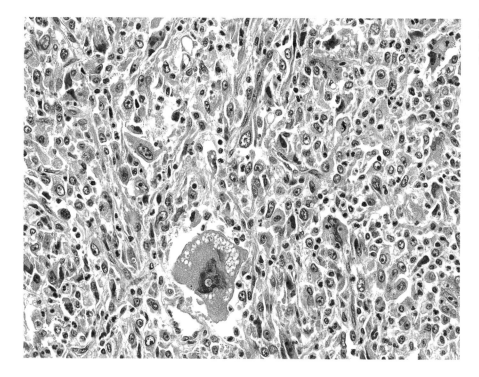

**Fig. 7-27.** Dedifferentiated liposarcoma. Most often, the non-lipogenic component overlaps morphologically with undifferentiated pleomorphic sarcoma.

gastrointestinal stromal tumors (GISTs) can be seen (Fig. 7-34). An additional fascinating morphologic feature is represented by heterologous differentiation that can be observed in about 5–10% of cases: Most often it is myogenic in type (leiomyosarcomatous or rhabdomyosarcomatous) (Fig. 7-35) or osteo/chondrosarcomatous (Fig. 7-36). A very peculiar morphologic presentation of DDLPS is represented by the presence of whorls of spindle cells somewhat reminiscent of neural or meningothelial structures (Fig. 7-37). This feature

is often associated with metaplastic bone formation and plasma cell infiltrates.

Importantly, contrary to common belief that dedifferentiation is always non-lipogenic, the dedifferentiated component may indeed exhibit lipogenic features overlapping morphologically with pleomorphic liposarcoma (Fig. 7-38). This morphologic presentation has been labeled "homologous dedifferentiation." Very rarely, an intense inflammatory infiltrate is observed to the extent that it may obscure the lipogenic

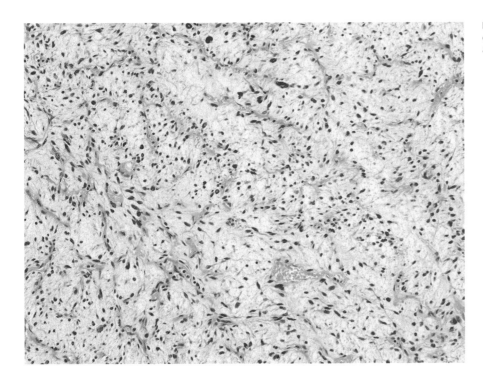

**Fig. 7-28.** Dedifferentiated liposarcoma. Often, the dedifferentiated component exhibits a myxofibrosarcoma-like appearance.

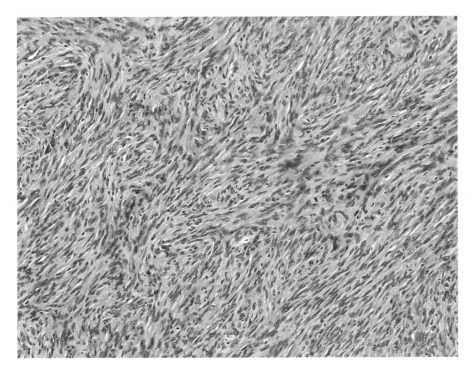

**Fig. 7-29.** Dedifferentiated liposarcoma. Sometimes a homogeneous, non-pleomorphic spindle cell proliferation organized in a "storiform" pattern of growth is seen.

nature of the neoplasm (Fig. 7-39). In the past, these cases have been regarded as inflammatory variants of malignant fibrous histiocytoma, but it is now broadly accepted (and genetically demonstrated) that they all represent examples of DDLPS.

The most relevant immunohistochemical feature is represented by the overexpression of MDM2 and CDK4 in both lipogenic and non-lipogenic components. When dealing with core biopsies of retroperitoneal pleomorphic mesenchymal neo-

plasm, the demonstration of MDM2 nuclear overexpression strongly supports the diagnosis of dedifferentiated liposarcoma (Fig. 7-40). In our experience, MDM2 immunohistochemistry exhibits high concordance with fluorescence in situ hybridization (FISH) analysis of *MDM2* gene status.

The presence of heterologous elements can be highlighted by use of appropriate differentiation markers. In particular, the combination of desmin/myogenin immunopositivity is

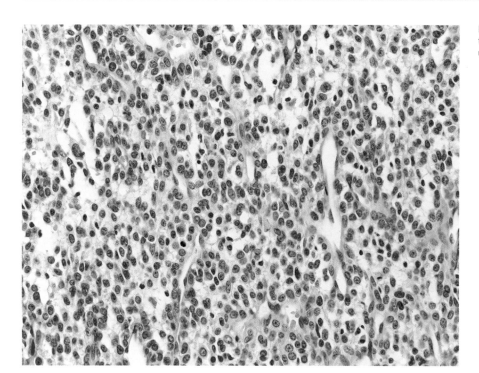

**Fig. 7-30.** Dedifferentiated liposarcoma. Rarely, the non-lipogenic component features an undifferentiated round cell morphology.

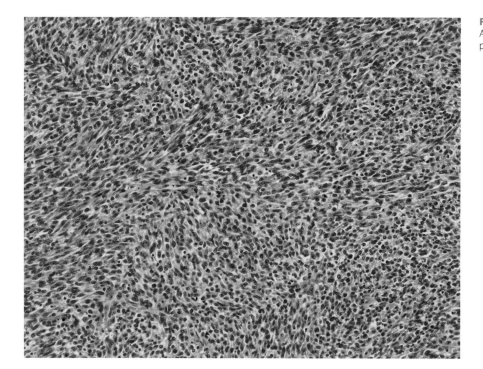

**Fig. 7-31.** Dedifferentiated liposarcoma. An undifferentiated high-grade spindle cell proliferation is rarely seen.

extremely helpful in proving the presence of rhabdomyoblastic differentiation that, as mentioned, appears to be associated with more aggressive clinical behavior.

## Genetics

Dedifferentiated liposarcoma usually shows the presence of ring and/or giant marker chromosomes, as in WD liposarcoma, although superimposed additional aberrations have been reported. At the molecular level, a significant increase of both overexpression and amplification of MDM2 in the high-grade areas has been observed, which may account for the tumor progression in this subset of sarcomas. MDM2 represents the main driver of the 12q amplicon (wherein also *CDK4* and *HMGA2* map). Co-amplification of c-JUN (mapping at 1p329) and of its activating kinase (mapping at 6q23) is observed. It has been suggested that the activation of the c-JUN pathway may be involved in tumor progression from well-differentiated to dedifferentiated liposarcoma; however, this concept still represents a source of debate. Interestingly, at variance with

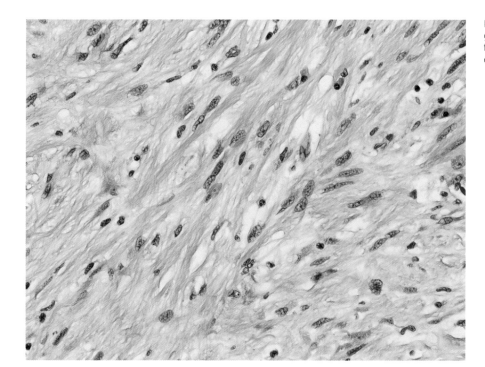

**Fig. 7-32.** Dedifferentiated liposarcoma, "low-grade variant." Often, the non-lipogenic areas feature a hypocellular, cytologically bland spindle cell proliferation.

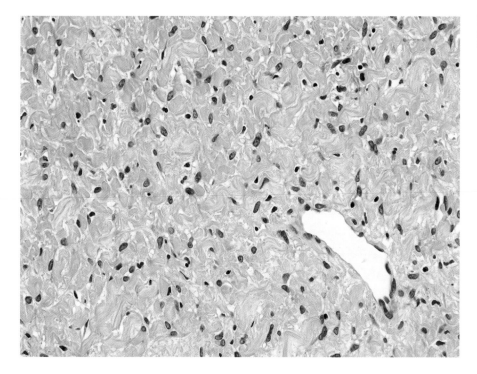

**Fig. 7-33.** Dedifferentiated liposarcoma, "low-grade variant." Rarely a paucicellular proliferation is set in a dense collagenous stroma.

high-grade pleomorphic sarcomas that most often present concomitant *MDM2* amplification and *TP53* mutations (being significantly related to poor clinical outcome), in DDLPS *TP53* is affected in less than 10% of cases. Very recently, amplification of *MDM4* has been observed in a case of dedifferentiated liposarcoma lacking *MDM2* gene amplification.

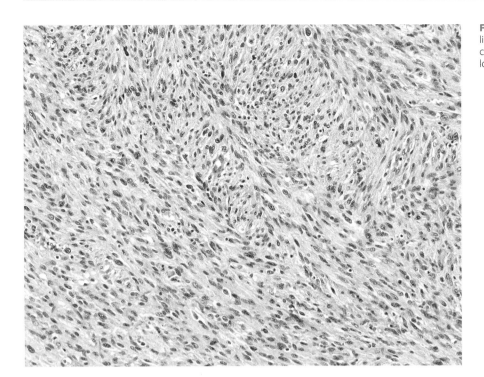

**Fig. 7-34.** Dedifferentiated liposarcoma. A GIST-like appearance can be rarely seen that, in consideration of the frequent intra-abdominal location, may represent a diagnostic challenge.

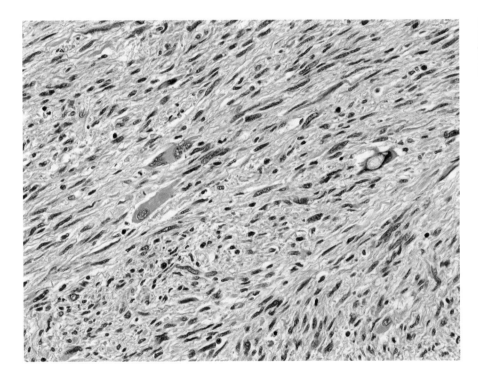

**Fig. 7-35.** Dedifferentiated liposarcoma. Rhabdomyoblasts featuring abundant eosinophilic cytoplasm are seen in this example showing heterologous differentiation. This component usually features nuclear expression of myogenin.

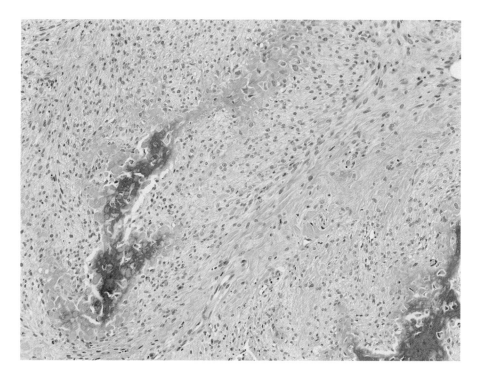

**Fig. 7-36.** Dedifferentiated liposarcoma. Heterologous osteogenic differentiation is seen very rarely.

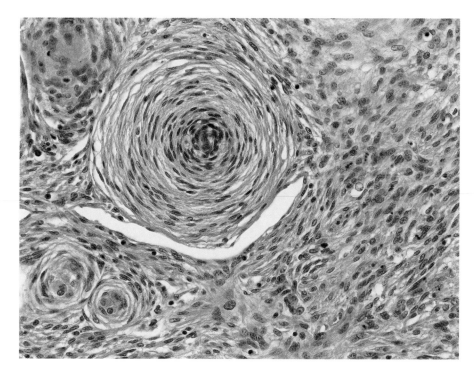

**Fig. 7-37.** Dedifferentiated liposarcoma. A very uncommon but distinctive morphology is represented by the presence of neural-like whorls.

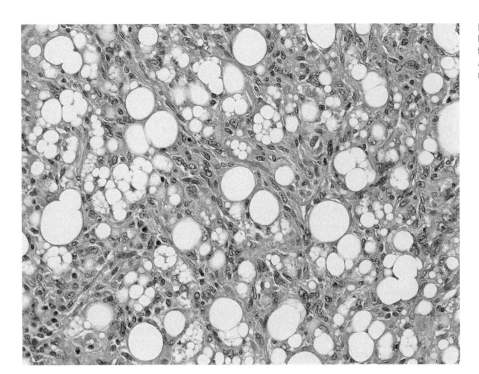

**Fig. 7-38.** Dedifferentiated liposarcoma, homologous type. The dedifferentiated component features the presence of pleomorphic lipoblasts. At variance with pleomorphic liposarcoma, neoplastic cells are MDM2 positive.

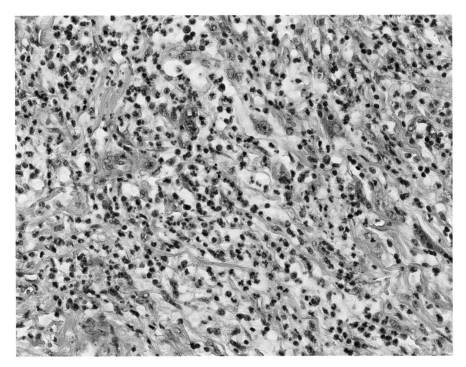

**Fig. 7-39.** Dedifferentiated liposarcoma. Rarely, an intense inflammatory infiltrate is present and may obscure the presence of neoplastic cells. In the past, these lesion were classified as "inflammatory MFH."

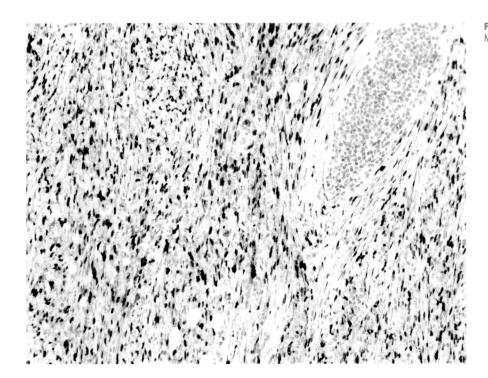

**Fig. 7-40.** Dedifferentiated liposarcoma. Diffuse MDM2 nuclear immunoreactivity is typically seen.

## Differential Diagnosis and Diagnostic Pitfalls

Dedifferentiated liposarcoma needs to be kept separate from other pleomorphic sarcomas (most often pleomorphic leiomyosarcoma and pleomorphic liposarcoma) occurring in the retroperitoneum as well as from non-sarcomatous lesions such as sarcomatoid carcinoma.

Pleomorphic liposarcoma and pleomorphic leiomyosarcoma are ruled out on the basis of the absence of MDM2 overexpression and/or *MDM2* gene amplification. As mentioned, dedifferentiated liposarcoma can express myogenic markers, generating significant morphologic overlaps with true myogenic neoplasms. Sarcomatoid carcinoma (particularly of renal origin) may also at times represent a major challenge; however, it almost always expresses cytokeratin and/or EMA.

Myxofibrosarcoma-like DDLPS may be mistaken for myxoid liposarcoma. As mentioned, myxoid liposarcoma arises primarily in the retroperitoneum only exceptionally, never features nuclear pleomorphism, and never expresses MDM2. MDM2 overexpression/amplification also differentiates homologous-type DDLPS from pleomorphic liposarcoma.

Inflammatory variants of DDLPS can easily be mistaken for hematolymphoid malignancies, in particular anaplastic large cell lymphoma (which consistently expresses CD30 and variably stains for ALK) and Castelman disease. Importantly, inflammatory cells may at times predominate, to the extent that neoplastic mesenchymal cells can be overlooked. Careful histologic examination most often allows the recognition of scattered atypical cells featuring enlarged hyperchromatic nuclei that are more easily picked up with MDM2 immunostaining.

In our experience, renal angiomyolipoma is at times mistaken for dedifferentiated liposarcoma. Co-expression of myogenic and melanocytic differentiation markers (HMB45 and/or Melan-A) allows proper classification in most cases.

As already mentioned, low-grade DDLPS enters the differential diagnosis chiefly with desmoid fibromatosis, solitary fibrous tumor, and GIST. Desmoid fibromatosis typically exhibits nuclear expression of beta-catenin and is generally MDM2/CDK4 negative. Solitary fibrous tumor may rarely exhibit focal MDM2 overexpression; however, in addition to CD34 immunopositivity, it characteristically features STAT6 nuclear staining, which is currently regarded as both sensitive and specific. GIST is relatively easily ruled out on the basis of KIT and/or DOG1 immunopositivity and the presence of *KIT/PDGFRA* gene mutations.

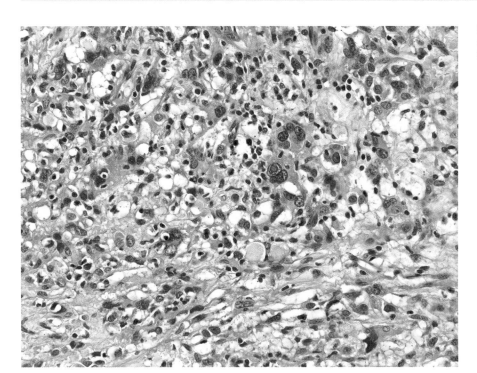

**Fig. 7-41.** Gastrointestinal stromal tumor. Very rarely, GIST may feature significant pleomorphism that represents a major diagnostic pitfall.

An important diagnostic pitfall is represented by dedifferentiated GIST, which, in addition to striking pleomorphism, may feature loss of KIT expression. It must also be remembered that aside from the extremely rare phenomenon of dedifferentiation, equally rare examples of GIST may feature significant pleomorphism that undoubtedly represents a diagnostic challenge (Fig. 7-41). These cases, however, express KIT and DOG1 as frequently as does conventional GIST.

**Key Points in Dedifferentiated Liposarcoma Diagnosis**

- Occurrence in the retroperitoneum and spermatic cord of adults
- Morphologic transition from well-differentiated liposarcoma to high-grade, most often non-lipogenic sarcoma
- Overexpression/amplification of MDM2
- Clinical behavior less aggressive than other pleomorphic sarcomas unless rhabdomyoblastic differentiation is present

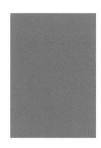

# Extraskeletal Osteosarcoma

## Definition and Epidemiology

Extraskeletal osteosarcoma (EOS) is an aggressive soft tissue sarcoma, the neoplastic cells of which produce osteogenic matrix. A relationship with the underlying bone must be excluded. Extraskeletal osteosarcoma accounts for approximately 1% of all sarcomas. Peak incidence is in the sixth and seventh decades of life, whereas it is extremely uncommon in the young population. Males outnumber females 2:1. Approximately 15% of cases arise in previously irradiated anatomic sites.

## Clinical Presentation and Outcome

Extraskeletal osteosarcoma occurs most frequently in the limbs of elderly patients. Most often, EOS is deep seated, with superficial locations accounting for no more than 10% of cases. Extraskeletal osteosarcoma is a very aggressive malignancy, with systemic spread to the lungs observed in most cases and a 5-year overall survival rate not exceeding 25%.

## Morphology and Immunohistochemistry

Grossly, EOS most often presents as a large, well-circumscribed, variably necrotic mass with hemorrhagic foci (Fig. 7-42). The presence of bone formation confers to the lesion a gritty cut surface. Microscopically, EOS almost always is high grade and exhibits significant nuclear pleomorphism (Fig. 7-43). The main diagnostic clue is the presence of

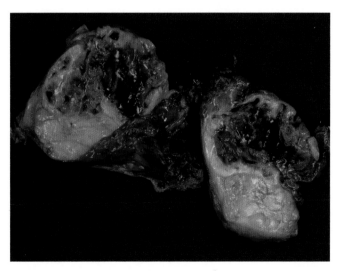

**Fig. 7-42.** Extraskeletal osteosarcoma. A well-circumscribed, fleshy mass featuring areas of necrosis and cystic degeneration and hemorrhage is seen.

**Fig. 7-43.** Extraskeletal osteosarcoma. A high-grade spindle and pleomorphic cell neoplasm featuring osteogenic matrix formation is seen.

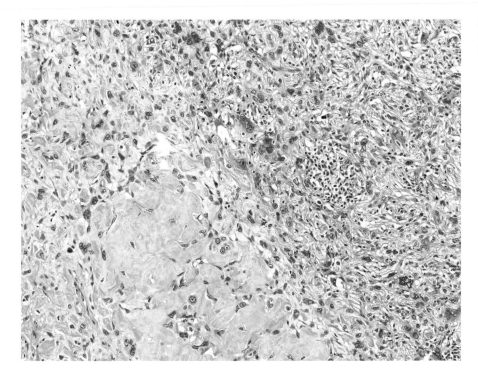

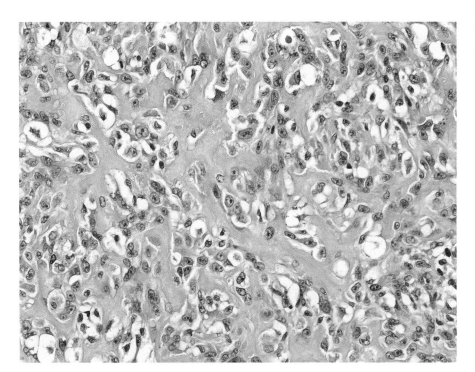

**Fig. 7-44.** Extraskeletal osteosarcoma. Higher magnification shows osteoid production by neoplastic cells.

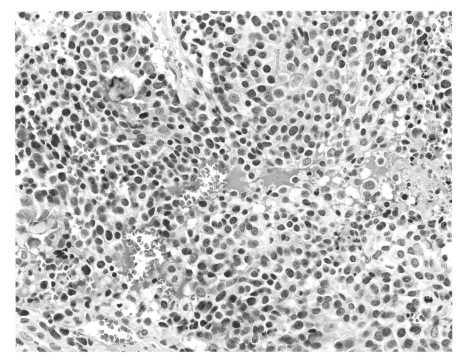

**Fig. 7-45.** Extraskeletal osteosarcoma. Very rarely, neoplastic cells feature a round cell morphology. Osteoid production can be, at times, very focal and therefore easily overlooked.

malignant osteoid produced by neoplastic cells (Fig. 7-44). The neoplastic cell population exhibits a variable morphology that includes spindle cell, round cell (Fig. 7-45), and epithelioid (Fig. 7-46) subtypes. High-grade osteoblastic features generally prevail; however, any osteosarcoma variant (fibroblastic, chondroblastic, telangiectatic, small cell, giant cell-rich) has been documented. The occurrence in the extraskeletal location of low-grade OS similar to parosteal osteosarcoma is regarded as extremely rare. Common immunohistochemical differentiation markers do not play a significant role. By contrast, the application in this context of the osteogenic differentiation marker SATB2 appears to be extremely helpful (Fig. 7-47). Importantly, SATB2 also decorates normal osteoblasts and therefore does not differentiate between neoplastic and metaplastic bone.

## Genetics

Data are very limited; however, specific genetic anomalies have not been reported so far.

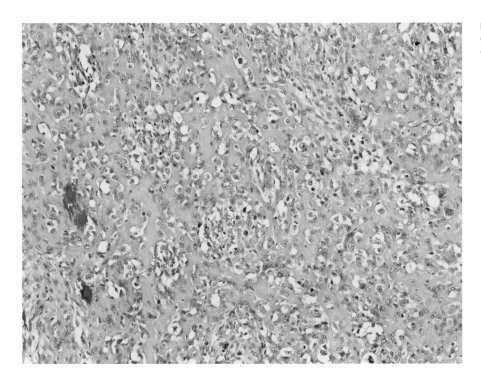

**Fig. 7-46.** Extraskeletal osteosarcoma. In some cases, neoplastic cells exhibit an epithelioid appearance. Abundant osteoid production is seen.

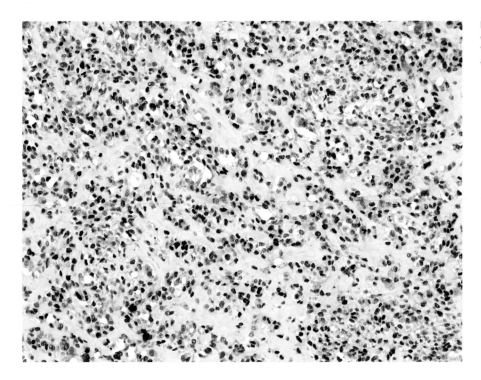

**Fig. 7-47.** Extraskeletal osteosarcoma. Nuclear expression of SATB2 is shown. SATB2 decorates the vast majority of osteosarcomas, including those that are extraskeletal.

## Differential Diagnosis and Diagnostic Pitfalls

When dealing with bone-forming neoplasms, it must be remembered that both dedifferentiated liposarcoma and malignant peripheral nerve sheath tumor may exhibit heterologous osteogenic differentiation. In both situations, it is important not merely to focus on the presence of bone formation but to identify the morphologic context in which osteogenic features occur.

One of the most important diagnostic pitfalls is presented by **myositis ossificans**. Myositis ossificans represents a benign, bone-forming myofibroblastic neoplasm occurring primarily in the limbs and the trunk of patients of variable age, from childhood to late adulthood (Fig. 7-48). Clinical history of trauma is reported in more than half of the cases. Even if radiologic findings are relatively distinctive, core biopsy at times may pose significant diagnostic difficulties. Grossly, it is generally well circumscribed, often soft and hemorrhagic at the center and firm and gritty at the periphery (Fig. 7-49). Well-formed examples exhibit a distinctive "zonal" pattern, featuring a peripheral shell of mature bone (Fig. 7-50) that merges into more immature, intermediate osteogenic areas (Fig. 7-51), and with a center composed of a hypercellular myofibroblastic proliferation almost indistinguishable from nodular fasciitis (Fig. 7-52). Immunohistochemically, lesional cells express abundantly smooth muscle actin. The presence of the typical "zonation" as well as the absence of nuclear atypia or pleomorphism represent the most important diagnostic clue in favor of myositis ossificans. Even if anecdotal cases of malignant transformation to osteosarcoma are reported, myositis ossificans is

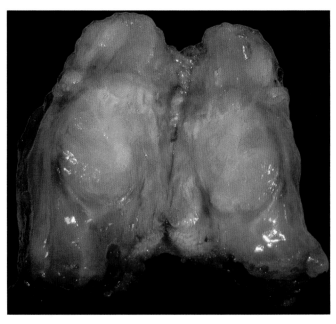

**Fig. 7-49.** Myositis ossificans. Grossly, a well-circumscribed mass is seen. Multifocal bone formation is seen at the periphery of the lesion.

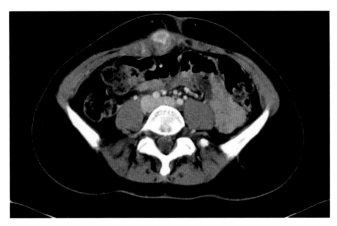

**Fig. 7-48.** Myositis ossificans. At imaging, a mass in the abdominal wall featuring a peripheral shell of bone is seen.

completely benign and simple excision is curative. Another rare mesenchymal neoplasm that may enter the differential diagnosis is ossifying fibromyxoid tumor (OFMT). This entity is discussed in detail in Chapter 8. In brief, OFMT most often features deposition of mature bone at the periphery of the lesion (only atypical cases may exhibit irregular deposition of osteoid), lacks pleomorphic cytomorphology, is often desmin and/or EMA positive, and features rearrangement of the *PHF1* gene.

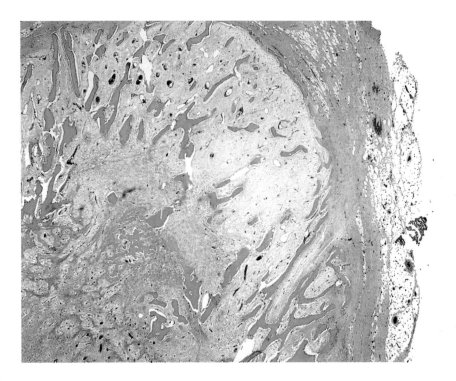

**Fig. 7-50.** Myositis ossificans. The "zoning phenomenon" represents a key feature. The mature bone located at the periphery gradually merges into an intermediate zone in which immature bone production is present but is absent at the center of the lesion.

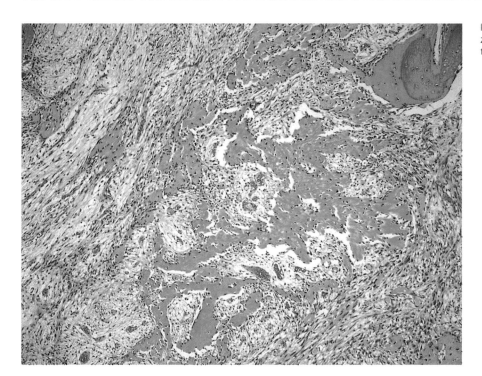

**Fig. 7-51.** Myositis ossificans. In the intermediate zone, immature bone production is seen, which at times causes an erroneous diagnosis of malignancy.

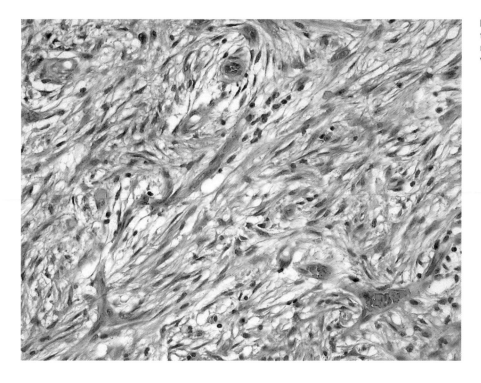

**Fig. 7-52.** Myositis ossificans. The central part of the lesion is composed of a spindle cell myofibroblastic proliferation that microscopically is virtually indistinguishable from nodular fasciitis.

**Key Points in Extraskeletal Osteosarcoma Diagnosis**

- Occurrence in the limbs of elderly patients
- Production of osteogenic matrix by neoplastic cells
- Most often high grade and pleomorphic
- Aggressive neoplasm with early metastatic spread to the lungs

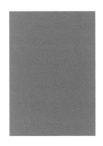

# Variants of Soft Tissue Sarcomas Featuring Pleomorphic Morphology

## Pleomorphic "High-Grade" Myxofibrosarcoma

Myxofibrosarcoma is discussed in more detail in Chapter 8. Myxoid malignant fibrous histiocytoma has been for decades the preferred synonym for myxofibrosarcoma (the term was actually coined by Angervall in 1977), based on the presence of pleomorphic, MFH-like morphology in high-grade examples.

The majority of these lesions arise in the limbs and limb girdles of elderly patients, while occurrence in the trunk, head and neck, and acral sites is comparatively much rarer. Approximately two-thirds tend to be superficially located and typically present as multinodular masses.

As mentioned, myxofibrosarcoma shows a broad spectrum of cellularity and pleomorphism. At the high-grade end of the spectrum, neoplastic cells exhibit remarkable pleomorphism and are invariably set in a variable amount of myxoid stroma (conventionally, at least 5% of the neoplasm) (Fig. 7-53). The presence of the characteristic thin-walled, archiform blood vessels (typically seen in low-grade myxofibrosarcoma) is usually also retained in high-grade myxofibrosarcoma (Fig. 7-54). Areas of lower grade are often present (Fig. 7-55). The metastatic rate of high-grade myxofibrosarcoma ranges between 30 and 35% and therefore appears lower than that observed in other subtypes of pleomorphic sarcomas. In contrast to local recurrences, metastatic spread is more reliably predicted by grading, to the extent that low-grade myxofibrosarcomas almost never metastasize.

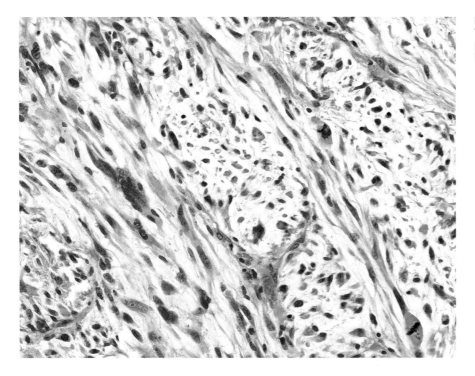

**Fig. 7-53.** High-grade myxofibrosarcoma. The tumor is composed of a spindle cell and pleomorphic cell proliferation set in a myxoid background.

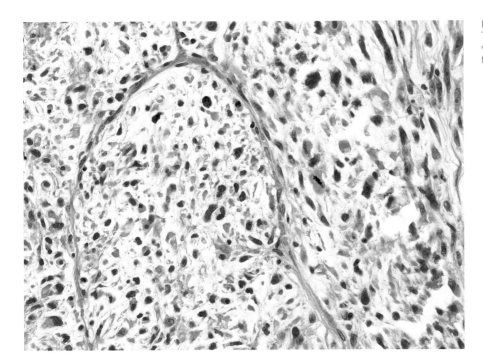

**Fig. 7-54.** High-grade myxofibrosarcoma. The presence of thin-walled, archiform blood vessels represents a very characteristic morphologic finding.

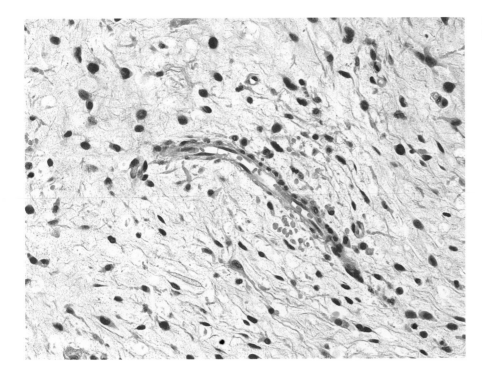

**Fig. 7-55.** High-grade myxofibrosarcoma. Lower-grade areas are often seen in the same lesion.

## Differential Diagnosis and Diagnostic Pitfalls

A high-grade myxofibrosarcoma-like appearance can be seen in other histotypes, most often in pleomorphic liposarcoma and dedifferentiated liposarcoma. Recognition of pleomorphic lipoblasts represents the key feature in favor of the diagnosis of pleomorphic liposarcomas. Dedifferentiated liposarcoma can also feature the presence of a myxofibrosarcoma-like morphology; however, MDM2 overexpression and/or amplification is consistently detected. An important caveat is represented by

the fact that myxofibrosarcoma may also exhibit MDM2 overexpression, but this is generally limited to a minority of cells, never matching the diffuse immunopositivity observed in dedifferentiated liposarcoma.

Myxoinflammatory fibroblastic sarcoma may enter the differential diagnosis; however, it most often occurs at acral sites and is characterized morphologically by the presence of variable amounts of pseudolipoblasts, spindle cells, and atypical neoplastic cells containing distinctive inclusion-like nucleoli

**395**

set in a myxoinflammatory background. Myxoinflammatory fibroblastic sarcoma is discussed in Chapter 8.

## Pleomorphic Leiomyosarcoma

Leiomyosarcoma (LMS) is discussed in detail in Chapter 4. Leiomyosarcoma most often represents a spindle cell neoplasm; however, approximately 20–30% of cases can display a pleomorphic phenotype. As with conventional LMS, pleomorphic LMS tends to occur in middle-aged or older patients and forms a significant subset of retroperitoneal sarcomas. It is also the most frequent sarcoma arising from large blood vessels;

it is somewhat less common in the limbs. From a clinical standpoint, pleomorphic LMS is associated with the poorest outcome among high-grade pleomorphic sarcomas, showing a 5-year metastatic rate ranging between 60 and 70%.

The recognition of pleomorphic LMS on histologic grounds alone may be challenging. Microscopically, a combination of spindle and pleomorphic cells is seen, associated with abundant necrosis and atypical mitotic figures (Fig. 7-56). The presence of better-differentiated areas composed of neoplastic cells featuring eosinophilic fibrillary cytoplasm and cigar-shaped nuclei represents the most helpful diagnostic clue (Fig. 7-57).

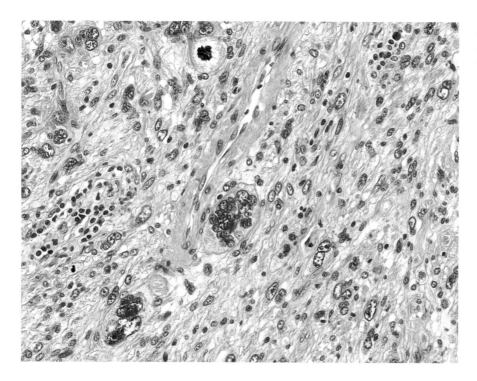

**Fig. 7-56.** Pleomorphic leiomyosarcoma. The tumor is composed of a combination of spindle cells and pleomorphic cells. Atypical mitotic figures represent a common finding.

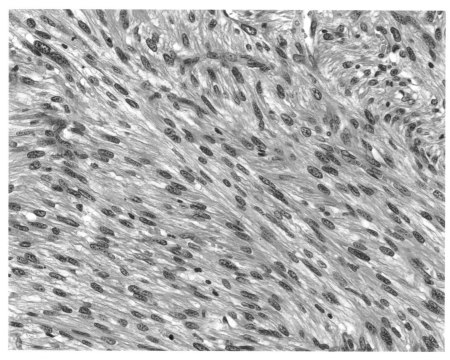

**Fig. 7-57.** Pleomorphic leiomyosarcoma. Most often, better differentiated areas featuring distinctive, blunt-ended nuclei and eosinophilic fibrillary cytoplasm are detected.

When LMS is purely pleomorphic, immunohistochemical stains play a key diagnostic role. Variable expression of smooth muscle actin, desmin, and h-caldesmon is observed in the vast majority of these lesions. Notably, expression of cytokeratins can be observed in approximately 20% of leiomyosarcomas. As previously discussed, absence of nuclear expression of myogenin helps in the differential diagnosis with pleomorphic rhabdomyosarcoma.

## Differential Diagnosis and Diagnostic Pitfalls

When dealing with retroperitoneal lesions, a clinically relevant differential diagnosis is with dedifferentiated liposarcoma that can relatively often exhibit a myogenic phenotype. Lack of expression/amplification of MDM2 represents the key diagnostic clue in favor of the diagnosis of leiomyosarcoma.

## Pleomorphic Malignant Peripheral Nerve Sheath Tumor

Malignant peripheral nerve sheath tumor is discussed in detail in Chapter 4 within the group of spindle cell neoplasms.

It accounts for approximately 5% of all sarcomas, and in half of the cases, it is associated with neurofibromatosis type 1 (NF1) syndrome (known eponymically as von Recklinghausen disease). Morphologically, most often MPNST features a homogeneous spindle cell morphology; however, a minority of cases may exhibit striking pleomorphism, which represents a real challenge (Fig. 7-58). Association with NF1 syndrome and/or origin from a nerve represent helpful clinical features. Morphologically, the most useful finding is the presence of conventional areas featuring a high-grade spindle cell neoplasm showing variation and perivascular accentuation of cellularity. However, close relationships with blood vessels are often seen in this rare variant (Fig. 7-59). Immunohistochemical analysis may not be that helpful, as S100 in this context is neither sensitive nor specific. Recently, nuclear expression of SOX10 has been suggested as a potentially useful neural differentiation marker, but further validation is needed. Loss of nuclear expression of H3K27me3 is observed in approximately half of the cases of MPNST.

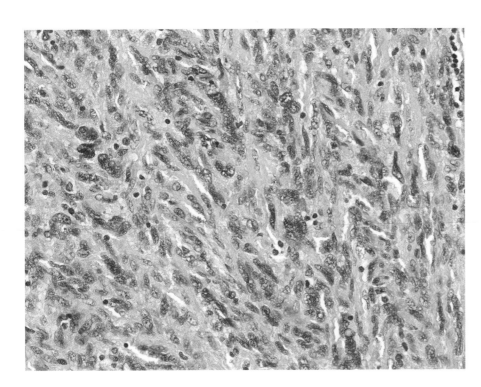

**Fig. 7-58.** Pleomorphic malignant peripheral nerve sheath tumor. The presence of significant pleomorphism is very rarely seen in MPNST. Note the presence of scattered pleomorphic cells within a spindle cell proliferation.

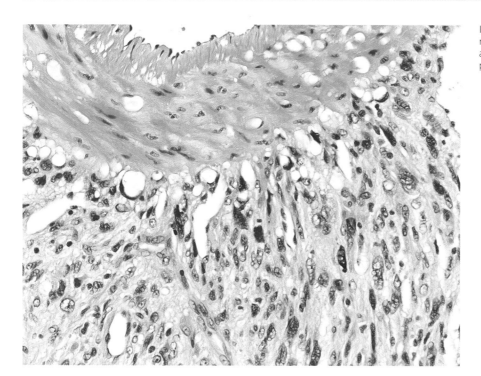

**Fig. 7-59.** Pleomorphic malignant peripheral nerve sheath tumor. The presence of perivascular accentuation of cellularity is also retained in pleomorphic variants.

## Differential Diagnosis and Diagnostic Pitfalls

As is discussed in more detail in the next section, when dealing with an S100-positive pleomorphic neoplasm, sarcomatoid (either primary or metastatic) melanoma should be considered first. Paradoxically, the presence of diffuse S100 positivity in a pleomorphic neoplasm should prompt (with exceedingly rare exceptions) reconsidering a diagnosis of pleomorphic MPNST.

## Undifferentiated Pleomorphic Sarcoma, Not Otherwise Specified

The 2013 WHO classification recognizes the existence of an undifferentiated, unclassifiable category of pleomorphic sarcoma, and defines it as a group of pleomorphic high-grade sarcomas in which any attempt to disclose their line of differentiation has failed. It has to be underlined that this is a diagnosis of exclusion following thorough sampling and judicious use of ancillary techniques. Most of these cases in the past have contributed to the category of storiform and pleomorphic MFH. Currently, undifferentiated pleomorphic sarcoma (UPS) accounts for no more than 20% of sarcomas occurring in adults.

Undifferentiated pleomorphic sarcomas tend to occur in the extremities (most often the lower limbs) of elderly patients (peak age is in the sixth and seventh decades). They present as deep-seated, progressively enlarging masses. Sometimes rapid growth is observed that may be associated with local pain. About 5% of patients exhibit distant metastases (primarily to the lungs) at presentation. Grossly, UPS most often is represented by a large, well-circumscribed mass featuring a variegated cut surface as a consequence of the presence of abundant necrosis and hemorrhage (Fig. 7-60). Microscopically,

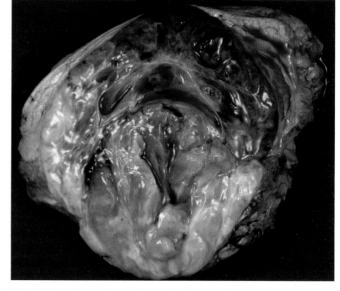

**Fig. 7-60.** Undifferentiated pleomorphic sarcoma. Gross specimen featuring a large, fleshy mass exhibiting abundant necrosis, hemorrhage, and cystic degeneration.

these lesions tend to be very heterogeneous; however, all share marked pleomorphism, often with bizarre giant cells, admixed with spindle cells and a variable (from many to none) number of foamy histiocytes. A high number of mitotic figures (including atypical ones) are seen (Fig. 7-61). Immunohistochemical analysis is most often disappointing, and specific lines of differentiation cannot be demonstrated (see Table 7.1). The presence of scattered SMA-positive cells should not be taken as evidence of myogenic differentiation. Genetically, UPS tends to exhibit complex karyotypes.

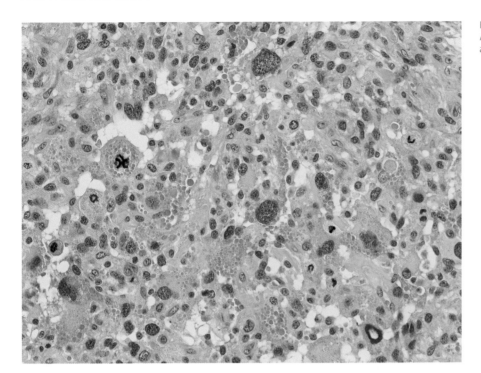

**Fig. 7-61.** Undifferentiated pleomorphic sarcoma. A highly pleomorphic cell population featuring atypical mitotic figures is typically seen.

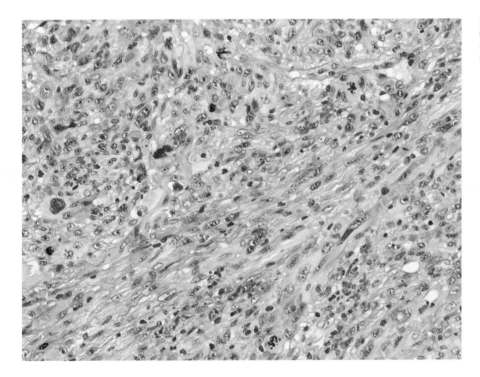

**Fig. 7-62.** Sarcomatoid amelanotic melanoma. Complete morphologic overlap with undifferentiated pleomorphic sarcomas can be seen.

## Differential Diagnosis and Diagnostic Pitfalls

Before rendering a diagnosis of UPS, it is important to exclude the specific sarcoma subtypes featuring pleomorphic morphology that have been discussed previously. In our experience, non-sarcomatous lesions that are frequently mistaken for UPS (or other pleomorphic sarcomas) are metastatic sarcomatoid carcinoma and metastatic sarcomatoid melanoma. Sarcomatoid carcinoma most often diffusely expresses pancytokeratins and EMA. Careful evaluation of the clinical history and application of organ-specific differentiation markers plays a fundamental role. Accurate scrutiny of the clinical history is fundamental when dealing with sarcomatoid melanoma. Importantly, in sarcomatoid amelanotic melanoma, helpful morphologic features, such as a nesting pattern of growth, can be totally absent (Fig. 7-62). In addition, melanocytic markers may be also negative. Diffuse S100 immunopositivity represents the most consistent immunohistochemical finding, and in the context of a pleomorphic malignancy should always prompt

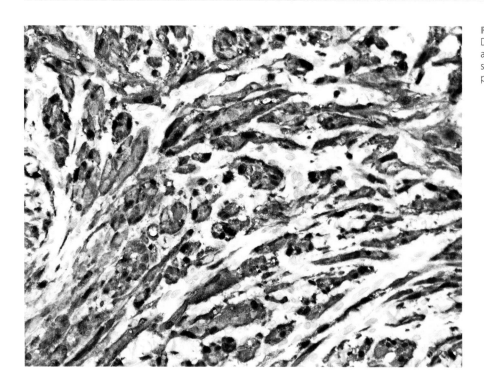

**Fig. 7-63.** Sarcomatoid amelanotic melanoma. Diffuse S100 immunopositivity represents a consistent finding and is helpful in differentiating sarcomatoid melanoma from non-melanocytic pleomorphic lesions.

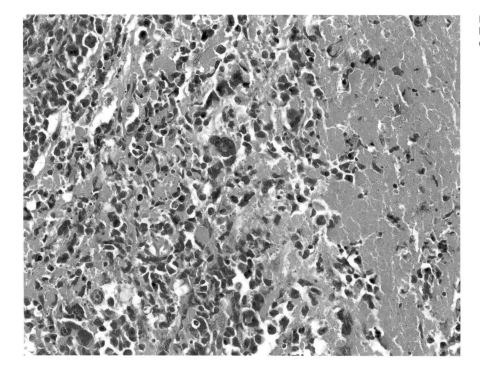

**Fig. 7-64.** Anaplastic large cell lymphoma. Extreme pleomorphism can be seen in ALCL that is often associated with abundant necrosis.

considering sarcomatoid melanoma (Fig. 7-63). As mentioned, the very exceptional examples of pleomorphic MPNSTs almost never feature abundant expression of S100 protein. Another neoplastic lesion that often is mistaken for a pleomorphic sarcoma is represented by anaplastic large cell lymphoma (ALCL) (Fig. 7-64). Expression of CD30 (ALK is also seen in approximately 60% of cases) in ALCL represents the key diagnostic clue (Fig. 7-65).

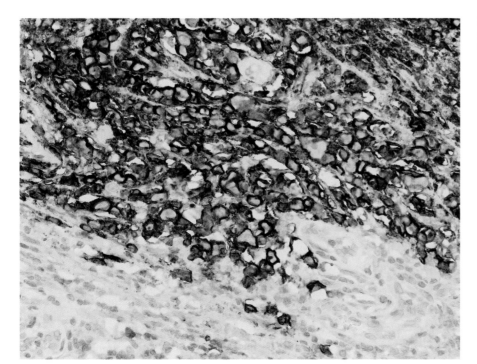

**Fig. 7-65.** Anaplastic large cell lymphoma. Positive membrane staining for CD30 represents an extremely helpful diagnostic finding.

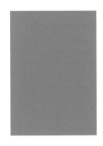

# Pleomorphic Mesenchymal Lesions, Not to Be Confused with High-Grade Pleomorphic Sarcomas

Pleomorphism is not per se an unquestionable indicator of extreme biologic aggression. There exist, in fact, neoplasms such as pleomorphic hyalinizing angiectatic tumor and atypical fibroxanthoma (AFX) that, despite featuring all the histologic hallmarks of pleomorphic mesenchymal malignancies, behave much less aggressively than expected. Furthermore, pleomorphism is also present in benign lesions, good examples being represented by the cytologic atypia of a degenerative/regressive nature commonly found in so-called ancient neurilemomas or in symplastic (bizarre) leiomyoma of the uterus.

## Atypical Fibroxanthoma

### Definition and Epidemiology

Atypical fibroxanthoma (AFX) represents a biologically fascinating dermal lesion that, despite extreme pleomorphism, is characterized by a benign clinical behavior. For many years, this distinct lesion was often regarded as the superficial, cutaneous non-metastasizing variant of so-called MFH. Currently, as a consequence of the conceptual evolution described above, AFX is no longer considered a fibrohistiocytic lesion, but rather

a dermal fibroblastic neoplasm generated by ultraviolet (UV)-induced genetic damage.

## Clinical Presentation and Outcome

Atypical fibroxanthoma presents as a solitary, polypoid, ulcerated lesion in sun-damaged skin, especially of the head and neck and much less commonly on the dorsum of the hands, of elderly patients. A clinical history of rapid growth is most often reported. Those cases reported in the past occurring in non-actinically damaged skin in the limbs of young adults most likely represent examples of atypical benign fibrous histiocytoma. When properly recognized on the basis of the adoption of strict diagnostic criteria, clinical behavior is uneventful and complete excision is generally curative. Local recurrence is uncommon and should prompt reconsideration of the initial diagnosis.

## Morphology and Immunohistochemistry

Histologically, all AFXs are centered in the dermis, quite often surrounded by an epidermal collarette (Fig. 7-66). Growth tends to be expansile with only limited infiltration of the subcutis (Fig. 7-67). Actinic degeneration of elastic fibers in the

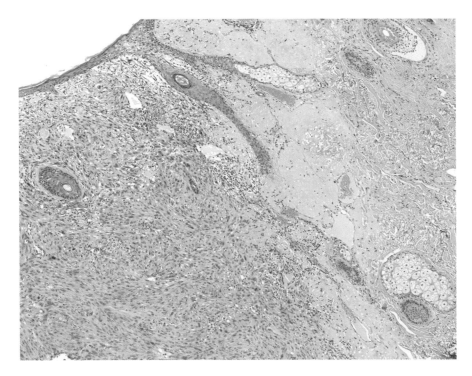

**Fig. 7-66.** Atypical fibroxanthoma. A dermal spindle and pleomorphic cell proliferation demarcated by an epidermal collarette is seen.

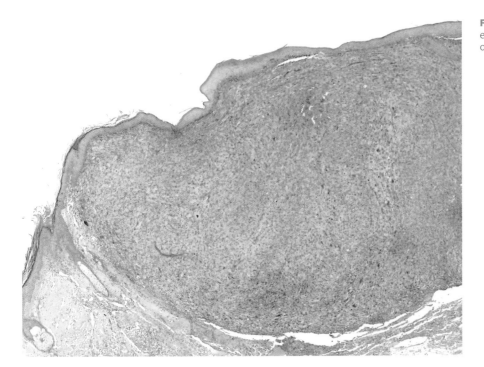

**Fig. 7-67.** Atypical fibroxanthoma. A pushing, expansile pattern of growth with minimal infiltration of the subcutis is typically seen.

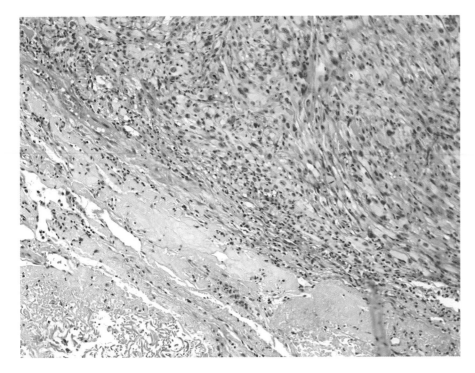

**Fig. 7-68.** Atypical fibroxanthoma. The presence of severe actinic damage of the dermis represents a consistent morphologic finding.

surrounding dermis is a prominent feature (Fig. 7-68). Classical AFX is composed of highly pleomorphic neoplastic cells, frequently featuring bizarre giant cells interspersed with a variable number of spindle-shaped cells and inflammatory cells (Fig. 7-69). Mitotic activity is usually very high and is associated with the presence of atypical mitotic figures (Fig. 7-70). The spindle cell (non-pleomorphic) variant of AFX is composed of fascicles of eosinophilic spindle cells with vesicular nuclei and

one or multiple eosinophilic nucleoli (Fig. 7-71). Mitotic figures, which are often atypical, are common but cytologic pleomorphism is focal or even absent in this subset of cases. Importantly, subcutaneous or deeper invasion, necrosis, or vascular or perineurial invasion should not be accepted as features of AFX, although there may exist focally very superficial invasion into fat.

Immunohistochemistry is essential for confirming the diagnosis of AFX. Approximately 30% of cases feature focal positivity

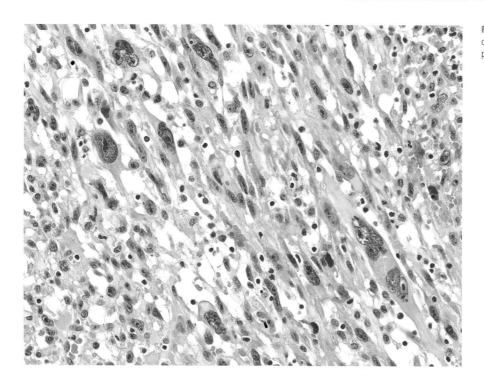

**Fig. 7-69.** Atypical fibroxanthoma. The tumor is composed of a combination of spindle cells, pleomorphic cells, and inflammatory elements.

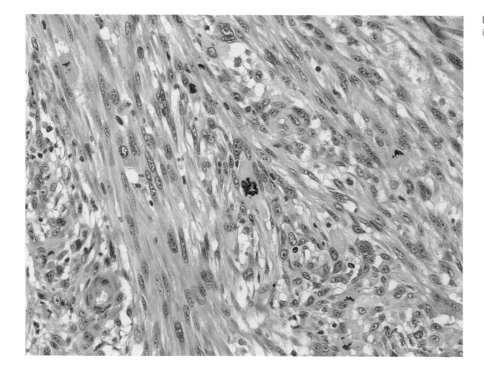

**Fig. 7-70.** Atypical fibroxanthoma. Mitotic activity is usually brisk and mitotic figures are often atypical.

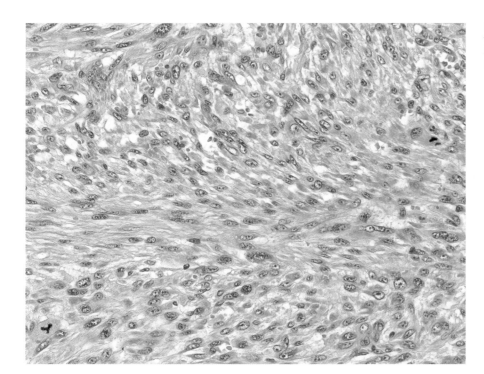

**Fig. 7-71.** Atypical fibroxanthoma, spindle cell variant. This variant of AFX is composed of a monomorphic spindle cell proliferation. Note the numerous as well as atypical mitotic figures.

for smooth muscle actin, suggestive of fibroblastic or myofibroblastic differentiation. Immunostains for keratins, S100 protein, and desmin are always negative and play a major role in ruling out the three main differential diagnoses, namely, spindle cell (sarcomatoid) squamous cell carcinoma, spindle cell melanoma, and leiomyosarcoma. Nuclear expression of p53 is consistently observed, however it is not specific for AFX.

## Genetics

Ultraviolet-induced TP53 mutations are typically seen in AFX. In addition, UV-induced TERT promoter mutations have also been recently reported.

## Differential Diagnosis and Diagnostic Pitfalls

With the advent of immunohistochemistry, AFX has become the prototypic diagnosis of exclusion, main differential diagnoses being represented by malignant melanoma, spindle cell (sarcomatoid) carcinoma, and leiomyosarcoma. As ulceration is present in most cases, making an evaluation for the presence of epidermal dysplasia or junctional activity is often difficult or even impossible. Application of pertinent melanocytic, epithelial, and myogenic differentiation markers allows proper classification in most cases. When dealing with spindle cell amelanotic melanoma, it must be remembered that only S100 protein is expressed consistently, whereas melanocytic markers such as HMB45 and Melan-A tend to be negative.

Cutaneous leiomyosarcoma may exhibit pleomorphic morphology (Figs. 7-72 and 7-73); however, it most often retains variable expression of common myogenic markers such as smooth muscle actin, h-caldesmon, and desmin. Importantly, cutaneous leiomyosarcoma limited to the dermis or with minimal infiltration of the subcutis most often pursues a benign clinical course, irrespective of grading.

Those lesions reported in the past as metastatic AFX were characterized by deep infiltrative growth and, taking into account the limited or absent immunohistochemical workup at that time, most probably represented examples of other high-grade sarcomas or non-mesenchymal malignancies, such as melanoma (Fig. 7-74) and sarcomatoid squamous cell carcinoma (Fig. 7-75). Undifferentiated pleomorphic sarcomas (pleomorphic dermal sarcoma) can obviously occur in the skin and need to be separated from AFX. Extensive involvement of the subcutis, vascular, or perineural invasion and necrosis, as well as the absence of expansile growth pattern, all represent major criteria of exclusion of AFX diagnosis, as they may be associated with adverse outcome.

The rare presence of pseudoangiomatous features may raise the differential diagnosis with spindle cell angiosarcoma that can be easily excluded on the base of ERG and CD31 immunonegativity.

Pleomorphic fibroma is a benign dermal lesion occurring anywhere in the body at any age. These polypoid lesions typically feature the presence of regressive nuclear pleomorphism. However, they are polypoid and distinctively hypocellular, therefore making confusion with AFX rather unlikely.

Eventually, as mentioned, those examples of AFX diagnosed in the past in sun-undamaged cutaneous locations are currently regarded as atypical variants of benign fibrous histiocytoma (Fig. 7-76).

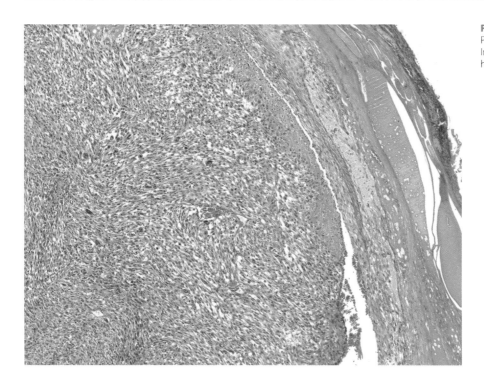

**Fig. 7-72.** Cutaneous leiomyosarcoma. Pleomorphic variant can mimic AFX. Immunostaining for desmin and h-caldesmon is helpful in differential diagnosis.

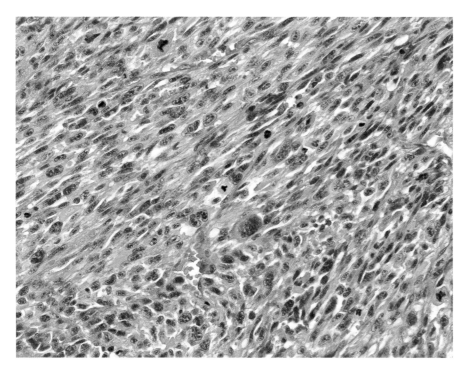

**Fig. 7-73.** Cutaneous leiomyosarcoma. Spindle and pleomorphic cells organized in a fascicular pattern of growth are seen.

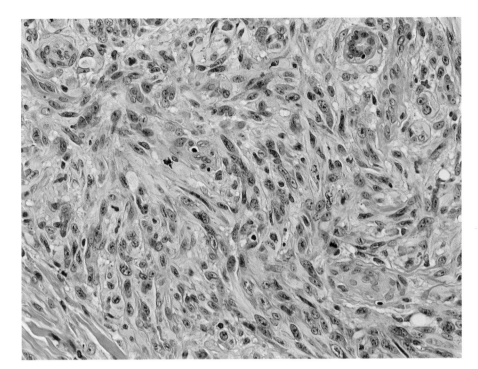

**Fig. 7-74.** Amelanotic sarcomatoid melanoma. Melanoma can feature a sarcomatoid morphology, creating complete overlap with AFX. S100 immunoreactivity represents the key diagnostic clue in favor of melanoma.

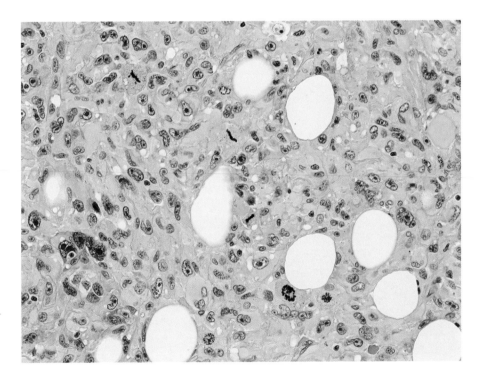

**Fig. 7-75.** Sarcomatoid squamous cell carcinoma. Pleomorphic neoplastic cells infiltrating the subcutaneous fat are seen. Cytoplasm tends to be abundant. Demonstration of even focal epithelial differentiation by immunohistochemistry (EMA and pankeratins) is mandatory to confirm diagnosis.

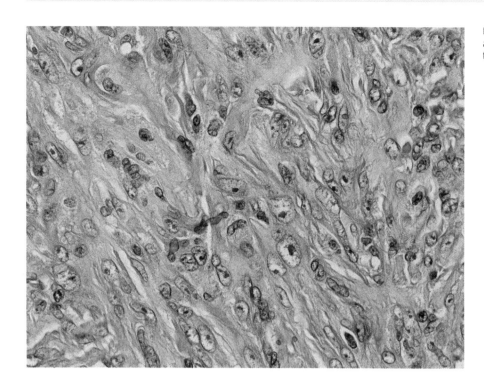

**Fig. 7-76.** Atypical fibrous histiocytoma. Scattered atypical cells are set in a lesion with the typical features of benign fibrous histiocytoma.

### Key Points in Atypical Fibroxanthoma Diagnosis

- Occurrence in sun-damaged skin of elderly patients
- Expansile silhouette
- Presence of epidermal collarette
- Minimal invasion of subcutis
- Absence of vascular and perineural invasion
- Absence of necrosis
- Indolent clinical behavior

# Pleomorphic Hyalinizing Angiectatic Tumor of Soft Parts

## Definition and Epidemiology

First reported in 1996, pleomorphic hyalinizing angiectatic tumor (PHAT) is a very uncommon, locally aggressive soft tissue neoplasm. It has been suggested that hemosiderotic fibrolipomatous tumor (HFLT) may represent a precursor of PHAT; however, genetic and clinicomorphologic findings would also indicate a possible relationship between HFLT and myxoinflammatory fibroblastic sarcoma.

## Clinical Presentation and Outcome

Pleomorphic hyalinizing angiectatic tumor occurs primarily in lower extremity subcutaneous tissue of middle-aged patients, with no sex predilection. Approximately one-third of cases experience local recurrences that are generally controlled by re-excision.

## Morphology and Immunohistochemistry

Pleomorphic hyalinizing angiectatic tumor is grossly non-encapsulated, often featuring hemorrhagic areas. Microscopically, PHAT presents as a proliferation of spindle and/or pleomorphic cells associated with ectatic, thin-walled blood vessels surrounded by prominent eosinophilic fibrin/collagen deposition (Fig. 7-77). Most often, the lesion exhibits infiltrative margins. Intratumoral hemosiderin deposits may be prominent (Fig. 7-78), and organized intravascular thrombi are commonly observed. Neoplastic cells possess bizarre hyperchromatic, pleomorphic nuclei often featuring intranuclear pseudoinclusions (Fig. 7-79), and inclusion-like nucleoli are rarely seen (Fig. 7-80). Mitoses are extremely rare (usually absent or less than 1 per 50 high-power fields). Chronic inflammatory cells can be found within or surrounding the lesion. The spindle/pleomorphic cells of PHAT exhibit CD34 immunopositivity in approximately half of the cases.

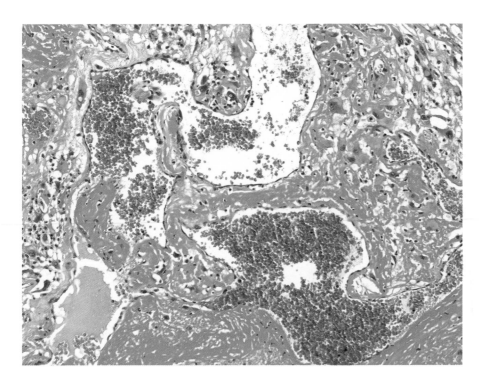

**Fig. 7-77.** Pleomorphic hyalinizing angiectatic tumor. At low power, the most striking feature is the presence of heavily hyalinized, dilated blood vessels.

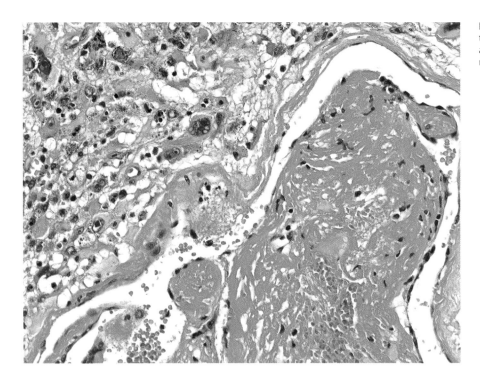

**Fig. 7-78.** Pleomorphic hyalinizing angiectatic tumor. At higher magnification, pleomorphic cells are easily detected. Deposition of hemosiderin represents a typical feature of PHAT.

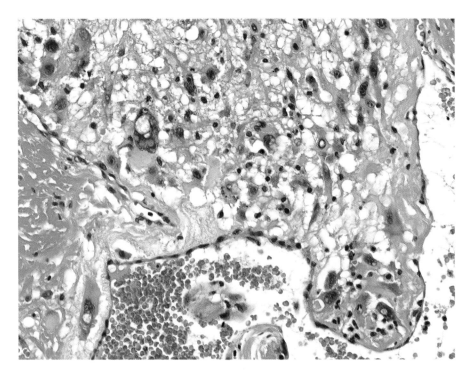

**Fig. 7-79.** Pleomorphic hyalinizing angiectatic tumor. Nuclear pseudoinclusions represent a common morphologic finding.

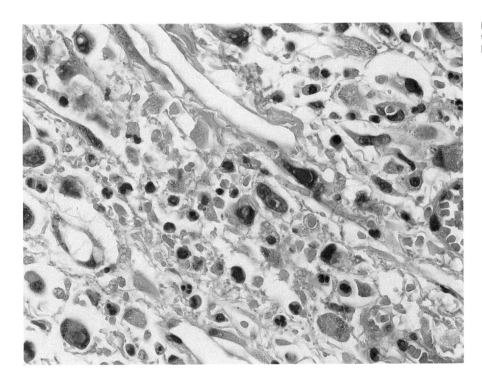

**Fig. 7-80.** Pleomorphic hyalinizing angiectatic tumor. The tumor cells occasionally show inclusion-like nucleoli.

## Genetics

The type of genetic abnormalities in PHAT represents a source of debate. Rearrangement of *TGFBR3* and *MGEA5* genes has been reported; however, others have not confirmed this finding.

## Differential Diagnosis and Diagnostic Pitfalls

Pleomorphic hyalinizing angiectatic tumor, particularly when featuring abundant intratumoral hemosiderin, is likely to be confused with ancient schwannoma or a long-standing hemangioma. Ancient schwannoma may exhibit significant "regressive" cytologic atypia that may represent a real challenge (Fig. 7-81). However, the presence of thick-walled blood vessels (very different from those that are heavily hyalinized, observed in PHAT) (Fig. 7-82) and diffuse S100 immunoreactivity both represent helpful diagnostic features (Fig. 7-83). Personal experience indicates that PHAT-like features can be observed in a variety of unrelated neoplasms such as meningiomas (Fig.7-84), myxofibrosarcoma, and solitary fibrous tumor (Fig. 7-85). As CD34 immunopositivity can be seen in both PHAT and solitary fibrous tumor, STAT6 nuclear immunoreactivity represents the most important diagnostic clue in favor of the latter (Fig. 7-86).

Because of the cellular pleomorphism, the hemorrhagic changes, and the occasional presence of prominent cytoplasmic intranuclear inclusions, the lesion may be confused with a high-grade pleomorphic sarcoma, although one should be alerted by the contrast between the extremely low mitotic rate and the marked pleomorphism of the lesion. By contrast, whenever significant mitotic activity is detected, a true pleomorphic sarcoma with PHAT-like features should be first considered.

**411**

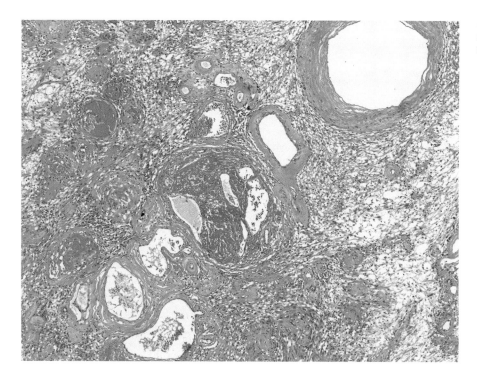

**Fig. 7-81.** Ancient schwannoma. Regressive changes may be seen in long-standing schwannomas that rarely mimic PHAT.

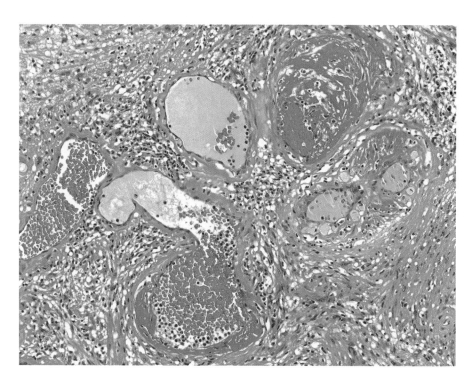

**Fig. 7-82.** Ancient schwannoma. PHAT-like deposits of fibrin within blood vessels are seen.

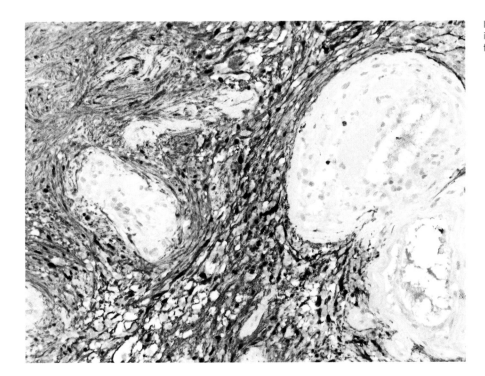

**Fig. 7-83.** Ancient schwannoma. Diffuse S100 immunopositivity represents a key diagnostic finding.

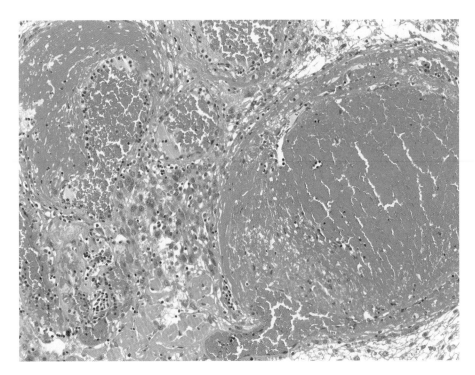

**Fig. 7-84.** Meningioma. PHAT-like features can be rarely seen in long-standing meningiomas.

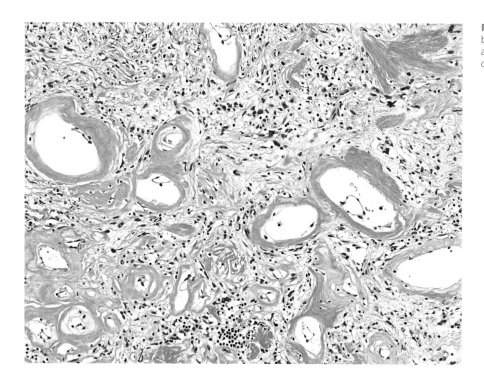

**Fig. 7-85.** Solitary fibrous tumor. Hyalinization of blood vessels (at times, associated with focal nuclear atypia) in solitary fibrous tumor may raise the differential diagnosis with PHAT.

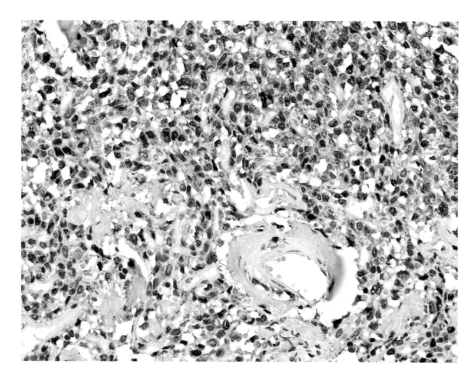

**Fig. 7-86.** Solitary fibrous tumor. As CD34 may be expressed in both solitary fibrous tumor and PHAT, nuclear expression of STAT6 represents an extremely helpful diagnostic finding.

---

### Key Points in Pleimorphic Hyalinizing Angiectatic Tumor Diagnosis

- Occurrence in the lower limbs of middle-aged patients
- Spindle and/or pleomorphic cell proliferation
- Presence of ectatic blood vessels surrounded by prominent eosinophilic fibrin/collagen deposition
- Minimal mitotic activity
- Indolent clinical behavior

# Chapter 7 Selected Key References

## MFH: The Conceptual Evolution

- Angervall L, Kindblom LG, Merck C. Myxofibrosarcoma. A study of 30 cases. *Acta Pathol Microbiol Scand A.* 1977;**85A**: 127–40.
- Cipriani NA, Kurzawa P, Ahmad RA, et al. Prognostic value of myogenic differentiation in undifferentiated pleomorphic sarcomas of soft tissue. *Hum Pathol.* 2014;**45**:1504–8.
- Coindre JM, Hostein I, Maire G, et al. Inflammatory malignant fibrous histiocytomas and dedifferentiated liposarcomas: histological review, genomic profile, and MDM2 and CDK4 status favour a single entity. *J Pathol.* 2004;**203**:822–30.
- Dahlin DC, Beabout JW. Dedifferentiation of low-grade chondrosarcomas. *Cancer.* 1971;**28**: 461–6.
- Dei Tos AP. Classification of pleomorphic sarcomas: where are we now? *Histopathology.* 2006; **48**:51–62.
- Deyrup AT, Haydon RC, Huo D, et al. Myoid differentiation and prognosis in adult pleomorphic sarcomas of the extremity: an analysis of 92 cases. *Cancer.* 2003;**15**(98):805–13.
- Enzinger FM. Angiomatoid malignant fibrous histiocytoma: a distinct fibrohistiocytic tumor of children and young adults simulating a vascular neoplasm. *Cancer.* 1979;**44**:2147–57.
- Enzinger FM. Malignant fibrous histiocytoma 20 years after Stout. *Am J Surg Pathol.* 1986;**10** Suppl 1:43–53.
- Evans HL. Liposarcoma: a study of 55 cases with a reassessment of its classification. *Am J Surg Pathol.* 1979;**3**: 507–23.
- Fletcher CD. Angiomatoid "malignant fibrous histiocytoma": an immunohistochemical study indicative of myoid differentiation. *Hum Pathol.* 1991;**22**:563–8.
- Fletcher CD. Pleomorphic malignant fibrous histiocytoma: fact or fiction? A critical reappraisal based on 159 tumors diagnosed as pleomorphic sarcoma. *Am J Surg Pathol.* 1992;**16**: 213–28.
- Fletcher CD, Gustafson P, Rydholm A, Willén H, Akerman M. Clinicopathologic re-evaluation of 100 malignant fibrous histiocytomas: prognostic relevance of subclassification. *J Clin Oncol.* 2001;**19**: 3045–50.

- Guccion JG, Enzinger FM. Malignant giant cell tumor of soft parts. An analysis of 32 cases. *Cancer.* 1972;**29**:1518–29.
- Mentzel T, Calonje E, Fletcher CD. Leiomyosarcoma with prominent osteoclast-like giant cells. Analysis of eight cases closely mimicking the so-called giant cell variant of malignant fibrous histiocytoma. *Am J Surg Pathol.* 1994;**18**:258–65.
- Merck C, Angervall L, Kindblom LG, et al. Myxofibrosarcoma. A malignant soft tissue tumor of fibroblastic-histiocytic origin. A clinicopathologic and prognostic study of 110 cases using multivariate analysis. *Acta Pathol Microbiol Immunol Scand Suppl.* 1983;**282**: 1–40.
- Ozzello L, Stout AP, Murray MR. Cultural characteristics of malignant histiocytomas and fibrous xanthomas. *Cancer.* 1963;**16**:331–44.
- Salm R, Sissons HA. Giant-cell tumours of soft tissues. *J Pathol.* 1972;**107**:27–39.
- Weiss SW, Enzinger FM. Myxoid variant of malignant fibrous histiocytoma. *Cancer.* 1977;**39**:1672–85.
- Weiss SW, Enzinger FM. Malignant fibrous histiocytoma: an analysis of 200 cases. *Cancer* 1978;**41**:2250–66.

## Pleomorphic Rhabdomyosarcoma

- de Jong AS, van Kessel-van Vark M, Albus-Lutter CE. Pleomorphic rhabdomyosarcoma in adults: immunohistochemistry as a tool for its diagnosis. *Hum Pathol.* 1987;**18**:298–303.
- Fadare O, Bonvicino A, Martel M, et al. Pleomorphic rhabdomyosarcoma of the uterine corpus: a clinicopathologic study of 4 cases and a review of the literature. *Int J Gynecol Pathol.* 2010;**29**:122–34.
- Furlong MA, Fanburg-Smith JC. Pleomorphic rhabdomyosarcoma in children: four cases in the pediatric age group. *Ann Diagn Pathol.* 2001;**5**:199–206.
- Furlong MA, Mentzel T, Fanburg-Smith JC. Pleomorphic rhabdomyosarcoma in adults: a clinicopathologic study of 38 cases with emphasis on morphologic variants and recent skeletal muscle-specific markers. *Mod Pathol.* 2001;**14**:595–603.
- Gaffney EF, Dervan PA, Fletcher CD. Pleomorphic rhabdomyosarcoma in adulthood. Analysis of 11 cases with definition of diagnostic criteria. *Am J Surg Pathol.* 1993;**17**:601–9.

- Gagné E, Têtu B, Blondeau L, Raymond PE, Blais R. Morphologic prognostic factors of malignant mixed müllerian tumor of the uterus: a clinicopathologic study of 58 cases. *Mod Pathol.* 1989;**2**:433–8.
- Keyhani A, Booher RJ. Pleomorphic rhabdomyosarcoma. *Cancer.* 1968;**22**: 956–67.
- Li G, Ogose A, Kawashima H, et al. Cytogenetic and real-time quantitative reverse-transcriptase polymerase chain reaction analyses in pleomorphic rhabdomyosarcoma. *Cancer Genet Cytogenet.* 2009;**192**:1–9.
- Noujaim J, Thway K, Jones RL, et al. Adult pleomorphic rhabdomyosarcoma: a multicentre retrospective study. *Anticancer Res.* 2015;**35**:6213–17.
- Sternberg WH, Clark WH, Smith RC. Malignant mixed müllerian tumor (mixed mesodermal tumor of the uterus); a study of twenty-one cases. *Cancer.* 1954;**7**:704–24.
- Stout AP. Rhabdomyosarcoma of the skeletal muscles. *Ann Surg.* 1946;**123**: 447–72.

## Pleomorphic Liposarcoma

- Creytens D, Mentzel T, Ferdinande L, et al. "Atypical" pleomorphic lipomatous tumor: a clinicopathologic, immunohistochemical and molecular study of 21 cases, emphasizing its relationship to atypical spindle cell lipomatous tumor and suggesting a morphologic spectrum (atypical spindle cell/pleomorphic lipomatous tumor). *Am J Surg Pathol.* 2017;**41**: 1443–55.
- Dei Tos AP. Liposarcomas: diagnostic pitfalls and new insights. *Histopathology.* 2014;**64**:38–52.
- Dei Tos AP, Mentzel T, Fletcher CDM. Primary liposarcoma of the skin: a rare neoplasm with unusual high grade features. *Am J Dermatopathol.* 1998;**20**: 332–8.
- Downes KA, Goldblum JR, Montgomery EA, Fisher C. Pleomorphic liposarcoma: a clinicopathologic analysis of 19 cases. *Mod Pathol.* 2001;**14**:179–84.
- Gardner JM, Dandekar M, Thomas D, et al. Cutaneous and subcutaneous pleomorphic liposarcoma: a clinicopathologic study of 29 cases with evaluation of MDM2 gene amplification in 26. *Am J Surg Pathol.* 2012;**36**:1047–51.
- Gebhard S, Coindre JM, Michels JJ, et al. Pleomorphic liposarcoma: clinicopathologic,

immunohistochemical, and follow-up analysis of 63 cases: a study from the French Federation of Cancer Centers Sarcoma Group. *Am J Surg Pathol.* 2002;**26**:601–16.

- Ghadimi MP, Liu P, Peng T, et al. Pleomorphic liposarcoma: clinical observations and molecular variables. *Cancer.* 2011;**117**:5359–69.

- Hornick JL, Bosenberg MW, Mentzel T, et al. Pleomorphic liposarcoma: clinicopathologic analysis of 57 cases. *Am J Surg Pathol.* 2004;**28**:1257–67.

- Mariño-Enríquez A, Fletcher CD, Dal Cin P, Hornick JL. Dedifferentiated liposarcoma with "homologous" lipoblastic (pleomorphic liposarcoma-like) differentiation: clinicopathologic and molecular analysis of a series suggesting revised diagnostic criteria. *Am J Surg Pathol.* 2010;**34**:1122–31.

- Miettinen M, Enzinger FM. Epithelioid variant of pleomorphic liposarcoma: a study of 12 cases of a distinctive variant of high-grade liposarcoma. *Mod Pathol.* 1999;**12**:722–8.

- Oliveira AM, Nascimento AG. Pleomorphic liposarcoma. *Semin Diagn Pathol.* 2001;**18**:274–85.

- Shmookler BM, Enzinger FM. Pleomorphic lipoma: a benign tumor simulating liposarcoma. A clinicopathologic analysis of 48 cases. *Cancer.* 1981;**1**(47):126–33.

- Tandon B, Hagemann IS, Maluf HM, Pfeifer JD, Al-Kateb H. Association of Li-Fraumeni syndrome with small cell carcinoma of the ovary, hypercalcemic type and concurrent pleomorphic liposarcoma of the cervix. *Int J Gynecol Pathol.* 2017;**36**:593–9.

# Dedifferentiated Liposarcoma

- Ambrosini G, Sambol EB, Carvajal D, et al. Mouse double minute antagonist Nutlin-3a enhances chemotherapy-induced apoptosis in cancer cells with mutant p53 by activating E2F1. *Oncogene.* 2007;**26**:3473–81.

- Binh MB, Guillou L, Hostein I, et al. Dedifferentiated liposarcomas with divergent myosarcomatous differentiation developed in the internal trunk: a study of 27 cases and comparison to conventional dedifferentiated liposarcomas and leiomyosarcomas. *Am J Surg Pathol.* 2007;**31**:1557–66.

- Binh MB, Sastre-Garau X, Guillou L, et al. MDM2 and CDK4 immunostainings are useful adjuncts in diagnosing

well-differentiated and dedifferentiated liposarcoma subtypes: a comparative analysis of 559 soft tissue neoplasms with genetic data. *Am J Surg Pathol.* 2005;**29**:1340–7.

- Coindre JM, Hostein I, Maire G, et al. Inflammatory fibrous histiocytoma and dedifferentiated liposarcoma: histological review, genomic profile, and MDM2 and CDK4 status favour a single entity. *J Pathol.* 2004;**203**:822–30.

- Dei Tos AP. Liposarcomas: diagnostic pitfalls and new insights. *Histopathology.* 2014;**64**:38–52.

- Dei Tos AP, Doglioni C, Piccinin S, et al. Molecular abnormalities of the p53 pathway in dedifferentiated liposarcoma. *J Pathol.* 1997;**181**:8–13.

- Evans HL. Liposarcoma: a study of 55 cases with a reassessment of its classification. *Am J Surg Pathol.* 1979;**3**:507–23.

- Evans HL. Atypical lipomatous tumor, its variants, and its combined forms: a study of 61 cases, with a minimum follow-up of 10 years. *Am J Surg Pathol.* 2007;**31**:1–14.

- Evans HL, Khurana KK, Kemp BL, Ahayla AG. Heterologous elements in the dedifferentiated component of dedifferentiated liposarcoma. *Am J Surg Pathol.* 1994;**18**:1150–7.

- Fanburg-Smith JC, Miettinen M. Liposarcoma with meningothelial-like whorls: a study of 17 cases of a distinctive histological pattern associated with dedifferentiated liposarcoma. *Histopathology.* 1998;**33**:414–24.

- Gronchi A, Collini P, Miceli R, et al. Myogenic differentiation and histologic grading are major prognostic determinants in retroperitoneal liposarcoma. *Am J Surg Pathol.* 2015;**39**:383–93.

- Gronchi A, Lo Vullo S, Fiore M, et al. Aggressive surgical policies in a retrospectively reviewed single-institution case series of retroperitoneal soft tissue sarcoma patients. *J Clin Oncol.* 2009;**27**:24–30.

- Huang HY, Brennan MF, Singer S, Antonescu CR. Distant metastasis in retroperitoneal dedifferentiated liposarcoma is rare and rapidly fatal: a clinicopathological study with emphasis on the low-grade myxofibrosarcoma-like pattern as an early sign of dedifferentiation. *Mod Pathol.* 2005;**18**:976–84.

- Le Guellec S, Chibon F, Ouali M, et al. Are peripheral purely undifferentiated pleomorphic sarcomas with MDM2 amplification dedifferentiated

liposarcomas? *Am J Surg Pathol.* 2014;**38**:293–304.

- Lucas DR, Shukla A, Thomas DG, et al. Dedifferentiated liposarcoma with inflammatory myofibroblastic tumor-like features. *Am J Surg Pathol.* 2010;**34**:844–51.

- Mariani O, Brennetot C, Coindre JM, et al. JUN oncogene amplification and overexpression block adipocytic differentiation in highly aggressive sarcomas. *Cancer Cell.* 2007;**11**:361–74.

- Mariño-Enríquez A, Fletcher CD, Dal Cin P, Hornick JL. Dedifferentiated liposarcoma with "homologous" lipoblastic (pleomorphic liposarcoma-like) differentiation: clinicopathologic and molecular analysis of a series suggesting revised diagnostic criteria. *Am J Surg Pathol.* 2010;**34**:1122–31.

- Mertens F, Fletcher CDM, Dal Cin P, et al. Cytogenetic analysis of 46 pleomorphic soft tissue sarcomas and correlation with morphologic and clinical features: a report of the CHAMP study group. CHromosomes And MorPhology. *Genes Chromosomes Cancer.* 1998;**22**:16–25.

- Mussi C, Collini P, Miceli R, et al. The prognostic impact of dedifferentiation in retroperitoneal liposarcoma: a series of surgically treated patients at a single institution. *Cancer.* 2008;**113**:1657–65.

- Nascimento AG: Dedifferentiated liposarcoma. *Sem Diagn Pathol.* 2001;**18**:263–6.

- Nascimento AG, Kurtin PJ, Guillou L, Fletcher CDM. Dedifferentiated liposarcoma. A report of nine cases with a peculiar neurallike whorling pattern associated with metaplastic bone formation. *Am J Surg Pathol.* 1998;**22**:945–55.

- Pissaloux D, Loarer FL, Decouvelaere AV, et al. MDM4 amplification in a case of de-differentiated liposarcoma and in-silico data supporting an oncogenic event alternative to MDM2 amplification in a subset of cases. *Histopathology.* 2017;**71**:1019–23.

- Ricciotti RW, Baraff AJ, Jour G, et al. High amplification levels of MDM2 and CDK4 correlate with poor outcome in patients with dedifferentiated liposarcoma: A cytogenomic microarray analysis of 47 cases. *Cancer Genet.* 2017;**218–219**:69–80.

- Saâda-Bouzid E, Burel-Vandenbos F, Ranchère-Vince D, et al. Prognostic value of HMGA2, CDK4, and JUN amplification in well-differentiated and dedifferentiated liposarcomas. *Mod Pathol*. 2015;**28**:1404–14.

- Singer S, Socci ND, Ambrosini G, et al. Gene expression profiling of liposarcoma identifies distinct biological types/ subtypes and potential therapeutic targets in well-differentiated and dedifferentiated liposarcoma. *Cancer Res*. 2007;**67**:6626–36.

- Snyder EL, Sandstrom DJ, Law K, et al. c-Jun amplification and overexpression are oncogenic in liposarcoma but not always sufficient to inhibit the adipocytic differentiation programme. *J Pathol*. 2009;**218**:292–300.

- Ware PL, Snow AN, Gvalani M, Pettenati MJ, Qasem SA. MDM2 copy numbers in well-differentiated and dedifferentiated liposarcoma: characterizing progression to high-grade tumors. *Am J Clin Pathol*. 2014;**141**: 334–41.

- Weiss SW, Rao VK. Well-differentiated liposarcoma (atypical lipoma) of deep soft tissue of the extremities, retroperitoneum and miscellaneous sites. A follow-up study of 92 cases with analysis of the incidence of dedifferentiation. *Am J Surg Pathol*. 1992;**16**:1051–8.

- Yamashita K, Kohashi K, Yamada Y, et al. Osteogenic differentiation in dedifferentiated liposarcoma: a study of 36 cases in comparison to the cases without ossification. *Histopathology*. 2018;**72**:729–38.

## Extraskeletal Osteosarcoma

- Berner K, Bjerkehagen B, Bruland ØS, Berner A. Extraskeletal osteosarcoma in Norway, between 1975 and 2009, and a brief review of the literature. *Anticancer Res*. 2015;**35**:2129–40.

- Conner JR, Hornick JL. SATB2 is a novel marker of osteoblastic differentiation in bone and soft tissue tumours. *Histopathology*. 2013;**63**:36–49.

- de Silva MV, Reid R. Myositis ossificans and fibroosseous pseudotumor of digits: a clinicopathological review of 64 cases with emphasis on diagnostic pitfalls. *Int J Surg Pathol*. 2003;**11**:187–95.

- Folpe AL, Weiss SW. Ossifying fibromyxoid tumor of soft parts: a clinicopathologic study of 70 cases with emphasis on atypical and malignant variants. *Am J Surg Pathol*. 2003;**27**: 421–31.

- Jones M, Chebib I, Deshpande V, Nielsen GP. Radiation-associated low-grade extraskeletal osteosarcoma of

the neck following treatment for thyroid cancer. *Int J Surg Pathol*. 2015;**23**:384–7.

- Lee JS, Fetsch JF, Wasdhal DA, et al. A review of 40 patients with extraskeletal osteosarcoma. *Cancer*. 1995;**1**(76): 2253–9.

- Lidang Jensen M, Schumacher B, Myhre Jensen O, Steen Nielsen O, Keller J. Extraskeletal osteosarcomas: a clinicopathologic study of 25 cases. *Am J Surg Pathol*. 1998;**22**:588–94.

## Pleomorphic "High-Grade" Myxofibrosarcoma

- Angervall L, Kindblom LG, Merck C. Myxofibrosarcoma. A study of 30 cases. *Acta Pathol Microbiol Scand A*. 1977;**85A**: 127–40.

- Merck C, Angervall L, Kindblom LG, et al. Myxofibrosarcoma. A malignant soft tissue tumor of fibroblastic-histiocytic origin. A clinicopathologic and prognostic study of 110 cases using multivariate analysis. *Acta Pathol Microbiol Immunol Scand Suppl*. 1983;**282**:1–40.

- Weiss SW, Enzinger FM. Myxoid variant of malignant fibrous histiocytoma. *Cancer*. 1977;**39**:1672–85.

- Willems SM, Debiec-Rychter M, Szuhai K, Hogendoorn PC, Sciot R. Local recurrence of myxofibrosarcoma is associated with increase in tumour grade and cytogenetic aberrations, suggesting a multistep tumour progression model. *Mod Pathol*. 2006;**19**:407–16.

## Pleomorphic Leiomyosarcoma

- Oda Y, Miyajima K, Kawaguchi K, et al. Pleomorphic leiomyosarcoma: clinicopathologic and immunohistochemical study with special emphasis on its distinction from ordinary leiomyosarcoma and malignant fibrous histiocytoma. *Am J Surg Pathol*. 2001;**25**: 1030–8.

## Atypical Fibroxanthoma

- Dei Tos AP, Maestro R, Doglioni C, et al. Ultraviolet-induced p53 mutations in atypical fibroxanthoma. *Am J Pathol*. 1994;**145**:11–17.

- Griewank KG, Schilling B, Murali R, et al. TERT promoter mutations are frequent in atypical fibroxanthomas and pleomorphic dermal sarcomas. *Mod Pathol*. 2014;**27**:502–8.

- Griewank KG, Wiesner T, Murali R, et al. Atypical fibroxanthoma and

pleomorphic dermal sarcoma harbor frequent NOTCH1/2 and FAT1 mutations and similar DNA copy number alteration profiles. *Mod Pathol*. 2018;**31**:418–28.

- Gru AA, Santa Cruz DJ. Atypical fibroxanthoma: a selective review. *Semin Diagn Pathol*. 2013;**30**:4–12.

- Kuwano H, Hashimoto H, Enjoji M. Atypical fibroxanthoma distinguishable from spindle cell carcinoma in sarcoma-like skin lesions. A clinicopathologic and immunohistochemical study of 21 cases. *Cancer*. 1985;**1**(55):172–80.

- Miller K, Goodlad JR, Brenn T. Pleomorphic dermal sarcoma: adverse histologic features predict aggressive behavior and allow distinction from atypical fibroxanthoma. *Am J Surg Pathol*. 2012;**36**:1317–26.

- Widemann BC, Italiano A. Biology and management of undifferentiated pleomorphic sarcoma, myxofibrosarcoma, and malignant peripheral nerve sheath tumors: state of the art and perspectives. *J Clin Oncol*. 2018;**36**:160–7.

## Pleomorphic Hyalinizing Angiectatic Tumor

- Antonescu CR, Zhang L, Nielsen GP, et al. Consistent t(1;10) with rearrangements of TGFBR3 and MGEA5 in both myxoinflammatory fibroblastic sarcoma and hemosiderotic fibrolipomatous tumor. *Genes Chromosomes Cancer*. 2011;**50**: 757–64.

- Boland JM, Folpe AL. Hemosiderotic fibrolipomatous tumor, pleomorphic hyalinizing angiectatic tumor, and myxoinflammatory fibroblastic sarcoma: related or not? *Adv Anat Pathol*. 2017;**24**: 268–77.

- Carter JM, Sukov WR, Montgomery E, et al. TGFBR3 and MGEA5 rearrangements in pleomorphic hyalinizing angiectatic tumors and the spectrum of related neoplasms. *Am J Surg Pathol*. 2014;**38**: 1182–992.

- Folpe AL, Weiss SW. Pleomorphic hyalinizing angiectatic tumor: analysis of 41 cases supporting evolution from a distinctive precursor lesion. *Am J Surg Pathol*. 2004;**28**:1417–25.

- Smith ME, Fisher C, Weiss SW. Pleomorphic hyalinizing angiectatic tumor of soft parts. A low-grade neoplasm resembling neurilemoma. *Am J Surg Pathol*. 1996;**20**:21–9.

# Myxoid Sarcomas

Marta Sbaraglia MD and Angelo Paolo Dei Tos MD

## Introduction

The presence of abundant extracellular myxoid matrix represents the most distinctive morphologic feature of a variety of benign and malignant mesenchymal lesions. This chapter will focus on those lesions in which a myxoid background represents a predominant morphologic finding. The many other mesenchymal tumors that may occasionally feature myxoid change of the stroma are discussed separately. In consideration of significant morphologic overlap, this heterogeneous group of lesions poses remarkable diagnostic challenges. Both immunohistochemistry and molecular genetics may provide important clues to correct diagnosis; however, their utility varies significantly depending on the histotype (Tables 8.1 and 8.2).

As always, it is important that ancillary diagnostic techniques are evaluated in strict context with morphology. As an example, when dealing with myxoid soft tissue tumors, key morphologic features are represented by the presence/absence of pleomorphism, architectural organization of the vascular network (plexiform versus curvilinear), and presence/absence of alternation between myxoid and collagenous stroma. As will be discussed in detail, the combination of the above-mentioned criteria would allow the recognition of at least three main myxoid malignancies: myxofibrosarcoma, low-grade fibromyxoid sarcoma, and myxoid liposarcoma. Of course, key diagnostic clues may be represented only focally; therefore, surgically the specimen should always be carefully sampled.

**Table 8.1** Immunophenotypic features of myxoid sarcomas

| Sarcoma type | S100 | MUC4 | Desmin | Myogenin | SMA | CD34 | EMA |
|---|---|---|---|---|---|---|---|
| Myxofibrosarcoma | – | – | – | – | 60% | 40% | –* |
| Myxoinflammatory fibroblastic sarcoma | – | – | – | – | 10% | 20% | – |
| Low-grade fibromyxoid sarcoma | – | >95% | – | – | – | – | 60% |
| Myxoid liposarcoma | 70% | – | – | – | – | – | – |
| Extraskeletal myxoid chondrosarcoma | <20% | – | – | – | – | – | 20% |
| Ossifying fibromyxoid tumor | 80% | – | 50% | – | – | – | <5% |
| Embryonal rhabdomyosarcoma | 5% | – | >95% | 100% | 10% | – | <5% |

* Positivity for EMA is observed in the epithelioid variant of myxofibrosarcoma

**Table 8.2** Genetics of round cell sarcomas (not including Ewing sarcoma)

| Sarcoma type | Cytogenetic alterations | Molecular alterations |
|---|---|---|
| Myxofibrosarcoma | Complex aberrations | *NF1* aberrations in 10% of cases |
| Myxoinflammatory fibroblastic sarcoma | t(1;10)(p22-23;q24-25) | *TGFBR3* and *MGEA5* |
| Low-grade fibromyxoid sarcoma | t(7;16)(q33;p11)<br>t(11;16)(p11;p11)<br>ring chromosomes | *FUS-CREB3L2*<br>*FUS-CREB3L1* |
| Myxoid liposarcoma | t(12;16)(q13;p11)<br>t(12;22)(q13;q12) | *DDIT3-FUS*<br>*DDIT3-EWSR1* |
| Extraskeletal myxoid chondrosarcoma | t(9;22)(q22;q12)<br>t(9;17)(q22;q11)<br>t(9;15)(q22;q21) | *NR4A3-EWSR1*<br>*NR4A3-TAF15*<br>*NR4A3-TCF12* |
| Ossifying fibromyxoid tumor | | *EPC1-PHF1; MEAF6-PHF1; ZC3H7B-BCOR* |
| Embryonal rhabdomyosarcoma | Complex aberrations | *IGF2, CDKN1C* |

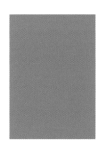

# Myxofibrosarcoma

## Definition and Epidemiology

Myxofibrosarcoma represents a morphologic spectrum of fibroblastic neoplasia, characterized by the presence of a variable amount of myxoid stroma. First reported in 1977 by Angervall, high-grade myxofibrosarcoma corresponds to the lesion designated by Enzinger as "myxoid malignant fibrous histiocytoma." Myxofibrosarcoma typically occurs in the elderly population (wherein it represents the most common mesenchymal malignancy), with a peak incidence in the seventh decade and a slight male predominance.

## Clinical Presentation and Outcome

Myxofibrosarcoma shows marked predilection for the subcutaneous tissue of the limbs and limb girdles. Two-thirds of the cases are superficially located, whereas one-third are deeply seated. Occurrence in the retroperitoneum and in the abdominal cavity is extremely rare. The treatment of choice for myxofibrosarcoma is wide surgical excision. Negative margins, however, are often difficult to obtain, because these tumors tend to have an infiltrative growth pattern and to extend along subcutaneous fibrous septa. The rate of local recurrence is about 50%, and importantly, it can be accompanied by morphologic progression to a higher grade. The risk of developing distant metastases (primarily to the lungs and bone) is about 30% and is generally limited to high-grade lesions. Metastatic spread to locoregional lymph nodes is sometimes observed. Overall survival ranges between 60 and 70%.

## Morphology and Immunophenotype

Grossly, superficially located lesions typically exhibit a multinodular gelatinous appearance(Fig. 8-1), whereas deep-seated lesions usually appear as large masses with myxoid and necrotic foci (Fig. 8-2). In general, myxofibrosarcoma tends to exhibit infiltrative margins. The microscopic spectrum of myxofibrosarcoma depends on its grade; however, there exist some morphologic features that tend to be invariably present. At low-power magnification, the most distinctive feature is the presence of multiple nodules separated by incomplete fibrous septa (Fig. 8-3). Low-grade lesions are remarkably hypocellular, composed of spindle and stellate neoplastic cells featuring atypical hyperchromatic nuclei and set in a prominent myxoid matrix (Fig. 8-4). Some neoplastic cells may exhibit univacuolated or multivacuolated, mucin-laden cytoplasm and are labeled "pseudolipoblasts" to distinguish them from true lipoblasts (Fig. 8-5). A very distinctive morphologic finding of myxofibrosarcoma (of any grade) is represented by the presence of curvilinear, thin-walled blood vessels (Fig. 8-6), around which tumor cells tend to cluster (Fig. 8-7). Mitotic activity in low-grade myxofibrosarcoma is generally low. As discussed in Chapter 7, the other extreme of the spectrum is formed by high-grade pleomorphic tumors, in which spindle and pleomorphic neoplastic cells grow in solid sheets and

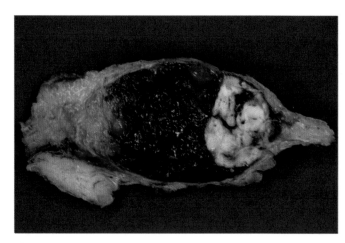

**Fig. 8-1.** Low-grade myxofibrosarcoma. Grossly, the tumor is superficially located and ill-defined, and exhibits a gelatinous appearance.

**Fig. 8-2.** High-grade myxofibrosarcoma. High-grade tumors present as large and deep-seated, featuring abundant necrosis and hemorrhage. Myxoid nodules are seen at the periphery of the lesion.

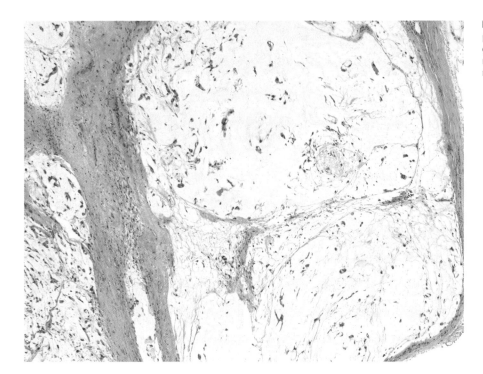

**Fig. 8-3.** Low-grade myxofibrosarcoma. At low power, the tumor shows a multinodular pattern of growth. Thick, fibrous septa separate the neoplastic nodules, which are composed of scattered atypical neoplastic cells set in a myxoid background.

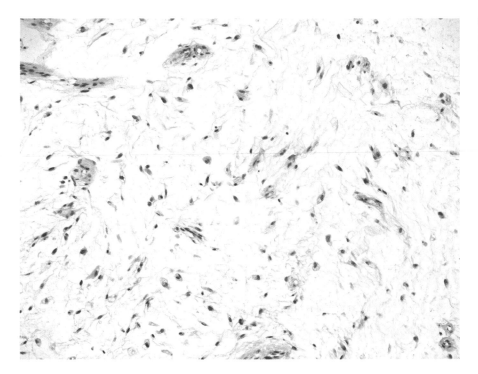

**Fig. 8-4.** Low-grade myxofibrosarcoma. The tumor is composed of a hypocellular proliferation of spindle cells with hyperchromatic nuclei, set in a highly vascularized, myxoid stroma.

fascicles, sometimes exhibiting a storiform arrangement (Fig. 8-8). Severe nuclear atypia, pleomorphism, high mitotic activity, hemorrhage, and necrosis all represent relatively common findings (Fig. 8-9). Often, a transition from low-grade to high-grade areas is encountered (Fig. 8-10). The amount of myxoid areas is very variable. Cases exist in which myxoid change can be minimal, and morphology may therefore entirely overlap with undifferentiated pleomorphic sarcomas. As outlined in Chapter 5, high-grade myxofibrosarcoma may rarely assume a striking epithelioid morphology that correlates with more aggressive clinical behavior (Fig. 8-11).

Immunohistochemically, neoplastic cells are often CD34 positive and may stain focally for smooth muscle actin, whereas all other differentiation markers are negative.

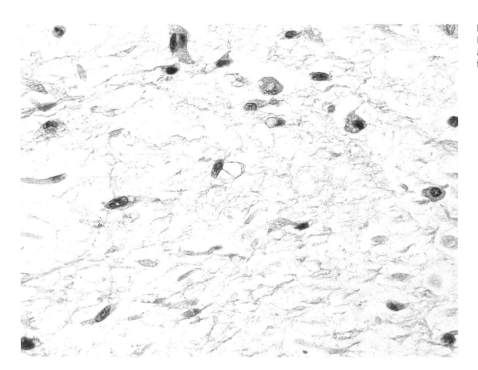

**Fig. 8-5.** Low-grade myxofibrosarcoma. Neoplastic cells featuring mucin-laden cytoplasm are labeled "pseudolipoblasts" to distinguish them from true lipoblasts.

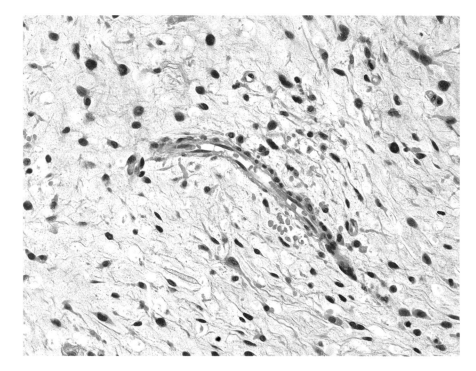

**Fig. 8-6.** Myxofibrosarcoma. One of the most distinctive morphologic features is represented by the presence of curvilinear, thin-walled blood vessels.

## Genetics

Cytogenetic analysis of myxofibrosarcoma has demonstrated several complex chromosomal aberrations, but no specific abnormality has emerged so far, the only exception being various NF1 aberrations observed in approximately 10% of cases.

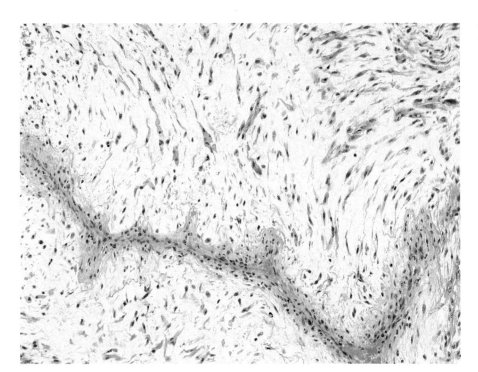

**Fig. 8-7.** Myxofibrosarcoma. Clusters of neoplastic cells are arranged around archiform blood vessels.

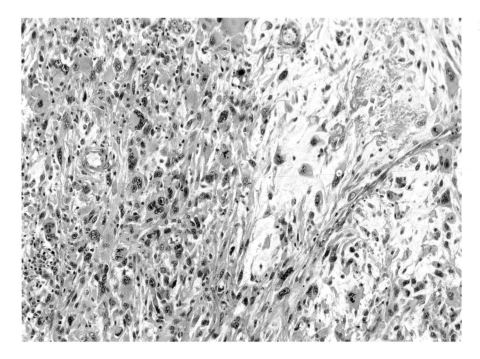

**Fig. 8-8.** High-grade myxofibrosarcoma. The tumor is composed of atypical spindle and pleomorphic cells arranged in solid sheets and fascicles with numerous atypical mitotic figures.

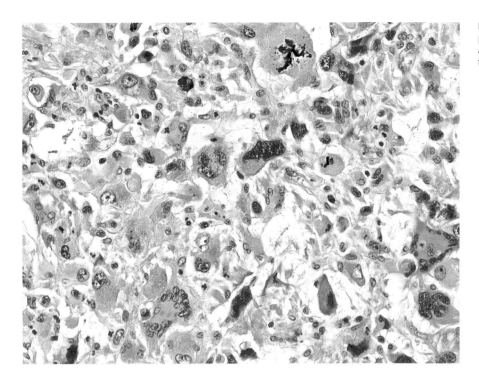

**Fig. 8-9.** High-grade myxofibrosarcoma. At high power, severe nuclear atypia, pleomorphism, and aberrant mitotic figures represent consistent features in high-grade tumors.

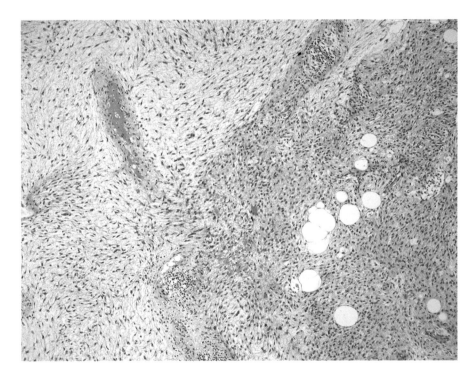

**Fig. 8-10.** Myxofibrosarcoma. The tumor shows a somewhat abrupt transition from low-grade (*left*) to high-grade (*right*) areas.

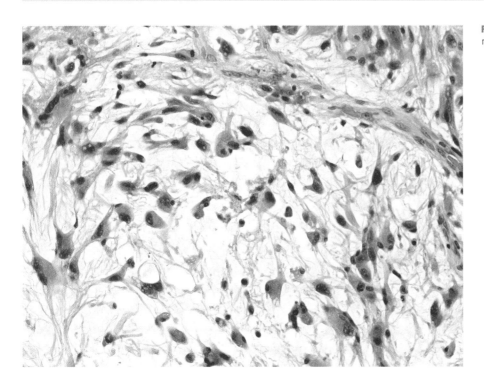

**Fig. 8-11.** Myxofibrosarcoma. High-grade tumors may show striking epithelioid morphology.

## Differential Diagnosis and Diagnostic Pitfalls

The differential diagnosis of myxofibrosarcoma depends on the grade of the lesion. Low-grade myxofibrosarcoma main differentials include superficial angiomyxoma, acral fibromyxoma, intramuscular and juxta-articular myxomas, deep "aggressive" angiomyxoma, reticular microcystic schwannoma, low-grade myxoid liposarcoma, and low-grade fibromyxoid sarcoma (Table 8.3).

**Superficial angiomyxoma** is a rare myxoid mesenchymal lesion, primarily occurring in middle-aged adults, characterized by a high tendency (up to 50%) for non-destructive local recurrences. The trunk, followed by the head and neck region, represents the most frequent anatomic location. Most cases occur as sporadic lesions; however, superficial angiomyxoma is also observed as part of the Carney complex. This is an autosomal dominant syndrome presenting with a variable combination of pigmentary disorders of the skin, myxomas, schwannomas, and endocrine abnormalities (pigmented nodular adrenocortical disease). Microscopically, superficial angiomyxoma is composed of hypocellular, ill-defined neoplastic lobules containing spindle and stellate cells set in a myxoid background (Fig. 8-12). Scattered neutrophils can be observed in approximately 50% of cases (Fig. 8-13). In consideration of the superficial location, epithelial inclusions may be frequently seen. Mild cytologic atypia is sometimes seen; however, in contrast to myxofibrosarcoma, overt nuclear hyperchromasia is not observed. Immunohistochemically, neoplastic cells may express focally smooth muscle actin and CD34.

**Acral (digital) fibromyxoma** is a rare cutaneous lesion occurring on fingers and toes of adults (peak incidence is in the fourth decade). The involvement of the nail bed is observed very frequently. Morphologically, the lesion is composed of

**Table 8.3** Differential diagnosis of low-grade myxofibrosarcoma

| Benign/locally aggressive | Malignant |
| --- | --- |
| Ganglion | Myxoid liposarcoma |
| Intramuscular myxoma | Myxoinflammatory fibroblastic sarcoma |
| Juxta-articular myxoma | Low-grade fibromyxoid sarcoma |
| Acral digital fibromyxoma | |
| Superficial angiomyxoma | |
| Myxoid nerve sheath tumor | |
| Reticula/microcystic schwannoma | |
| Deep "aggressive" angiomyxoma | |

spindle and/or stellate fibroblasts set in a myxocollagenous matrix (Fig. 8-14). Occasionally, moderate atypia can be observed, raising some concern. Immunohistochemically, CD34 immunopositivity is seen in most cases (Fig. 8-15). Acral fibromyxoma pursues an invariably benign clinical course; however, local recurrences are observed in approximately 20% of cases.

**Intramuscular myxoma** is a benign lesion that most often occurs in the limbs and limb girdles of adults (peak incidence is between the fifth and seventh decade) with significant female predominance. The thigh is the most commonly affected anatomic site, followed by the arm and the buttock. The association of intramuscular myxomas and polyostotic

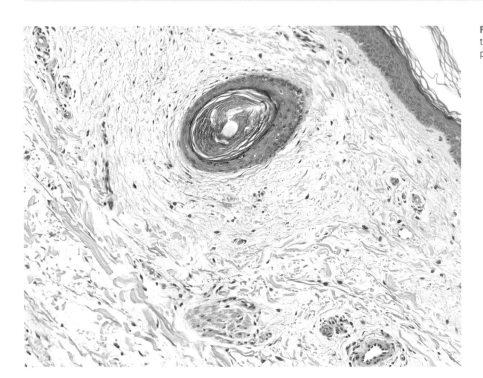

**Fig. 8-12.** Superficial angiomyxoma. At low power, the tumor shows an infiltrative growth. Note the presence of epithelial inclusions.

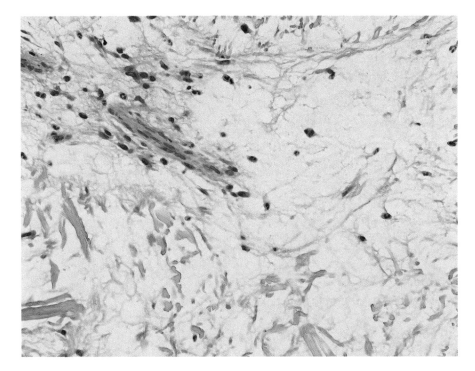

**Fig. 8-13.** Superficial angiomyxoma. The tumor is composed of bland spindle cells set in abundant myxoid stroma. The presence of scattered neutrophils represents a distinctive morphologic feature.

skeletal fibrous dysplasia represents a syndromic disorder known as Mazabraud syndrome. At variance with low-grade myxofibrosarcoma, intramuscular myxoma is always deep seated and uninodular (Fig. 8-16). Microscopically, myxomas are composed of a hypocellular spindle cell and/or stellate cell population set in an abundant myxoid matrix (Fig. 8-17). Vascularization in most cases is limited to a few capillary-sized blood vessels. Infiltration of the surrounding skeletal muscle fibers represents a relatively common phenomenon.

One major diagnostic pitfall is represented by the presence of increased cellularity (so-called cellular myxoma) that is often associated with an increased number of blood vessels (Fig. 8-18). Cellular myxomas are also benign; however, they seem to exhibit a greater risk of local recurrence. The absence of nuclear atypia remains the most important diagnostic clue to exclude low-grade myxofibrosarcoma (Fig. 8-19). Genetically, intramuscular myxomas are characterized by point mutations of the *GNAS* gene. Interestingly, this genetic

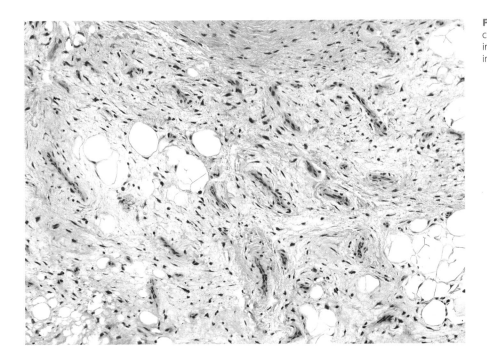

**Fig. 8-14.** Acral fibromyxoma. The tumor is composed of spindle to stellate neoplastic cells set in myxocollagenous stroma. Fat tissue can be included within the lesion.

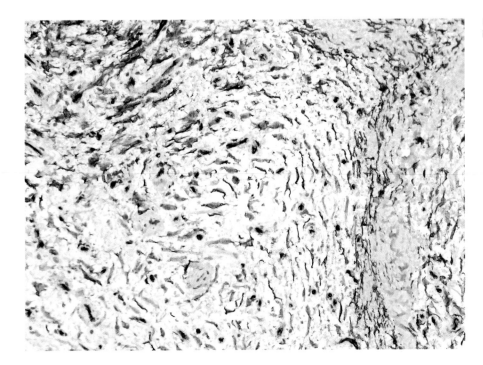

**Fig. 8-15.** Acral fibromyxoma. CD34 immunopositivity is often seen.

aberration seems to be absent in the closely related entity called "juxta-articular myxomas." Juxta-articular myxomas (as the name implies) occur close to the large joints (most often the knee and shoulder) of adult patients. Morphologically, they exhibit almost complete overlap with cellular myxoma. At variance with intramuscular myxomas that most often do not recur, juxta-articular myxomas often feature local, even multiple local, recurrence.

**Deep "aggressive" angiomyxoma** represents a rather unique mesenchymal lesion primarily occurring in the genital areas of young to middle-aged female patients. Similar lesions may be occasionally encountered in males. Deep angiomyxoma is typically ill defined, always exhibiting infiltrative margins. Microscopically, a hypocellular spindle cell population is observed, associated with hyalinized small to medium-sized blood vessels (Fig. 8-20). A relatively common as well as distinctive morphologic finding is represented by the so-called spinning off of smooth muscle cells from the wall of blood vessels (Fig. 8-21). Immunohistochemically, neoplastic cells show positivity for desmin and smooth muscle actin.

Interestingly, deep angiomyxoma may feature a recurrent genetic abnormality represented by the rearrangement of the *HMGA2* gene. Deep "aggressive angiomyxoma" exhibits a remarkable tendency to recur locally; however, there exists growing evidence that complete excision (certainly difficult to achieve in some cases) may be curative.

Myxoid change of the stroma can be encountered in basically all benign neural neoplasms; however, there exists one variant, **reticular/microcystic schwannoma**, in which myxoid change is typically prominent. Reticular/microcystic schwannoma is benign; even if it may occur at any anatomic location, it shows a distinctive tropism for visceral locations, particularly

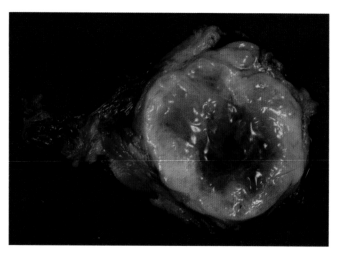

**Fig. 8-16.** Intramuscular myxoma. Grossly, the tumor is typically a uninodular, intramuscular mass featuring a gelatinous cut surface.

in the gastrointestinal tract. Neoplastic cells are spindled and cytologically bland, and exhibit a distinctive reticular pattern of growth (Fig. 8-22). The presence of abundant myxoid stroma generates the formation of the microcystic spaces that contribute to the name of the lesion (Fig. 8-23). Similar to any other schwannoma variant, reticular/microcystic schwannoma is diffusely S100 positive (Fig. 8-24).

Another neural lesion that, in consideration of both its distinctive multinodularity and superficial location, enters the differential diagnosis with low-grade myxofibrosarcoma is **dermal nerve sheath myxoma**. Nerve sheath myxoma is a benign, well-circumscribed lesion, most often occurring in the distal extremities of adults (peak incidence is in the third decade) with no sex predominance. Microscopically, the lesion is composed of a multinodular proliferation of spindle cells, set in an abundant myxoid matrix (Figs. 8-25 and 8-26). Immunohistochemically, as a further proof of schwannian differentiation, lesional cells diffusely express S100, which can be also associated with the expression of glial fibrillary acid protein (GFAP). Dermal nerve sheath myxoma is currently regarded as unrelated to **cellular neurothekeoma**, a cutaneous lesion that chiefly occurs in the head and neck region, is not well circumscribed, and exhibits a distinctive nesting pattern of growth (Fig. 8-27). Occasionally, cellular neurothekeoma features myxoid areas that raise diagnostic confusion with nerve sheath myxoma (Fig. 8-28). However, cellular neurothekeoma (with or without myxoid change) is characterized by an S100-negative/CD63-positive immunophenotype. Occasionally, cellular neurothekeoma may exhibit atypical features such as the presence of nuclear pleomorphism and even atypical mitotic figures that,

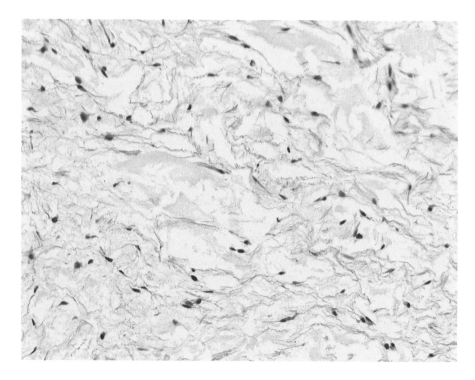

**Fig. 8-17.** Myxoma. A hypocellular tumor composed of non-atypical spindle cells is shown. In classic examples, the stroma exhibits abundant myxoid matrix and poor vascularization.

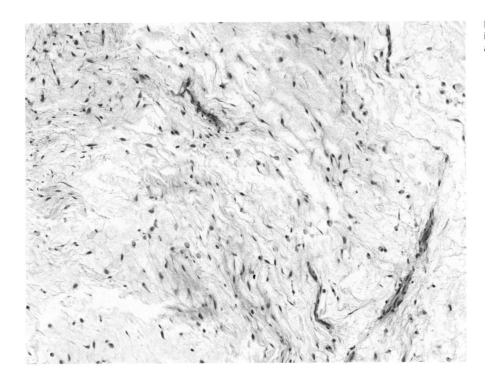

**Fig. 8-18.** Cellular myxoma. The tumor shows increased cellularity. Neoplastic cells are not atypical and blood vessels tend to be more numerous.

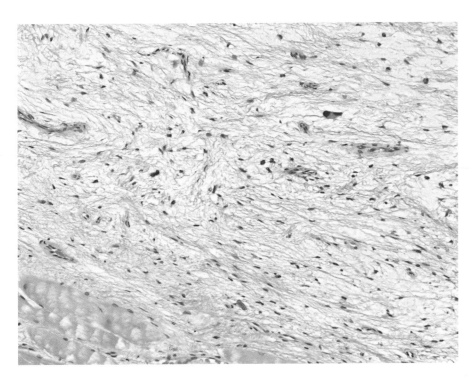

**Fig. 8-19.** Intramuscular low-grade myxofibrosarcoma. The presence of atypical cells featuring hyperchromatic nuclei represent the key diagnostic clue.

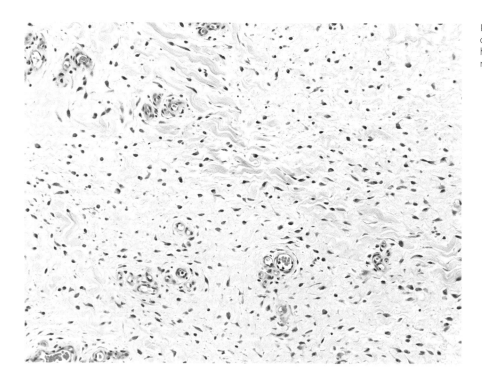

**Fig. 8-20.** Deep angiomyxoma. The tumor is composed of spindle cells associated with hyalinized, small blood vessels. The stroma is myxoid and contains eosinophilic collagen bundles.

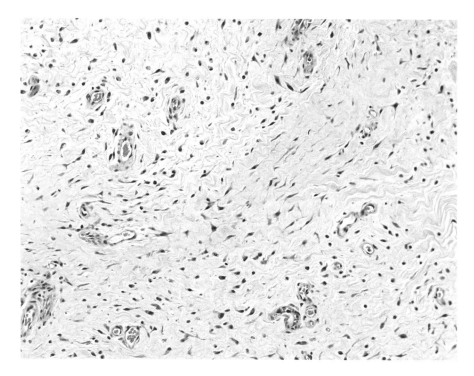

**Fig. 8-21.** Deep angiomyxoma. Note the abundance of blood vessels and the "spinning off" of smooth muscle cells.

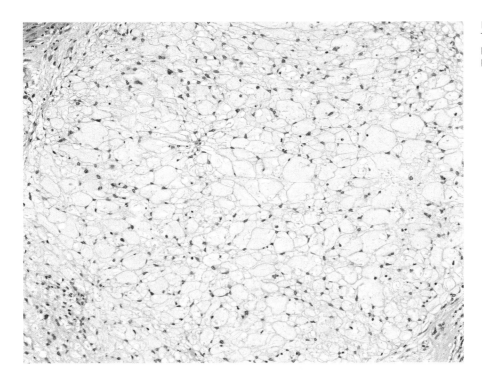

**Fig. 8-22.** Reticular/microcystic schwannoma. The tumor is composed of a spindle cell proliferation organized in a distinctive reticular pattern of growth.

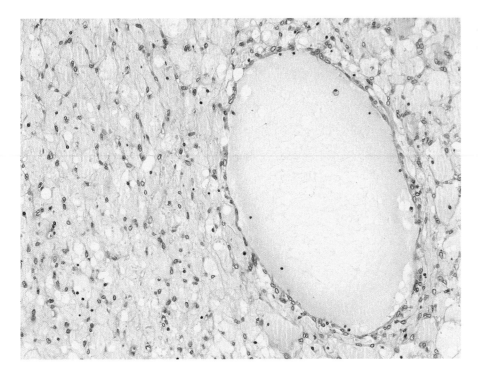

**Fig. 8-23.** Reticular/microcystic schwannoma. The formation of microcystic spaces represents a characteristic morphologic feature of the lesion.

however, do not seem to have an impact on the clinical outcome (Fig. 8-29).

Low-grade myxoid liposarcoma is discussed in detail in this chapter and may also enter in the differential diagnosis. Its characteristic capillary network, organized in a plexiform pattern (instead of the curvilinear vessels observed in myxofibrosarcoma), represents the key diagnostic clue. True lipoblasts (most often univacuolated) can be seen more often in the proximity of capillaries and need to be distinguished from mucin-laden pseudolipoblasts.

Low-grade fibromyxoid sarcoma is also discussed in this chapter and can be distinguished from myxofibrosarcoma because of the presence of the cytologically bland spindle cell proliferation set in a collagen-rich hyalinized matrix, juxtaposed with myxoid areas.

High-grade myxofibrosarcoma needs to be separated from other high-grade pleomorphic sarcomas as well as from non-

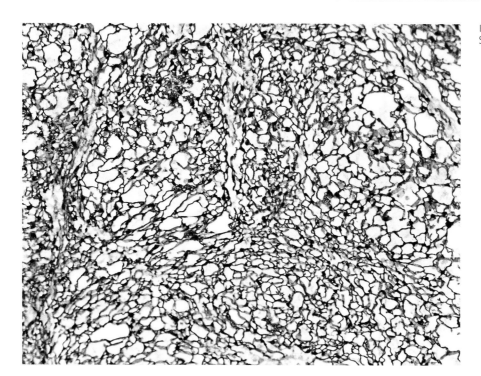

Fig. 8-24. Reticular/microcystic schwannoma. S100 immunopositivity is always appreciated.

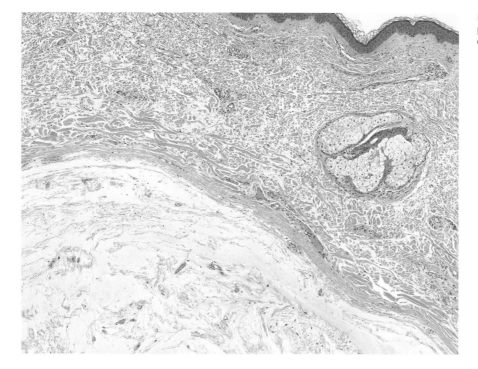

Fig. 8-25. Dermal nerve sheath myxoma. At low power, the tumor is dermal seated, well circumscribed, and unencapsulated.

sarcomatous malignancies, such as melanoma and metastatic carcinoma. As discussed in Chapter 7, pleomorphic liposarcoma may feature abundant myxofibrosarcoma-like areas. The differential diagnosis is based mainly on the presence of true lipoblasts. Careful sampling is mandatory, as lipoblasts can be scanty and therefore easily overlooked. The differential diagnosis with undifferentiated pleomorphic sarcoma is based on the presence of any amount of low-grade myxofibrosarcoma-like areas. Interestingly, high-grade myxofibrosarcoma may feature cytoplasmic eosinophilia, which may raise the differential diagnosis with myogenic pleomorphic sarcomas. However, with the notable exception of focal immunopositivity for smooth muscle actin, both desmin and myogenin are consistently negative. Sarcomatoid melanoma is ruled out on the basis of the absence of S100 and melanoma marker immunoreactivity. As discussed in

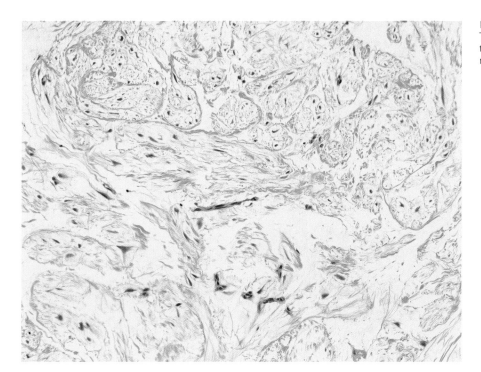

**Fig. 8-26.** Dermal nerve sheath myxoma. The presence of abundant myxoid stroma is typically seen. Neoplastic cells exhibit minimal nuclear atypia.

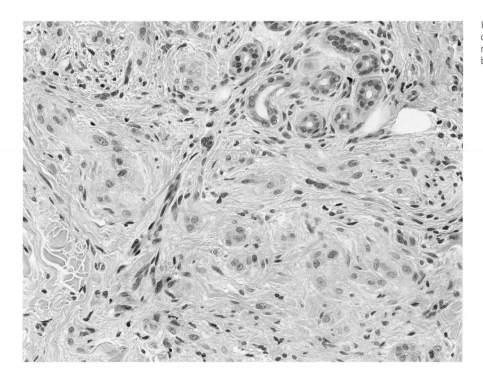

**Fig. 8-27.** Cellular neurothekeoma. The tumor is ill defined. The neoplastic cells are organized in small nests separated by collagen bundles and grow in between cutaneous appendages.

Chapter 5, epithelioid myxofibrosarcoma (which is always high grade) may express EMA; however, it generally lacks diffuse positivity for cytokeratin as is frequently seen in metastatic carcinoma.

A final comment should be reserved for "myxofibrosarcoma" arising in the retroperitoneum. This represents an extremely rare event and, in fact, most of these lesions actually represent examples of myxofibrosarcoma-like dedifferentiated liposarcoma. Demonstrations of diffuse MDM2 immunoreactivity (in contrast to the multifocal immunopositivity commonly observed in myxofibrosarcoma) or of MDM2 amplification represent key confirmatory findings.

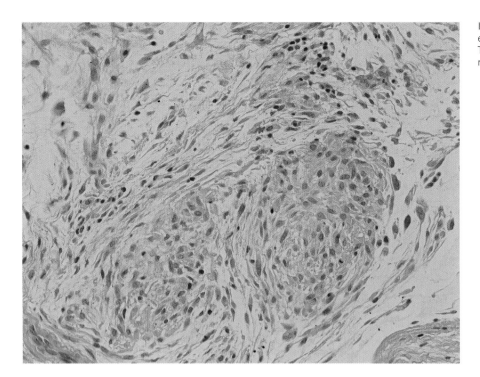

**Fig. 8-28.** Cellular neurothekeoma. This lesion exhibits significant myxoid change of the stroma. The typical nesting pattern of growth is, however, retained.

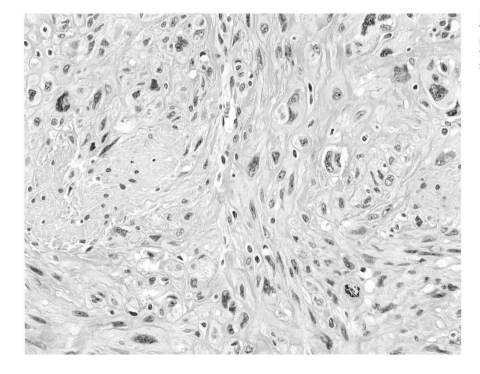

**Fig. 8-29.** Atypical cellular neurothekeoma. The tumor features the presence of atypical, pleomorphic cells set in collagenous stroma. Note the atypical mitotic figure. These findings do not seem to have an impact over clinical outcome.

### Key Points in Myxofibrosarcoma Diagnosis

- Occurrence in the superficial soft tissues of elderly patients
- Multinodular pattern of growth
- Presence of myxoid matrix
- Presence of curvilinear, thin-walled blood vessels
- Presence of nuclear hyperchromasia independently of grade
- Frequent transition from low-grade to high-grade morphology
- Aggressive behavior in high-grade tumors

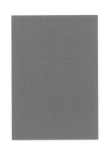

# Myxoinflammatory Fibroblastic Sarcoma

## Definition and Epidemiology

Myxoinflammatory fibroblastic sarcoma (MFS) is a locally aggressive neoplasm characterized by the presence of distinctive neoplastic cells harboring inclusion-like nucleoli, set in a myxoinflammatory background. The lesion was first reported independently by Montgomery (who labeled the lesion "inflammatory myxohyaline tumor of the distal extremities with virocyte or Reed-Sternberg-like cells"), and by Meis and Kindblom (who coined the term "acral myxoinflammatory fibroblastic sarcoma") in 1998. This tumor occurs predominantly in adults; it has no sex predominance.

## Clinical Presentation and Outcome

Clinically, most cases tend to occur in the distal extremities with more than two-thirds involving hand and wrist and the remaining the foot and ankle. Occurrence in non-acral sites has been documented but is comparatively very rare. Most patients present with a long-lasting lesion, which is often interpreted clinically as a benign process. Repeated local recurrences vary from 30 to 70% and are most probably related to inadequate surgery. In fact, it has to be considered that when dealing with lesions occurring primarily at acral sites, radical excision is not easy to achieve. Metastatic spread seems to be exceedingly rare (less than 2% of cases) and is observed only in regional lymph nodes. Complete surgery tends to be curative; however, it should be limited to those situations in which it can be achieved without involving mutilating procedures.

## Morphology and Immunophenotype

Grossly, MFS tends to be poorly circumscribed and multinodular and features both firm and gelatinous areas (Fig. 8-30). Microscopically, it exhibits an infiltrative growth pattern with extension into joints, tendons, and dermis. The classic morphologic picture is represented by the presence of a dense inflammatory infiltrate that includes both chronic and acute elements (Fig. 8-31), set in a stroma characterized by a varying admixture of collagenous areas, myxoid areas, and

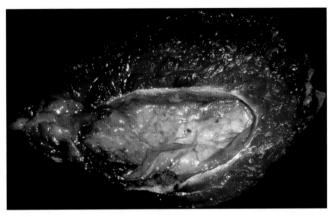

**Fig. 8-30.** Myxoinflammatory fibroblastic sarcoma. Macroscopically, the tumor is poorly circumscribed. The cut surface features both firm and gelatinous areas.

hemosiderin deposition (Fig. 8-32). The neoplastic cell population is represented by a combination of spindle cells, large polygonal and bizarre ganglion-like cells containing distinctive inclusion-like nucleoli (Fig. 8-33), and pseudolipoblasts (Fig. 8-34). Neoplastic cells may feature bi-nucleation and, in consideration of the presence of the large nucleoli, somewhat mimic Reed-Sternberg cells (Fig. 8-35) or virally infected cells (Fig. 8-36). Immunohistochemistry has not proved truly helpful in showing variable positivity for CD34, smooth muscle actin, and CD68. Weak expression of cytokeratin has also been reported in rare cases.

## Genetics

Myxoinflammatory fibroblastic sarcoma may feature a balanced or unbalanced t(1;10)(p22-23;q24-25) translocation, often associated with loss of material from chromosome region 3p. The genes involved are *TGFBR3* and *MGEA5*. Interestingly, the same chromosome aberration is observed in hemosiderotic fibrolipomatous tumor (HFLT). *BRAF* gene rearrangement has been recently observed in cases lacking a *TGFBR3/MGEA5* fusion gene.

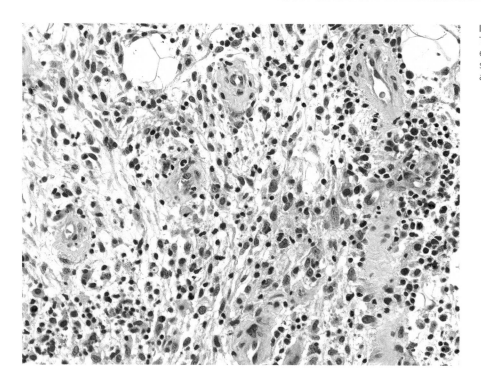

**Fig. 8-31.** Myxoinflammatory fibroblastic sarcoma. The tumor typically shows infiltrative margins with extension into the fat. It is composed of spindle cells set in a variably myxoid stroma and associated with abundant inflammatory infiltrate.

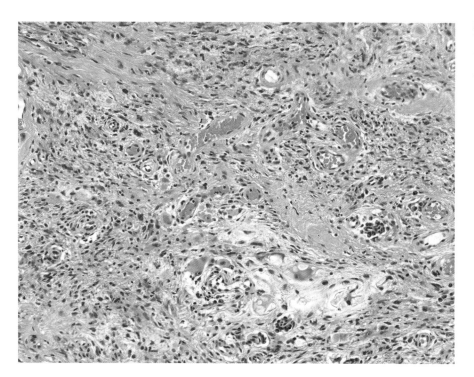

**Fig. 8-32.** Myxoinflammatory fibroblastic sarcoma. The background is remarkably heterogeneous, showing a variable combination of myxoinflammatory and fibrous areas. Hemosiderin deposition is also present.

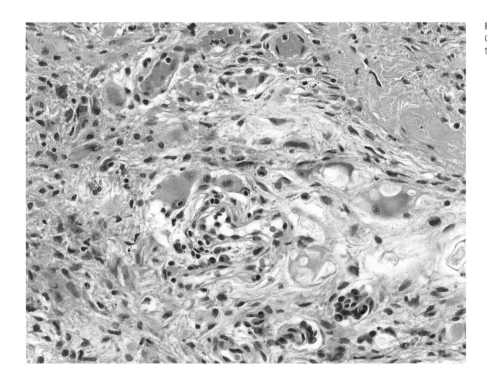

**Fig. 8-33.** Myxoinflammatory fibroblastic sarcoma. One of the most distinctive morphologic features is the presence of large polygonal, ganglion-like cells.

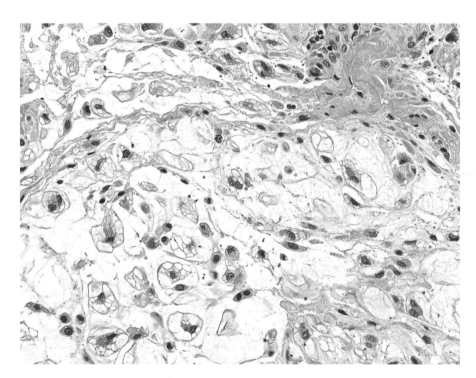

**Fig. 8-34.** Myxoinflammatory fibroblastic sarcoma. The presence of a variable amount of pseudolipoblasts represents an additional characteristic finding.

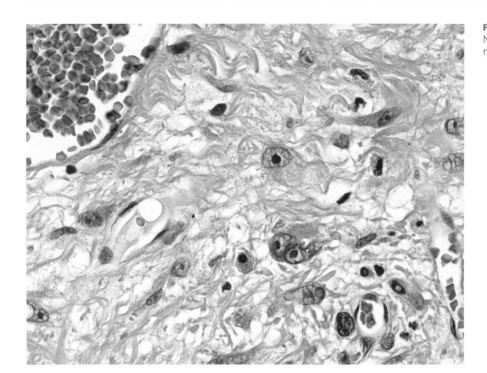

**Fig. 8-35.** Myxoinflammatory fibroblastic sarcoma. Neoplastic cells feature distinctive inclusion-like nucleoli somewhat mimicking Reed-Sternberg cells.

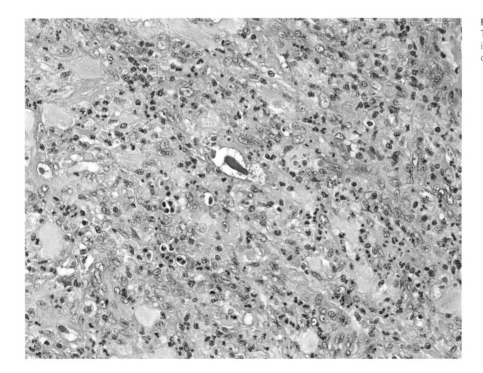

**Fig. 8-36.** Myxoinflammatory fibroblastic sarcoma. The presence of large nucleoli similar to those seen in virally infected cells is one of the most important diagnostic clues.

## Differential Diagnosis and Diagnostic Pitfalls

The differential diagnosis of MFS is rather broad and includes both benign and malignant entities. Among benign lesions, **ganglion cyst**, in consideration of its acral location, is certainly to be considered. Ganglion cysts represent a problem whenever they rupture and, through extravasation in the surrounding soft tissue, can elicit variably intense inflammatory reactions. Importantly, the distinctive macronucleolated lesional cells of MFS are never seen (Fig. 8-37).

**Proliferative fasciitis** and **proliferative myositis**, two fibroblastic/myofibroblastic benign entities somewhat related to nodular fasciitis, also enter the differential diagnosis. Proliferative fasciitis most often occurs in the subcutis of the upper and lower limbs. Adult patients are most often affected, with a peak incidence in the sixth decade. The lesion is composed of a proliferation of spindle cells set in a fibromyxoid background and associated with an extremely variable amount of distinctive "ganglion-like" cells

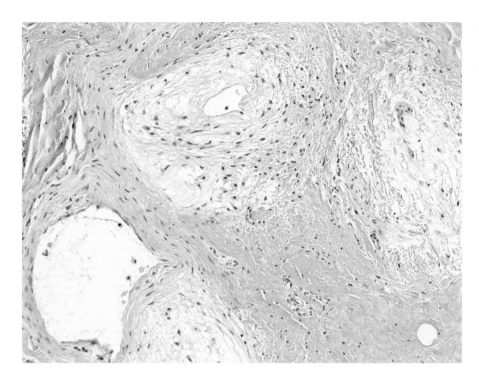

**Fig. 8-37.** Ganglion cyst. The lesion shows a variable admixture of collagenous and myxoid areas with scattered fibroblastic and inflammatory cells. Typically, the presence of cysts filled by mucin is observed.

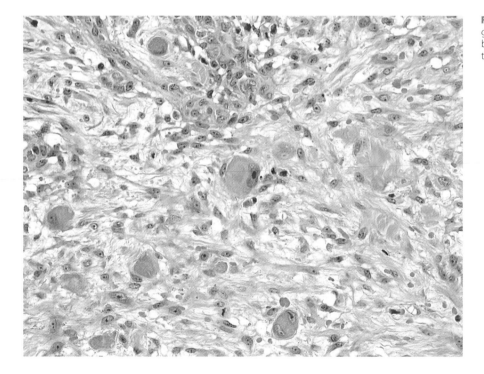

**Fig. 8-38.** Proliferative fasciitis. The presence of ganglion-like cells set in variably myxoid background represents the key diagnostic feature of this benign lesion.

(Fig. 8-38). The presence of macronucleoli may raise the differential diagnosis with myxoinflammatory fibroblastic sarcoma. However, proliferative fasciitis usually lacks both a prominent inflammatory infiltrate and the presence of pseudolipoblasts. Immunohistochemically, the spindle cell component (similar to nodular fasciitis) exhibits diffuse expression of smooth muscle actin. Proliferative myositis basically corresponds to an intramuscular form of proliferative fasciitis. It tends to affect the muscles of the shoulder girdle and trunk of middle-aged patients. Microscopically, proliferative myositis extends in between muscle fibers, leaving them almost unaffected and therefore generating the distinctive "checkerboard" appearance (Fig. 8-39). The cell population overlaps morphologically that of proliferative fasciitis, in particular the presence of large, ganglion-like cells (Fig. 8-40).

Myxofibrosarcoma represents the main differential diagnosis. Superficial location, multinodular growth pattern,

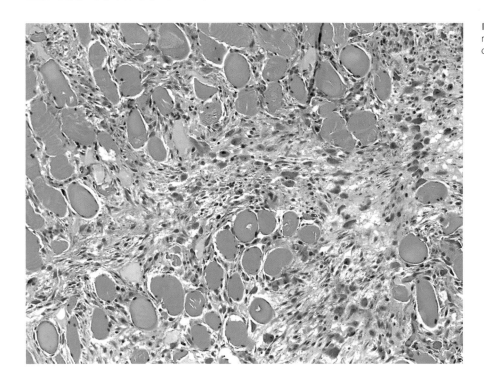

Fig. 8-39. Proliferative myositis. At low magnification, the typical checkerboard appearance of this lesion is better appreciated.

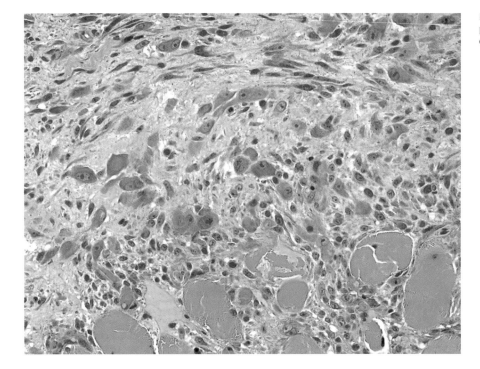

Fig. 8-40. Proliferative myositis. At high power, the presence of the distinctive ganglion-like cells is easily appreciated.

presence of distinctive archiform, thin-walled blood vessels, much less prominent or absent inflammatory infiltrate, and absence of inclusion-like nucleoli in neoplastic cells represent the key differential diagnostic clues.

The fact that MFS shares the same genetic abnormalities with **hemosiderotic fibrolipomatous tumor** (HFLT) has raised the question of whether the two lesions are actually related. Hemosiderotic fibrolipomatous tumor is a locally aggressive lesion that also occurs acrally (most often, dorsum of the feet and dorsum of the hands) in middle-aged females. Microscopically, the lesion is poorly circumscribed, composed of adipocytes, hemosiderin-laden spindle cells associated with a chronic inflammatory infiltrate (Fig. 8-41). Interestingly, examples of lesions exhibiting mixed features of both HFLT and MFS have been observed, further supporting the existence of a morphologic spectrum (Fig. 8-42). It has to be noted that this view has been challenged by other authors, who instead believe that HFLT is related to pleomorphic hyalinizing angiectatic tumor (PHAT).

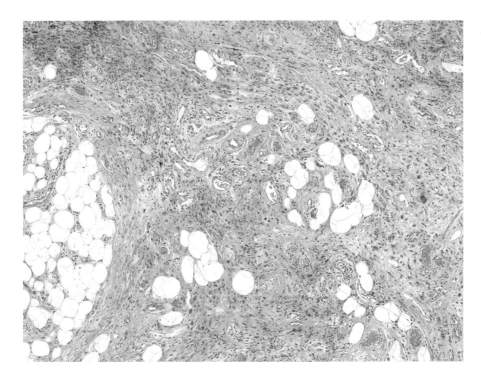

**Fig. 8-41.** Hemosiderotic fibrolipomatous tumor. The tumor shows ill-defined margins and it is composed of adipocytes, hemosiderin-laden spindle cells associated with a chronic inflammatory infiltrate.

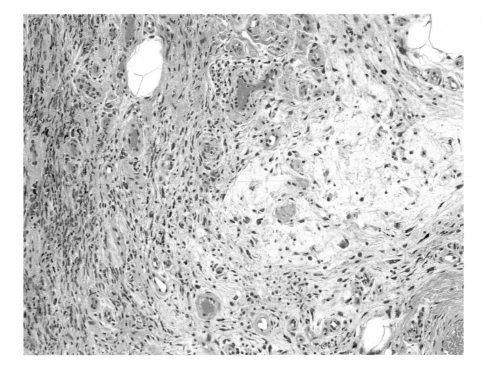

**Fig. 8-42.** Myxoinflammatory fibroblastic sarcoma/Hemosiderotic fibrolipomatous tumor. Rare cases show mixed features of both tumors, supporting the existence of a close relationship.

The presence of inclusion-like nucleoli also raises the differential diagnosis with hematologic malignancies. Negativity within large cells of both B- and T-cell markers as well as of CD30 and ALK represents useful diagnostic findings. In consideration of the acral location, the presence of cytokeratin may in principle raise the differential diagnosis with epithelioid sarcoma. However, MFS lacks the presence of sheets of spindle and epithelioid neoplastic cells and always features complete preservation of INI1 nuclear immunoreactivity.

**Key Points in Myxoinflammatory Fibroblastic Sarcoma Diagnosis**
- Occurrence at acral sites of adult patients
- Presence of myxoid matrix associated with variably prominent chronic inflammatory infiltrate
- Presence of pseudolipoblasts
- Presence of large cells containing inclusion-like nucleoli
- Locally aggressive

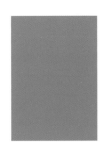

# Low-Grade Fibromyxoid Sarcoma

## Definition and Epidemiology

Low-grade fibromyxoid sarcoma (LGFMS) represents a cytologically bland, fibroblastic malignant neoplasm, showing a distinctive fibromyxoid stroma and characterized by aggressive clinical behavior. First reported by Evans in 1987, classic forms of LGFMS tend to occur in young adults, with a peak incidence in the third decade. However, approximately 20% of cases occur in patients younger than 18 years of age. Both sexes are equally affected.

## Clinical Presentation and Outcome

The proximal extremities and the trunk represent the most frequently affected anatomic sites for LGFMS. Rare cases occurring at visceral locations have been recently reported. Clinical presentation is relatively non-specific, characterized by the occurrence of a slowly growing, deep-seated, painless soft tissue mass, most often attaining a size ranging between 6 and 10 cm. Low-grade fibromyxoid sarcoma, in stark contrast to its bland morphology, actually represents an aggressive neoplasm. In fact, on long-term follow-up, it shows a local recurrence rate of approximately 65%, a metastatic rate of 45% (most common in the lungs and pleura), and a mortality of 42%. Patients often present with a recurrence of a previously excised (up to 10 years earlier) "benign" mesenchymal neoplasm. At the opposite end of the clinical spectrum, there exist patients in which systemic spread is observed at onset.

From the therapeutic standpoint, radical surgery with free margins represents a key step in trying to reduce local recurrences and subsequent metastatic spread.

An additional point of recent interest is represented by the occurrence of LGFMS in the pediatric population. At least in one series, LGFMS in children tends to be more superficial and smaller in size. As a consequence of easier surgical removal, prognosis of LGFMS seems to be more favorable in this age-group.

## Morphology and Immunophenotype

Grossly, LGFMS tends to be relatively well circumscribed, with a firm, whitish cut surface (Fig. 8-43). Microscopically, LGFMS is characterized by a cytologically bland spindle cell proliferation, set in a stroma that alternates collagenized hypocellular areas (Fig. 8-44) and more cellular myxoid foci (Fig. 8-45). Such an exquisitely distinctive architecture is better appreciated at low magnification (Fig. 8-46). The vascular network

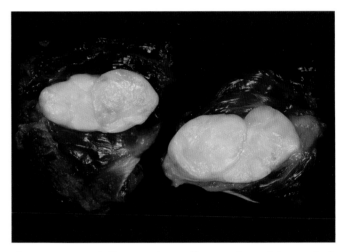

**Fig. 8-43.** Low-grade fibromyxoid tumor. The tumor is a well-circumscribed mass with firm and whitish cut surface.

is composed of small, capillary-sized blood vessels, often exhibiting a curvilinear or branching configuration, somewhat reminiscent of the vascular architecture exhibited by low-grade myxofibrosarcoma (Fig. 8-47). Mitotic activity is usually low, and cellularity at times can be deceptively low (Fig. 8-48). Interestingly, a minority of cases shows multiple foci of increased cellularity, which can be associated with moderate pleomorphism. This phenomenon appears to be observed more frequently when dealing with local recurrences and metastases (Fig. 8-49). Transition to genuine high-grade pleomorphic sarcoma is seen very rarely, as in the case reported by Evans that "dedifferentiated" 30 years after initial surgery. Those lesions reported under the descriptive term "hyalinizing spindle cell tumor with giant collagen rosettes" actually represent part of the morphologic spectrum of LGFMS. In fact, it has subsequently become evident that approximately 30% of LGFMS sarcomas, in addition to the classic morphology, may feature the presence of variably formed, large pseudorosettes (Fig. 8-50) composed of hyalinized collagen demarcated by a palisade of epithelioid lesional cells (Fig. 8-51). As a further confirmation of the existence of a morphologic continuum, the clinical presentation also overlaps with that of conventional forms of LGFMS.

Immunohistochemically, the most useful marker is represented by MUC4, which is expressed by the vast majority of LGFMS (Fig. 8-52). Occasional expression of smooth muscle

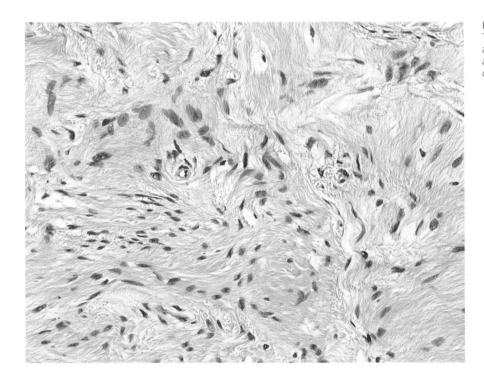

**Fig. 8-44.** Low-grade fibromyxoid tumor. The tumor is characterized by alternation of myxoid and collagenized areas. The neoplastic cells feature a spindle morphology and are characterized by mild cytologic atypia.

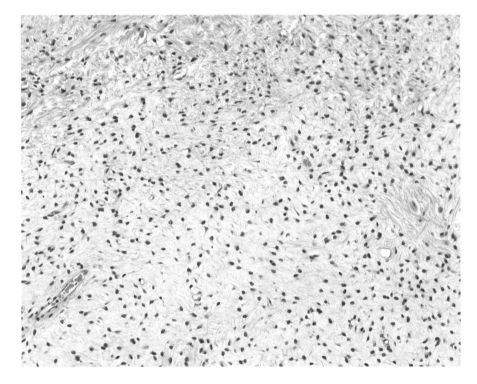

**Fig. 8-45.** Low-grade fibromyxoid tumor. Myxoid areas tend to show increased cellularity.

actin and/or muscle specific actin is seen. Desmin, keratin, and CD34 immunopositivity has been reported only exceptionally. Approximately 60% of cases of LGFMS may express epithelial membrane antigen (EMA).

As mentioned in Chapter 5, LGFMS shares with a numerically significant subset of sclerosing epithelioid fibrosarcoma (SEF) morphologic (i.e., a transition from LGFMS to SEF can

be observed), immunophenotypic (MUC4 immunopositivity), and genetic features (Fig. 8-53).

## Genetics

In approximately 95% of cases, genetic analyses have demonstrated the presence of a recurrent balanced translocation, t(7;16)(q33;p11), fusing the gene *FUS* with *CREB3L2*. More

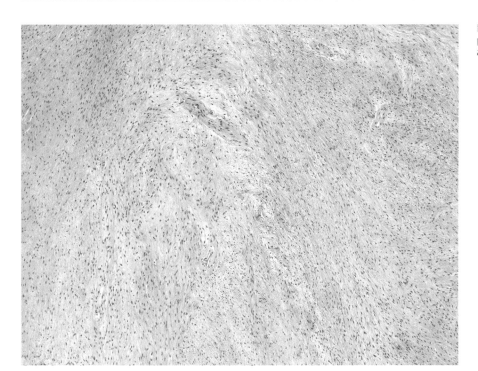

**Fig. 8-46.** Low-grade fibromyxoid tumor. At low power, the distinctive alternation of myxoid stroma and collagenous stroma is better appreciated.

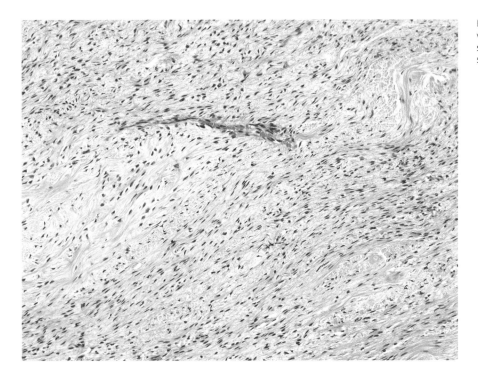

**Fig. 8-47.** Low-grade fibromyxoid tumor. A rich vascular network is present, composed of small-sized blood vessels somewhat resembling those seen in low-grade myxofibrosarcoma.

rarely, the *FUS* gene fuses with the *CREB3L1* gene. Both *CREB3L1* and *CREB3L2* encode for proteins belonging to the leucine-zipper family of transcription factors and show significant sequence homology in their DNA-binding domains. A supernumerary ring chromosome is seen in approximately 25% of cases.

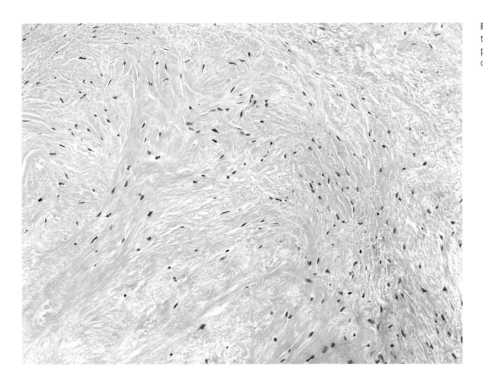

**Fig. 8-48.** Low-grade fibromyxoid tumor. At times, tumors may be remarkably hypocellular. This phenomenon is generally associated with increased collagen deposition in the stroma.

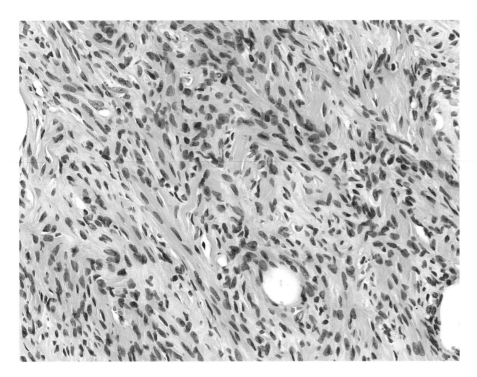

**Fig. 8-49.** Low-grade fibromyxoid tumor. Increased cellularity and atypia can be observed in recurrences or metastases.

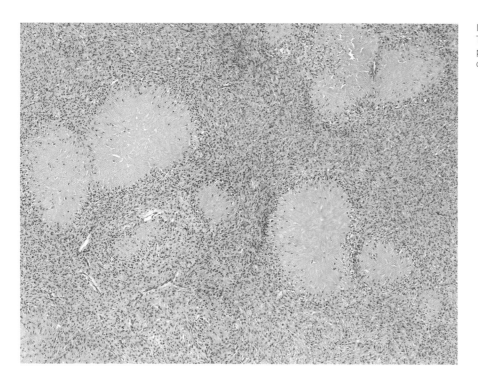

**Fig. 8-50.** Low-grade fibromyxoid tumor. The presence of distinctive, large collagenous pseudorosettes can be observed in a subset of cases.

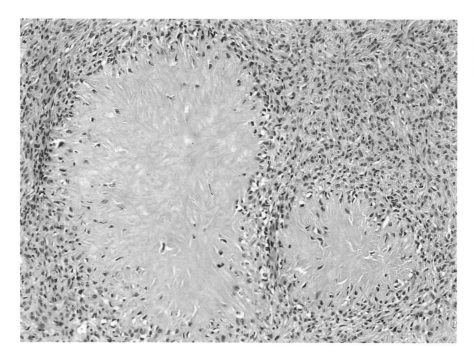

**Fig. 8-51.** Low-grade fibromyxoid tumor. Giant pseudorosettes are composed of a central area of hyalinized collagen surrounded by a palisade of neoplastic cells that tend to assume an epithelioid morphology.

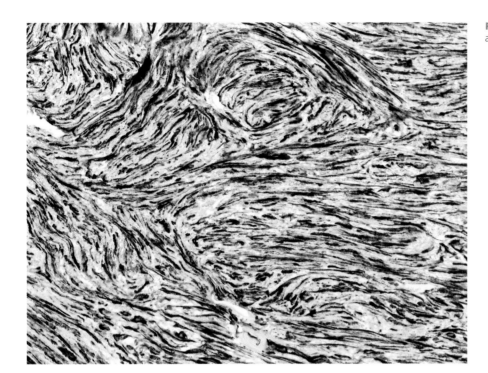

**Fig. 8-52.** Low-grade fibromyxoid tumor. Almost all cases are strongly MUC4 immunopositive.

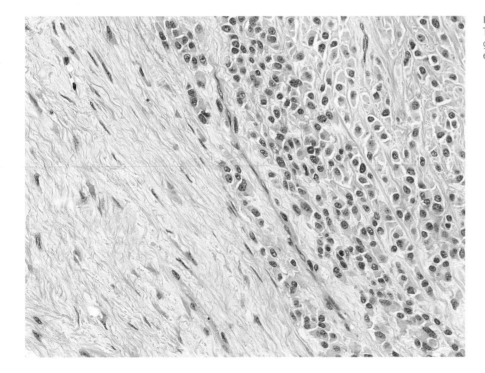

**Fig. 8-53.** Low-grade fibromyxoid tumor. The tumor presents areas of transition from low-grade fibromyxoid tumor (*left*) to sclerosing epithelioid fibrosarcoma (*right*).

## Differential Diagnosis and Diagnostic Pitfalls

The differential diagnosis of LGFMS includes several benign and low-grade entities. **Nodular fasciitis** represents a benign myofibroblastic lesion, in most cases characterized genetically by a *MYH9-USP6* gene fusion. More rarely, *USP6* fuses with alternative partners. Some of its morphologic features not infrequently may generate diagnostic confusion with a sarcoma. Typically, nodular fasciitis presents as a fast-

growing lump (duration most often is less than 2 months), most often located in the upper extremities, trunk, or head and neck region of young individuals. Most cases are located superficially; however, approximately 10% of cases are intramuscular. Rare variants are represented by intravascular, periosteal, intradermal, intra-articular, and cranial fasciitis. The latter typically occurs in the outer table of the skull of male patients younger than 2 years. Relatively often, cranial fasciitis may extend through the bone into the meninges.

Grossly, nodular fasciitis is either well circumscribed or infiltrative (Fig. 8-54). Microscopically, the lesion is typically composed of cytologically bland spindle cells organized in intersecting fascicles, set in a variably myxoid matrix (Fig. 8-55) that, with time, tend to become more collagenized and, in long-standing lesions, may acquire a keloid-like morphology (Fig. 8-56). Mitotic activity is distinctively brisk; however, atypical figures are never seen (Fig. 8-57). In early lesions, the overall morphologic picture somewhat recalls that of fibroblasts in culture (Fig. 8-58). Extravasated erythrocytes along with a modest, chronic inflammatory infiltrate are often seen, which may be associated with the presence of osteoclast-like giant cells (Fig. 8-59). Rarely (although particularly in the pediatric age-group), nodular fasciitis exhibits a striking myxoid change of the stroma that can certainly represent a potential diagnostic challenge (Fig. 8-60). Immunohistochemically, nodular fasciitis exhibits smooth muscle actin positivity, while all other myogenic markers tend to be negative. As mentioned, nodular fasciitis frequently generates major diagnostic anxiety based on the presence of both hypercellularity and high mitotic activity. The distinctive cell culture appearance and the absence of cytologic atypia represent the key diagnostic features. Nodular fasciitis is entirely benign and exhibits a tendency to regress spontaneously if left untreated. Local marginal excision is curative, and in the presence of local recurrence (in less than 2% of cases, most often following incomplete excision), the initial diagnosis should be immediately reconsidered.

The most challenging differential diagnosis is certainly represented by **perineurioma**, a benign lesion that shares with LGFMS both morphologic and immunophenotypic features. Perineurioma most often occurs in the limbs and trunk of middle-aged patients, with a female predominace. Approximately 10% of perineuriomas occur in the skin. Microscopically, perineurioma is composed of a spindle cell proliferation, characterized by the presence of long, bipolar cytoplasmic processes organized in intersecting fascicles and perivascular whorls (Figs. 8-61 and 8-62). A collagen matrix is most often seen; however, myxoid change of the stroma can be detected in approximately 20% of cases. The vasculature is much less prominent than in LGFMS. Immunohistochemically, perineurioma shares with LGFMS immunopositivity for EMA that also highlights the typical cytoplasmic processes (Fig. 8-63). CD34 is expressed in half of the cases. MUC4 is consistently negative and represents a key diagnostic finding.

**Desmoid fibromatosis** also represents a very important differential diagnosis, as actually occurred in the very first

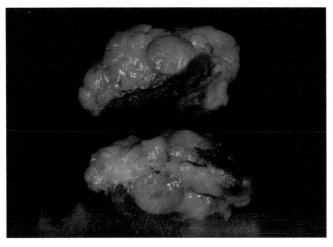

**Fig. 8-54.** Nodular fasciitis. The tumor is represented by a well-circumscribed, suprafascial nodule featuring a myxoid cut surface.

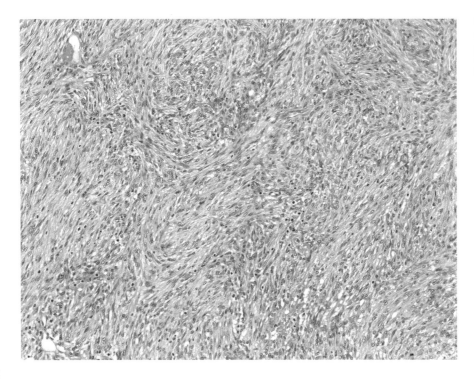

**Fig. 8-55.** Nodular fasciitis. Intersecting fascicles of non-atypical spindle cells set in a fibromyxoid stroma represent the typical feature of the tumor. Extravasated red blood cells are the other consistent elements in this tumor.

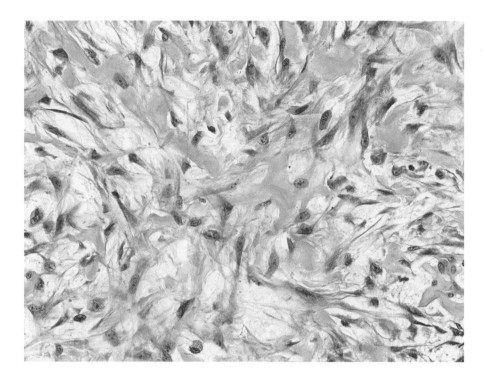

**Fig. 8-56.** Nodular fasciitis. Long-standing lesions may show abundant collagen deposition and assume a keloid-like morphology.

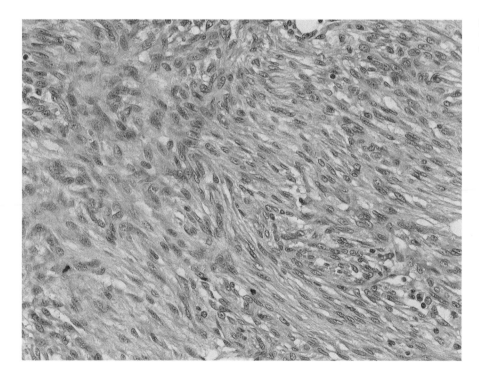

**Fig. 8-57.** Nodular fasciitis. Mitotic activity is typically brisk and should not be regarded as evidence of malignancy.

two cases initially reported by Evans. Desmoid fibromatosis represents a locally aggressive, non-metastasizing myofibroblastic neoplasm that may occur at any extra-abdominal (60%), abdominal (25%), or intra-abdominal anatomic site (15%). Clinical presentation varies with anatomic site. The most common extra-abdominal location is represented by the shoulder, followed by chest wall, back, thigh, and head and neck region. Abdominal wall lesions most often occur in pregnant women or up to 1 year after gestation, most often within the rectum muscle. Intra-abdominal desmoids are usually located in the

pelvis or in the mesentery. Mesenteric desmoids can be sporadic or associated with familial adenomatous polyposis (FAP; Gardner syndrome). There exists a subset of desmoids that occurs in the pediatric age-group that exhibits a tendency to develop in the head and neck region. Desmoid fibromatosis typically shows poor circumscription, often with infiltration of the surrounding soft tissues (Fig. 8-64). Microscopically, a monotonous spindle cell proliferation set in a collagenous background is most often seen (Fig. 8-65). A useful diagnostic clue is represented by the fact that neoplastic cells often exhibit

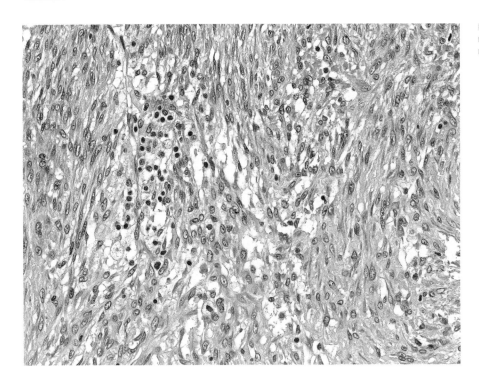

**Fig. 8-58.** Nodular fasciitis. The neoplastic cells resemble fibroblasts in culture. The stroma shows multifocal myxoid changes.

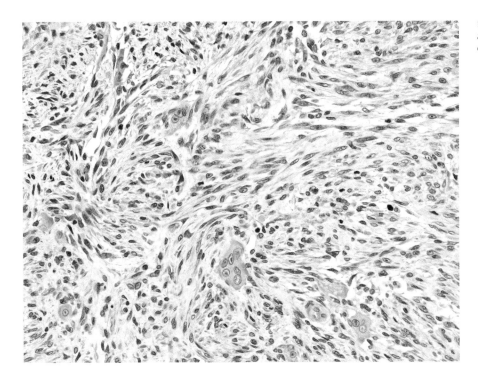

**Fig. 8-59.** Nodular fasciitis. Scattered lymphocytes are frequently seen, sometimes associated with osteoclast-like giant cells.

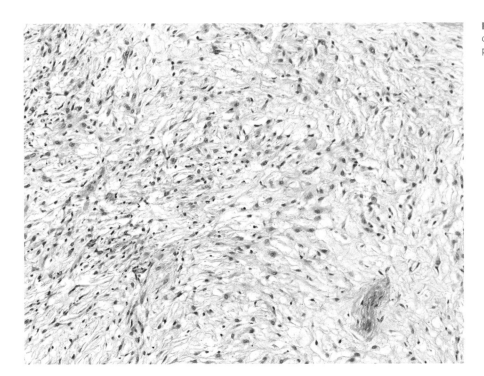

**Fig. 8-60.** Nodular fasciitis with extreme myxoid change of the stroma is shown. Interestingly, this phenomenon is often seen in pediatric cases.

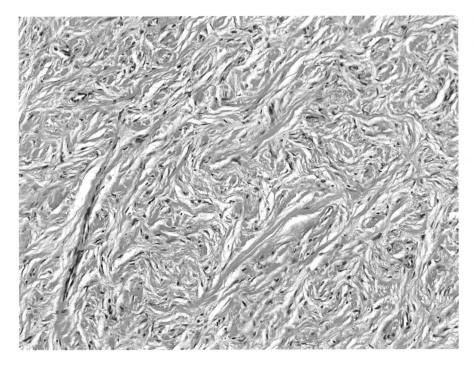

**Fig. 8-61.** Perineurioma. The tumor is composed of cytologically bland, from slender to more plump spindle cells, set in collagen-rich stroma.

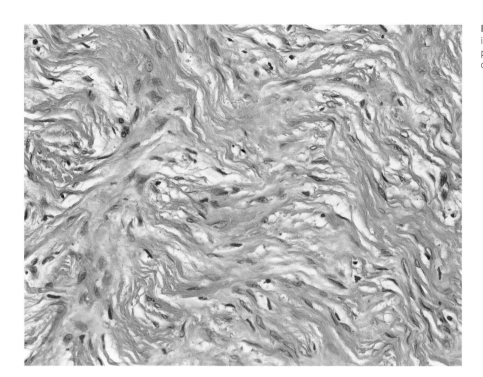

**Fig. 8-62.** Perineurioma. The neoplastic cells have indistinct, pale cytoplasm with long bipolar processes and tapering nuclei. Focal myxoid change of the stroma is appreciable.

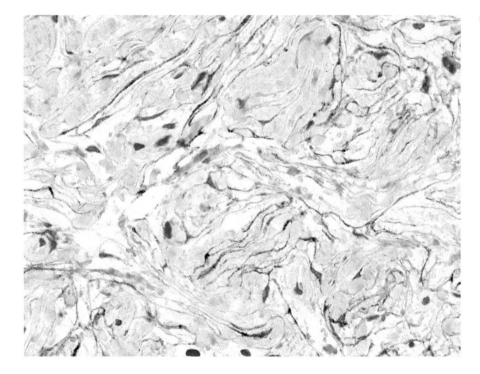

**Fig. 8-63.** Perineurioma. EMA immunopositivity highlights the long bipolar cytoplasmic processes of neoplastic cells.

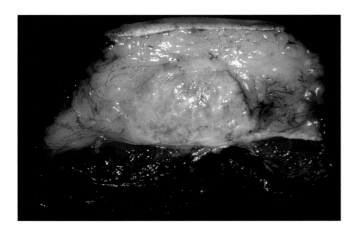

**Fig. 8-64.** Desmoid fibromatosis. Grossly, the tumor most often presents as a firm, solitary mass with ill-defined margins and a tendency to infiltrate the surrounding soft tissue.

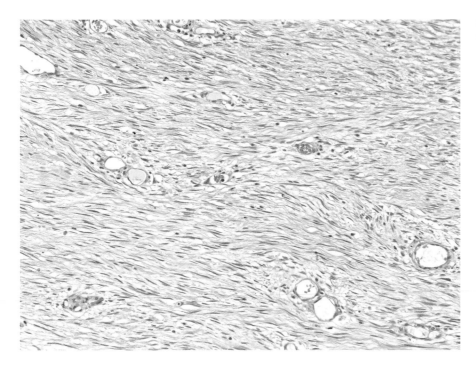

**Fig. 8-65.** Desmoid fibromatosis. The tumor is composed of monotonous, cytologically bland spindle cells, associated with numerous medium-sized vessels and set in a fibrous background.

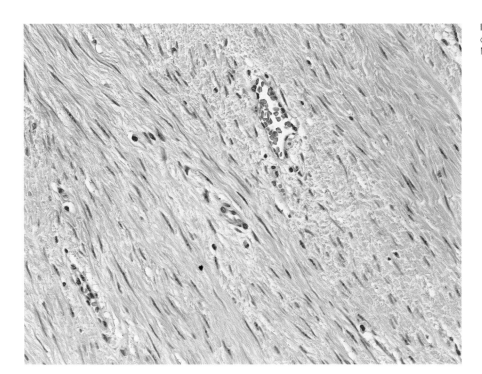

**Fig. 8-66.** Desmoid fibromatosis. The neoplastic cells exhibit a regular, evenly spaced distribution. Nuclear atypia is absent or mild.

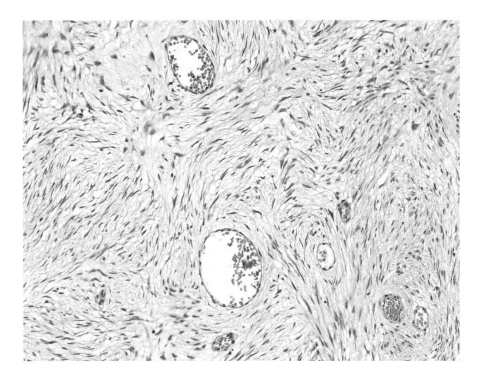

**Fig. 8-67.** Desmoid fibromatosis. Sometimes, prominent myxoid change of the stroma may occur.

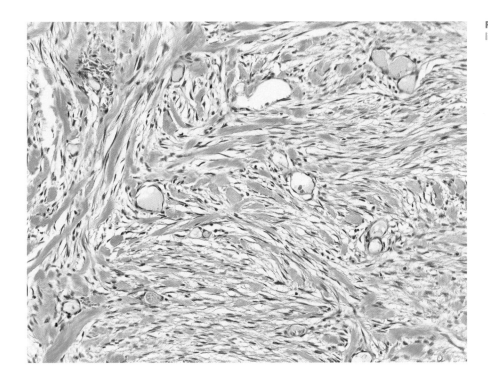

**Fig. 8-68.** Desmoid fibromatosis. Extensive, keloid-like hyalinization of the stroma is seen in some cases.

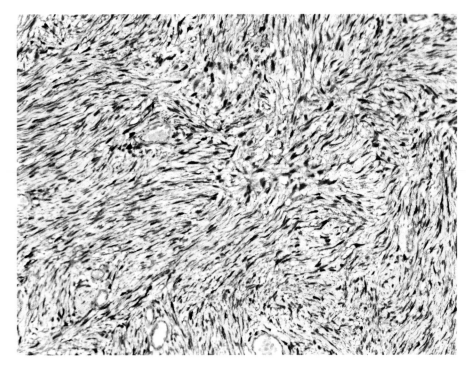

**Fig. 8-69.** Desmoid fibromatosis. Nuclear staining for beta-catenin represents a major diagnostic clue.

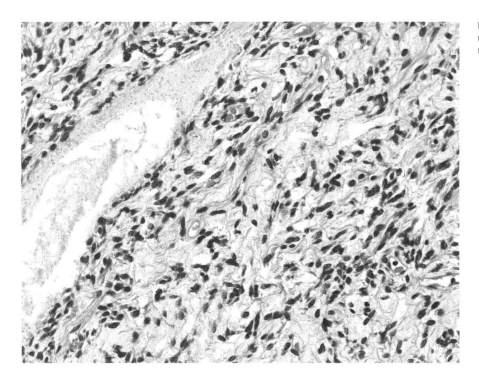

**Fig. 8-70.** Solitary fibrous tumor. Abundant myxoid stroma with formation of mucin pools is rarely seen.

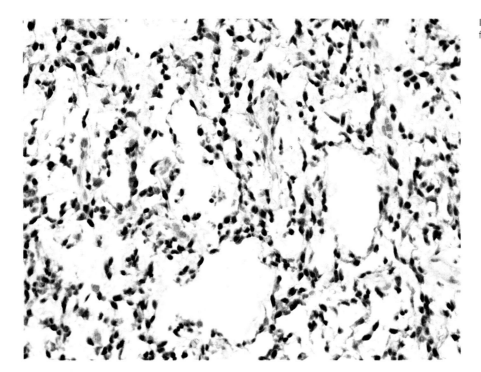

**Fig. 8-71.** Solitary fibrous tumor. Nuclear staining for STAT6 represents a key diagnostic tool.

a relatively regular disposition (Fig. 8-66). Nuclear atypia is absent, and mitotic figures may vary in number but are usually not numerous. A major cause of diagnostic confusion with LGFMS is represented by the occurrence of myxoid change of the matrix (Fig. 8-67), a finding most often encountered in intra-abdominal desmoids. At the opposite end of the morphologic spectrum, desmoids can feature extensive, keloid-like hyalinization (Fig. 8-68). Importantly, desmoid fibromatosis always lacks MUC4 immunopositivity, and by contrast exhibits nuclear immunopositivity for beta-catenin (Fig. 8-69). Nuclear accumulation of beta-catenin protein represents the consequence of mutations of the *CTNNB1* gene that occur in approximately 85% of sporadic cases. In Gardner syndrome–associated cases, the same phenomenon is determined by the mutation of the *APC* gene. A sharp debate surrounds the potential prognostic meaning of *CTNNB1* gene mutations (it has been suggested that the 45F mutation is associated with higher rates of local recurrences) that is still unresolved. In the past, the therapeutic approach to desmoid fibromatosis has been dominated by surgical excision. The use of radiotherapy as well as of systemic treatments (which include hormone antagonists, tyrosine kinase inhibitors, and low-dose cytotoxic chemotherapy) has been suggested for progressive lesions. More recently, in consideration that, in a significant subset of patients, repeated surgery may lead to increased recurrence rates, a "wait and see" approach has been suggested unless clear clinical progression is observed.

**Solitary fibrous tumor** represents another important differential diagnosis, particularly when dealing with cases showing myxoid change of the stroma (Fig. 8-70). Solitary fibrous tumor is discussed in detail in Chapter 4. The main differences with LGFMS are represented by the presence of more obvious alternation of hypercellular and hypocellular zones, presence of a distinctive hemangiopericytoma-like vascularization, absence of MUC4 immunopositivity, and presence of CD34 and STAT6 nuclear immunoreactivity (Fig. 8-71).

### Key Points in Low-Grade Fibromyxoid Sarcoma Diagnosis

- Occurrence in the deep soft tissues of young adults
- Cytologically bland spindle cell proliferation
- Alternation of collagenized and myxoid areas
- MUC4 immunopositivity
- Aggressive behavior despite bland cytology

# Myxoid Liposarcoma

## Definition and Epidemiology

Myxoid liposarcoma is a malignant adipocytic tumor composed of spindle cells and monovacuolated lipoblasts set in a myxoid stroma. Myxoid liposarcoma forms a morphologic continuum, which includes hypercellular neoplasms composed of oval to round neoplastic cells, formerly know as "round cell liposarcoma" (also discussed in Chapter 6). Myxoid liposarcoma represents the second-largest group of adipocytic malignancies, accounting for about 30–35% of all liposarcomas. Peak incidence is between the third and fifth decade, and both sexes are equally affected.

## Clinical Presentation and Outcome

Clinically, myxoid and round cell liposarcomas occur predominantly in the limbs, the thigh being by far the most common location. The presence of hypercellularity or round cell differentiation is associated with a worsening prognosis. Different cut-off values, ranging between 5 and 25%, have been set by independent studies. A reliable assessment of the percentage of hypercellular areas is difficult to achieve, as it may be hampered by inadequate sampling as well as by that degree of subjectivity that is an intrinsic part of morphologic evaluation. For the time being, it appears safer to consider any amount of hypercellularity (conventionally, more than 5–10%) as prognostically relevant.

Myxoid liposarcoma tends to recur repeatedly and to metastasize to both bone and soft tissue locations, including the retroperitoneum, even in the absence of lung dissemination. Standard treatment is represented by wide surgical resection. In high-grade lesions, adjuvant therapy (radiotherapy and/or chemotherapy) may be associated. Myxoid liposarcoma ranks among the most chemosensitive (and also radiosensitive) soft tissue sarcomas. Recent data have shown that the marine-derived drug trabectedin appears to be a highly active treatment for metastatic myxoid liposarcoma.

## Morphology and Immunophenotype

Grossly, myxoid liposarcoma is most often a deep-seated, well-circumscribed, multinodular gelatinous mass (Fig. 8-72). The presence of high-grade areas may confer a more fleshy appearance (Fig. 8-73). Microscopically, purely myxoid (low-grade) liposarcoma is composed of a hypocellular, cytologically bland spindle cell proliferation set in a myxoid background (Fig. 8-74), often featuring mucin pooling (Fig. 8-75). Lipoblasts are most often monovacuolated and tend to cluster around vessels or at the periphery of the lesion (Fig. 8-76). The most distinctive morphologic clue is represented by the presence of a capillary network organized in a plexiform pattern (Fig. 8-77). This very peculiar vascular configuration has been variably labeled as "crow's feet" (Fig. 8-78) or "chicken

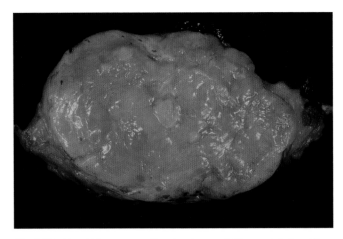

**Fig. 8-72.** Myxoid liposarcoma. Grossly, a large, gelatinous, relatively well-circumscribed, deep-seated mass is appreciated.

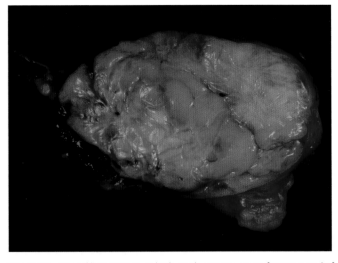

**Fig. 8-73.** Myxoid liposarcoma. In high-grade tumors, areas of necrosis and of a firmer appearance are most often seen.

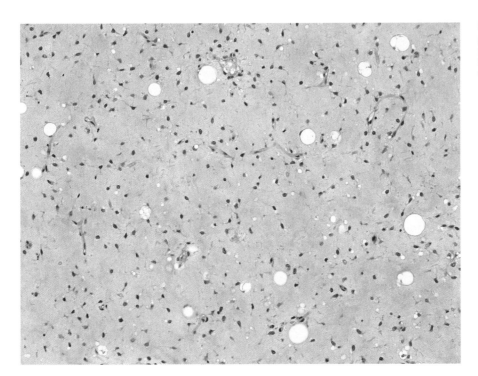

**Fig. 8-74.** Myxoid liposarcoma, low grade. At low power, the tumor is hypocellular and composed of a few spindle cells set in abundant myxoid stroma with characteristic branching, capillary-sized blood vessels, and rare lipoblasts.

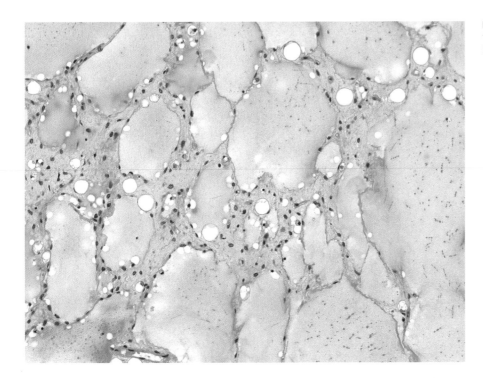

**Fig. 8-75.** Myxoid liposarcoma, low grade. This tumor shows an extensive area of mucin pooling, producing a "pulmonary edema–like" pattern.

wire" (Fig. 8-79). Rarely, extensive adipocytic "maturation" can be observed (Fig. 8-80).

As mentioned in Chapter 6, round cell liposarcoma is defined by the presence of hypercellular areas (which most frequently begin to form in a perivascular distribution) featuring an undifferentiated round cell morphology (Fig. 8-81); however, neoplastic cells may retain a spindle cell cytology (Fig. 8-82). As mentioned, several independent studies have

set different thresholds of hypercellularity (more than 5% or more than 25%) as predictors of outcome. A pragmatic approach (one based more on experience than on evidence-based data) may consider any lesion with more than 25% hypercelluarity as high grade and those with less than 5% as low grade. There exists, therefore, an intermediate group in which there is a significant risk of systemic spread, but its accurate quantification is still unclear. Pure round cell

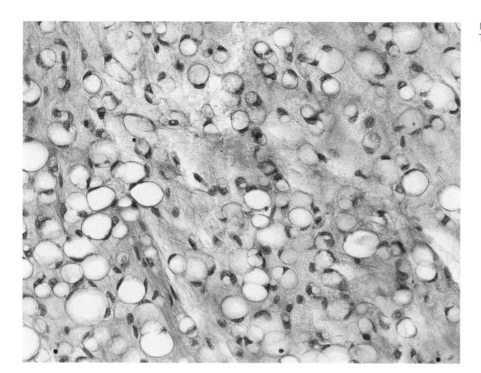

**Fig. 8-76.** Myxoid liposarcoma, low grade. The lipoblasts are typically monovacuolated.

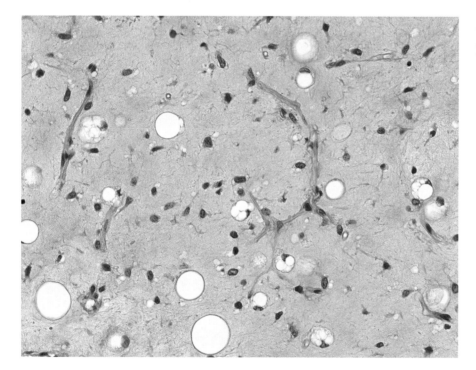

**Fig. 8-77.** Myxoid liposarcoma, low grade. The presence of a prominent plexiform vascular network represents a major diagnostic clue. Note the presence of scattered lipoblasts.

liposarcoma is a rare neoplasm and again is conventionally defined as a lesion in which hypercellularity or round cell differentiation accounts for more than 80% of tumor tissue (Figs. 8-83 and 8-84). Transition to hypercellular/round cell areas is commonly observed in myxoid liposarcoma, therefore providing strong evidence in favor of the concept that myxoid and round cell liposarcomas represent a morphologic continuum of myxoid adipocytic neoplasia (Fig. 8-85). Myxoid

liposarcoma usually exhibits S100 immunopositivity that also tends to be retained in the hypercellular/round cell areas.

More and more, pathologists are exposed to pretreated surgical specimens. Interestingly, the microscopic analysis of tumors treated with neoadjuvant chemotherapy shows extensive maturation with full-blown adipocytic differentiation. This phenomenon is observed both with cytotoxic agents and after administration of trabectedin (Fig. 8-86). Very rarely,

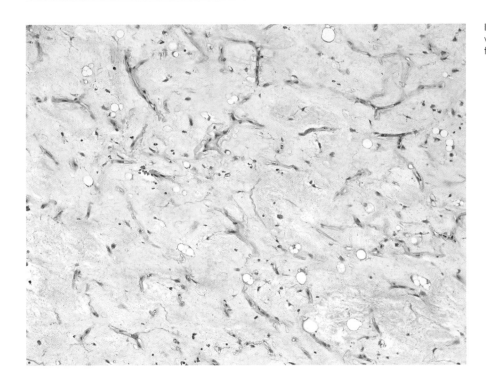

**Fig. 8-78.** Myxoid liposarcoma. The plexiform vascular network may assume the so-called crow's feet configuration.

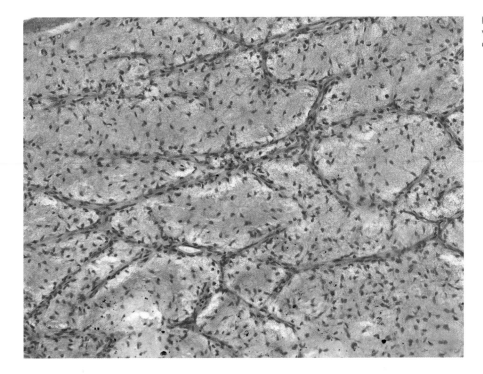

**Fig. 8-79.** Myxoid liposarcoma. The rich vasculature may assume the so-called chicken wire configuration.

post-chemotherapy effects may generate overt pleomorphism (Fig. 8-87).

## Genetics

Myxoid liposarcoma is characterized by two main karyotypic aberrations: a t(12;16)(q13;p11) that fuses the *CHOP/DDIT3* gene on 12q13 (a member of the CCAAT/enhancer-binding protein family involved in adipocyte differentiation), with the *FUS* (or *TLS*) gene on 16p11 (95%), and a t(12;22)(q13; q12) that fuses *CHOP/DDIT3* with *EWSR1* on 22q12 (5%). The normal function of the *CHOP/DDIT3* gene is to promote growth arrest by inducing terminal adipocytic differentiation. One of the functional consequences of the translocation is the loss of anti-proliferative activity exerted by wild-type *CHOP/DDIT3*. Trisomy 8 has also been observed as a non-random secondary change.

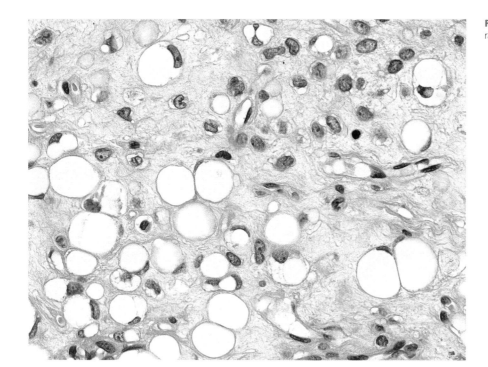

**Fig. 8-80.** Myxoid liposarcoma. The tumor may rarely feature extensive adipocytic "maturation."

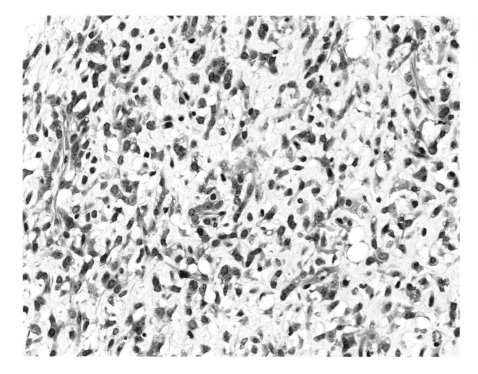

**Fig. 8-81.** Myxoid liposarcoma, high grade. The tumor is highly cellular and composed of atypical round cells, predominantly organized in a perivascular distribution.

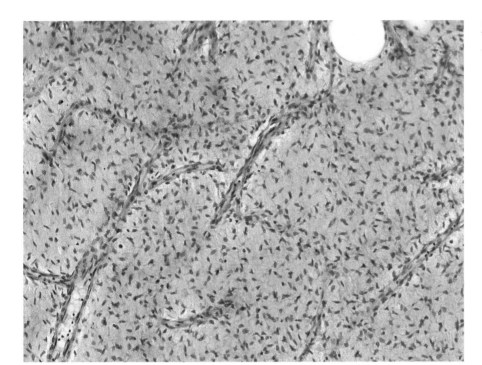

**Fig. 8-82.** Myxoid liposarcoma, high grade. The hypercellular component may maintain a spindle cell morphology.

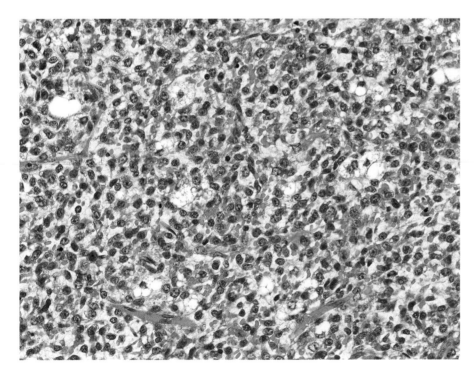

**Fig. 8-83.** Myxoid liposarcoma, high grade. When the round cell component predominates, the adipocytic nature of the lesion can be obscured.

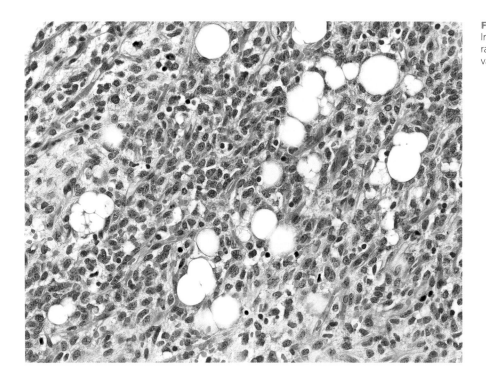

**Fig. 8-84.** Myxoid liposarcoma, high grade. In predominantly round cell tumors, the presence of rare lipoblasts associated with the characteristic vasculature represents diagnostic clues.

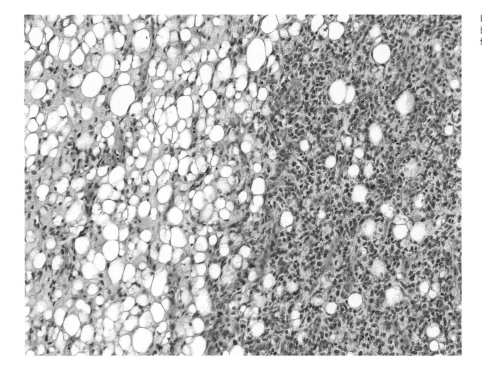

**Fig. 8-85.** Myxoid liposarcoma. The transition between low-grade to high-grade areas is frequently seen.

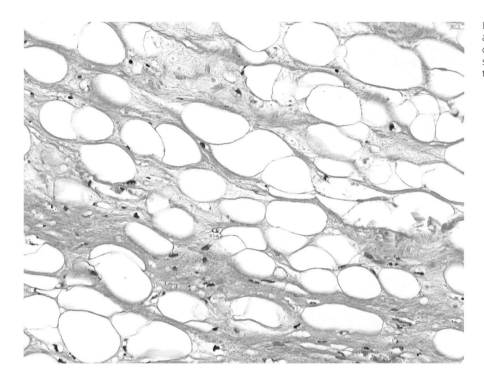

**Fig. 8-86.** Myxoid liposarcoma. Extensive mature adipocytic differentiation associated with fibrous change of the stroma is often seen in surgical specimens excised following neoadjuvant systemic treatments.

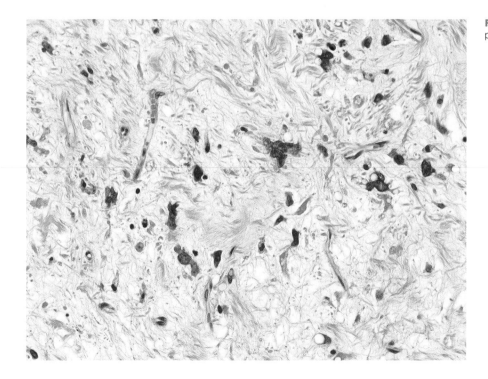

**Fig. 8-87.** Myxoid liposarcoma. Post-treatment pleomorphism represents a relatively rare event.

## Differential Diagnosis and Diagnostic Pitfalls

Among benign neoplasms, the lesion that is often misdiagnosed as myxoid liposarcoma is represented by **spindle cell lipoma** with myxoid change of the stroma. Spindle cell lipoma occurs primarily in the head and neck region of middle-aged males. Classical examples of spindle cell lipoma are composed of a cytologically bland spindle cell proliferation associated with a variable number of adipocytes (from many to almost nil), set in a background rich in distinctive eosinophilic, broad collagen fibers (Fig. 8-88A). When myxoid degeneration of the stroma occurs, spindle cell lipoma appears remarkably hypocellular and may somewhat mimic low-grade myxoid liposarcoma (Fig. 8-88B). The most important diagnostic clues are represented by the absence of a plexiform vascular pattern as well as by the presence of the typical coarse, eosinophilic collagen fibers (Fig. 8-89). Interestingly, loss of nuclear expression of RB1 is often observed.

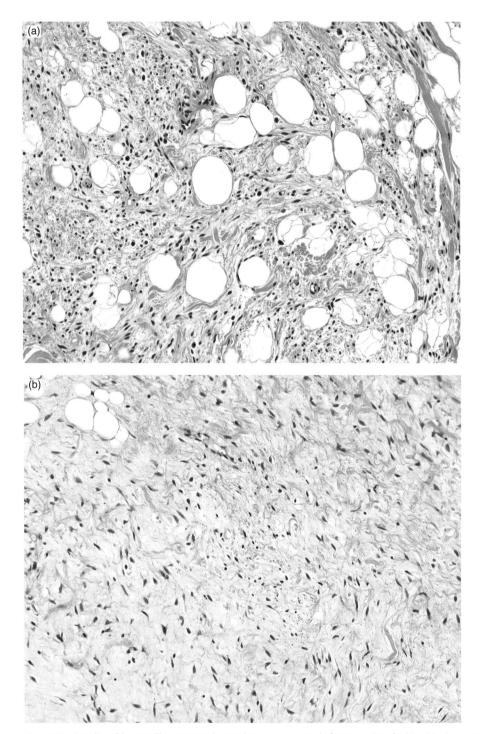

**Fig. 8-88.** Spindle cell lipoma. This common benign lesion is composed of mature white fat, bland-looking spindle cells and eosinophilic, coarse collagen bundles. (A) Myxoid spindle cell lipoma. At low power, a hypocellular tumor composed of uniform, cytologically bland spindle cells set in a myxoid stroma with minimal adipocytic component is seen (B).

Spindle cell lipoma is benign. Local recurrences are rare and most often represent persistence following incomplete excision.

Another relevant differential diagnosis among benign adipocytic lesions is represented by **lipoblastoma**. Lipoblastoma tends to occur predominantly in young patients (most often in boys younger than 3 years) and is characterized by a very distinctive lobular growth pattern (Fig. 8-90). A rare diffuse form exists that is characterized by infiltration of subcutis and

muscles and is termed "lipoblastomatosis." Genetically, lipoblastoma features a rearrangement most often involving the 8q11-13 chromosome region and leading to *PLAG1* gene rearrangement. Lipoblastoma features the presence of neoplastic lobules composed of a variable combination of spindle cells, adipocytes, and lipoblasts, set in a myxoid background. Overall, the morphology of lipoblastoma recapitulates the process of maturation of normal fat tissues. At high magnification,

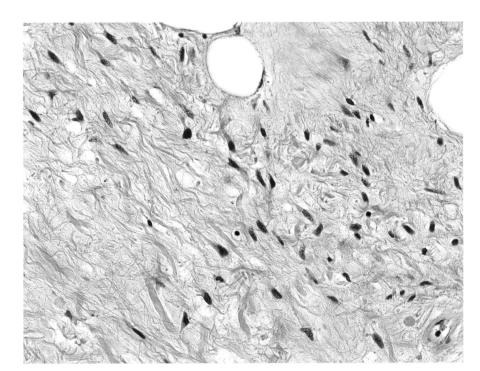

**Fig. 8-89.** Myxoid spindle cell lipoma. A key diagnostic clue is represented by the presence of eosinophilic, refractile, collagenous bundles.

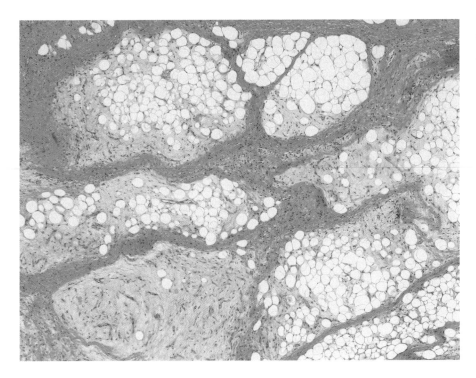

**Fig. 8-90.** Lipoblastoma. The tumor shows a characteristic lobular pattern of growth. Tumor nodules are divided by thick septa and are composed of an admixture of mature adipocytes, spindle cells, and lipoblasts.

lipoblastoma can be indistinguishable from myxoid liposarcoma, as it also features the presence of a plexiform vascular network (Fig. 8-91). However, low-magnification observation allows the recognition of the lobular pattern, facilitating a correct diagnosis in most cases. Certainly there exist situations in which the safest approach is represented by molecular genetic analysis demonstrating the absence of *CHOP/DDIT3* gene rearrangements. An extremely rare entity morphologically related to lipoblastoma that can be confused with

myxoid liposarcoma is represented by so-called lipoblastoma-like tumor of the vulva (LLTV). However, lack of PLAG1 and HMGA2 expression in the majority of LLTV suggests that these lesions are distinct from "true" lipoblastoma.

Intramuscular myxoma is excluded on the basis of the absence of a plexiform vascularization as well as the absence of adipocytic differentiation. Cellular myxoma may feature an increased vascular network; however, it never matches the

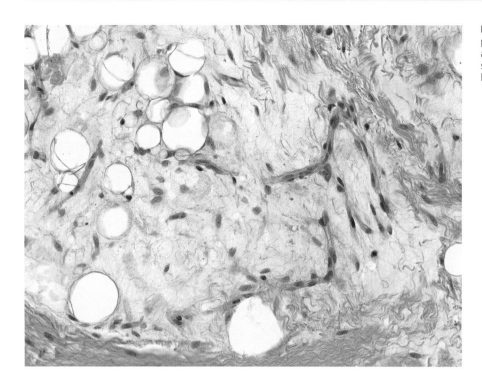

**Fig. 8-91.** Lipoblastoma. At high power, the presence of myxoid stroma associated with a plexiform vasculature represents a significant source of diagnostic confusion with myxoid liposarcoma.

distinctive "chicken wire" configuration of myxoid liposarcoma.

Among malignant neoplasms, the differential diagnosis includes well-differentiated/dedifferentiated liposarcoma with myxoid change of the stroma and myxofibrosarcoma. A fundamental caveat is represented by the fact that when dealing with a neoplasm in a retroperitoneal location, myxoid liposarcoma always represents the less likely diagnostic option. Primary myxoid liposarcoma of the retroperitoneum is exceedingly rare and, unless it represents a metastasis, well-differentiated liposarcoma with myxoid change of the stroma or dedifferentiated liposarcoma (myxofibrosarcoma-like variant) is most often the correct diagnosis. The presence of MDM2 overexpression and/or amplification represents a key confirmatory finding.

Myxofibrosarcoma, as discussed earlier in this chapter, is recognized on the basis of a different vascular pattern (archiform versus plexiform), the presence of nuclear hyperchromasia/pleomorphism (most often absent in myxoid liposarcoma), and the absence of true lipoblasts (only mucin-laden pseudolipoblasts are in fact seen in myxofibrosarcoma).

As discussed in Chapter 6, purely round cell liposarcoma enters the differential diagnosis with all other round cell malignancies, and most often, in addition to the presence of rare lipoblasts as well as the distinctive vascular network, molecular genetic data play a key confirmatory diagnostic role.

**Key Points in Myxoid Liposarcoma Diagnosis**

- Occurrence in the lower limbs of adults
- Presence of abundant myxoid matrix
- Presence of a distinctive plexiform capillary network
- Presence of predominantly monovacuolated lipoblasts
- Transition to high-grade hypercellular tumors
- Outcome related to the amount of high-grade areas

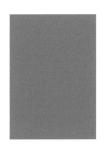

# Extraskeletal Myxoid Chondrosarcoma

## Definition and Epidemiology

Extraskeletal myxoid chondrosarcoma (EMCHS) is a malignant soft tissue tumor of uncertain differentiation characterized by a multinodular architecture and abundant myxoid matrix. Despite the name, there is no convincing evidence of cartilaginous differentiation. Extraskeletal myxoid chondrosarcoma is very rare, representing less than 3% of all soft tissue sarcomas. It usually occurs in adults, with a peak incidence in the fifth decade. There exists a male predominance, with a male-to-female ratio of 2:1.

## Clinical Presentation and Outcome

Extraskeletal myxoid chondrosarcoma mainly involves the deep soft tissues of the proximal extremities and limb girdles. Thigh and popliteal fossa are the most commonly involved sites, followed by the trunk, paraspinal region, foot, and head and neck region. It has also been rarely reported in the finger, retroperitoneum, pleura, bone, and even intracranially. Extraskeletal myxoid chondrosarcoma presents as a slow-growing, soft tissue-enlarging mass, with pain and tenderness. Skin ulceration and hemorrhage have been rarely reported. The duration of symptoms varies from a few weeks to several years. Extraskeletal myxoid chondrosarcoma is associated with prolonged survival; however, there are local recurrences and metastases (usually to the lungs) in half of the cases, generally more than 10 years after diagnosis. Long-term survival in the presence of metastases is reported. Large tumor size (in particular, larger than 10 cm) and high-grade morphology (in particular, in the presence of pleomorphism or rhabdoid cytology) are adverse prognostic factors. Complete surgery represents the current treatment modality.

## Morphology and Immunophenotype

Grossly, EMCHS is usually large and well demarcated by a fibrous pseudocapsule. It appears multinodular on cut section, with gelatinous nodules separated by fibrous septa. Hemorrhage, necrosis, and cystic degeneration can be present (Fig. 8-92). Highly cellular tumors are fleshy. Microscopically, EMCHS is characterized by a multinodular architecture with fibrous septa delimiting areas filled with strikingly hypovascular myxoid or chondromyxoid matrix (Fig. 8-93). The cellularity is often higher at the periphery of nodules (Fig. 8-94). Cells are eosinophilic, with granular to vacuolated scant cytoplasm and uniform, round to oval nuclei (Fig. 8-95). In some cases, neoplastic cells may feature a predominantly spindle cell morphology (Fig. 8-96). The formation of cords or clusters (Fig. 8-97), and sometimes the organization in a filigree or cribriform pattern, is observed (Fig. 8-98). Approximately 10% of cases may contain, at least focally, neoplastic cells featuring an eosinophilic "rhabdoid" cytoplasm (Fig. 8-99). Mitoses are usually not numerous. Areas of hemorrhage are frequently seen. In contrast to the name, true cartilaginous differentiation is never encountered. A minority of cases exhibits increased cellularity associated with minimal myxoid stroma (Fig. 8-100). Neoplastic cells tend to feature an epithelioid morphology that is generally associated with remarkable nuclear atypia (Fig. 8-101) and with significantly higher mitotic activity. In contrast to initial reports, immunohistochemical analysis demonstrates S100 protein in less than 20% of cases. Neuroendocrine differentiation, with chromogranin and synaptophysin immunoreactivity, has been reported in a few cases and correlates with gene profiling data. INI1 also seems to be lost in a subset of cases.

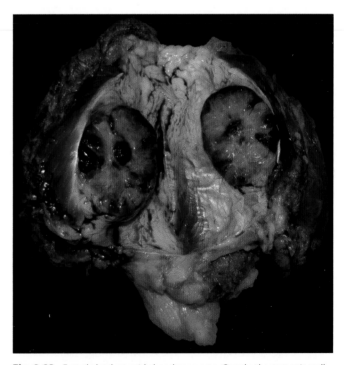

**Fig. 8-92.** Extraskeletal myxoid chondrosarcoma. Grossly, the tumor is well demarcated with a multinodular, gelatinous cut surface. Hemorrhagic foci are frequently observed.

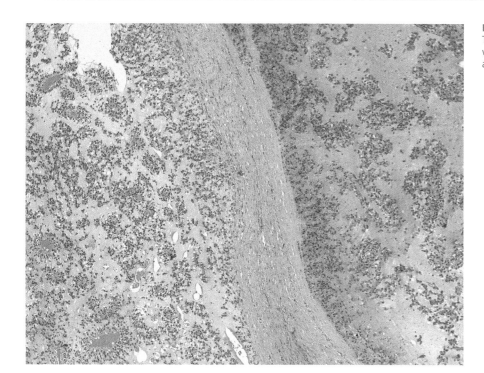

**Fig. 8-93.** Extraskeletal myxoid chondrosarcoma. Thick collagenous septa divides neoplastic lobules, which are composed of neoplastic cells set in abundant chondromyxoid matrix.

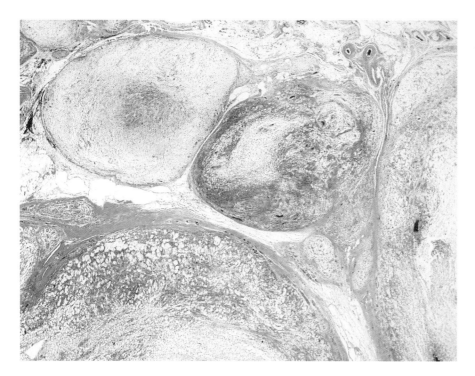

**Fig. 8-94.** Extraskeletal myxoid chondrosarcoma. At low power, the multinodular architecture of the tumor is better appreciated. Note the higher cellularity at the periphery of the nodules.

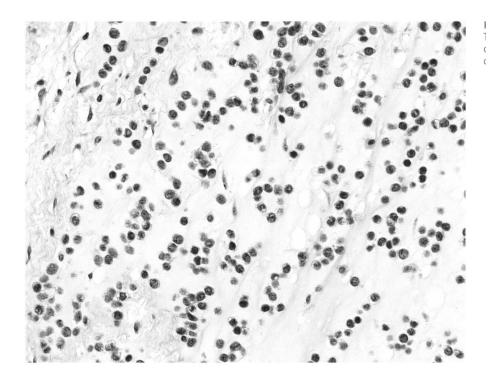

**Fig. 8-95.** Extraskeletal myxoid chondrosarcoma. The neoplastic cells are epithelioid with round to oval nuclei, small nucleoli, and scant eosinophilic cytoplasm.

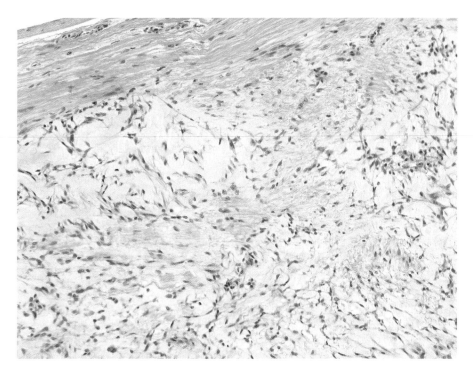

**Fig. 8-96.** Extraskeletal myxoid chondrosarcoma. Sometimes a spindle cell morphology predominates.

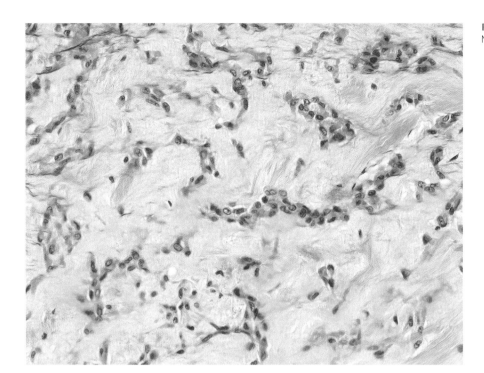

**Fig. 8-97.** Extraskeletal myxoid chondrosarcoma. Neoplastic cells typically grow in cords and strands.

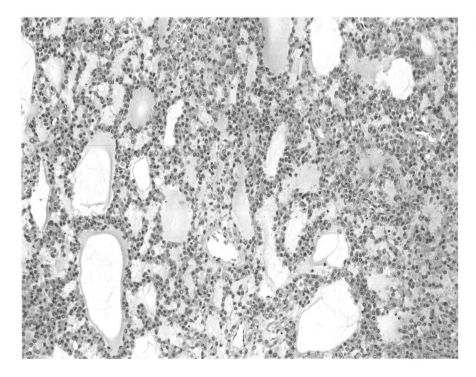

**Fig. 8-98.** Extraskeletal myxoid chondrosarcoma. This tumor shows higher cellularity organized in a cribriform pattern of growth.

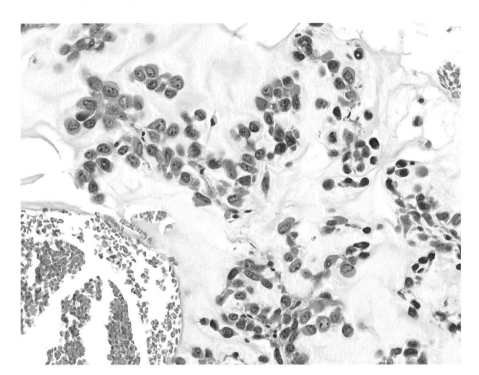

**Fig. 8-99.** Extraskeletal myxoid chondrosarcoma. The tumor is composed of epithelioid cells featuring eccentric nuclei with eosinophilic "rhabdoid" cytoplasm.

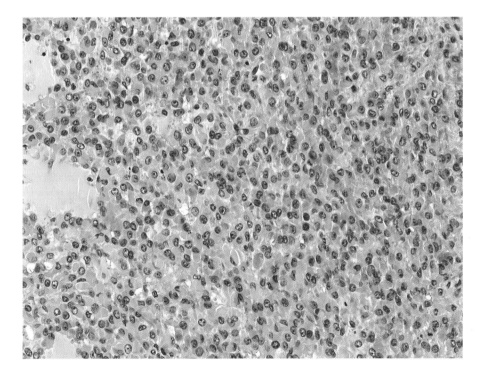

**Fig. 8-100.** Extraskeletal myxoid chondrosarcoma. In this "high-grade" example, a hypercellular epithelioid tumor with minimal myxoid stroma is seen.

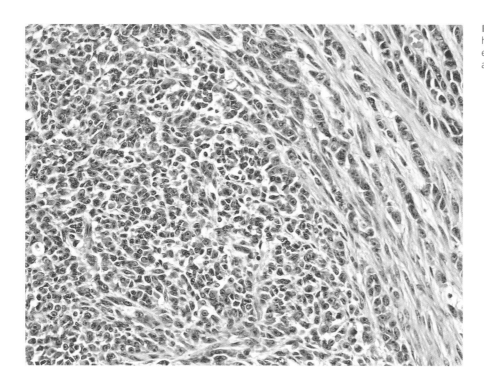

**Fig. 8-101.** Extraskeletal myxoid chondrosarcoma, high grade. The tumor consists of atypical, large epithelioid cells with discernible nucleoli set in a collagenous stroma.

## Genetics

Extraskeletal myxoid chondrosarcoma contains a t(9;22)(q22; q12) translocation and, less frequently, a t(9;17)(q22;q11) and a t(9;15)(q22;q21), fusing the *NR4A3* gene with *EWSR1, TAF15*, and *TCF12*, respectively. Recently, it has been shown that *HSPA8* represents a further fusion partner.

## Differential Diagnosis and Diagnostic Pitfalls

Myoepithelioma of soft tissue certainly represents the most challenging differential diagnosis. This entity is discussed in detail in Chapter 5. As mentioned, myoepithelioma of soft tissue may exhibit almost complete morphologic overlap with EMCHS, to the extent that at times only genetic analysis may ascertain the differential diagnosis. Immunophenotypic analysis also plays an important role. S100 immunopositivity (limited to approximately 20% of cases of EMCHS) is usually present and associated with a variable expression of cytokeratin EMA and GFAP. It is important to underline that EMA can also be seen in approximately 30% of genetically proven EMCHS. Loss of nuclear expression of INI1 is also not very helpful, as it can be rarely seen in both entities, in particular when rhabdoid cytology is present. The presence of ductal differentiation (a situation in which the term "mixed tumor" can be used) obviously speaks in favor of the diagnosis of

myoepithelioma. Both metastatic as well as the exceedingly rare extra-axial chordoma, in addition to the classic morphology, which includes the presence of the characteristic physaliphorous cells, exhibits a variable combination of S100 and cytokeratin, and most important, shows nuclear expression of brachyury. It seems likely that so-called parachordoma merely represents the aggregation of extra-axial chordomas, myoepitheliomas, and EMCHS.

High-grade EMCHS needs to be distinguished from epithelioid malignant peripheral nerve sheath tumor (MPNST), which rarely may exhibit myxoid change of the stroma and is also discussed in Chapter 5. Epithelioid MPNST, in addition to a frank epithelioid, melanoma-like cytology, typically features diffuse S100 immunopositivity, most often associated with loss of nuclear expression of INI1.

---

**Key Points in Extraskeletal Myxoid Chondrosarcoma Diagnosis**

- Occurrence in the deep soft tissues of adults
- Multinodular pattern of growth
- Cords and strands of round to oval cells set in an abundant myxoid matrix
- Presence of *NR4A3* gene rearrangement
- Prolonged survival, with late metastatic spread

---

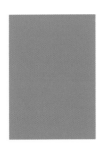

# Ossifying Fibromyxoid Tumor

## Definition and Epidemiology

Ossifying fibromyxoid tumor (OFMT) is a tumor of unknown differentiation characterized by a distinctive histologic appearance that includes cords and nests of monomorphic round cells set in an abundant fibromyxoid stroma, and most often surrounded by an incomplete shell of mature bone. First reported by Enzinger in 1989, OFMT is a rare tumor, with a peak incidence in the fifth decade, and a slight male predominance.

## Clinical Presentation and Outcome

Ossifying fibromyxoid tumor presents most often as a slowly growing, firm, and painless mass, usually 5 to 10 cm in diameter. It occurs primarily in the proximal limbs, limb girdles, and head and neck, and it is more often subcutaneous, with only about 20% of cases being subfascial. Some debate surrounds the existence of malignant forms of OFMT. Lesions featuring severe nuclear atypia, high cellularity, and mitotic activity more than 2 mitoses/50HPF seems to have a substantial risk of metastasis and may be labeled as atypical

or malignant OFMT. The vast majority of OFMT pursues a benign clinical course. The overall recurrence and metastatic rates of typical OFMT are about 15% and 5%, respectively. Surgical excision with a margin of normal tissue is therefore the treatment of choice.

## Morphology and Immunophenotype

Grossly, the lesion is usually well circumscribed and encapsulated and of hard consistency in its outer aspect. The cut surface is lobulated, tan-white, and glistening. Histologically, the tumor is composed of lobules of small round and spindled bland cells arranged in cords and set in a fibromyxoid stroma (Fig. 8-102). Rarely, the stroma is more collagenized (Fig. 8-103). Areas of ossification are characteristically present in most lesions, being localized primarily at the periphery (Fig. 8-104). In typical cases, pleomorphism is absent, mitoses are extremely rare, and necrosis is not seen. The presence of hypercellularity, more than 2 mitoses/50HPF (Fig. 8-105), irregular distribution of bone throughout the lesion (Fig. 8-106), severe atypia (Fig. 8-107), and necrosis (Fig. 8-108) seems to be

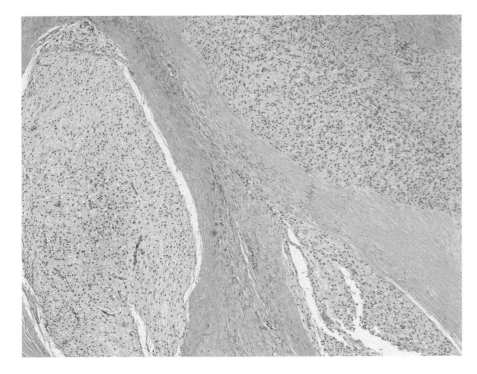

**Fig. 8-102.** Ossifying fibromyxoid tumor. The tumor is typically multilobulated. The lobules are composed of small, cytologically bland ovoid cells, organized in cords and nests and set in a fibromyxoid stroma.

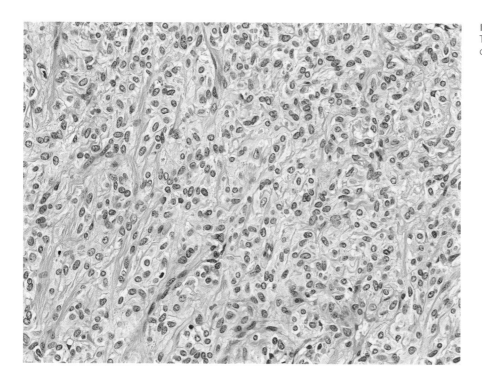

**Fig. 8-103.** Ossifying fibromyxoid tumor. The nests of neoplastic cells are lined by subtle collagen fibers.

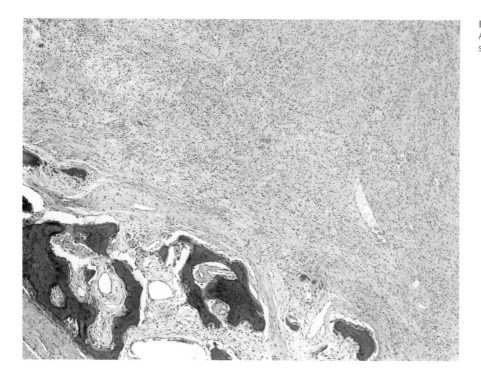

**Fig. 8-104.** Ossifying fibromyxoid tumor. A characteristic incomplete shell of lamellar bone is seen at the periphery of lobules.

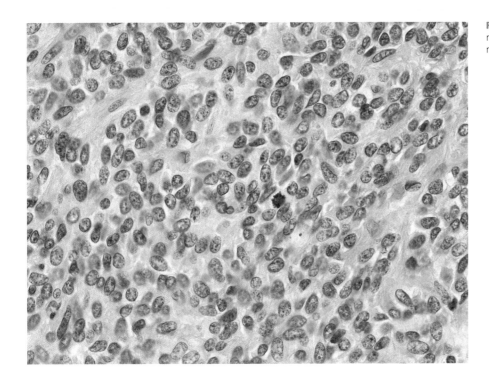

**Fig. 8-105.** Ossifying fibromyxoid tumor, atypical/malignant. Increased cellularity and significant mitotic activity are seen.

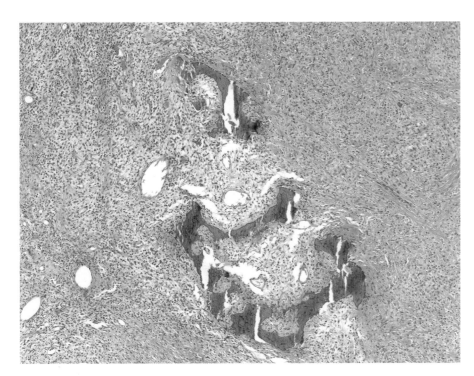

**Fig. 8-106.** Ossifying fibromyxoid tumor, atypical/malignant. In the atypical form, ossification can be seen throughout the tumor.

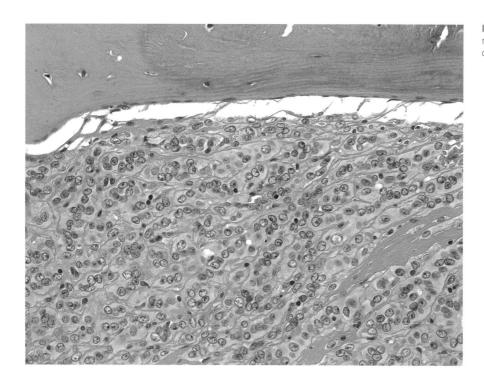

**Fig. 8-107.** Ossifying fibromyxoid tumor, atypical/malignant. The tumor presents epithelioid atypical cells featuring macronucleoli.

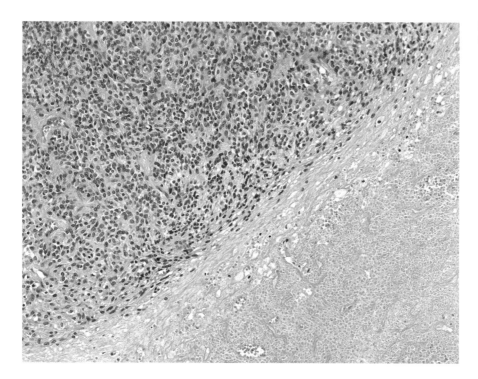

**Fig. 8-108.** Ossifying fibromyxoid tumor, atypical/malignant. Abundant coagulative necrosis is seen.

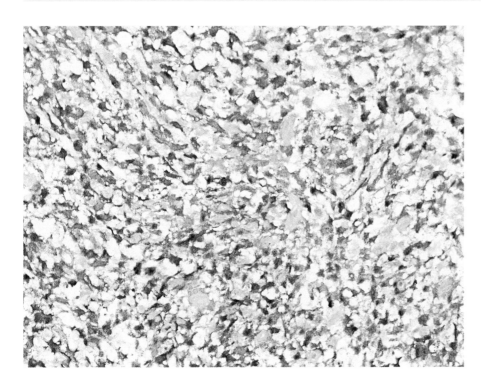

**Fig. 8-109.** Ossifying fibromyxoid tumor. S100 immunostaining is appreciable in approximately 80% of cases.

associated with significant metastatic potential (primarily to the lungs); however, in consideration of the extreme rarity of OFMT, experience is rather limited. Immunohistochemically, tumor cells more frequently stain positive for S100 protein (about 80% of cases) (Fig. 8-109) and desmin (approximately 50% of cases) and less frequently for actin, GFAP, neuron-specific enolase (NSE), and Leu-7. Epithelial markers are usually negative. Bona fide examples of OFMT totally lack bone formation and are therefore labeled as non-ossifying variants of OFMT.

## Genetics

Ossifying fibromyxoid tumor exhibits rearrangement of the *PHF1* gene with *MEAF6* and *EPC1* genes. The same aberration has been observed in both conventional and atypical/malignant cases. CREBBP-BCOLRL1 and KDM2A-WWTR1 represent alternative, recently described fusions.

## Differential Diagnosis and Diagnostic Pitfalls

Differential diagnosis is limited to only a few entities. Mature examples of myositis ossificans share with OFMT the presence of a shell of mature bone; however, as discussed in Chapter 7, mature bone merges into more immature intermediate osteogenic areas, creating a distinctive "zonal" pattern. Extraskeletal myxoid chondrosarcoma is usually deep seated, features a more prominent myxoid matrix, and lacks the peripheral

bony shell. Myoepithelioma of soft tissue may exhibit significant morphologic overlap, including the presence of metaplastic bone and expression of S100. It can, however, be separated on the basis of the expression of epithelial markers as well as the presence of *EWSR1* gene rearrangement (and absence of *PHF1* aberrations). Sclerosing epithelioid fibrosarcoma exhibits more striking stromal hyalinization and, in contrast to OFMT, is almost always strongly and diffusely MUC4 positive. Atypical/malignant variants of OFMT with bone formation in the central portion of the lesion should be distinguished from extraskeletal osteosarcoma, which, however, is far more pleomorphic, lacks the distinctive lobular architecture of OFMT, and diffusely expresses SATB2.

---

**Key Points in Ossifying Fibromyxoid Tumor Diagnosis**

- Occurrence in the superficial soft tissues of the limbs and limb girdles of adults
- Cytologically monotonous spindle cell proliferation set in fibromyxoid stroma
- Usually, presence of an incomplete shell of mature bone
- Alternation of collagenized and myxoid areas
- Variable combination of desmin and S100 immunopositivity
- Presence of *PHF1* gene rearrangement.
- Benign behavior unless atypical morphologic features occur

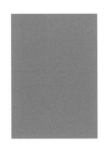

# Embryonal Rhabdomyosarcoma

## Definition and Epidemiology

Embryonal rhabdomyosarcoma (ERMS) is a pediatric soft tissue sarcoma that recapitulates the phenotypic and biologic features of embryonic skeletal muscle. In addition to the classic type, a botryoid type and an anaplastic type are recognized.

Malignant tumors showing skeletal muscle differentiation represent the most frequent soft tissue sarcomas in children and adolescents. Embryonal rhabdomyosarcoma is the most frequent rhabdomyosarcoma subtype and accounts for about 75% of all pediatric rhabdomyosarcomas. It occurs predominantly in children under 10 years of age. Classic ERMS represents about 85% of all ERMS, with a peak incidence at 7 years. Botryoid ERMS represents about 10% of all ERMS cases, with a mean age at diagnosis of about 5 years. Anaplastic ERMS represents the rarest subtype and accounts for about 5% of all ERMS, with a mean age at diagnosis of 6 years.

## Clinical Presentation and Outcome

Embryonal rhabdomyosarcoma occurs most frequently in the head and neck region (about 50%), genitourinary tract (about 30%), and extremities (about 9%). The most common primary site for botryoid ERMS is the genitourinary system (80%), followed by the head and neck region, the gastrointestinal tract, and the perianal region. Patients usually present with obstruction and bleeding. Anaplastic ERMS occurs most frequently in the lower extremities (25%), followed by the paratesticular region, head and neck, retroperitoneum, and pelvis. Overall survival of ERMS patients has improved to 70% with multimodal therapies. Localized neoplasms have a better prognosis. The most common sites for metastases are the lungs (about 60%), lymph nodes (33%), liver (22%), and brain (20%). The botryoid variant is associated with a more favorable outcome. Anaplastic ERMS is characterized by poor prognosis, in particular when diffuse anaplasia is present. Recent studies also indicate that anaplasia is associated with drug resistance. Prognosis is also dependent on tumor stage (as from the Intergroup Rhabdomyosarcoma Study grouping), tumor location (favorable: orbit, genitourinary non-bladder and prostate, and non-parameningeal head and neck region), size, and age (favorable in up to 5 cm and up to 10 years).

## Morphology and Immunophenotype

Grossly, embryonal rhabdomyosarcoma is represented by a poorly circumscribed, fleshy to solid, white to tan mass, with a mean size of 5 cm. Areas of hemorrhage and necrosis can be present. The botryoid variant shows a typical polypoid, soft, and gelatinous appearance, with clusters of small, sessile or pedunculated, grape-like vesicles that abut an epithelial surface and protrude into the lumen of viscera, i.e., urinary bladder, vagina, extrahepatic biliary tract, pharynx, conjunctiva, and auditory canal.

Microscopically, ERMS tends to mimic the various stages of embryonic striated muscle cell development. Architecturally, ERMS resembles embryonic muscle. Areas composed of neoplastic spindle cells, organized in sheets or fascicles, alternate with more primitive round cells set in a prominent myxoid or fibrotic stroma (Fig. 8-110).

The most undifferentiated cells most often exhibit a spindled morphology, featuring scanty amphophilic cytoplasm and centrally located round to oval nuclei (Fig. 8-111). With maturation, neoplastic cells tend to acquire cytoplasmic eosinophilia (Fig. 8-112) and assume various shapes, variably named tadpole, strap, tennis racquet, and spider cells (Fig. 8-113). Differentiated cells show multinucleation and giant cell transformation (Fig. 8-114), bright eosinophilia (Fig. 8-115), and cytoplasmic cross striation (terminally differentiated myoblasts are observed in less than 30% of cases) (Fig. 8-116). Interestingly, extensive maturation can be observed following systemic treatment.

As mentioned, the botryoid variant of ERMS arises beneath the epithelial surface of mucosae, most often of the urinary bladder, vagina, extrahepatic biliary tract, pharynx, conjunctiva, and auditory canal. It is characterized by the presence of a hypercellular layer of undifferentiated, mitotically active, short, spindled and round cells clustering beneath the surface epithelium (cambium layer) (Figs. 8-117 and 8-118). Beneath the cambium layer, hypocellularity predominates. Rare neoplastic cells are set in an abundant myxoid stroma, somewhat mimicking a benign process (Fig. 8-119).

The anaplastic variant of ERMS is characterized by the presence of atypical cells with enlarged, hyperchromatic nuclei and atypical, multipolar mitoses (Fig. 8-120). Anaplasia is defined as focal when only isolated anaplastic cells are seen. Diffuse anaplasia requires the presence of clusters or large sheets of anaplastic cells.

Immunohistochemically, ERMS is reactive for desmin (Fig. 8-121), MyoD1, and myogenin (Fig. 8-122). Usually, myogenin reactivity is far less diffuse than in alveolar RMS

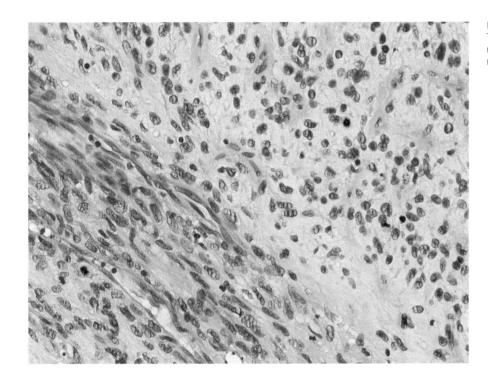

**Fig. 8-110.** Embryonal rhabdomyosarcoma. The tumor presents variations in cellularity, with more dense areas juxtaposed with hypocellular myxoid areas.

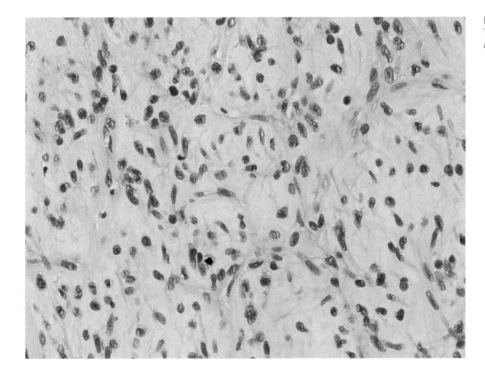

**Fig. 8-111.** Embryonal rhabdomyosarcoma. The tumor is composed of ovoid to spindle cells associated with abundant myxoid stroma.

and tends to stain approximately 30% of neoplastic cells. Other myogenic makers can also be expressed, i.e., smooth muscle actin. There can be focal expression of cytokeratins, CD99, S100 protein, and neurofilaments.

## Genetics

Embryonal rhabdomyosarcoma shows no distinct molecular signature. Allelic loss in chromosomal region 11p15 is reported in most ERMS, with the possible inactivation of putative tumor suppressor genes such as *IGF2, H19,* and *CDKN1C.* Importantly, a relevant subset of cases exhibits aberrations of the FGFR4/RAS/AKT pathway.

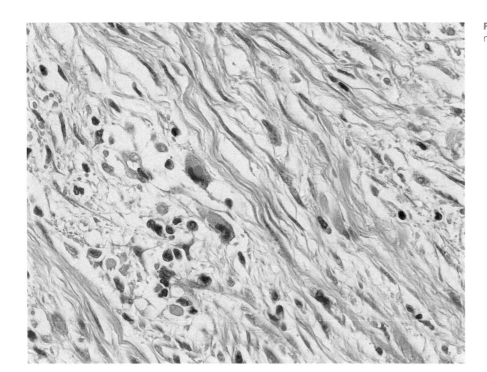

**Fig. 8-112.** Embryonal rhabdomyosarcoma. Some neoplastic cells show larger, eosinophilic cytoplasm.

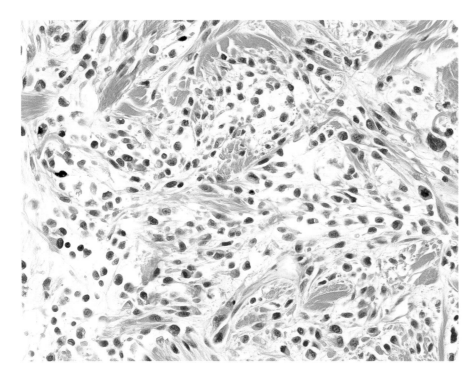

**Fig. 8-113.** Embryonal rhabdomyosarcoma. Maturation of neoplastic cells is associated with acquisition of eosinophilic cytoplasm.

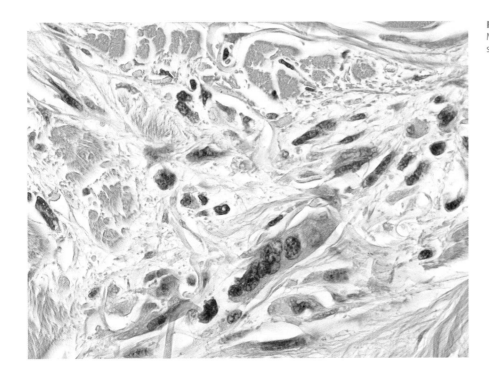

**Fig. 8-114.** Embryonal rhabdomyosarcoma. Multinucleated neoplastic giant cells mimic mature skeletal muscle cells.

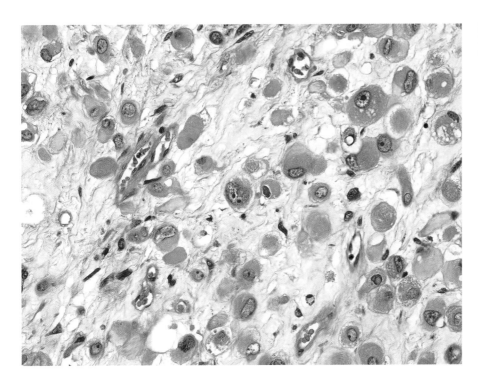

**Fig. 8-115.** Embryonal rhabdomyosarcoma. Large neoplastic cells featuring cytoplasmic eosinophilia are seen more often after chemotherapy.

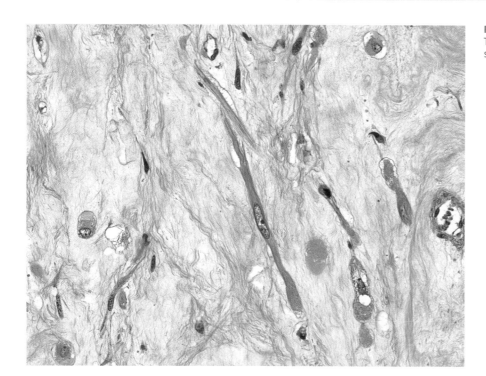

Fig. 8-116. Embryonal rhabdomyosarcoma. The similarity with muscle fibers sometimes can be striking.

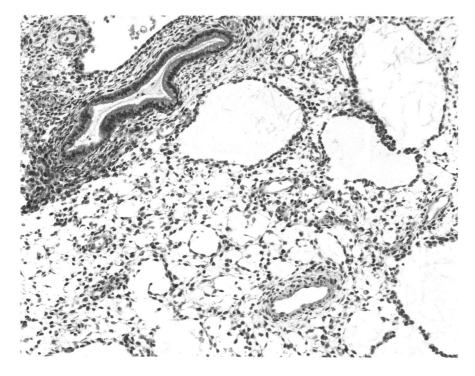

Fig. 8-117. Embryonal rhabdomyosarcoma, botryoid variant. The distinctive subepithelial accentuation of cellularity (cambium layer) is seen in this tumor of the uterine cervix.

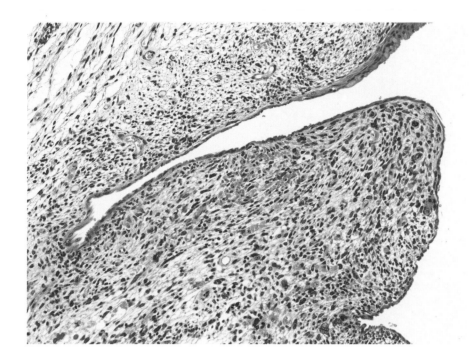

**Fig. 8-118.** Embryonal rhabdomyosarcoma, botryoid variant. Primitive neoplastic cells condense beneath the surface epithelium.

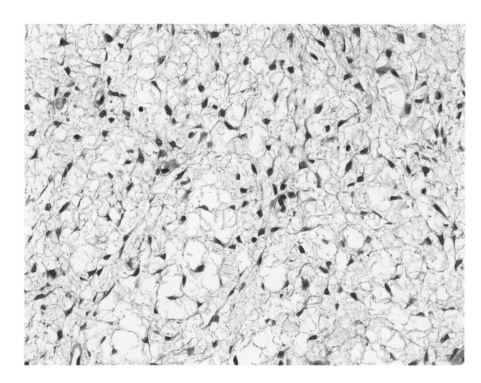

**Fig. 8-119.** Embryonal rhabdomyosarcoma, botryoid variant. The tumor can be remarkably hypocellular and composed of cytologically bland spindle cells set in a loose myxoid matrix.

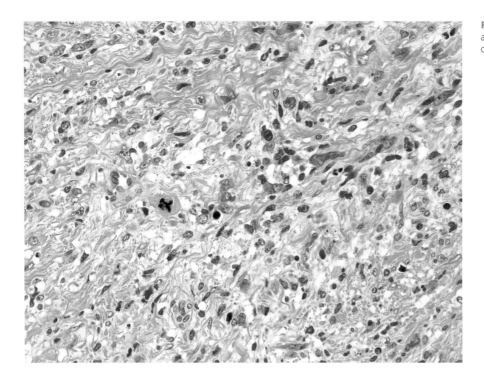

**Fig. 8-120.** Embryonal rhabdomyosarcoma, anaplastic variant. The presence of anaplasia correlates with more aggressive behavior.

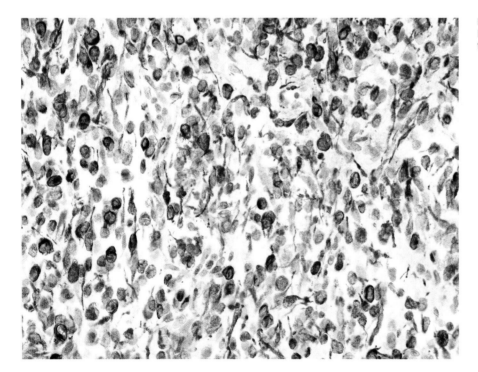

**Fig. 8-121.** Embryonal rhabdomyosarcoma. Desmin immunopositivity represents a consistent finding.

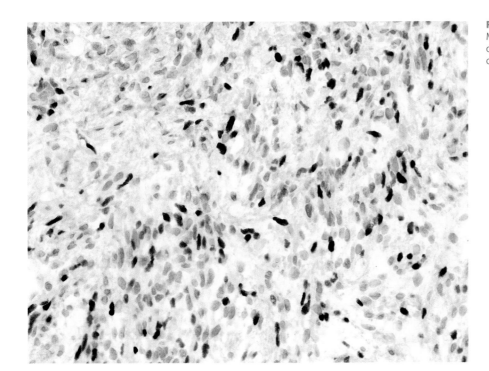

**Fig. 8-122.** Embryonal rhabdomyosarcoma. Myogenin immunostaining represents a key diagnostic clue. Interestingly, nuclear positivity is observed only in a subset of neoplastic cells.

## Differential Diagnosis and Diagnostic Pitfalls

Differential diagnosis is rather broad; however, in consideration of a young patient's age and the existence of specific markers of striated muscle differentiation, chances of misdiagnosis are relatively low. Paradoxically, the other two variants of rhabdomyosarcoma, alveolar and pleomorphic RMS, enter the differential diagnosis quite rarely. Alveolar rhabdomyosarcoma is a round cell neoplasm featuring a distinctive pseudoalveolar (rarely solid) pattern of growth, characteristically exhibits diffuse nuclear expression of myogenin, and harbors *FOXO1* gene rearrangement. A potential pitfall is between the anaplastic form of ERMS and pleomorphic rhabdomyosarcoma (PRMS); however, PRMS almost never occurs in the pediatric population, the morphologic features of myogenic differentiation are limited to the presence of intense cytoplasmic eosinophilia, and the expression of myogenin is typically very focal.

Malignant peripheral tumors with heterologous rhabdomyoblastic differentiation are exceptional in the pediatric age-group, and in half of these, patients are associated with neurofibromatosis type 1 (NF1) syndrome. Myogenic features may include the presence of cytoplasmic cross striations but are generally limited in amount and set in the context of a purely spindle cell sarcoma characterized by variation in cellularity that tends to accentuate at perivascular locations.

---

**Key Points in Embryonal Rhabdomyosarcoma Diagnosis**

- Occurrence in the deep soft tissues or hollow viscera of children
- Heterogeneous cell population set in a myxoid stroma
- Variable amounts of striated muscle differentiation
- Positivity for desmin and myogenin
- Aggressive neoplasm; however, multimodal therapy has led to significant improvement in overall survival

---

## Chapter 8 Selected Key References

### Myxofibrosarcoma and Its Differential Diagnosis

- Angervall L, Kindblom LG, Merck C. Myxofibrosarcoma. A study of 30 cases. *Acta Pathol Microbiol Scand A.* 1977;**85A:** 127–40.
- Busam KJ, Mentzel T, Colpaert C, Barnhill RL, Fletcher CD. Atypical or worrisome features in cellular neurothekeoma: a study of 10 cases. *Am J Surg Pathol.* 1998;**22:**1067–72.
- Calonje E, Guerin D, McCormick D, Fletcher CD. Superficial angiomyxoma: clinicopathologic analysis of a series of distinctive but poorly recognized cutaneous tumors with tendency for recurrence. *Am J Surg Pathol.* 1999;**23:**910–17.
- Fetsch JF, Laskin WB, Lefkowitz M, Kindblom LG, Meis-Kindblom JM. Aggressive angiomyxoma: a clinicopathologic study of 29 female patients. *Cancer.* 1996;**78:**79–90.
- Fletcher CD, Chan JK, McKee PH. Dermal nerve sheath myxoma: a study of three cases. *Histopathology.* 1986;**10:** 135–45.
- Graadt van Roggen JF, Hogendoorn PC, Fletcher CD. Myxoid tumours of soft tissue. *Histopathology.* 1999;**35:**291–312.
- Graadt van Roggen JF, McMenamin ME, Fletcher CD. Cellular myxoma of soft tissue: a clinicopathological study of 38 cases confirming indolent clinical behaviour. *Histopathology.* 2001;**39:** 287–97.

- Heitzer E, Sunitsch S, Gilg MM, et al. Expanded molecular profiling of myxofibrosarcoma reveals potentially actionable targets. *Mod Pathol.* 2017;**30**:1698–1709.

- Hollmann TJ, Bovée JV, Fletcher CD. Digital fibromyxoma (superficial acral fibromyxoma): a detailed characterization of 124 cases. *Am J Surg Pathol.* 2012;**36**:789–98.

- Hornick JL, Fletcher CD. Cellular neurothekeoma: detailed characterization in a series of 133 cases. *Am J Surg Pathol.* 2007;**31**:329–40.

- Huang H-Y, Lal P, Qin J, et al. Low-grade myxofibrosarcoma: a clinicopathologic analysis of 49 cases treated at a single institution with simultaneous assessment of the efficacy of 3-tier and 4-tier grading systems. *Hum Pathol.* 2004;**35**:612–21.

- Liegl B, Bennett MW, Fletcher CD. Microcystic/reticular schwannoma: a distinct variant with predilection for visceral locations. *Am J Surg Pathol.* 2008;**32**:1080–7.

- Meis JM, Enzinger FM. Juxta-articular myxoma: a clinical and pathologic study of 65 cases. *Hum Pathol.* 1992;**23**:639–46.

- Mentzel T, Brown LF, Dvorak HF, et al. The association between tumor progression and vascularity in myxofibrosarcoma and myxoid/round cell liposarcoma. *Virchows Arch.* 2001;**438**:13–22.

- Mentzel T, Calonje E, Wadden C, et al. Myxofibrosarcoma. Clinicopathologic analysis of 75 cases with emphasis on the low-grade variant. *Am J Surg Pathol.* 1996;**20**: 391–405.

- Merck C, Angervall L, Kindblom LG, et al. Myxofibrosarcoma. A malignant soft tissue tumor of fibroblastic-histiocytic origin. A clinicopathologic and prognostic study of 110 cases using multivariate analysis. *Acta Pathol Microbiol Immunol Scand Suppl.* 1983;**282**:1–40.

- Nascimento AF, Bertoni F, Fletcher CDM. Epithelioid variant of myxofibrosarcoma: expanding the clinicomorphologic spectrum of myxofibrosarcoma in a series of 17 cases. *Am J Surg Pathol.* 2007;**31**:99–105.

- Nielsen GP, O'Connell JX, Rosenberg AE. Intramuscular myxoma: a clinicopathologic study of 51 cases with emphasis on hypercellular and hypervascular variants. *Am J Surg Pathol.* 1998;**22**:1222–7.

- Nucci MR. Mesenchymal lesions of the lower genital tract. *Surg Pathol Clin.* 2009;**2**:603–23.

- Nucci MR, Weremowicz S, Neskey DM, et al. Chromosomal translocation t(8;12) induces aberrant HMGIC expression in aggressive angiomyxoma of the vulva. *Genes Chromosomes Cancer.* 2001;**32**: 172–6.

- Steeper TA, Rosai J. Aggressive angiomyxoma of the female pelvis and perineum. Report of nine cases of a distinctive type of gynecologic soft-tissue neoplasm. *Am J Surg Pathol.* 1983;**7**: 463–75.

- Weiss SW, Enzinger FM. Myxoid variant of malignant fibrous histiocytoma. *Cancer.* 1977;**39**:1672–85.

- Willems SM, Debiec-Rychter M, Szuhai K, Hogendoorn PC, Sciot R. Local recurrence of myxofibrosarcoma is associated with increase in tumour grade and cytogenetic aberrations, suggesting a multistep tumour progression model. *Mod Pathol.* 2006;**19**:407–16.

- Willems SM, Mohseny AB, Balog C, et al. Cellular/intramuscular myxoma and grade I myxofibrosarcoma are characterized by distinct genetic alterations and specific composition of their extracellular matrix. *J Cell Mol Med.* 2009;**13**:1291–301.

## Myxoinflammatory Fibroblastic Sarcoma and Its Differential Diagnosis

- Antonescu CR, Zhang L, Nielsen GP, et al. Consistent t(1;10) with rearrangements of TGFBR3 and MGEA5 in both myxoinflammatory fibroblastic sarcoma and hemosiderotic fibrolipomatous tumor. *Genes Chromosomes Cancer.* 2011;**50**:757–64.

- Boland JM, Folpe AL. Hemosiderotic fibrolipomatous tumor, pleomorphic hyalinizing angiectatic tumor, and myxoinflammatory fibroblastic sarcoma: related or not? *Adv Anat Pathol.* 2017;**24**:268–77.

- Chung EB, Enzinger FM. Proliferative fasciitis. *Cancer.* 1975;**36**:1450–8.

- Elco CP, Mariño-Enríquez A, Abraham JA, Dal Cin P, Hornick JL. Hybrid myxoinflammatory fibroblastic sarcoma/hemosiderotic fibrolipomatous tumor: report of a case providing further evidence for a pathogenetic link. *Am J Surg Pathol.* 2010;**34**:1723–7.

- Enzinger FM, Dulcey F. Proliferative myositis. Report of thirty-three cases. *Cancer.* 1967;**20**:2213–23.

- Hallor KH, Sciot R, Staaf J, et al. Two genetic pathways, t(1;10) and amplification of 3p11-12, in myxoinflammatory fibroblastic sarcoma, haemosiderotic fibrolipomatous tumour, and morphologically similar lesions. *J Pathol.* 2009;**217**:716–27.

- Jurčić V, Zidar A, Montiel MD, et al. Myxoinflammatory fibroblastic sarcoma: a tumor not restricted to acral sites. *Ann Diagn Pathol.* 2002;**6**:272–80.

- Kao YC, Ranucci V, Zhang L, et al. Recurrent BRAF gene rearrangements in myxoinflammatory fibroblastic sarcomas, but not hemosiderotic fibrolipomatous tumors. *Am J Surg Pathol.* 2017;**4**:1456–65.

- Laskin WB, Fetsch JF, Miettinen M. Myxoinflammatory fibroblastic sarcoma: a clinicopathologic analysis of 104 cases, with emphasis on predictors of outcome. *Am J Surg Pathol.* 2014;**38**:1–12.

- Lucas DR. Myxoinflammatory fibroblastic sarcoma: review and update. *Arch Pathol Lab Med.* 2017;**141**:1503–7.

- Marshall-Taylor C, Fanburg-Smith JC. Hemosiderotic fibrohistiocytic lipomatous lesion: ten cases of a previously undescribed fatty lesion of the foot/ankle. *Mod Pathol.* 2000;**13**:1192–9.

- Meis-Kindblom JM, Kindblom LG. Acral myxoinflammatory fibroblastic sarcoma: a low-grade tumor of the hands and feet. *Am J Surg Pathol.* 1998;**22**: 911–24.

- Montgomery EA, Devaney KO, Giordano TJ, Weiss SW. Inflammatory myxohyaline tumor of distal extremities with virocyte or Reed-Sternberg-like cells: a distinctive lesion with features simulating inflammatory conditions, Hodgkin's disease, and various sarcomas. *Mod Pathol.* 1998;**11**:384–91.

- Solomon DA, Antonescu CR, Link TM, et al. Hemosiderotic fibrolipomatous tumor, not an entirely benign entity. *Am J Surg Pathol.* 2013;**37**:1627–30.

## Low-Grade Fibromyxoid Sarcoma and Its Differential Diagnosis

- Allen PW. Nodular fasciitis. *Pathology.* 1972;**4**:9–26.

- Allen PW. The fibromatoses: a clinicopathologic classification based on 140 cases. *Am J Surg Pathol.* 1977;**1**: 255–70.

- Bhattacharya B, Dilworth HP, Iacobuzio-Donahue C, et al. Nuclear beta-catenin expression distinguishes deep fibromatosis from other benign and malignant fibroblastic and myofibroblastic lesions. *Am J Surg Pathol.* 2005;**29**:653–9.

- Burke AP, Sobin LH, Shekitka KM, Federspiel BH, Helwig EB. Intra-abdominal fibromatosis. A pathologic analysis of 130 tumors with comparison of clinical subgroups. *Am J Surg Pathol.* 1990;**14**:335–41.

- Coffin CM, Davis JL, Borinstein SC. Syndrome-associated soft tissue tumours. *Histopathology.* 2014;**64**:68–87.

- Colombo C, Bolshakov S, Hajibashi S, et al. 'Difficult to diagnose' desmoid tumours: a potential role for CTNNB1 mutational analysis. *Histopathology.* 2011;**59**:336–40.

- de Feraudy S, Fletcher CD. Intradermal nodular fasciitis: a rare lesion analyzed in a series of 24 cases. *Am J Surg Pathol.* 2010;**34**:1377–81.

- de Saint Aubain Somerhausen N, Rubin BP, Fletcher CD. Myxoid solitary fibrous tumor: a study of seven cases with emphasis on differential diagnosis. *Mod Pathol.* 1999;**12**:463–71.

- De Wever I, Dal Cin P, Fletcher CD, et al. Cytogenetic, clinical, and morphologic correlations in 78 cases of fibromatosis: a report from the CHAMP Study Group. *Mod Pathol.* 2000;**3**: 1080–5.

- Doyle LA, Möller E, Dal Cin P, et al. MUC4 is a highly sensitive and specific marker for low-grade fibromyxoid sarcoma. *Am J Surg Pathol.* 2011;**35**: 733–41.

- Erickson-Johnson MR, Chou MM, Evers BR, et al. Nodular fasciitis: a novel model of transient neoplasia induced by MYH9-USP6 gene fusion. *Lab Invest.* 2011;**91**:1427–33.

- Evans HL. Low-grade fibromyxoid sarcoma. A report of two metastasizing neoplasms having a deceptively benign appearance. *Am J Clin Pathol.* 1987;**88**: 615–19.

- Evans HL. Low-grade fibromyxoid sarcoma. A report of 12 cases. *Am J Surg Pathol.* 1993;**17**: 595–600.

- Evans HL. Low-grade fibromyxoid sarcoma: a clinicopathologic study of 33 cases with long-term follow-up. *Am J Surg Pathol.* 2011;**35**:1450–62.

- Folpe AL, Lane KL, Paull G, Weiss SW. Low-grade fibromyxoid sarcoma and hyalinizing spindle cell tumor with giant rosettes: a clinicopathologic study of 73 cases supporting their identity and assessing the impact of high-grade areas. *Am J Surg Pathol.* 2000;**24**:1353–60.

- Gardner EJ. Follow-up study of a family group exhibiting dominant inheritance for a syndrome including intestinal polyps, osteomas, fibromas and epidermal cysts. *Am J Hum Genet.* 1962;**14**:376–90.

- Goodlad JR, Mentzel T, Fletcher CD. Low grade fibromyxoid sarcoma: clinicopathological analysis of eleven new cases in support of a distinct entity. *Histopathology.* 1995;**26**:229–37.

- Gronchi A, Colombo C, Le Péchoux C, et al. Sporadic desmoid-type fibromatosis: a stepwise approach to a non-metastasising neoplasm–a position paper from the Italian and the French Sarcoma Group. *Ann Oncol.* 2014;**25**:578–83.

- Guillou L, Benhattar J, Gengler C, et al. Translocation-positive low-grade fibromyxoid sarcoma: clinicopathologic and molecular analysis of a series expanding the morphologic spectrum and suggesting potential relationship to sclerosing epithelioid fibrosarcoma: a study from the French Sarcoma Group. *Am J Surg Pathol.* 2007;**31**:1387–402.

- Honeyman JN, Theilen TM, Knowles MA, et al. Desmoid fibromatosis in children and adolescents: a conservative approach to management. *J Pediatr Surg.* 2013;**48**:62–6.

- Hornick JL, Fletcher CD. Soft tissue perineurioma: clinicopathologic analysis of 81 cases including those with atypical histologic features. *Am J Surg Pathol.* 2005;**29**:845–58.

- Hornick JL, Fletcher CD. Intraarticular nodular fasciitis – a rare lesion: clinicopathologic analysis of a series. *Am J Surg Pathol.* 2006;**30**:237–41.

- Lane KL, Shannon RJ, Weiss SW. Hyalinizing spindle cell tumor with giant rosettes: a distinctive tumor closely resembling low-grade fibromyxoid sarcoma. *Am J Surg Pathol.* 1997;**21**: 1481–8.

- Lau PP, Lui PC, Lau GT, et al. EWSR1-CREB3L1 gene fusion: a novel alternative molecular aberration of low-grade fibromyxoid sarcoma. *Am J Surg Pathol.* 2013;**37**:734–8.

- Lazar AJ, Tuvin D, Hajibashi S, et al. Specific mutations in the beta-catenin gene (CTNNB1) correlate with local recurrence in sporadic desmoid tumors. *Am J Pathol.* 2008;**173**: 1518–27.

- Le Guellec S, Soubeyran I, Rochaix P, et al. CTNNB1 mutation analysis is a useful tool for the diagnosis of desmoid tumors: a study of 260 desmoid tumors and 191 potential morphologic mimics. *Mod Pathol.* 2012;**25**:1551–8.

- Linos K, Bridge JA, Edgar MA. MUC 4-negative FUS-CREB3L2 rearranged low-grade fibromyxoid sarcoma. *Histopathology.* 2014;**65**:722–4.

- Matsuyama A, Hisaoka M, Shimajiri S, et al. Molecular detection of FUS-CREB3L2 fusion transcripts in low-grade fibromyxoid sarcoma using formalin-fixed, paraffin-embedded tissue specimens. *Am J Surg Pathol.* 2006;**30**: 1077–84.

- Mentzel T, Dei Tos AP, Fletcher CD. Perineurioma (storiform perineurial fibroma): clinico-pathological analysis of four cases. *Histopathology.* 1994;**25**: 261–7.

- Mertens F, Fletcher CD, Antonescu CR, et al. Clinicopathologic and molecular genetic characterization of low-grade fibromyxoid sarcoma, and cloning of a novel FUS/CREB3L1 fusion gene. *Lab Invest.* 2005;**85**:408–15.

- Mohamed M, Fisher C, Thway K. Low-grade fibromyxoid sarcoma: clinical, morphologic and genetic features. *Ann Diagn Pathol.* 2017;**28**:60–7.

- Montgomery EA, Meis JM. Nodular fasciitis. Its morphologic spectrum and immunohistochemical profile. *Am J Surg Pathol.* 1991;**15**:942–8.

- Ng TL, Gown AM, Barry TS, et al. Nuclear beta-catenin in mesenchymal tumors. *Mod Pathol.* 2005; **18**:68–74.

- Patel NR, Chrisinger JSA, Demicco EG, et al. USP6 activation in nodular fasciitis by promoter-swapping gene fusions. *Mod Pathol.* 2017;**30**:1577–88.

- Penel N, Le Cesne A, Bonvalot S, et al. Surgical versus non-surgical approach in primary desmoid-type fibromatosis patients: A nationwide prospective cohort from the French Sarcoma Group. *Eur J Cancer.* 2017;**83**:125–31.

- Reid R, de Silva MV, Paterson L, Ryan E, Fisher C. Low-grade fibromyxoid sarcoma and hyalinizing spindle cell tumor with giant rosettes share a common t(7;16)(q34;p11) translocation. *Am J Surg Pathol.* 2003;**27**:1229–36.

- Wirman JA. Nodular fasciitis, a lesion of myofibroblasts: an ultrastructural study. *Cancer.* 1976;**38**:2378–89.

## Myxoid Liposarcoma and Its Differential Diagnosis

- Åman P, Ron D, Mandahl N, et al. Rearrangement of the transcript factor gene CHOP in myxoid liposarcomas with t(12;16)(q13;p11). *Genes Chromosomes Cancer.* 1992;**5**:278–85.

- Antonescu CR, Tschernyavsky SJ, Decuseara R, et al. Prognostic impact of P53 status, TLS-CHOP fusion transcript structure, and histological grade in myxoid liposarcoma: a molecular and clinicopathologic study of 82 cases. *Clin Cancer Res.* 2001;7:3977–87.

- Bolen JW, Thorning D. Benign lipoblastoma and myxoid liposarcoma: a comparative light- and electron-microscopic study. *Am J Surg Pathol.* 1980;4:163–74.

- Chen BJ, Mariño-Enríquez A, Fletcher CD, Hornick JL. Loss of retinoblastoma protein expression in spindle cell/pleomorphic lipomas and cytogenetically related tumors: an immunohistochemical study with diagnostic implications. *Am J Surg Pathol.* 2012;36:1119–28.

- Creytens D. Lipoblastoma-like tumor of the vulva, an important benign mimic of myxoid liposarcoma. *Int J Gynecol Pathol.* 2018 Jan 3. [Epub ahead of print]

- Dal Cin P, Sciot R, Panagopoulos I, et al. Additional evidence of a variant translocation t(12;22) with EWS/CHOP fusion in myxoid liposarcoma: clinicopathological features. *J Pathol.* 1997;182:437–41.

- Dei Tos AP. Liposarcomas: diagnostic pitfalls and new insights. *Histopathology.* 2014;64:38–52.

- Dei Tos AP, Piccinin S, Doglioni C, et al. Molecular aberrations of the G1-S checkpoint in myxoid and round cell liposarcoma. *Am J Pathol.* 1997;151: 1531–9.

- Demetri GD, von Mehren M, Jones RL, et al. Efficacy and safety of trabectedin or dacarbazine for metastatic liposarcoma or leiomyosarcoma after failure of conventional chemotherapy: results of a phase III randomized multicenter clinical trial. *J Clin Oncol.* 2016;34:786–93.

- de Saint Aubain Somerhausen N, Coindre JM, Debiec-Rychter M, Delplace J, Sciot R. Lipoblastoma in adolescents and young adults: report of six cases with FISH analysis. *Histopathology.* 2008;52: 294–8.

- de Vreeze RS, de Jong D, Tielen IH, et al. Primary retroperitoneal myxoid/round cell liposarcoma is a nonexisting disease: an immunohistochemical and molecular biological analysis. *Mod Pathol.* 2009;22: 223–31.

- Enzinger FM, Harvey DA. Spindle cell lipoma. *Cancer.* 1975;36:1852–9.

- Fletcher CD, Martin-Bates E. Spindle cell lipoma: a clinicopathological study with some original observations. *Histopathology.* 1987;11:803–17.

- Fritchie KJ, Goldblum JR, Tubbs RR, et al. The expanded histologic spectrum of myxoid liposarcoma with an emphasis

on newly described patterns: implications for diagnosis on small biopsy specimens. *Am J Clin Pathol.* 2012;137:229–39

- Gronchi A, Ferrari S, Quagliuolo V, et al. Histotype-tailored neoadjuvant chemotherapy versus standard chemotherapy in patients with high-risk soft-tissue sarcomas (ISG-STS 1001): an international, open-label, randomised, controlled, phase 3, multicentre trial. *Lancet Oncol.* 2017;18:812–22.

- Grosso F, Jones RL, Demetri GD, et al. Efficacy of trabectedin (ecteinascidin-743) in advanced pretreated myxoid liposarcomas: a retrospective study. *Lancet Oncol.* 2007;8:595–602.

- Hawley IC, Krausz T, Evans DJ, Fletcher CD. Spindle cell lipoma – a pseudoangiomatous variant. *Histopathology.* 1994;24(6):565–9.

- Hibbard MK, Kozakewich HP, Dal Cin P, et al. PLAG1 fusion oncogenes in lipoblastoma. *Cancer Res.* 2000;60: 4869–72.

- Kilpatrick SE, Doyon J, Choong PFM, et al. The clinicopathologic spectrum of myxoid and round cell liposarcoma. A study of 95 cases. *Cancer.* 1996;77:1450–8.

- Knight JC, Renwick PJ, Dal Cin P, Van den Berghe H, Fletcher CD. Translocation t(12;16)(q13;p11) in myxoid liposarcoma and round cell liposarcoma: molecular and cytogenetic analysis. *Cancer Res.* 1995;55:24–7.

- Lee ATJ, Thway K, Huang PH, Jones RL. Clinical and molecular spectrum of liposarcoma. *J Clin Oncol.* 2018;10(36): 151–9.

- Mentzel T, Calonje E, Fletcher CD. Lipoblastoma and lipoblastomatosis: a clinicopathological study of 14 cases. *Histopathology.* 1993;23:527–33.

- Mirkovic J, Fletcher CD. Lipoblastoma-like tumor of the vulva: further characterization in 8 new cases. *Am J Surg Pathol.* 2015;39:1290–5.

- Moreau LC, Turcotte R, Ferguson P, et al; Canadian Orthopaedic Oncology Society (CANOOS). Myxoid\round cell liposarcoma (MRCLS) revisited: an analysis of 418 primarily managed cases. *Ann Surg Oncol.* 2012;19: 1081–8.

- Orvieto E, Furlanetto A, Laurino L, Dei Tos AP. Myxoid and round cell liposarcoma: a spectrum of myxoid adipocytic neoplasia. *Semin Diagn Pathol.* 2001;18:267–73.

- Smith TA, Easley KA, Goldblum JR. Myxoid/round cell liposarcoma of the

extremities: a clinicopathologic study of 29 cases with particular attention to extent of round cell liposarcoma. *Am J Surg Pathol.* 1996;20:171–80.

- Tallini G, Akerman M, Dal Cin P, et al. Combined morphologic and karyotypic study of 28 myxoid liposarcomas. Implications for a revised morphologic typing, (a report from the CHAMP Group). *Am J Surg Pathol.* 1996;20: 1047–55.

- ten Heuvel SE, Hoekstra HJ, van Ginkel RJ, et al. Clinicopathologic prognostic factors in myxoid liposarcoma: a respective study of 49 patients with long-term follow-up. *Ann Surg Oncol.* 2007;14:222–9.

# Extraskeletal Myxoid Chondrosarcoma

- Agaram NP, Zhang L, Sung YS, Singer S, Antonescu CR. Extraskeletal myxoid chondrosarcoma with non-EWSR1-NR 4A3 variant fusions correlate with rhabdoid phenotype and high-grade morphology. *Hum Pathol.* 2014 45: 1084–91.

- Antonescu CR, Argani P, Erlandson RA, et al. Skeletal and extraskeletal myxoid chondrosarcoma: a comparative clinicopathologic, ultrastructural, and molecular study. *Cancer.* 1998 15;83: 1504–21.

- Attwooll C, Tariq M, Harris M, et al. Identification of a novel fusion gene involving hTAFII68 and CHN from a t(9;17)(q22;q11.2) translocation in an extraskeletal myxoid chondrosarcoma. *Oncogene.* 1999;18:7599–601.

- Broehm CJ, Wu J, Gullapalli RR, Bocklage T. Extraskeletal myxoid chondrosarcoma with a t(9;16)(q22; p11.2) resulting in a NR4A3-FUS fusion. *Cancer Genet.* 2014;207:276–80.

- Demicco EG, Wang WL, Madewell JE, et al. Osseous myxochondroid sarcoma: a detailed study of 5 cases of extraskeletal myxoid chondrosarcoma of the bone. *Am J Surg Pathol.* 2013;37:752–62.

- Enzinger FM, Shiraki M. Extraskeletal myxoid chondrosarcoma. An analysis of 34 cases. *Hum Pathol.* 1972;3:421–35.

- Flucke U, Tops BB, Verdijk MA, et al. NR4A3 rearrangement reliably distinguishes between the clinicopathologically overlapping entities myoepithelial carcinoma of soft tissue and cellular extraskeletal myxoid chondrosarcoma. *Virchows Arch.* 2012;460:621–8.

- Hirabayashi Y, Ishida T, Yoshida MA, et al. Translocation (9;22)(q22;q12). A recurrent chromosome abnormality in extraskeletal myxoid chondrosarcoma. *Cancer Genet Cytogenet.* 1995;**81**:33–7.

- Hisaoka M, Hashimoto H. Extraskeletal myxoid chondrosarcoma: updated clinicopathological and molecular genetic characteristics. *Pathol Int.* 2005;**55**:453–63.

- Hisaoka M, Ishida T, Imamura T, Hashimoto H. TFG is a novel fusion partner of NOR1 in extraskeletal myxoid chondrosarcoma. *Genes Chromosomes Cancer.* 2004;**40**:325–8.

- Kohashi K, Oda Y, Yamamoto H, et al. SMARCB1/INI1 protein expression in round cell soft tissue sarcomas associated with chromosomal translocations involving EWS: a special reference to SMARCB1/INI1 negative variant extraskeletal myxoid chondrosarcoma. *Am J Surg Pathol.* 2008;**32**:1168–74.

- Okamoto S, Hisaoka M, Ishida T, et al. Extraskeletal myxoid chondrosarcoma: a clinicopathologic, immunohistochemical, and molecular analysis of 18 cases. *Hum Pathol.* 2001;**32**:1116–24.

- Panagopoulos I, Mertens F, Isaksson M, et al. Molecular genetic characterization of the EWS/CHN and RBP56/CHN fusion genes in extraskeletal myxoid chondrosarcoma. *Genes Chromosomes Cancer.* 2002;**35**:340–52.

- Smith MT, Farinacci CJ, Carpenter HA, Bannayan GA. Extraskeletal myxoid chondrosarcoma: a clinicopathological study. *Cancer.* 1976;**37**:821–7.

- Stacchiotti S, Pantaleo MA, Astolfi A, et al. Activity of sunitinib in extraskeletal myxoid chondrosarcoma. *Eur J Cancer.* 2014;**50**:1657–64.

- Urbini M, Astolfi A, Pantaleo MA, et al. HSPA8 as a novel fusion partner of NR4A3 in extraskeletal myxoid chondrosarcoma. *Genes Chromosomes Cancer.* 2017;**56**:582–6.

## Ossifying Fibromyxoid Tumor and Its Differential Diagnosis

- Antonescu CR, Sung YS, Chen CL, et al. Novel ZC3H7B-BCOR, MEAF6-PHF1, and EPC1-PHF1 fusions in ossifying fibromyxoid tumors–molecular characterization shows genetic overlap with endometrial stromal sarcoma. *Genes Chromosomes Cancer.* 2014;**53**:183–93.

- Atanaskova Mesinkovska N, Buehler D, McClain CM, et al. Ossifying fibromyxoid tumor: a clinicopathologic analysis of 26 subcutaneous tumors with emphasis on differential diagnosis and prognostic factors. *J Cutan Pathol.* 2015;**42**:622–31.

- de Silva MV, Reid R. Myositis ossificans and fibroosseous pseudotumor of digits: a clinicopathological review of 64 cases with emphasis on diagnostic pitfalls. *Int J Surg Pathol.* 2003;**11**:187–95.

- Enzinger FM, Weiss SW, Liang CY. Ossifying fibromyxoid tumor of soft parts. A clinicopathological analysis of 59 cases. *Am J Surg Pathol.* 1989;**13**: 817–27.

- Folpe AL, Weiss SW. Ossifying fibromyxoid tumor of soft parts: a clinicopathologic study of 70 cases with emphasis on atypical and malignant variants. *Am J Surg Pathol.* 2003; **27**:421–31.

- Gebre-Medhin S, Nord KH, Möller E, et al. Recurrent rearrangement of the PHF1 gene in ossifying fibromyxoid tumors. *Am J Pathol.* 2012;**181**:1069–77.

- Graham RP, Dry S, Li X, et al. Ossifying fibromyxoid tumor of soft parts: a clinicopathologic, proteomic, and genomic study. *Am J Surg Pathol.* 2011;**35**:1615–25.

- Kawashima H, Ogose A, Umezu H, et al. Ossifying fibromyxoid tumor of soft parts with clonal chromosomal aberrations. *Cancer Genet Cytogenet.* 2007; **176**:156–60.

- Kilpatrick SE, Ward WG, Mozes M, et al. Atypical and malignant variants of ossifying fibromyxoid tumor. Clinicopathologic analysis of six cases. *Am J Surg Pathol.* 1995; **19**:1039–46.

- Miettinen M. Ossifying fibromyxoid tumor of soft parts. Additional observations of a distinctive soft tissue tumor. *Am J Clin Pathol.* 1991; **95**:142–9.

- Miettinen M, Finnell V, Fetsch JF. Ossifying fibromyxoid tumor of soft parts–a clinicopathologic and immunohistochemical study of 104 cases with long-term follow-up and a critical review of the literature. *Am J Surg Pathol.* 2008;**32**:996–1005.

- Min KW, Seo IS, Pitha J. Ossifying fibromyxoid tumor: modified myoepithelial cell tumor? Report of three cases with immunohistochemical and electron microscopic studies. *Ultrastruct Pathol.* 2005; **29**:535–48.

- Nishio J, Iwasaki H, Ohjimi Y, et al. Ossifying fibromyxoid tumor of soft parts. Cytogenetic findings. *Cancer Genet Cytogenet.* 2002; **133**:124–8.

- Schneider N, Fisher C, Thway K. Ossifying fibromyxoid tumor: morphology, genetics, and differential diagnosis. *Ann Diagn Pathol.* 2016;**20**:52–8.

- Schofield JB, Krausz T, Stamp GW, et al. Ossifying fibromyxoid tumour of soft parts: immunohistochemical and ultrastructural analysis. *Histopathology.* 1993; **22**:101–12.

- Zamecnik M, Michal M, Simpson RH, et al. Ossifying fibromyxoid tumor of soft parts: a report of 17 cases with emphasis on unusual histological features. *Ann Diagn Pathol.* 1997; **1**:73–81.

## Embryonal Rhabdomyosarcoma

- Asmar L, Gehan EA, Newton WA, et al. Agreement among and within groups of pathologists in the classification of rhabdomyosarcoma and related childhood sarcomas. Report of an international study of four pathology classifications. *Cancer.* 1994; **74**:2579–88,.

- Dias P, Parham DM, Shapiro DN, Webber BL, Houghton PJ. Myogenic regulatory protein (MyoD1) expression in childhood solid tumors: diagnostic utility in rhabdomyosarcoma. *Am J Pathol.* 1990; **137**:1283–91.

- Huang SC, Alaggio R, Sung YS, et al. Frequent HRAS mutations in malignant ectomesenchymoma: overlapping genetic abnormalities with embryonal rhabdomyosarcoma. *Am J Surg Pathol.* 2016;**40**:876–85.

- Kumar S, Perlman E, Harris CA, Raffeld M, Tsokos, M. Myogenin is a specific marker for rhabdomyosarcoma: an immunohistochemical study in paraffin-embedded tissues. *Mod Pathol.* 2000;**13**:988–93.

- Langenau DM, Keefe MD, Storer NY, et al. Effects of RAS on the genesis of embryonal rhabdomyosarcoma. *Genes Dev.* 2007;**21**:1382–95.

- Newton WA Jr, Gehan EA, Webber B, et al. Classification of rhabdomyosarcomas and related sarcomas. Pathologic aspects and proposal for a new classification–an Intergroup Rhabdomyosarcoma Study. *Cancer.* 1995;**76**:1073–85.

- Parham DM, Barr FG. Classification of rhabdomyosarcoma and its molecular basis. *Adv Anat Pathol* 2013;**20**:387–97.

- Parham DM, Ellison DA. Rhabdomyosarcomas in adults and children. An update. *Arch Pathol Lab Med.* 2006;**130**:1454–65.

- Parham DM, Webber B, Holt H, Williams WK, Maurer H. Immunohistochemical study of childhood rhabdomyosarcomas and related neoplasms. Results of an Intergroup Rhabdomyosarcoma study project. *Cancer.* 1991; **67**:3072–80.

- Qualman S, Lynch J, Bridge J, et al. Prevalence and clinical impact of anaplasia in childhood rhabdomyosarcoma : a report from the Soft Tissue Sarcoma Committee of the Children's Oncology Group. *Cancer.* 2008;**113**:3242–7.

- Rudzinski ER, Anderson JR, Hawkins DS, et al. The World Health Organization Classification of Skeletal Muscle Tumors in Pediatric Rhabdomyosarcoma: a report from the Children's Oncology Group. *Arch Pathol Lab Med.* 2015;**139**: 1281–7.
- Seki M, Nishimura R, Yoshida K, et al. Integrated genetic and epigenetic analysis defines novel molecular subgroups in rhabdomyosarcoma. *Nat Commun.* 2015;**6**:7557.
- Stratton MR, Fisher C, Gusterson BA, Cooper CS. Detection of point mutations in N-ras and K-ras genes of human embryonal rhabdomyosarcomas using oligonucleotide probes and the polymerase chain reaction. *Cancer Res.* 1989;**49**:6324–7.
- Tobar A, Avigad S, Zoldan M, et al. Clinical relevance of molecular diagnosis in childhood rhabdomyosarcoma. *Diagn Mol Pathol.* 2000; **9**:9–13.
- Wijnaendts LC, van der Linden JC, van Unnik AJ, et al. Histopathological classification of childhood rhabdomyosarcomas: relationship with clinical parameters and prognosis. *Hum Pathol.* 1994; **25**:900–7.

# Intermediate Malignant and Malignant Tumors of Soft Tissue Featuring an Inflammatory Background

Angelo Paolo Dei Tos MD

## Introduction

The presence of a variably abundant inflammatory infiltrate represents a relatively common phenomenon in soft tissue tumors. Interestingly, since the advent of immune therapies based on checkpoint inhibitors, this morphologic finding has often been undervalued. It is therefore possible that, in the future, identification and subtyping of immune infiltrate may become therapeutically relevant. From the diagnostic standpoint, however, there exists a group of entities in which the presence of a prominent inflammatory infiltrate represents part of the typical morphologic spectrum of the specific tumor entity. Good examples are represented by the rare tumors originating from (or, it may be better to say, differentiated toward) the specialized dendritic cells of the immune system, in which the presence of scattered lymphocytes represents an important clue to the correct diagnosis. The same concept applies to inflammatory myofibroblastic tumor, which contains a heterogeneous infiltrate that includes a variable proportion of lymphocytes, plasma cells, and eosinophils that contributes significantly to raising the diagnostic suspect.

A different situation occurs when relatively common soft tissue sarcoma subtypes present that are associated with an inflammatory component. This may happen in leiomyosarcoma, which at times may exhibit a prominent osteoclast-like giant cell population.

However, the presence of a prominent inflammatory infiltrate may also represent the source of diagnostic error, as its presence may obscure the real nature of the neoplastic process. The best example is certainly represented by well-differentiated/dedifferentiated liposarcoma in which the neoplastic proliferation may be totally overshadowed by a reactive inflammatory component. As always, a diagnostic approach that integrates clinical, morphologic, immunohistochemical, and molecular findings enables a correct diagnosis to be made in most instances. In this context, with the exception of inflammatory myofibroblastic tumor, it has to be admitted that molecular diagnostics seems not to be as useful as in other histologies.

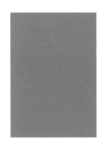

# Plexiform Fibrohistiocytic Tumor

## Definition and Epidemiology

Plexiform fibrohistiocytic tumor (PFHT) is a locally aggressive, rarely metastasizing soft tissue neoplasm, occurring preferentially in the pediatric age-group (peak incidence is in the first decade), with female predominance.

## Clinical Presentation and Outcome

Plexiform fibrohistiocytic tumor more often involves the superficial soft tissues of the upper extremities (65%), particularly the hands and wrists, and the lower limbs (25%). The trunk and the head and neck region represent less frequently affected anatomic locations. Most often, PFHT presents as an ill-defined mass or thickening of the dermis and subcutis. Deeper locations are comparatively very rare and lesions usually do not exceed 2 to 3 cm in size. Wide surgical excision represents the best therapeutic option. Local recurrences are seen in approximately 30% of cases, but it is most often related to incomplete excision. Systemic spread to locoregional lymph nodes and lung metastases is observed in approximately 5% of cases. It is, however, possible that

"referral center" series may be biased, leading to an overestimation of the real metastatic potential of PFHT.

## Morphology and Immunophenotype

Grossly, plexiform fibrohistiocytic tumor usually appears as a poorly circumscribed, infiltrative, multinodular lesion involving the dermis or the subcutis, measuring 0.3 to 6 cm (most lesions are smaller than 3 cm) Microscopically, PFHT exhibits a distinctive plexiform, multinodular architecture, being composed of several interconnected nodules of varying size (Fig. 9-1). Neoplastic nodules are composed of a uniform population of mononuclear histiocyte-like cells (Fig. 9-2) featuring mild nuclear atypia associated with a variable number of scattered multinucleated, osteoclast-like giant cells (Fig. 9-3). Most often, low to absent mitotic activity (usually fewer than 3 mitoses/10 high-power fields [HPF]) is observed. At the periphery of the nodules and in the spaces between the nodules, short fascicles of elongated fibroblast-like cells are present (Fig. 9-4). As mentioned, the presence of significant cytologic atypia represents an extremely rare morphologic finding (Fig. 9-5). In the so-called

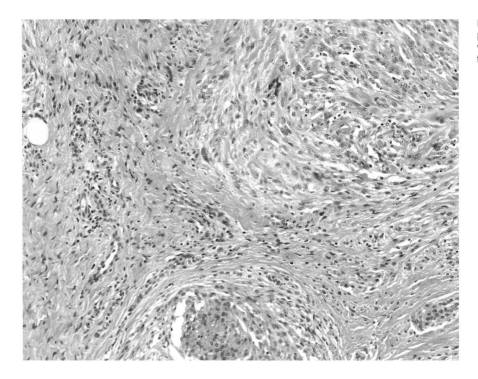

**Fig. 9-1.** Plexiform fibrohistiocytic tumor. At low power, the distinctive multinodular architecture, in which neoplastic nodules are partially separated by fibrous septa, is better appreciated.

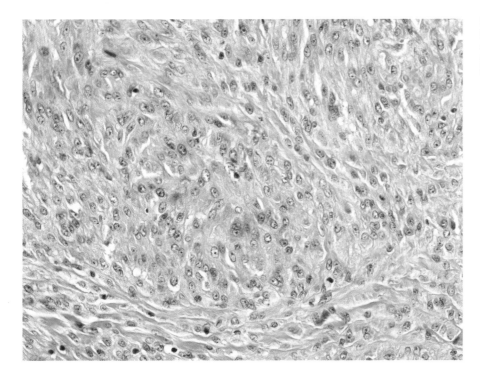

**Fig. 9-2.** Plexiform fibrohistiocytic tumor. Neoplastic nodules are composed of a proliferation of mononuclear "histiocyte-like" cells that at high power appear fairly uniform. Nuclear atypia tends to be mild.

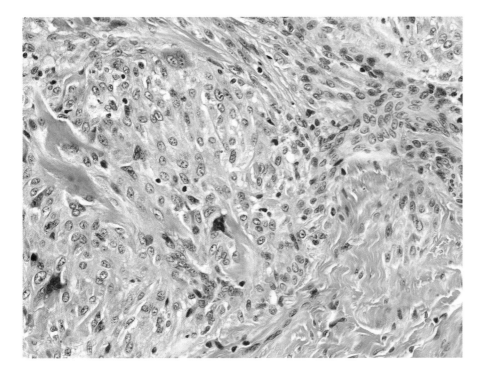

**Fig. 9-3.** Plexiform fibrohistiocytic tumor. The presence of multinucleated giant cells represents a common morphologic finding.

fibroblastic variant, the lesion is composed of fascicles of spindle cells arranged in a plexiform architecture that predominates over the fibrohistiocytic nodules (Fig. 9-6). Cases exist in which giant cells tend to be more prominent. Immunohistochemically, both mononuclear histiocyte-like cells and multinucleated cells stain intensely for CD68. Smooth muscle actin positivity can be detected in the fibroblast-like component. CD10 and CD63 immunopositivity is also reported.

## Genetics

Karyotypic analysis has been conducted in only a few lesions and no recurrent chromosome abnormalities have been detected.

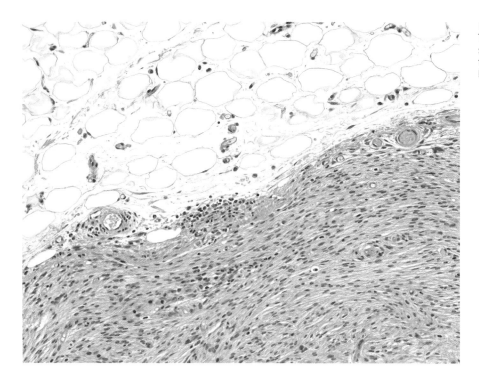

**Fig. 9-4.** Plexiform fibrohistiocytic tumor. The typical morphology includes the presence of short fascicles of elongated fibroblast-like cells that tend to predominate at the periphery of or in between the nodules.

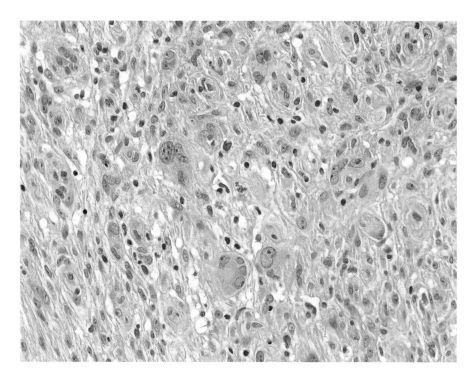

**Fig. 9-5.** Plexiform fibrohistiocytic tumor. Multifocal significant nuclear atypia can occasionally be observed.

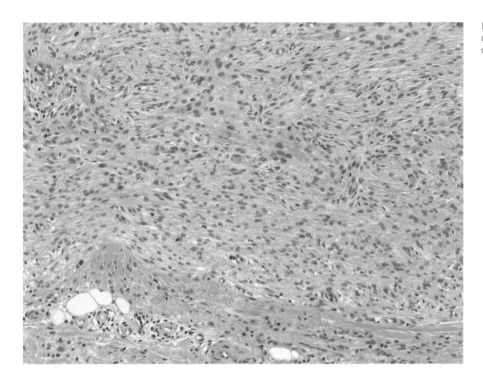

**Fig. 9-6.** Plexiform fibrohistiocytic tumor. In the so-called fibroblastic variant, cellular fascicle of spindle cells predominate.

## Differential Diagnosis and Diagnostic Pitfalls

The differential diagnosis of PFHT includes inflammatory processes, as well as benign, locally aggressive, and malignant mesenchymal lesions.

**Deep-seated granuloma anulare** may feature a multinodular architecture. However, CD68-positive mononuclear histiocytes organize in palisades around areas of degenerated collagen of variable size (Figs. 9-7 and 9-8). **Cellular neurothekeoma** has been linked to PFHT, and in small biopsies there might be some morphologic as well as immunophenotypic overlap. However, the two lesions maintain distinctive clinicopathologic features and should therefore be kept separated. **Giant cell tumor of soft tissues** is discussed in detail in this chapter, but it can be anticipated that unless it undergoes regressive changes, it generally lacks the biphasic pattern determined by the presence of the spindle cell component. Moreover, osteoclast-like multinucleated giant cells are far more

numerous. **Fibrous hamartoma of infancy** is discussed in Chapter 4. It typically occurs in the first 2 years of life and exhibits a triphasic, organoid architecture composed of mature adipose tissue, fascicles of spindle cells, and cellular nodules composed of immature spindle cells set in a myxoid background.

The fibroblastic variant of PFHT may raise the differential diagnosis with **desmoid fibromatosis**, which can be distinguished because of the organization of neoplastic cells in longer and wider fascicles and consistent nuclear expression of beta-catenin. **Epithelioid sarcoma (classical types)** also tends to occur acrally in young adults. As reported in Chapter 5, it features a multinodular architecture and is composed of a spindle and epithelioid atypical cell population that is often associated with central geographic necrosis. Consistent expressions of cytokeratins and loss of nuclear expression of INI1 both represent helpful diagnostic clues.

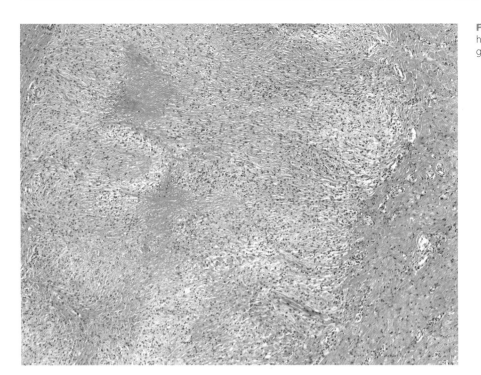

**Fig. 9-7.** Granuloma anulare. At low power, histiocytes surround areas of degenerated collagen, generating a "geographic" pattern of growth.

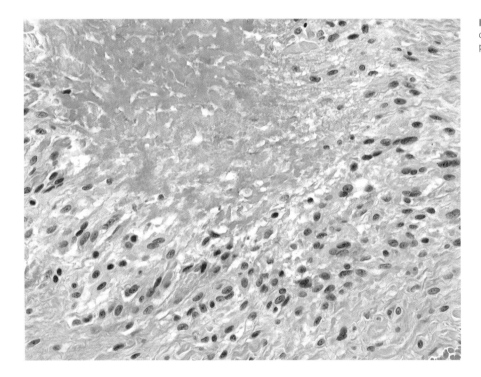

**Fig. 9-8.** Granuloma anulare. Non-atypical, cytologically uniform mononuclear cells organize in palisades around masses of degenerated collagen.

### Key Points in Plexiform Fibrohistiocytic Tumor Diagnosis

- Young age
- Occurrence at acral sites
- Infiltrative, multinodular pattern of growth
- Combination of mononuclear histiocyte-like cells, multinucleated giant cells, and spindle cells
- Expression of CD68/CD163 in histiocytes and SMA in spindle cells
- Indolent clinical behavior with extremely rare metastatic dissemination

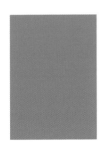

# Giant Cell Tumor of Soft Tissue

## Definition and Epidemiology

Giant cell tumor of soft tissue (GCT-ST) is a locally aggressive, rarely metastasizing primary soft tissue lesion morphologically overlapping with giant cell tumor of bone. It tends to occur predominantly in middle-aged patients, with a peak incidence in the fifth decade, but it actually can be observed at any age. Males and females are equally affected. Interestingly, Salm and Sissons first reported GCT-ST in 1972. However, it was subsequently buried (along with extraskeletal osteosarcoma and giant cell-rich leiomyosarcoma) within the now-abandoned label "giant cell malignant fibrous histiocytoma." This entity was not revived until 2000.

## Clinical Presentation and Outcome

The superficial soft tissues of the lower extremities represent the most frequently affected anatomic location. Less than one-third of cases arise in the trunk and in the head and neck region. Giant cell tumor of soft tissue tends to exhibit a benign clinical behavior with a recurrence rate of approximately 10–15%; however, as may happen with giant cell tumor of bone (that parenthetically exhibits complete morphologic overlap with GCT of soft tissue), it has to be expected that rare cases (in the range of 2%) will metastasize to the lungs. Unfortunately, no morphologic features can reliably predict systemic spread. Importantly, even in those rare cases associated with lung spread, the clinical course tends to remain indolent. When dealing with GCT-ST, the most important task is to set apart those sarcomas featuring osteoclast-like giant cells in order to avoid either inadequate or excessive treatment. Whether anti-RANKL therapy (denosumab) could also be used in the setting of giant cell tumor arising primarily in the soft tissues is still a matter of debate.

## Morphology and Immunophenotype

Grossly, GCT-ST is usually well circumscribed with a fleshy, brown to red cut surface (Fig. 9-9). Microscopically, this lesion is often organized in a multinodular growth pattern with nodules measuring up to 2 cm. In approximately 15% of cases, GCT-ST presents as a single lesion of variable size. The nodules are composed of a double cell population: mononuclear eosinophilic round cells (Fig. 9-10) and multinucleated osteoclast-like giant cells set in a richly vascularized stroma

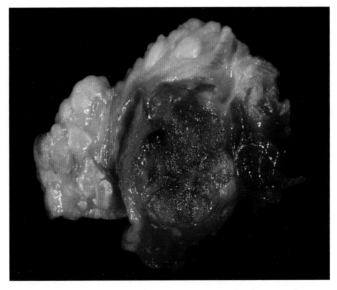

**Fig. 9-9.** Giant cell tumor of soft tissue. Macroscopically, the cut surface appears fleshy, featuring brown to red color.

(Fig. 9-11). The nodules are separated by fibrous septa containing hemosiderin-laden macrophages. Mitotic activity is variable but most often very brisk, with cases showing up to 30 mitoses/10HPF. Interestingly, similar to what is seen in giant cell tumor of bone, GCT-ST frequently undergoes aneurysmal bone cyst-like secondary changes represented by cellular spindling, presence of pseudovascular spaces, and metaplastic bone formation (Figs. 9-12 and 9-13). Regressive changes represented by fibrosis and stromal hemorrhages are seen relatively often. Immunohistochemistry plays its major role in the differential diagnosis with other mesenchymal lesions featuring giant cells. CD68 and CD163 decorate giant cells and, focally, also mononuclear cells. Variable staining for smooth muscle actin, S100, and even cytokeratin has been observed.

## Genetics

Very recently, driver mutations of the *H3F3-A* gene have been reported in giant cell tumor of bone. Recent molecular data tend to demonstrate that giant cell tumor of soft tissue seems not to harbor the same aberration.

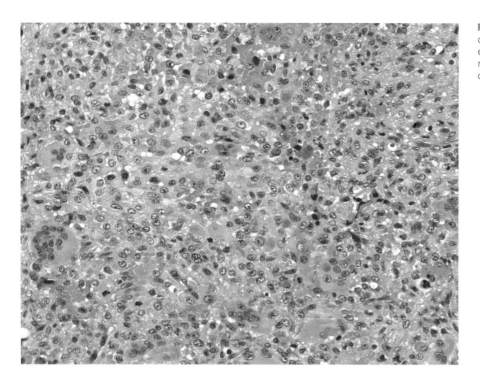

**Fig. 9-10.** Giant cell tumor of soft tissue. A double cell population represented by mononuclear eosinophilic round cells and a variable number of multinucleated osteoclast-like giant cells are observed.

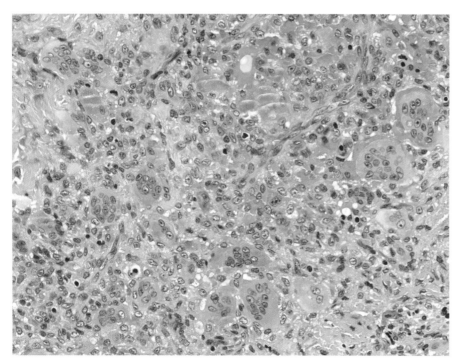

**Fig. 9-11.** Giant cell tumor of soft tissue. The number of giant cells can vary from area to area. A rich, capillary-sized vascular network is consistently detected.

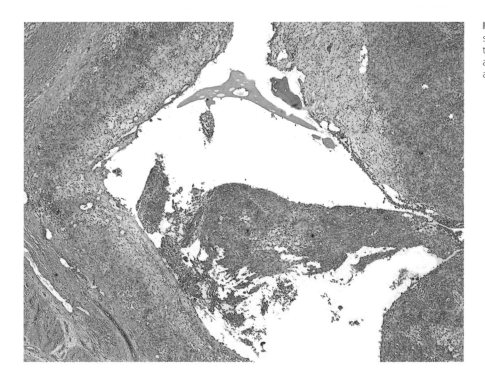

**Fig. 9-12.** Giant cell tumor of soft tissue. In long-standing lesions (as happens with bone lesions), the tumor may undergo pseudocystic degeneration associated with hemorrhage, therefore mimicking an aneurysmal bone cyst (i.e., ABC-like changes).

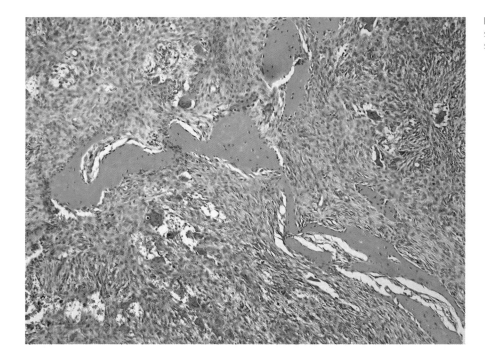

**Fig. 9-13.** Giant cell tumor of soft tissue. Long-standing lesions may also feature significant cellular spindling as well as formation of metaplastic bone.

## Differential Diagnosis and Diagnostic Pitfalls

Giant cell tumor of soft tissue certainly represents a significant proportion of the cases that in the past have been classified as "giant cell malignant fibrous histiocytoma" (GC-MFH). In fact, among those examples of GC-MFH included in Guccion and Enzinger's original paper, there was a subset of cases that exhibited a very indolent clinical behavior. Giant cell tumor of soft tissue has undergone the same critical reappraisal that has reshaped the entity known as pleomorphic and storiform MFH. As discussed in Chapter 7, pleomorphic MFH (once the most frequently diagnosed sarcoma) at best is now considered as an obsolete synonym for undifferentiated high-grade pleomorphic sarcoma and accounts for approximately 5% of mesenchymal malignancies. Similarly, it is now broadly accepted that GC-MFH represents a heterogeneous category that includes relatively indolent diseases such as GCT-ST and a variety of unrelated malignancies featuring the presence of osteoclast-like giant cells. This phenomenon is in fact observed in leiomyosarcoma (Fig. 9-14), giant

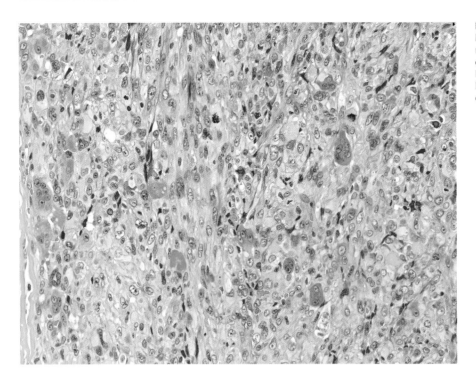

**Fig. 9-14.** Leiomyosarcoma. Rarely, leiomyosarcoma may feature the presence of multinucleated osteoclast-like giant cells. Overt cytologic atypia and atypical mitoses are observed. Neoplastic cells are organized in fascicles and, in the better-differentiated areas, feature distinctive eosinophilic fibrillary cytoplasm.

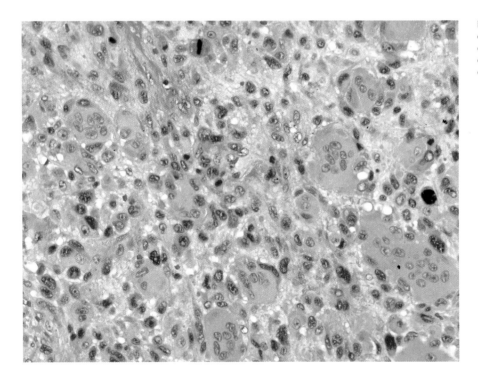

**Fig. 9-15.** Extraskeletal osteosarcoma. Neoplastic cells are associated with a high number of osteoclast-like giant cells. Importantly, giant cell-rich osteosarcoma may feature a minimal amount of osteogenic matrix, making extensive sampling of paramount importance.

cell-rich extraskeletal osteosarcoma (Fig. 9-15), osteoclast-rich carcinoma, and even in gastrointestinal stromal tumor (GIST). Clinically, at variance with GCT-ST, both leiomyosarcoma and extraskeletal osteosarcoma tend to arise in the deep soft tissues. Histologically, most often both neoplasms represent high-grade malignancies featuring severe cytologic atypia, necrosis, and atypical mitotic figures. Variable expression of myogenic markers (smooth muscle actin, desmin, and h-caldesmon) in leiomyosarcoma as well as the presence of malignant osteoid in extraskeletal osteosarcoma, most often associated with the expression of SATB2 (Fig. 9-16), represent helpful diagnostic clues. It has to be underlined that both in bone and soft tissue giant cell-rich osteosarcoma, malignant osteoid may be minimally represented, making SATB2 immunostaining even more important. Interestingly, very rare examples of undifferentiated pleomorphic sarcomas may also occasionally contain osteoclast-like giant cells (Fig. 9-17).

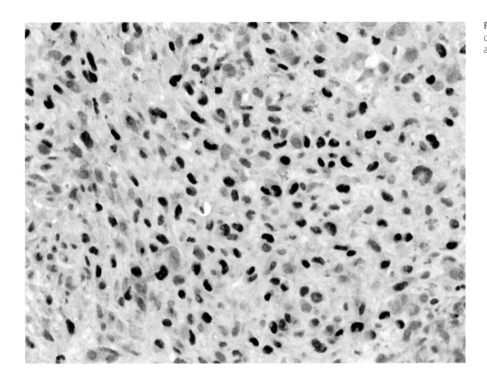

**Fig. 9-16.** Extraskeletal osteosarcoma. Strong and diffuse nuclear expression of SATB2 supports a morphologic diagnosis of osteogenic malignancy.

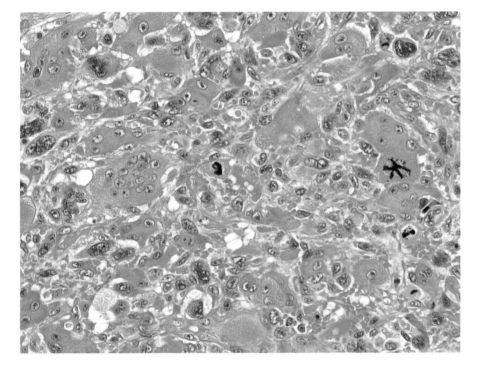

**Fig. 9-17.** Undifferentiated pleomorphic sarcomas. Very rarely, high-grade undifferentiated sarcomas may feature the presence of giant cells.

A lesion that potentially can be confused with GCT-ST is represented by those rare examples of **giant cell tumor of tendon sheath** (GCTTS) occurring at an extra-articular location. The main morphologic features of extra-articular GCTTS are represented by a composite proliferation of variably admixed mononuclear cells, osteoclast-like giant cells, and foamy macrophages set in a very variable amount (from minimal to abundant) of fibrous stroma (Fig. 9-18). Mononuclear cells are round to oval with irregular nuclei and pale cytoplasm (Fig. 9-19). In some cases, a population of desmin-positive, larger mononuclear cells featuring glassy cytoplasm and dendritic cytoplasmic processes is seen (Fig. 9-20). The diffuse form of giant cell tumor of tendon sheath, despite its benign nature, particularly in its articular diffuse form, can

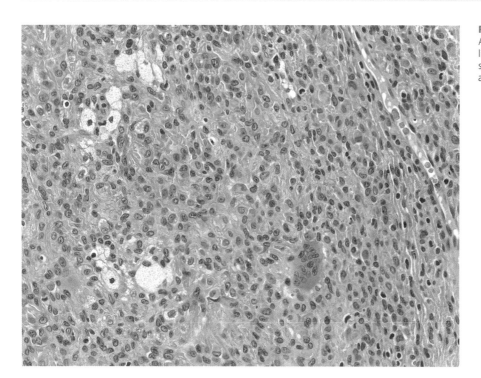

**Fig. 9-18.** Giant cell tumor of tendon sheath. A variable mixture of mononuclear cells, osteoclast-like giant cells, and foamy macrophages is observed, set in a very variable amount (from minimal to abundant) of fibrous stroma.

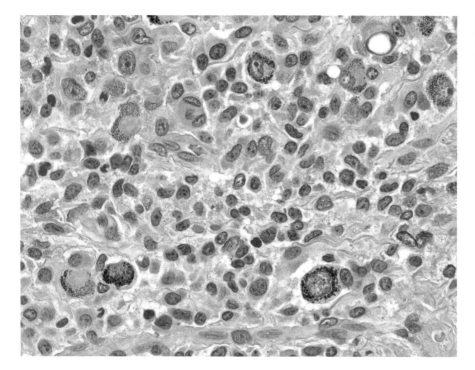

**Fig. 9-19.** Giant cell tumor of tendon sheath. Mononuclear cells are round to oval with irregular nuclei and pale cytoplasm. Single cells may feature the presence of intracytoplasmic hemosiderin (i.e., ladybug cells).

cause significant morbidity determined by repeated local recurrences, and in rare cases, even leading to amputation. However, the presence of translocations involving the gene *CSF1* and most often the *COL6A3* gene represents the preclinical rationale for successfully treating this disease with imatinib and, more recently, with anti-CSF1 monoclonal antibody. An exceedingly rare malignant variant of GCTTS has been reported in which an overt sarcomatous component is present.

Another benign soft tissue lesion that may enter the differential diagnosis with GCT-ST is represented by those examples of **deep-seated fibrous histiocytoma** (FH) that contains osteoclast-like giant cells (Fig. 9-21). The most relevant diagnostic clue is represented by the fact that the mononuclear cell population exhibits the typical polymorphic cytomorphology observed in most variants of benign fibrous histiocytoma (Fig. 9-22).

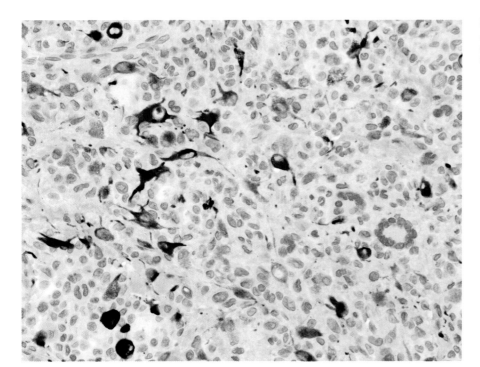

**Fig. 9-20.** Giant cell tumor of tendon sheath. A subpopulation of mononuclear cells exhibits abundant glassy cytoplasm, dendritic processes, and immunopositivity for desmin.

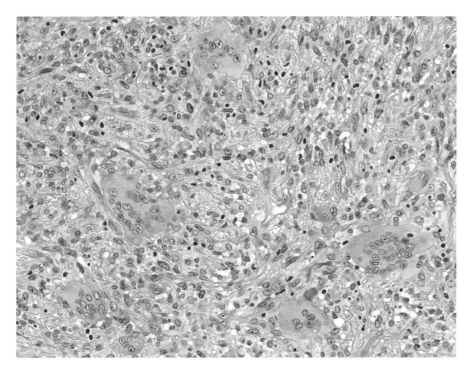

**Fig. 9-21.** Deep-seated fibrous histiocytoma. Giant cells can be observed in approximately 20% of deep-seated benign FH.

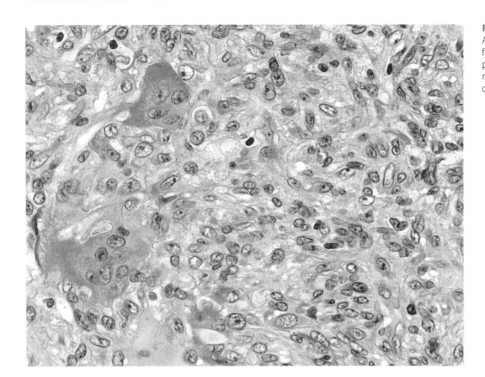

**Fig. 9-22.** Deep-seated fibrous histiocytoma. An important diagnostic clue is represented by the fact that the mononuclear cell population is polymorphic, therefore contrasting with the monomorphic quality most often observed in giant cell tumor of soft tissue.

### Key Points in Giant Cell Tumor of Soft Tissue Diagnosis

- Occurrence in the extremities of adults
- Multinodular pattern of growth
- Combination of mononuclear cells and multinucleated osteoclast-like giant cells, set in a richly vascularized stroma
- ABC-like changes observed in a subset of cases
- Indolent clinical behavior with extremely rare dissemination to the lungs

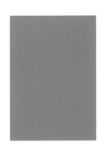

# Inflammatory Myofibroblastic Tumor

## Definition and Epidemiology

Inflammatory myofibroblastic tumor (IMT), also known as "inflammatory pseudotumor or plasma cell granuloma," represents a distinctive entity whose morphologic hallmark is most often represented by the coexistence of a spindle cell fibroblastic/myofibroblastic proliferation with an inflammatory infiltrate, which is mainly composed of plasma cells, lymphocytes, and eosinophils. Lymphocytes and plasma cells tend to predominate in most cases. Inflammatory myofibroblastic tumor most likely represents a spectrum of lesions with different biologic potential. The entity presented under the label "inflammatory fibrosarcoma" actually is part of the clinicopathologic spectrum of IMT. Inflammatory myofibroblastic tumor tends to occur in both children and young adults, with most cases occurring within the first two decades; however, it can be observed in the adult population.

## Clinical Presentation and Outcome

The lungs, the mesentery, and the omentum represent the most frequently affected sites of occurrence of IMT. Inflammatory myofibroblastic tumor has been reported at virtually any site; however, soft tissue and the gastrointestinal and the genitourinary tracts (particularly the uterus) are also relatively frequently involved. Extrapulmonary forms primarily occur in children and adolescents. The modality of IMT clinical presentation is obviously related to the site of origin.

The prediction of the biologic behavior of IMT represents a difficult task. There is local recurrence in approximately 25% of cases; however, the recurrence rate really depends on anatomic site and resectability. It has been suggested that the presence of nuclear atypia may correlate with malignant behavior. ALK expression has been associated with better outcome. Lesions located in the abdominopelvic region exhibit a significantly higher risk of recurrence. Distant metastases seem to be rare, occurring in less than 5% of cases. The presence of epithelioid morphology (predominantly observed at visceral locations) is associated with markedly aggressive behavior. When occurring in surgically amenable locations, complete surgery represents the best treatment; however, in some cases good control has also been reported using steroids or non-steroidal anti-inflammatory drugs. Relatively recently, the use of the ALK/ROS1 inhibitor crizotinib has proved effective in treating the very rare, locally advanced/metastatic IMT.

## Morphology and Immunophenotype

Grossly, IMT usually presents as a well-circumscribed, sometimes multinodular mass (Fig. 9-23). Rarely, the presence of central scarring is reported.

The microscopic features of IMT depend on the predominance of the three main cellular components: myofibroblasts, fibroblasts, and inflammatory cells.

A first morphologic presentation is represented by the presence of a relatively hypocellular spindled myofibroblastic proliferation set in a fibromyxoid background (Fig. 9-24). A rich vascular network is usually seen, along with a prominent inflammatory infiltrate variably composed of lymphocytes, plasma cells, and eosinophils. Plasma cells tend to predominate in most cases (Fig. 9-25). These morphologic findings may somewhat mimic a reactive process. Neoplastic cells are most often spindle shaped, featuring indistinct cytoplasmic borders and variably atypical nuclei (Fig. 9-26). Immunostaining with smooth muscle actin often highlights myofibroblastic features such as peripheral condensation of actin filaments within the cytoplasm of neoplastic cells (so-called tram track configuration) (Fig. 9-27).

A second morphologic option is represented by the presence of a cellular spindle cell proliferation set in a stroma that can be either collagenous or myxoid (Fig. 9-28). An inflammatory infiltrate as described above is invariably present. A relatively distinctive morphologic finding that is observed in these cellular examples is represented by the

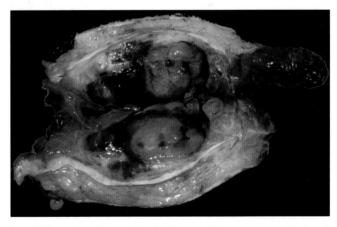

**Fig. 9-23.** Inflammatory myofibroblastic tumor. Tumor mass is relatively well circumscribed. Cut surface appears fleshy with areas of hemorrhage and necrosis.

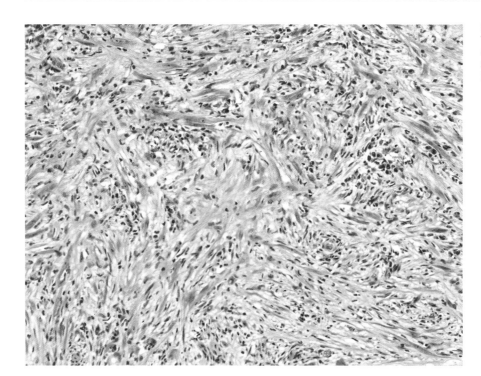

Fig. 9-24. Inflammatory myofibroblastic tumor. Typical low-power morphology features a spindle cell proliferation set in a fibromyxoid background and associated with a chronic inflammatory infiltrate.

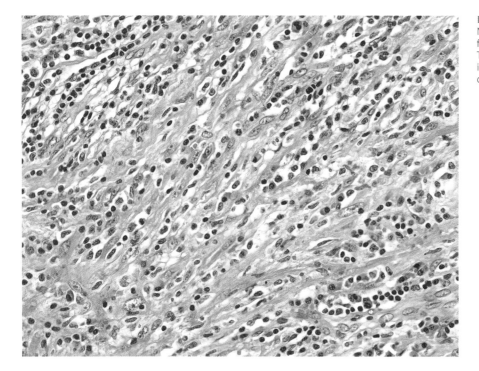

Fig. 9-25. Inflammatory myofibroblastic tumor. Neoplastic cells exhibit a spindled morphology and feature mild to moderate nuclear atypia. The presence of an abundant chronic inflammatory infiltrate represents an important clue to the diagnosis.

presence of ganglion-like cells featuring abundant eosinophilic cytoplasm (Fig. 9-29).

The last pattern somewhat recalls a scar, showing less cellularity and featuring the presence of a densely collagenous stroma (Figs. 9-30 and 9-31). The inflammatory infiltrate tends to be sparser.

In IMT, cellular atypia is usually mild to moderate; however, cases have been reported in which significant nuclear atypia (Fig. 9-32) is associated with mitotic activity and even the presence of atypical mitoses. These cases most likely represent what have been called "inflammatory fibrosarcoma."

As discussed in Chapter 5, an epithelioid variant of IMT has recently been described. These lesions tend to occur at visceral locations and feature the presence of a striking epithelioid morphology (Figs. 9-33 and 9-34). As epithelioid IMT seems to behave aggressively, it has been wisely suggested to label it "epithelioid inflammatory myofibroblastic sarcoma."

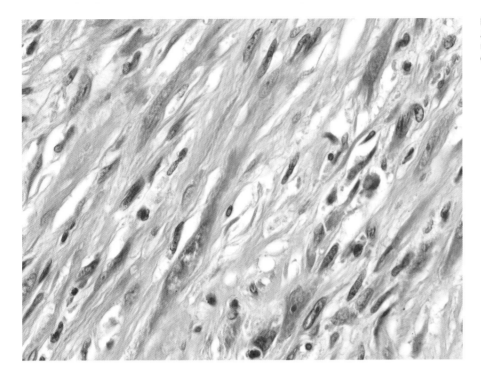

**Fig. 9-26.** Inflammatory myofibroblastic tumor. At high power, neoplastic cells exhibit elongated nuclei and abundant, poorly circumscribed cytoplasm.

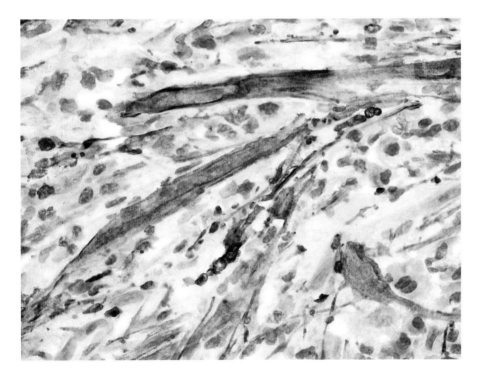

**Fig. 9-27.** Inflammatory myofibroblastic tumor. Smooth muscle actin immunostaining highlights some myofibroblastic features such as the peripheral condensation of actin filaments (i.e., "tram track" configuration).

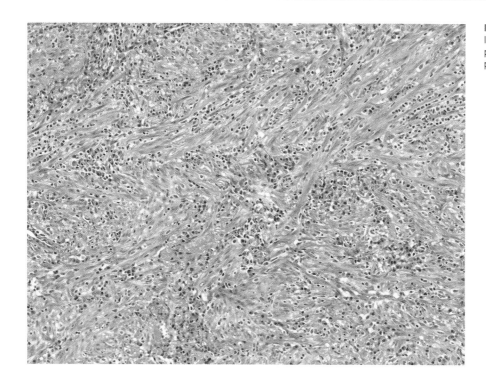

**Fig. 9-28.** Inflammatory myofibroblastic tumor. IMT at times may be more cellular. Note the presence of a rich inflammatory component that plays a key role in raising the diagnostic suspect.

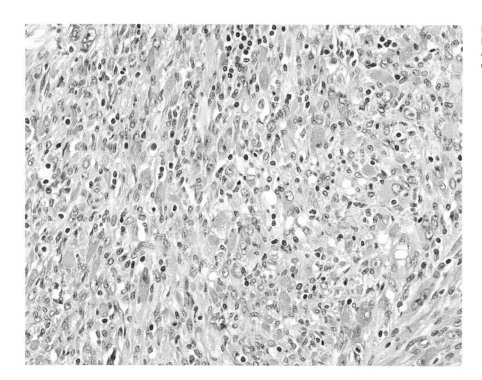

**Fig. 9-29.** Inflammatory myofibroblastic tumor. Relatively often, neoplastic cells tend to assume a ganglion-like appearance, featuring the presence of abundant, palely eosinophilic cytoplasm.

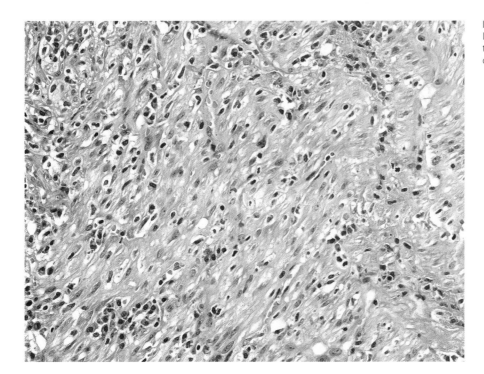

**Fig. 9-30.** Inflammatory myofibroblastic tumor. In hypocellular forms of IMT, the background tends to be more fibrous and the inflammatory component tends to predominate.

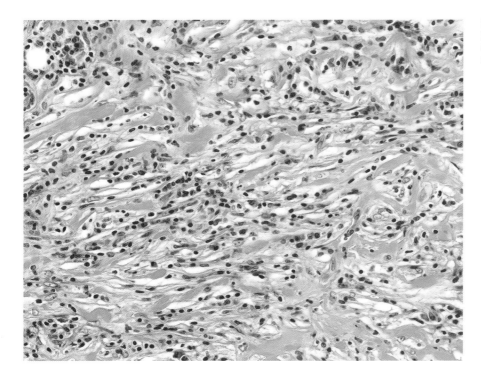

**Fig. 9-31.** Inflammatory myofibroblastic tumor. In this hypocellular variant of IMT, coarse bundles of collagen are observed. The inflammatory component includes eosinophils.

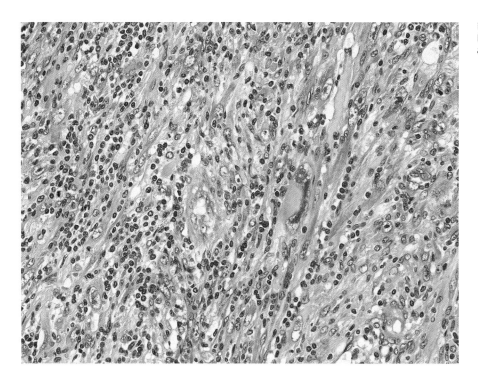

**Fig. 9-32.** Inflammatory myofibroblastic tumor. Rarely, IMT may feature the presence of markedly atypical neoplastic cells.

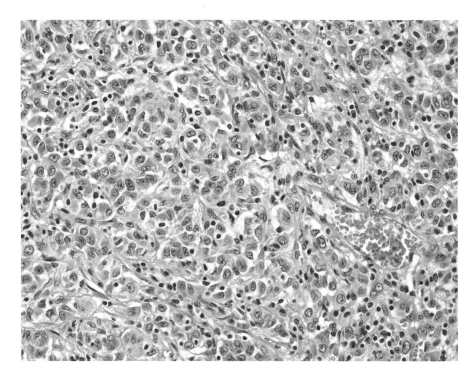

**Fig. 9-33.** Epithelioid inflammatory myofibroblastic tumor. Neoplastic cells exhibit a distinctive epithelioid morphology and are characterized by a solid pattern of growth. Scattered lymphocytes and eosinophils are seen.

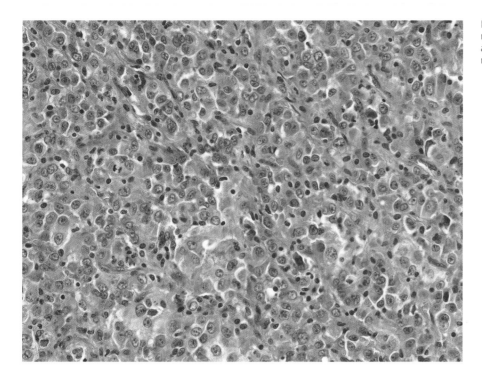

**Fig. 9-34.** Epithelioid inflammatory myofibroblastic tumor. Neoplastic cells feature abundant eosinophilic cytoplasm and large atypical nuclei. Mitotic activity tends to be brisk.

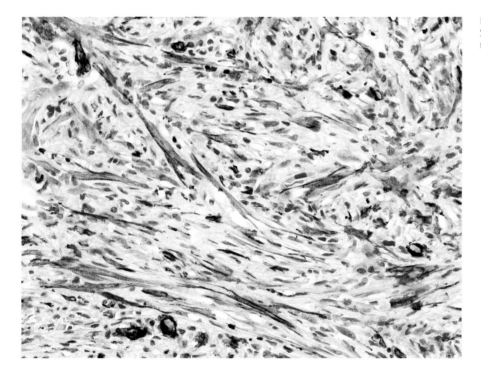

**Fig. 9-35.** Inflammatory myofibroblastic tumor. Smooth muscle actin most often decorates neoplastic myofibroblasts.

Immunohistochemically, in addition to vimentin, the spindle cell component exhibits positivity for smooth muscle actin (Fig. 9-35), muscle specific actin, and desmin in many cases. However, immunopositivity may be focal and therefore easily overlooked. Approximately one-third of cases will stain positively with cytokeratin. Half of the cases also stain positively for ALK (Fig. 9-36). This finding correlates with the presence of ALK gene rearrangement. Rarely, ROS1 immunoreactivity (which is mutually exclusive with ALK) is observed.

## Genetics

*ALK* genomic rearrangement is more frequently observed in pediatric cases and leads to constitutive activation and overexpression of the ALK protein. *ALK* fuses with an increasing variety of partner genes that includes *TPM3, TPM4, CLTC, RANBP2*, and *ATIC*. The *ALK-RAMP2* fusion transcript appears to be associated with an epithelioid morphology. More recently, a novel *RRBP1-ALK* fusion was reported that was also associated with epithelioid morphology, perinuclear

513

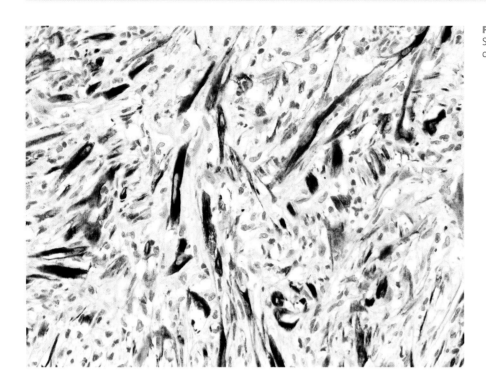

**Fig. 9-36.** Inflammatory myofibroblastic tumor. Strong cytoplasmic ALK immunopositivity is observed in approximately half of all IMTs.

accentuation of cytoplasmic ALK immunopositivity, and aggressive clinical behavior. Importantly, this aberration is restricted to the myofibroblastic component of IMT. Interestingly, a subset of IMT lacking ALK rearrangements presents with an aberration of the *HMGA2* gene on chromosome 12. It is also of interest that ALK abnormalities are extremely uncommon in IMT diagnosed in patients over 40 years of age. ROS1 represents a rare (an alternative to ALK but equally targetable) molecular aberration.

## Differential Diagnosis and Diagnostic Pitfalls

The term **pseudosarcomatous myofibroblastic proliferation** (PMP) describes a group of myofibroblastic lesions occurring most often in the genitourinary tract and, despite an infiltrative growth pattern, tends to behave in a very indolent fashion. Clinical presentation of PMP can be impressive, as it may form a large exophytic, often ulcerated mass that may even extend transmurally through the affected viscera, erroneously suggestive of aggressive clinical behavior. Morphologically, PMP is composed of a spindle cell proliferation admixed with a variably abundant inflammatory component, most often less prominent than that seen in IMT. Mitotic activity is very variable but, importantly, cytologic atypia is usually absent (Fig. 9-37), as is the presence of atypical mitoses. Very importantly, as the differential diagnosis herein includes leiomyosarcoma and sarcomatoid spindle cell carcinoma, any significant atypia should lead to a reconsideration of the diagnosis of PMP. Immunohistochemically, PMP exhibits smooth muscle actin positivity that is relatively often associated with expression of pancytokeratins (Fig. 9-38). Approximately half of the cases of PMP express ALK. Such expression is most often not associated with *ALK* gene rearrangement; however, this

finding is still a source of debate, as is the biologic relationship with IMT.

The differential diagnosis of inflammatory myofibroblastic tumor also depends on the site, morphologic characteristics of an individual tumor, and the nature of the specimen available for examination. Other spindle cell tumors featuring a prominent inflammatory infiltrate that may mimic the histologic appearance of inflammatory myofibroblastic tumor include sarcomatoid anaplastic large cell lymphoma, dendritic cell neoplasms, inflammatory leiomyosarcoma, well-differentiated liposarcoma, and dedifferentiated liposarcoma with inflammation.

As mentioned in Chapter 7, **dedifferentiated liposarcoma** (as well as well-differentiated liposarcoma) may at times feature the presence of a prominent inflammatory infiltrate that can obscure the lipogenic nature of the lesion. The presence of large atypical cells featuring hyperchromatic nuclei represents a key diagnostic clue (Fig. 9-39); however, diagnosis can be very challenging when dedifferentiated liposarcoma does not exhibit overt pleomorphism (Fig. 9-40). The immunodetection of MDM2 (and/or CDK4) is extremely helpful, as it highlights the neoplastic cell population independently from the histologic grade (Fig. 9-41). A minor caveat is that IMT may also occasionally exhibit MDM2 overexpression, which, however, is most often limited to a small percentage of neoplastic cells.

**Myxoinflammatory fibroblastic sarcoma** also enters the differential diagnosis. This entity (discussed in detail in Chapter 8) tends to occur acrally and is composed of a spindle cell proliferation associated with pseudolipoblasts, set in variably abundant myxoid matrix, and associated with a prominent chronic inflammatory infiltrate. The diagnostic hallmark is represented by the presence of inclusional macronucleoli harbored by enlarged neoplastic cells.

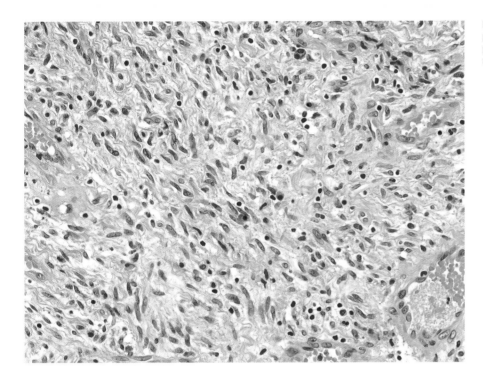

**Fig. 9-37.** Pseudosarcomatous myofibroblastic proliferation. A variably cellular spindle cell proliferation is observed. Importantly, lesional cells never feature cytologic atypia.

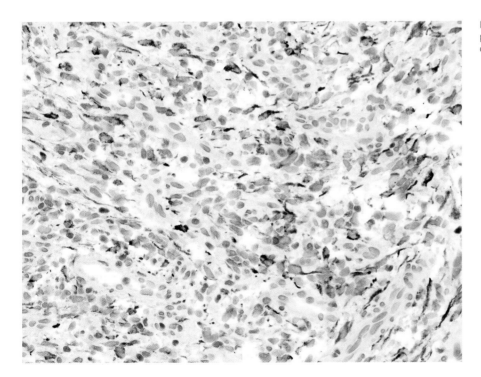

**Fig. 9-38.** Pseudosarcomatous myofibroblastic proliferation. Multifocal immunopositivity for cytokeratin is frequently observed.

The differential diagnosis of IMT also includes a group of fibroinflammatory idiopathic disorders that can simulate a neoplasm. These include **sclerosing mesenteritis** (SM), **idiopathic retroperitoneal fibrosis** (IRF), and **IgG4-related sclerosing disease**. All these entities share the presence of a variable combination of fibrosis and chronic inflammation.

Patients affected by sclerosing mesenteritis are most often middle aged and can be symptomatic (abdominal pain) or asymptomatic. In consideration of the intra-abdominal location, the lesion can attain a large size (up to 20–25 cm). Sclerosing mesenteritis is a non-recurrent, sometimes self-healing condition. Morphologically, in addition to the fibrous and inflammatory lymphohistiocytic components, SM features variably abundant areas of fat necrosis.

Idiopathic retroperitoneal fibrosis also affects middle-aged patients and is characterized by male predominance.

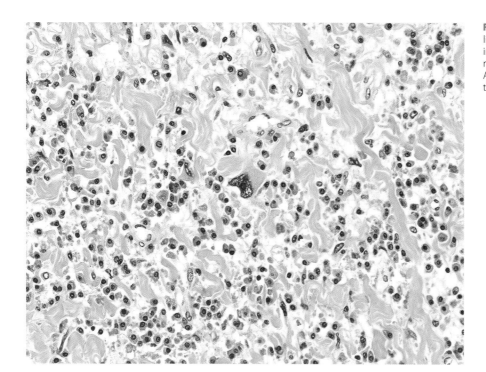

**Fig. 9-39.** Inflammatory well-differentiated liposarcoma. In this example, the inflammatory infiltrate predominates to the extent that the neoplastic nature of the lesion can be overlooked. A careful search of scattered atypical cells represents the most important diagnostic clue.

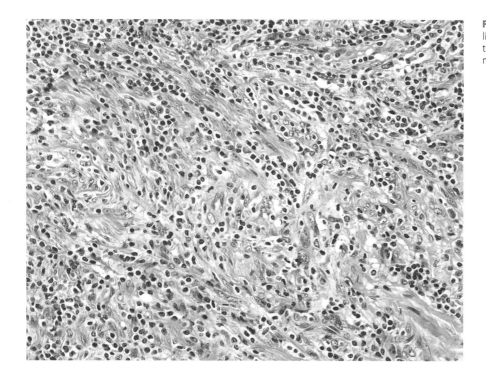

**Fig. 9-40.** Inflammatory dedifferentiated liposarcoma. The absence of overt atypia along with the presence of intense inflammatory background makes diagnosis particularly challenging.

It typically involves the retroperitoneum bilaterally, relatively often causing obstruction of the ureters that may potentially lead to secondary hydronephrosis. The therapeutic mainstay is based on administration of steroids. Diagnosis is usually based on the combination of clinical (primarily radiologic) and histopathologic findings. Microscopically, IRF is composed of a diffuse chronic inflammatory infiltrate in which T lymphocytes predominate, set in a densely sclerotic background (Fig. 9-42). Lymphocytes also may cluster around blood vessels wherein a B-cell component is also observed. Immunohistochemistry plays a role only in ruling out the main differential diagnosis that is represented by lymphomas.

IgG4-related sclerosing disease represents a recently described disorder that combines the presence of visceral masses with serum elevation of IgG4. IgG4-related sclerosing diseases has been described anywhere in the body (and may be

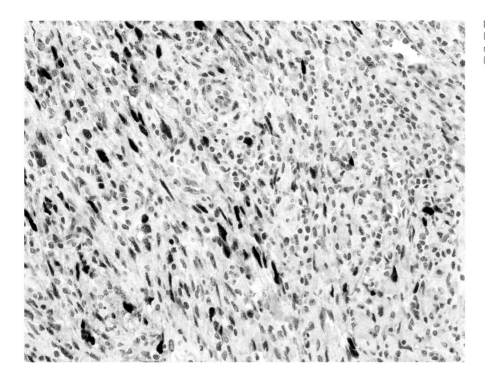

**Fig. 9-41.** Inflammatory dedifferentiated liposarcoma. MDM2 immunopositivity plays a key role in the recognition of dedifferentiated liposarcoma.

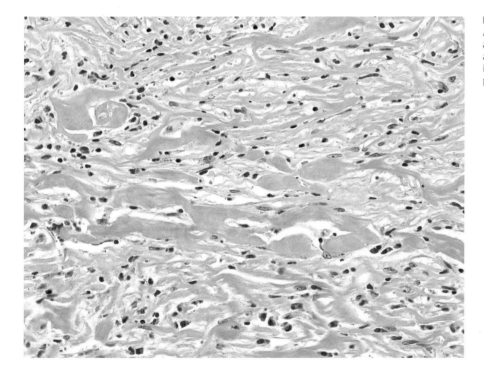

**Fig. 9-42.** Idiopathic retroperitoneal fibrosis. A dense sclerotic background contains a hypocellular myofibroblastic proliferation associated with variably abundant inflammatory infiltrate that includes lymphocytes, macrophages, plasma cells, and eosinophils.

overdiagnosed based on the mere immunohistochemical detection of increased IgG4-positive elements); however, the most commonly affected anatomic sites are the pancreas and the liver, followed by the orbit and the salivary glands. Again, there is a tendency for IgG4-related sclerosing disease to occur in middle-aged males. As in IRF, therapy is based on steroids. Histomorphology, it is characterized by a variable combination

of fibrosis with a prominent lymphoplasmacytic inflammatory infiltrate (Figs. 9-43 and 9-44). The process exhibits the tendency to infiltrate the surrounding tissues. The diagnostic cut-off of IgG4-positive plasma cells (Fig. 9-45) is still the object of sharp debate. It seems that instead of simply counting the number of IgG4-positive elements, the ratio of IgG4-positive to IgG-positive plasma cells should be evaluated. With regard

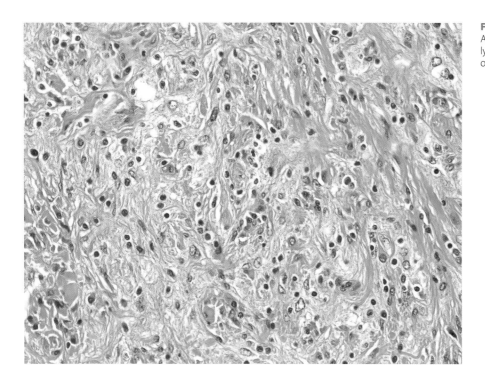

**Fig. 9-43.** IgG4-related sclerosing disease. A variable combination of fibrosis with a prominent lymphoplasmacytic inflammatory infiltrate is usually observed.

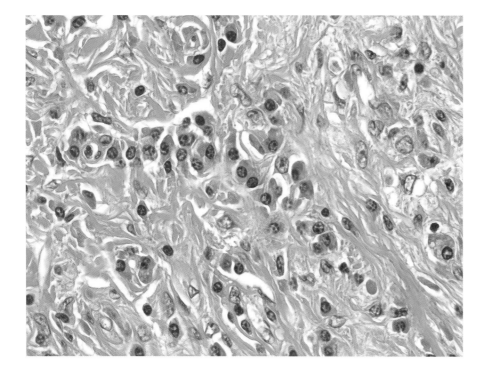

**Fig. 9-44.** IgG4-related sclerosing disease. Plasma cells may aggregate in small clusters.

to the differential diagnosis with IMT, it should also be remembered that IMT may show elevated numbers of IgG4-positive plasma cells. This further underlines the basic rule of evaluating immunohistochemical results strictly in context with morphology.

It has been suggested that the rare benign condition **calcifying fibrous pseudotumor** represents an end stage of IMT; however, morphologic, clinical, and molecular evidence is not supportive of this hypothesis.

A final important warning is related to the fact that ALK expression is also observed in anaplastic large cell lymphoma (ALCL) and in a small subset of lung adenocarcinoma. The differential diagnosis with ALCL is particularly challenging when dealing with the epithelioid variant of IMT.

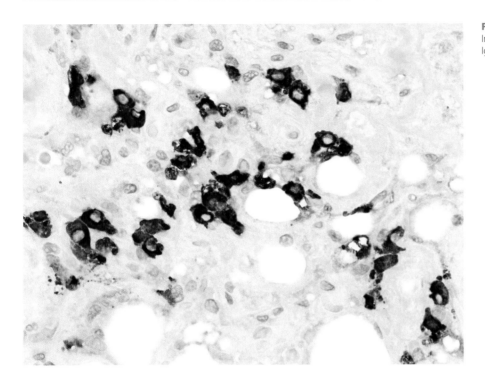

**Fig. 9-45.** IgG4-related sclerosing disease. Immunohistochemistry is helpful in highlighting the IgG4-positive population.

**Key Points in Inflammatory Myofibroblastic Tumor Diagnosis**

- Occurrence in children and young adults
- Frequent visceral location
- Proliferation of mildly atypical myofibroblasts intermingled with variably abundant inflammatory cell population (plasma cells, lymphocytes, and eosinophils)
- Immunohistochemical expression of smooth muscle actin (and other myogenic markers)
- Immunohistochemical expression of ALK in a subset of cases
- Rather indolent clinical behavior with the notable exception of the epithelioid variant

# Follicular Dendritic Cell Sarcoma

## Definition and Epidemiology

Follicular dendritic cell (FDC) sarcoma is a neoplasm originating from/differentiating toward follicular dendritic cells, which represent accessory cells located in the B region of lymphoid follicles. Therein, they provide architectural support and play a key role in the process of antigen presentation and recognition, therefore regulating B-cell adaptive immune response. Steinman and colleagues coined the term "follicular dendritic cells" in 1978 to highlight the presence of a rich network of cytoplasmic processes encircling follicular lymphoid cells. Follicular dendritic cell sarcoma primarily occurs in the adult population and has no gender predilection. The first description of neoplasms composed of follicular dendritic cells dates back to 1986, when Monda and Rosai reported the first series of four cases arising in the lymph nodes of the head and neck region. Distinctive variants of accessory cell neoplasms are represented by interdigitating reticulum cell sarcoma and fibroblastic reticulum cell sarcoma, discussed separately.

## Clinical Presentation and Outcome

Follicular dendritic cell sarcoma can occur in approximately 30% of cases as a nodal lesion. Even if FDC sarcoma was originally described in the lymph nodes of the head and neck region and subsequently in the groin, it seems that abdominal, axillary, and mediastinal involvement is relatively more common. The groin represents the second-most common anatomic site for nodal presentation. Extranodal locations are comparatively more common (approximately 70% of cases) and include the gastrointestinal tract (the liver being the most common anatomic site) and the lungs, as well as other immune organs such as the spleen and the tonsils. Interestingly, less than 10% of FDC sarcomas can arise in the context of hyaline-vascular Castleman disease. Most cases arise in adult patients, with a peak incidence occurring in the fourth decade. An extremely rare variant of FDC sarcoma is represented by the so-called inflammatory myofibroblastic tumor-like FDC, a lesion that tends to occur most often in the liver and spleen, exhibits a preference for the female gender, and is associated with Epstein-Barr virus (EBV) infection.

The outcome of FDC sarcomas appears to be extremely variable. While nodal lesions tend to exhibit a rather indolent clinical behavior, extranodal tumors tend to be significantly aggressive, with systemic spread (primarily to liver and lungs) being observed in approximately 40% of cases. In consideration of its rarity, best systemic treatments have not yet been established.

## Morphology and Immunophenotype

The gross appearance of FDC sarcoma depends on size. Larger masses tend to be fleshy with multiple foci of necrosis. Microscopically, FDC sarcoma is most often composed of a spindle cell proliferation, featuring light cytoplasmic eosinophilia (Fig. 9-46) organized in fascicular, whorled, or short storiform patterns of growth (Figs. 9-47 and 9-48). Nuclei usually harbor small nucleoli. In some cases, cytoplasm can be more abundant (Fig. 9-49) and sometimes assumes a remarkably epithelioid morphology that often is associated with the presence of round nuclei with larger nucleoli (Fig. 9-50). The presence of significant nuclear pleomorphism represents an uncommon but certainly observed morphologic variation and is often associated with higher mitotic activity (Figs. 9-51 and 9-52). One of the distinctively common features of FDC sarcoma is represented by the presence of scattered lymphocytes (more rarely, plasma cells are also seen), the amount of which is remarkably variable (Fig. 9-53). Perivascular clustering of lymphoid cells is sometimes observed and represents an important clue to the diagnosis of FDC (Figs. 9-54 and 9-55). In the rare IMT-like variant of FDC sarcoma, a more abundant inflammatory infiltrate is seen (at times obscuring the neoplastic component) and is mainly composed of lymphocytes and plasma cells (Figs. 9-56 and 9-57). As mentioned, approximately 10% of FDCs arise in association with hyaline vascular Castleman disease (Figs. 9-58 and 9-59).

Immunohistochemistry plays a major diagnostic role. Most FDC sarcomas variably express CD21 (Fig. 9-60), CD23 (Fig. 9-61), and CD35. In addition, neoplastic cells tend to consistently exhibit strong immunopositivity for clusterin (Fig. 9-62), podoplanin (D2-40), and CXCL-13 (Fig. 9-63). CXCL-13 represents a chemokine that is normally secreted by FDC and plays a major role in lymphoid organ development by attracting B cells expressing its receptor CXCR5. Importantly, the IMT-like variant of FDC sarcoma tends to exhibit weaker expression of conventional FDC markers and, in addition, is characterized by intense EBER (EBV-encoded RNA) positivity (Fig. 9-64). Focal EMA immunopositivity is observed in approximately half of the cases.

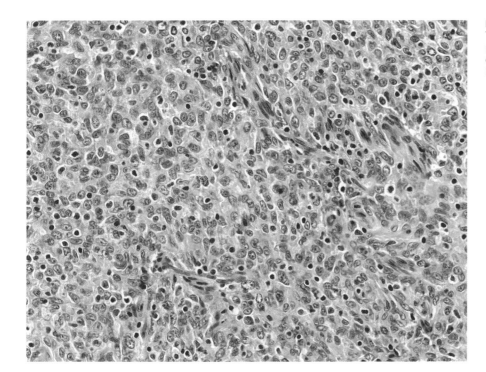

**Fig. 9-46.** Follicular dendritic cell sarcoma. The typical morphology is represented by the presence of a relatively uniform spindle to epithelioid cell proliferation, featuring scattered lymphocytes.

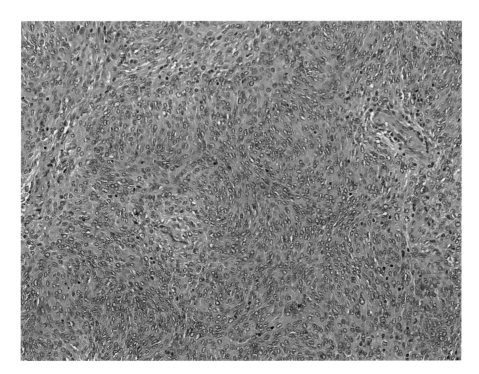

**Fig. 9-47.** Follicular dendritic cell sarcoma. A storiform pattern of growth is better appreciated at low power.

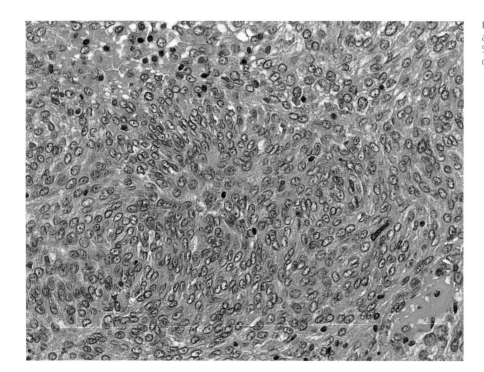

**Fig. 9-48.** Follicular dendritic cell sarcoma. Nuclei are monomorphous and harbor small nucleoli. Small lymphocytes are seen in between neoplastic cells.

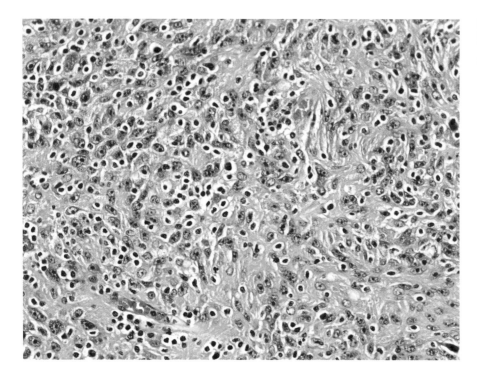

**Fig. 9-49.** Follicular dendritic cell sarcoma. In some cases, cytoplasm can be more abundant. The presence of interspersed small lymphocytes represents an important diagnostic clue.

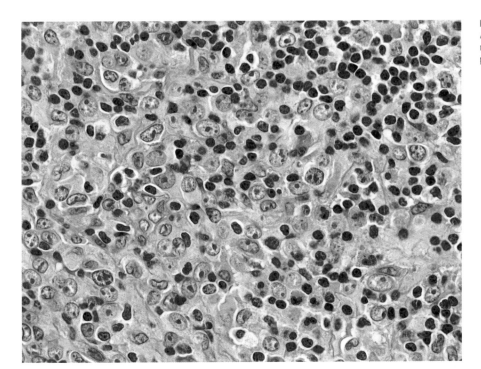

**Fig. 9-50.** Follicular dendritic cell sarcoma. At times neoplastic cells may assume an epithelioid morphology that often is associated with the presence of round nuclei harboring larger nucleoli.

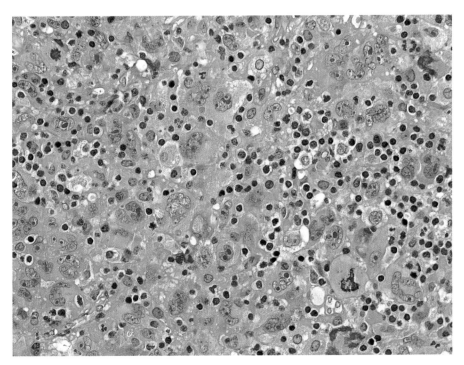

**Fig. 9-51.** Follicular dendritic cell sarcoma. Significant cytologic atypia is sometimes observed that may be associated with the presence of high mitotic activity.

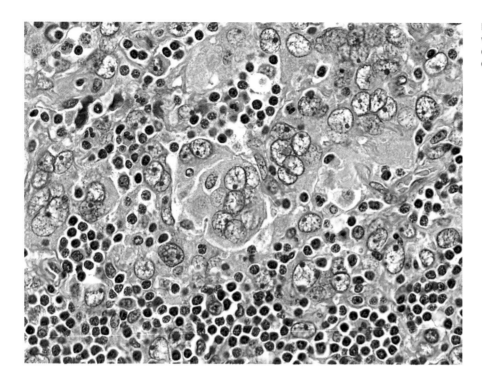

**Fig. 9-52.** Follicular dendritic cell sarcoma. Even when dealing with significant atypia, the presence of scattered lymphocytes is helpful in raising the diagnostic suspicion.

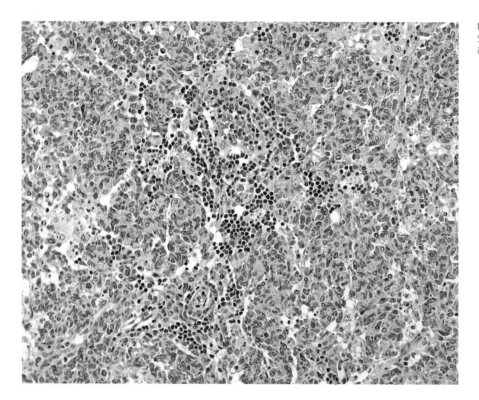

**Fig. 9-53.** Follicular dendritic cell sarcoma. Sometimes lymphocytes aggregate in small clusters instead of percolating between tumor cells.

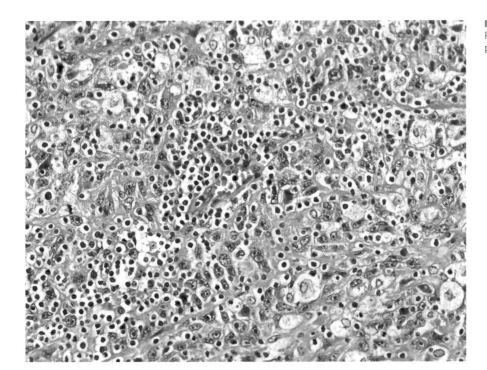

**Fig. 9-54.** Follicular dendritic cell sarcoma. Perivascular cuffing represents a relatively common phenomenon.

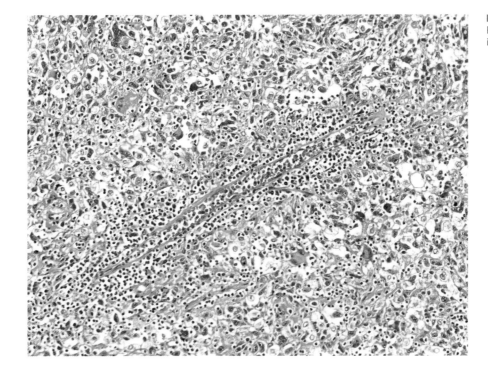

**Fig. 9-55.** Follicular dendritic cell sarcoma. Perivascular organization of lymphocytes is striking in the markedly pleomorphic example of FDC.

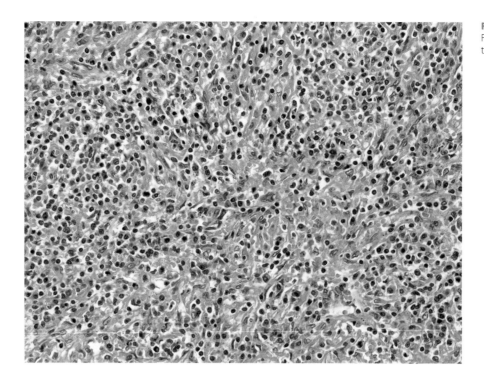

**Fig. 9-56.** IMT-like variant of FDC sarcoma. In this FDC subtype, the inflammatory component tends to be more abundant.

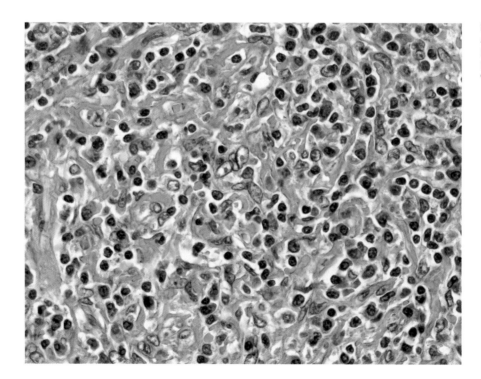

**Fig. 9-57.** IMT-like variant of FDC sarcoma. At higher power, the presence of a spindle proliferation featuring the presence of delicate pericellular collagen is seen. The inflammatory component is abundant.

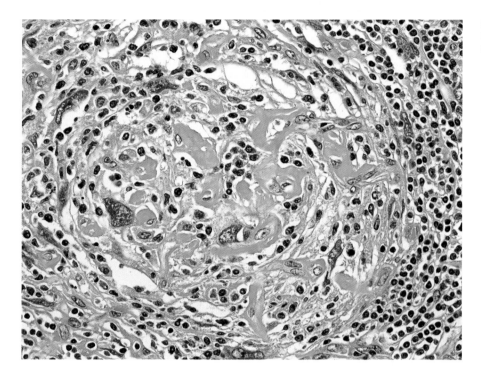

**Fig. 9-58.** Follicular dendritic cell sarcoma. When associated with Castleman disease, FDC sarcoma develops within the diseased follicle.

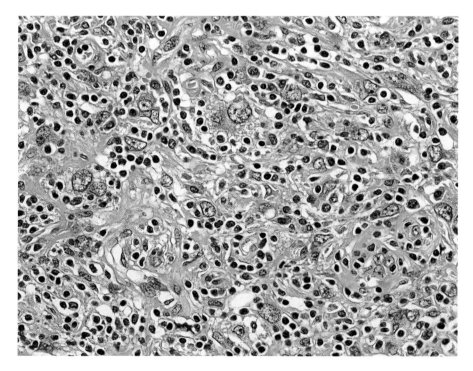

**Fig. 9-59.** Follicular dendritic cell sarcoma. Neoplastic cells spread out from the center of the follicle, colonizing interfollicular areas.

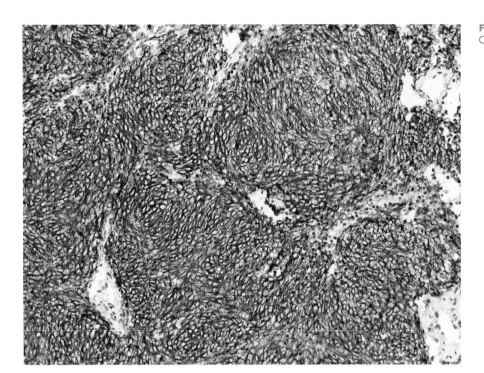

**Fig. 9-60.** Follicular dendritic cell sarcoma. Diffuse CD21 immunopositivity is seen.

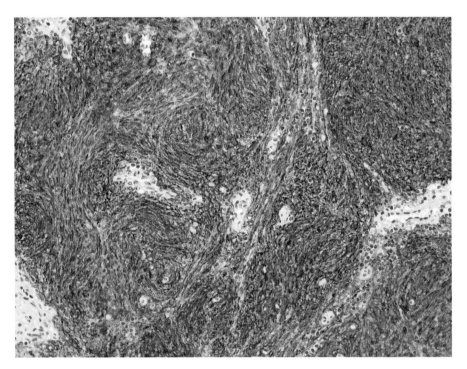

**Fig. 9-61.** Follicular dendritic cell sarcoma. CD23 decorates diffusely neoplastic cells.

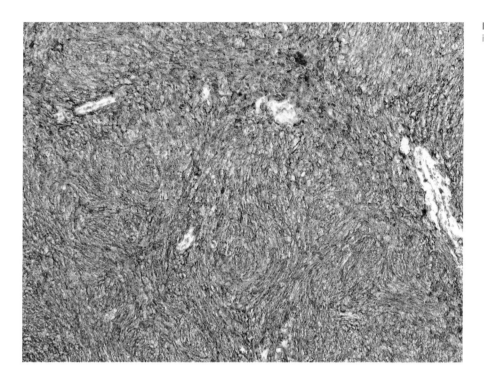

**Fig. 9-62.** Follicular dendritic cell sarcoma. Diffuse immunopositivity for clusterin is seen.

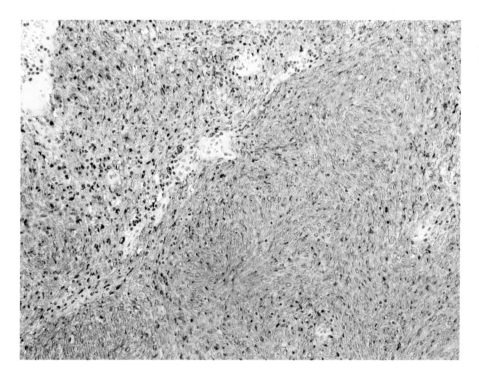

**Fig. 9-63.** Follicular dendritic cell sarcoma. CXCL-13 represents a novel immunohistochemical marker for FDC sarcoma. The pattern of expression is cytoplasmic.

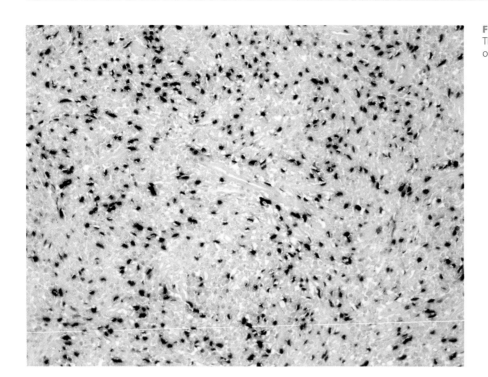

**Fig. 9-64.** IMT-like variant of FDC sarcoma. The presence of EBV-encoded RNA is typically observed (in situ hybridization).

## Genetics

Recent data have shown that miRNA profiling may split FDC-sarcoma into two subgroups: one related to perivascular fibroblasts and one apparently more related to Castleman disease. *BRAF* gene mutations have been found in approximately 20% of cases.

## Differential Diagnosis and Diagnostic Pitfalls

Main differential diagnoses include a group of related accessory cell neoplasms (interdigitating dendritic cell sarcoma and fibroblastic reticular cell sarcoma) and true histiocytic sarcomas. All entities are discussed separately in this chapter. As summarized in Table 9.1, immunohistochemistry plays a major role in recognizing the different tumor entities. As FDC may arise in the gastrointestinal tract, a clinically relevant differential diagnosis is represented by **gastrointestinal stromal tumors** (GISTs) that may exhibit significant overlap. However, the variable combination of KIT and DOG1 immunopositivity allows separation in the vast majority of cases. As discussed in Chapter 4, rare examples of GIST may lack KIT expression (approximately 20% of gastric GST) and, extremely rarely, DOG1 expression. In this situation, molecular analysis of *KIT* and *PDGFRA* genes is extremely helpful in achieving correct classification.

### Key Points in Follicular Dendritic Cell Sarcoma Diagnosis

- Occurrence in adults at nodal and extranodal locations
- Proliferation of mildly atypical spindle cells associated with scattered lymphocytes
- Cytologic pleomorphism comparatively rare
- Immunohistochemical expression of CD21, CD23, CD35, clusterin, podoplanin (D2-40), and CXCL-13
- EBER positivity in IMT-like variant of FDC sarcoma
- Variable clinical behavior from indolent to very aggressive

**Table 9.1** Immunohistochemical profile of inflammatory infiltrate-associated neoplasms/disorders

| | CK | CD68 | CD163 | S100 | CD1A | Clusterin | CXCL-13 | CD21/CD35 | ALK | IgG4 | MDM2 |
|---|---|---|---|---|---|---|---|---|---|---|---|
| FDC-S | – | – | – | – | – | + | + | + | – | – | – |
| IDC-S | – | +/– | – | + | – | – | – | – | – | – | – |
| FRC-S | + | – | – | – | – | – | – | – | – | – | – |
| H-S | – | + | + | – | – | – | – | – | – | – | – |
| LC-S | – | +/– | +/– | + | + | – | – | – | – | – | – |
| RDD | – | +/– | +/– | + | – | – | – | – | – | – | – |
| IMT | +/– | – | – | – | – | – | – | – | + | + | Focally + |
| IgG4-RSD | – | – | – | – | – | – | – | – | – | + | – |
| WD/DDLPS | – | – | – | – | – | – | – | – | – | – | + |

**Legends:**
FDC-S: Follicular dendritic cell sarcoma
IDC-S: Interdigitating dendritic cell sarcoma
FRC-S: Fibroblastic reticular cell sarcoma
H-S: Histiocytic sarcoma
LC-S: Langerhans cell sarcoma
RDD: Rosai-Dorfman disease
IMT: Inflammatory myofibroblastic tumor
IgG4-RSD: IgG4-related sclerosing disease
WD/DDLPS: Well-differentiated/dedifferentiated liposarcoma

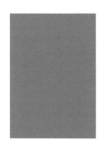

# Interdigitating Dendritic Cell Sarcoma

## Definition and Epidemiology

Interdigitating dendritic cell (IDC) sarcoma represents an extremely rare neoplasm hypothetically originating from antigen-presenting accessory cells normally populating the paracortex of lymph nodes.

## Clinical Presentation and Outcome

Interdigitating dendritic cell sarcoma occurs most often in the lymph nodes of adult patients, with striking male predominance. Occurrence in the pediatric age-group has been exceptionally reported. The spleen, the skin, and the gastrointestinal tract represent other, relatively common anatomic locations. Some patients (approximately 20%) develop IDC sarcoma in association with or following a low-grade B-cell lymphoma. Considering the rarity of the lesion, solid prognostic data are difficult to obtain. It seems that most tumors behave aggressively, with early onset of lung and liver metastases and with a median overall survival of only 15 months. In patients presenting with localized nodal disease, IDC sarcoma seems to pursue a rather indolent clinical course. Morphology does not

seem to provide strong prognostic indicators even if the presence of high mitotic rates as well as of high-grade "sarcoma-like" morphology has been associated with poor outcome. As for FDC sarcoma, data on efficacy of systemic treatment are very limited.

## Morphology and Immunophenotype

Interdigitating dendritic cell sarcoma microscopically recalls FDC sarcoma because of the presence of a variable number (from few to prominent) of scattered lymphocytes (Fig. 9-65). Neoplastic cells are most often ovoid, featuring abundant, poorly defined eosinophilic cytoplasm. Nuclei are vesicular and harbor small nucleoli (Fig. 9-66). Pleomorphism (Fig. 9-67) and an epithelioid morphology (Fig. 9-68) both tend to be very rare. Considering the significant morphologic overlap with FDC sarcoma, the most important finding is represented by expression of S100 protein that also tends to decorate the dendritic processes of neoplastic cells (Fig. 9-69). Variable expression of lymphoid markers such as LCA and CD45RO is observed, whereas classic FDC markers are usually negative.

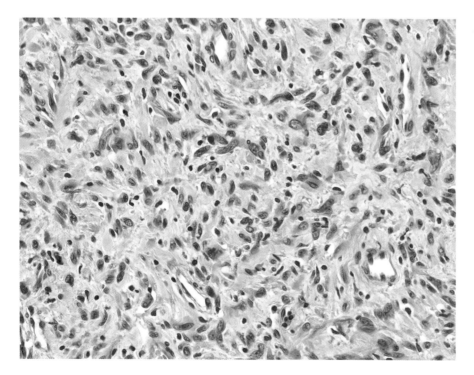

**Fig. 9-65.** Interdigitating dendritic cell sarcoma. The presence of scattered small lymphocytes contributes to morphologic overlap with FDC sarcoma. In this example, neoplastic cells are embedded in a fibrous background.

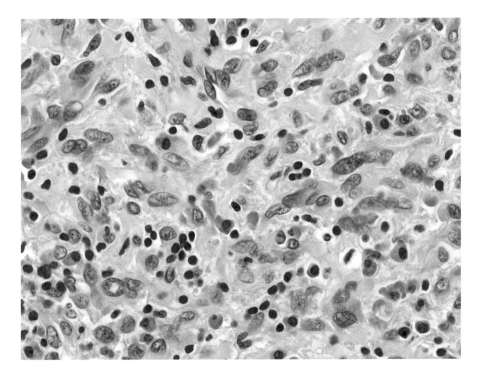

**Fig. 9-66.** Interdigitating dendritic cell sarcoma. The neoplastic cell population exhibits an ovoid shape. Poorly defined eosinophilic cytoplasm contain vesicular, somewhat irregular nuclei, with small nucleoli.

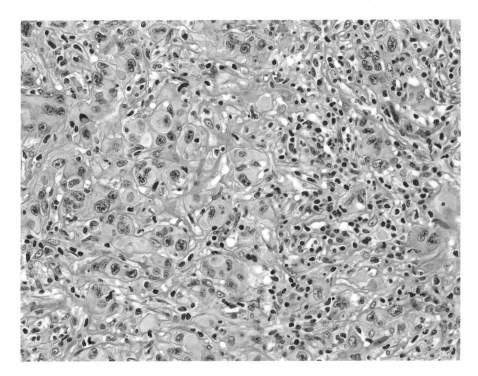

**Fig. 9-67.** Interdigitating dendritic cell sarcoma. Rare cases may exhibit striking nuclear pleomorphism.

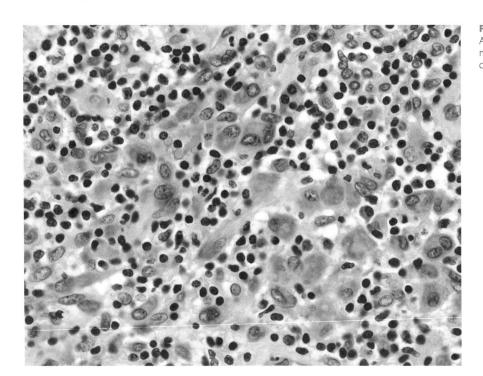

**Fig. 9-68.** Interdigitating dendritic cell sarcoma. At times, neoplastic cells assume an epithelioid morphology featuring more abundant eosinophilic cytoplasm.

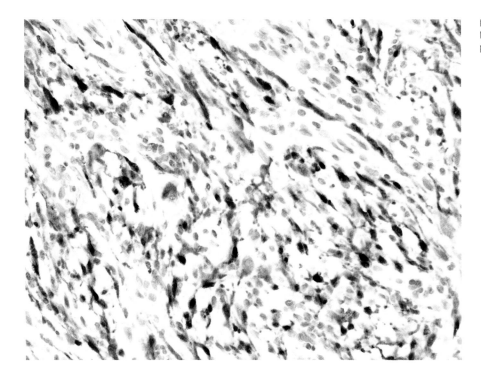

**Fig. 9-69.** Interdigitating dendritic cell sarcoma. Neoplastic cells exhibit immunopositivity for S100 protein of variable intensity.

## Genetics

No major recurrent genetic aberrations have been reported thus far.

## Differential Diagnosis and Diagnostic Pitfalls

In consideration of S100 immunopositivity, when dealing with nodal locations (and also in soft tissue locations) the most important differential diagnosis is with metastatic melanoma. In particular, spindle cell "sarcomatoid" melanoma represents the greatest challenge, as it often does not express common melanocytic markers such as HMB45 and Melan-A. The main problem is that spindle cell melanoma may not exhibit diffuse cytologic atypia (Fig. 9-70). Careful examination of histology will allow identification of scattered atypical cells that may be

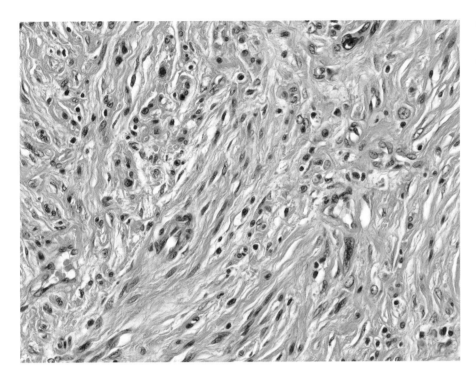

**Fig. 9-70.** Spindle cell amelanotic melanoma. Neoplastic cells are embedded in a densely fibrous background. The presence of multifocal nuclear atypia represents a consistent finding.

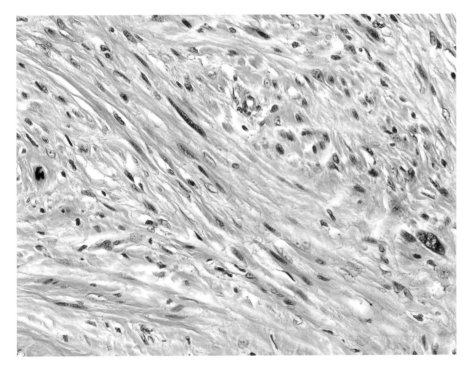

**Fig. 9-71.** Spindle cell amelanotic melanoma. Striking multifocal cytologic atypia is seen and is associated with mitotic figures.

associated with mitotic activity (Fig. 9-71). Importantly, S100 positivity tends to be more diffuse than normally seen in IDC sarcoma. *BRAF* gene mutations are much less common in sarcomatoid melanoma, therefore hampering the diagnostic utility of molecular testing in this context. In any case, careful clinical information regarding a previous history of melanoma should always be obtained, and if negative, patients should always be examined for the presence of regressed cutaneous or mucosal melanocytic malignancies.

**Key Points in Interdigitating Dendritic Cell Sarcoma Diagnosis**

- Occurrence in adults at nodal and extranodal locations
- Proliferation of ovoid neoplastic cells associated with scattered lymphocytes
- Immunohistochemical expression of S100 protein and CD45RO
- No expression of FDC differentiation markers
- Variable clinical behavior from indolent to very aggressive

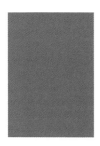

# Fibroblastic Reticular Cell Sarcoma

## Definition and Epidemiology

Fibroblastic reticular cell (FRC) sarcoma represents an exceedingly rare neoplasm hypothetically originating from keratin-positive dendritic cells that are seen in lymphoid organs such as lymph node, spleen, and tonsils. The incidence of FRC sarcoma is difficult to establish because of the very few cases reported.

## Clinical Presentation and Outcome

Fibroblastic reticular cell sarcoma occurs most often in the lymph nodes of adults. The spleen and the soft tissue are among other reported anatomic sites. Clinical behavior again is very variable, from an indolent course to widespread metastatic dissemination. As for FDC sarcoma and IDC sarcoma, data on efficacy of systemic treatment are very limited.

## Morphology and Immunophenotype

Fibroblastic reticular cell sarcoma microscopically exhibits some morphologic overlap with FDC sarcoma and IDC sarcoma, mainly because of the presence of scattered lymphocytes interspersed among lesional cells (Fig. 9-72). Neoplastic cells are most often spindled, featuring pale cytoplasm and irregular nuclei (Fig. 9-73). Cellularity may be variable, with some cases featuring increased fibrous background (Fig. 9-74) and others exhibiting moderate hypercellularity (Fig. 9-75). Rarely, nuclear pleomorphism can be observed that can be associated with increased mitotic activity (Fig. 9-76). Immunohistochemically, the most important finding is represented by expression of both cytokeratin (Fig. 9-77) and, less consistently, desmin (Fig. 9-78), which highlights cytoplasmic dendritic processes. Smooth muscle actin is also frequently positive. Importantly, S100 as well as FDC differentiation markers are consistently negative.

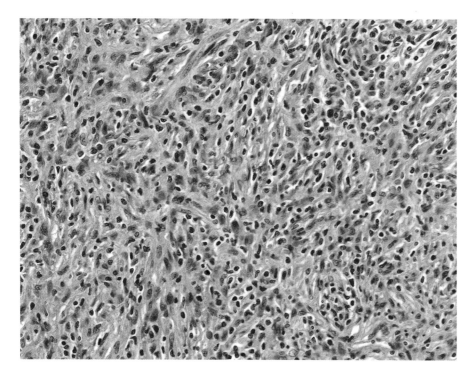

**Fig. 9-72.** Fibroblastic reticular cell sarcoma. Often, the morphologic overlap with both FDC sarcoma and IDC sarcoma is striking. At low power, an ovoid cell population associated with scattered small lymphocytes is seen.

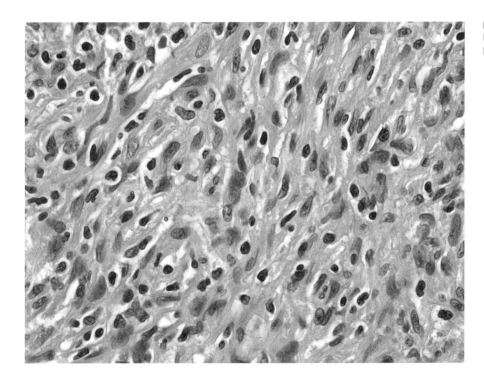

**Fig. 9-73.** Fibroblastic reticular cell sarcoma. Neoplastic cells are most often spindled, featuring pale cytoplasm and irregular nuclei.

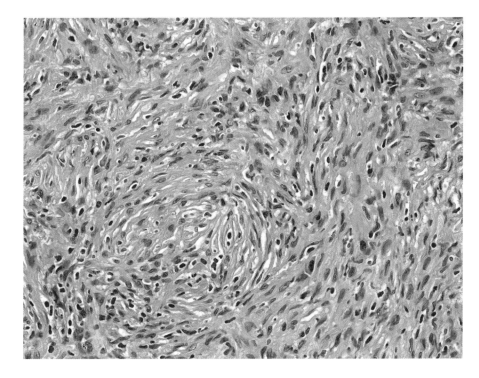

**Fig. 9-74.** Fibroblastic reticular cell sarcoma. Some cases exhibit an increased amount of intercellular collagenous matrix.

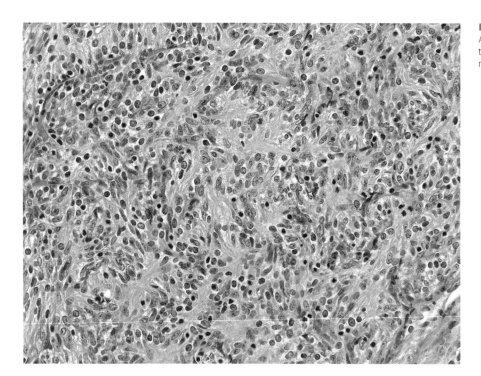

**Fig. 9-75.** Fibroblastic reticular cell sarcoma. At times, increased cellularity is observed, which in this example is associated with a rich vascular network.

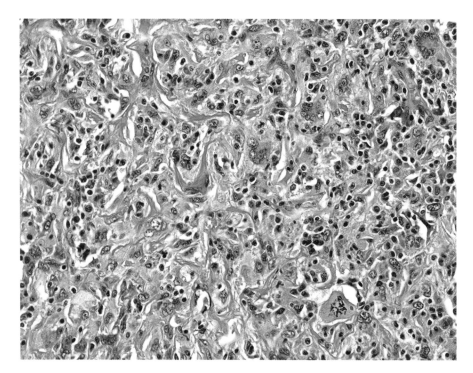

**Fig. 9-76.** Fibroblastic reticular cell sarcoma. The presence of striking pleomorphism, as observed occasionally in all other accessory cell lesions, is possible but comparatively rare.

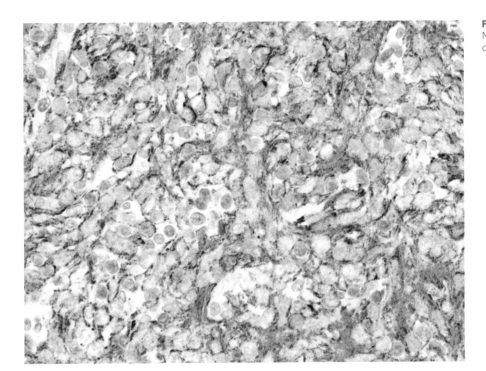

**Fig. 9-77.** Fibroblastic reticular cell sarcoma. Neoplastic cells exhibit strong expression of cytokeratin.

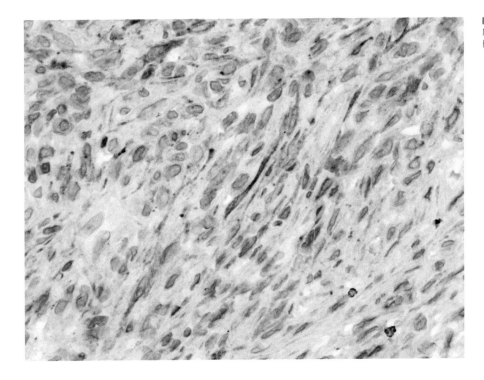

**Fig. 9-78.** Fibroblastic reticular cell sarcoma. Multifocal desmin positivity is seen, which tends to highlight the presence of cytoplasmic processes.

## Genetics

No major genetic aberrations have been reported thus far.

## Differential Diagnosis and Diagnostic Pitfalls

In addition to the differential diagnosis with FDC sarcoma and IDC sarcoma, wherein immunohistochemical findings represent an extremely helpful diagnostic clue, when dealing with nodal locations the most challenging differential is with metastatic sarcomatoid carcinoma (Fig. 9-79). Of course, clinical workup is extremely helpful; however, the presence of significantly less cytologic atypia, the presence of scattered lymphocytes (which actually may also be seen in sarcomatoid carcinoma), and the presence of dendritic morphology

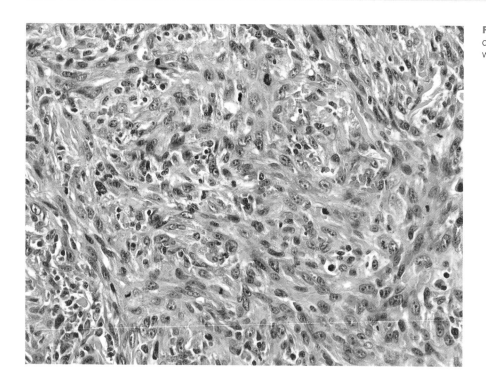

**Fig. 9-79.** Sarcomatoid carcinoma. Obvious diffuse cytologic atypia is present and is associated with a high number of atypical mitotic figures.

highlighted by both desmin and cytokeratin are all very important diagnostic features.

### Key Points in Fibroblastic Reticular Cell Sarcoma Diagnosis

- Occurrence in adults in lymph nodes, spleen, and soft tissue
- Proliferation of neoplastic spindle cells associated with scattered lymphocytes
- Immunohistochemical expression of cytokeratin and desmin
- No expression of FDC differentiation markers
- Variable clinical behavior, from indolent to very aggressive

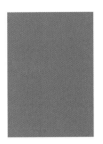

# Histiocytic Sarcoma

## Definition and Epidemiology

Histiocytic sarcoma represents an exceedingly rare, aggressive neoplasm, entirely composed of immunohistochemically proven malignant histiocytes. Incidence is very difficult to predict because of its rarity. Even if a rather broad age range is observed, most patients are adults, with a peak incidence occurring in the fourth decade.

## Clinical Presentation and Outcome

Histiocytic sarcoma may occur in lymphoid organs such as the lymph nodes and the spleen; however, it is relatively more common at extranodal locations such as the soft tissue and bone, the gastrointestinal tract, the skin, and the central nervous system. It can occur as a primary lesion or secondary neoplasm following various hematolymphoid malignancies. Histiocytic sarcoma most often pursues a very aggressive clinical course with the exception of those very rare cases exhibiting a low-grade morphology. Early dissemination (lymph nodes, lungs, and bone) is frequently observed, and chemotherapy seems to be of limited efficacy.

## Morphology and Immunophenotype

Histiocytic sarcoma often presents as large masses featuring a fleshy cut surface. Histiocytic sarcoma is most often composed of a proliferation of epithelioid cells, organized in a diffuse pattern of growth (Fig. 9-80) and featuring abundant eosinophilic cytoplasm harboring irregular nuclei (Figs. 9-81 and 9-82). Nuclear pleomorphism can often be observed (Fig. 9-83). The presence of variably numerous scattered lymphocytes (Fig. 9-84) is a typical feature. Immunohistochemically, histiocytic sarcomas consistently express classic histiocytic markers such as CD68, CD163, CD4 (Fig. 9-85), and lysozyme. FDC differentiation markers are negative. Importantly, focal expression of S100 and consistent expression of CD31 are observed, representing a potential diagnostic pitfall.

## Genetics

Somatic mutations of *BRAF* and *HRAS* have been reported recently.

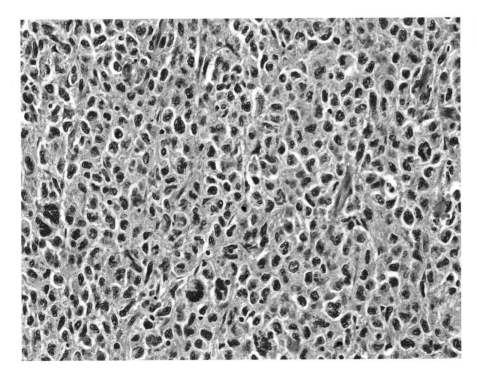

**Fig. 9-80.** Histiocytic sarcoma. Most often, a proliferation of epithelioid neoplastic cells, organized in a diffuse pattern of growth, is seen.

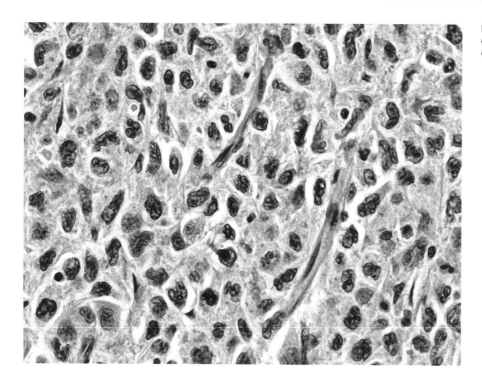

**Fig. 9-81.** Histiocytic sarcoma. Neoplastic cells exhibit abundant eosinophilic, somewhat granular cytoplasm harboring irregular nuclei.

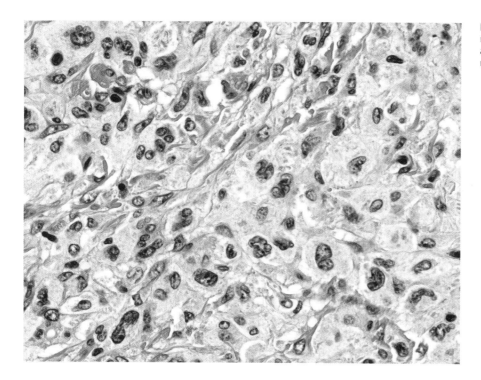

**Fig. 9-82.** Histiocytic sarcoma. Nuclei with remarkably irregular contours embedded in abundant cytoplasm represent consistent morphologic findings.

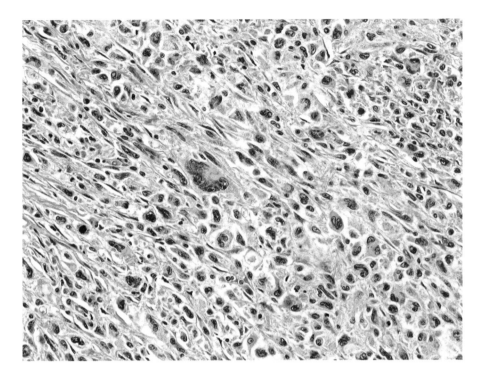

**Fig. 9-83.** Histiocytic sarcoma. Nuclear pleomorphism can be observed.

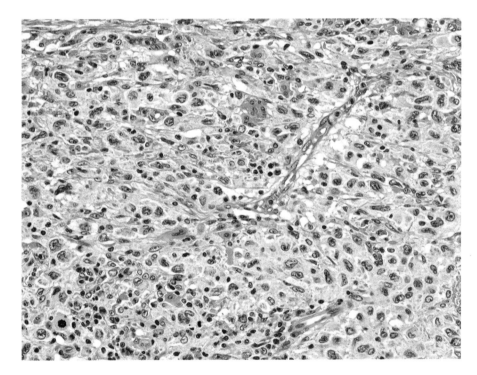

**Fig. 9-84.** Histiocytic sarcoma. Scattered lymphocytes can be observed (associated with eosinophils, in this case); however, their presence is usually far less striking than in accessory cell sarcoma.

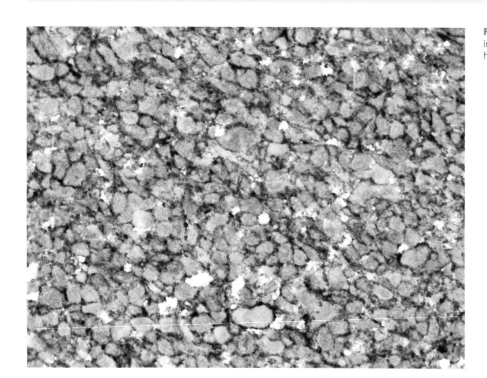

**Fig. 9-85.** Histiocytic sarcoma. Strong CD4 immunopositivity is most often observed in histiocytic sarcoma.

## Differential Diagnosis and Diagnostic Pitfalls

Histiocytic sarcoma represents a true diagnostic challenge, and the differential diagnosis includes several epithelioid malignancies. Undifferentiated carcinoma is easily ruled out on the basis of the expression of cytokeratin and EMA. Metastatic melanoma can enter the differential diagnosis. As histiocytic sarcoma can multifocally express S100 protein, application of a broader panel of melanocytic markers is generally recommended. Diffuse, large B-cell lymphoma and anaplastic large cell lymphoma can be excluded on the basis of negativity for B and T differentiation markers (with the exception of CD4) and of both CD30 and ALK. Immunopositivity for CD31, in combination with the epithelioid morphology, may raise diagnostic confusion with solid forms of epithelioid angiosarcoma. Angiosarcoma, however, exhibits higher nuclear atypia that is most often associated with the presence of large eosinophilic nucleoli (Fig. 9-86). Moreover, epithelioid angiosarcoma consistently shows nuclear expression of ERG, which has never been reported in histiocytic sarcoma.

An extremely rare entity that can enter the differential diagnosis is represented by **Langerhans cell sarcoma**. Langerhans cell sarcoma most often occurs in the soft tissue, the skin, and the gastrointestinal tract of adult patients.

As observed in the comparatively more common **Langerhans cell histiocytosis**, the presence of a variably prominent eosinophilic inflammatory infiltrate represents an important diagnostic clue (Fig. 9-87). Neoplastic cells are also epithelioid; however, cytoplasm is less abundant than generally observed in histiocytic sarcoma (Fig. 9-88). Whereas S100 protein is expressed diffusely, Langerhans cell differentiation markers such as CD1a and CD207 (langerin) may be more limited.

**Rosai-Dorfman disease** is part of the group of S100 protein-positive histiocytic proliferations. First reported as "sinus histiocytosis with massive lymphadenopathy," it may occur anywhere, both at nodal and extranodal locations. Most often it affects children and young adults and is characterized by a rather indolent clinical course. Microscopically, Rosai-Dorfman disease is composed of a proliferation of S100-positive histiocytes featuring abundant pale cytoplasm (Fig. 9-89). A key diagnostic feature is represented by intracytoplasmic engulfment of intact inflammatory cells (so-called emperipolesis) (Fig. 9-90). The histiocytic proliferation is generally associated with a prominent inflammatory infiltrate that includes neutrophils, lymphocytes, and plasma cells. In addition to the expression of S100 protein (Fig. 9-91), the expression of common histiocytic markers such as CD68 and CD163 is commonly observed.

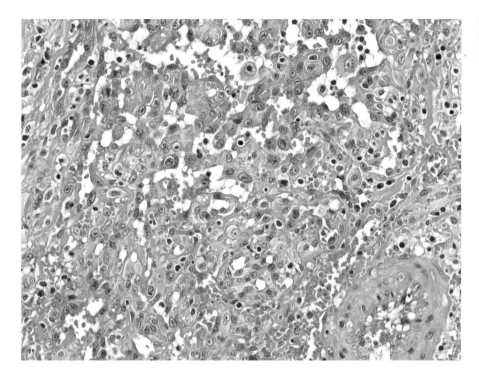

**Fig. 9-86.** Epithelioid angiosarcoma. The presence of vesicular nuclei harboring eosinophilic macronucleoli represents a key morphologic clue to the diagnosis of epithelioid angiosarcoma.

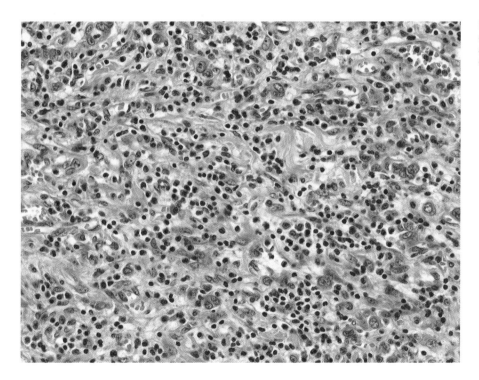

**Fig. 9-87.** Langerhans cell sarcoma. Neoplastic cells exhibit large atypical, convoluted nuclei associated with the presence of an abundant eosinophilic inflammatory infiltrate.

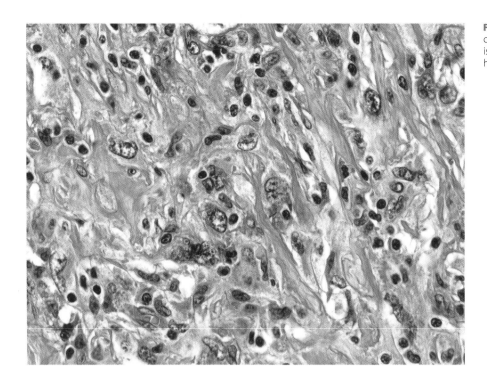

**Fig. 9-88.** Langerhans cell sarcoma. Neoplastic cells are somewhat epithelioid; however, cytoplasm is less abundant than generally observed in histiocytic sarcoma.

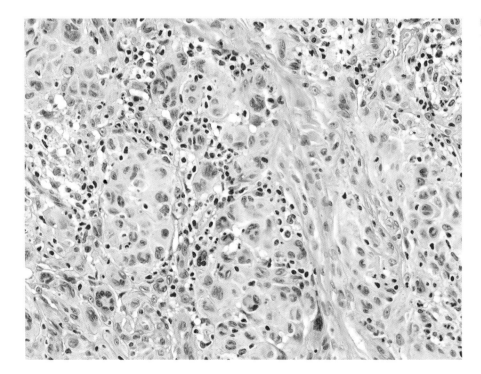

**Fig. 9-89.** Rosai-Dorfman disease. A proliferation of histiocytes featuring abundant pale cytoplasm and associated with chronic inflammatory cells is seen.

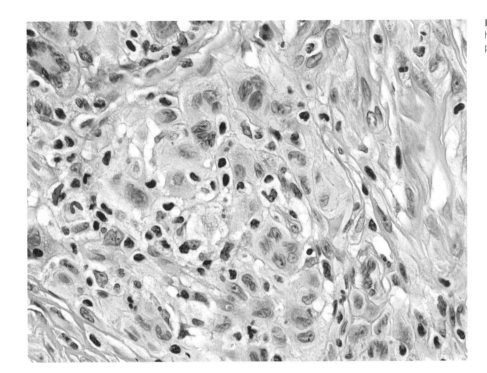

**Fig. 9-90.** Rosai-Dorfman disease. Large histiocytes tend to engulf inflammatory cells. This phenomenon is known as "emperipolesis."

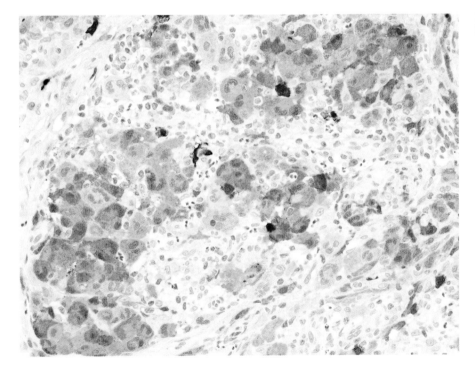

**Fig. 9-91.** Rosai-Dorfman disease. Diffuse S100 immunopositivity is invariably seen in lesional cells.

**Key Points in Histiocytic Sarcoma Diagnosis**

- Occurrence in lymph node, spleen, soft tissue, and bone of adults
- Proliferation of epithelioid neoplastic cells associated with scattered lymphocytes
- Immunohistochemical expression of CD68, CD163, CD4, lysozyme, CD31, and S100 (focal)
- FDC differentiation markers negative
- Aggressive clinical behavior with early metastatic dissemination

## Chapter 9 Selected Key References

### Plexiform Fibrohistiocytic Tumor

- Ehrenstein V, Andersen SL, Qazi I, et al. Tenosynovial giant cell tumor: incidence, prevalence, patient characteristics, and recurrence. A registry-based cohort study in Denmark. *J Rheumatol.* 2017;**44**(10):1476–83.
- Enzinger FM, Zhang RY. Plexiform fibrohistiocytic tumor presenting in children and young adults. An analysis of 65 cases. *Am J Surg Pathol.* 1988;**12**:818–26.
- Fox MD, Billings SD, Gleason BC, et al. Expression of MiTF may be helpful in differentiating cellular neurothekeoma from plexiform fibrohistiocytic tumor (histiocytoid predominant) in a partial biopsy specimen. *Am J Dermatopathol.* 2012;**34**:157–60.
- Hollowood K, Holley MP, Fletcher CD. Plexiform fibrohistiocytic tumour: clinicopathological, immunohistochemical and ultrastructural analysis in favour of a myofibroblastic lesion. *Histopathology.* 1991;**19**:503–13.
- Jaffer S, Ambrosini-Spaltro A, Mancini AM, Eusebi V, Rosai J. Neurothekeoma and plexiform fibrohistiocytic tumor: mere histologic resemblance or histogenetic relationship? *Am J Surg Pathol.* 2009;**33**:905–13.
- Moosavi C, Jha P, Fanburg-Smith JC. An update on plexiform fibrohistiocytic tumor and addition of 66 new cases from the Armed Forces Institute of Pathology, in honor of Franz M. Enzinger, MD. *Ann Diagn Pathol.* 2007;**11**:313–19.
- Redlich GC, Montgomery KD, Allgood GA, Joste NE. Plexiform fibrohistiocytic tumor with a clonal cytogenetic anomaly. *Cancer Genet Cytogenet.* 1999;**108**:141–3.
- Remstein ED, Arndt CA, Nascimento AG. Plexiform fibrohistiocytic tumor: clinicopathologic analysis of 22 cases. *Am J Surg Pathol.* 1999;**23**:662–70.
- Salomao DR, Nascimento AG. Plexiform fibrohistiocytic tumor with systemic metastases: a case report. *Am J Surg Pathol.* 1997;**21**:469–76.
- Zelger B, Weinlich G, Steiner H, Zelger BG, Egarter-Vigl E. Dermal and subcutaneous variants of plexiform fibrohistiocytic tumor. *Am J Surg Pathol.* 1997;**21**:235–41.

### Giant Cell Tumor of Soft Tissue and Its Differential Diagnosis

- Cupp JS, Miller MA, Montgomery KD, et al. Translocation and expression of CSF1 in pigmented villonodular synovitis, tenosynovial giant cell tumor, rheumatoid arthritis and other reactive synovitides. *Am J Surg Pathol.* 2007;**31**:970–6.
- Folpe AL, Morris RJ, Weiss SW. Soft tissue giant cell tumor of low malignant potential: a proposal for the reclassification of malignant giant cell tumor of soft parts. *Mod Pathol.* 1999;**12**:894–902.
- Gleason BC, Fletcher CD. Deep "benign" fibrous histiocytoma: clinicopathologic analysis of 69 cases of a rare tumor indicating occasional metastatic potential. *Am J Surg Pathol.* 2008;**32**:354–62.
- Guccion JC, Enzinger FM. Malignant giant cell tumor of soft parts. An analysis of 32 cases. *Cancer.* 1972;**29**:1518–29.
- Lee JC, Liang CW, Fletcher CD. Giant cell tumor of soft tissue is genetically distinct from its bone counterpart. *Mod Pathol.* 2017;**30**:728–33.
- Mancini I, Righi A, Gambarotti M, et al. Phenotypic and molecular differences between giant-cell tumour of soft tissue and its bone counterpart. *Histopathology.* 2017;**71**:453–60.
- Mentzel T, Calonje E, Fletcher CD. Leiomyosarcoma with prominent osteoclast-like giant cells. Analysis of eight cases closely mimicking the so-called giant cell variant of malignant fibrous histiocytoma. *Am J Surg Pathol.* 1994;**18**:258–65.
- O'Connell XJ, Wehrli BM, Nielsen GP, Rosenberg AE. Giant cell tumors of soft tissue: a clinicopatologic study of 18 benign and malignant tumors. *Am J Surg Pathol.* 2000;**24**:386–95.
- Oliveira AM, Dei Tos AP, Fletcher CDM, Nascimento AG. Primary giant cell tumor of soft tissue: a study of 22 cases. *Am J Surg Pathol.* 2000;**24**:248–56.
- Rubin BP. Tenosynovial giant cell tumor and pigmented villonodular synovitis: a proposal for unification of these clinically distinct but histologically and genetically identical lesions. *Skeletal Radiol.* 2007;**6**:267–8.
- Salm R, Sissons HA. Giant-cell tumours of soft tissues. *J Pathol.* 1972;**107**:27–39.
- Sciot R, Rosai J, Dal Cin P, et al. Analysis of 35 cases of localized and diffuse tenosynovial giant cell tumor: a report from the Chromosomes and Morphology (CHAMP) study group. *Mod Pathol.* 1999;**12**:576–9.
- Tap WD, Wainberg ZA, Anthony SP, et al. Structure-guided blockade of CSF1R kinase in tenosynovial giant-cell tumor. *N Engl J Med.* 2015;**373**:428–37.

### Inflammatory Myofibroblastic Tumor

- Akram S, Pardi DS, Schaffner JA, Smyrk TC. Sclerosing mesenteritis: clinical features, treatment, and outcome in ninety-two patients. *Clin Gastroenterol Hepatol.* 2007;**5**:589–96.
- Albores-Saavedra J, Manivel JC, Essenfeld H, et al. Pseudosarcomatous myofibroblastic proliferations in the urinary bladder of children. *Cancer.* 1990;**66**:1234–41.
- Bennett JA, Nardi V, Rouzbahman M, et al. Inflammatory myofibroblastic tumor of the uterus: a clinicopathological, immunohistochemical, and molecular analysis of 13 cases highlighting their broad morphologic spectrum. *Mod Pathol.* 2017;**30**:1489–1503.
- Bridge JA, Kanamori M, Ma Z, et al. Fusion of the ALK gene to the clathrin heavy chain gene, CLTC, in inflammatory myofibroblastic tumor. *Am J Pathol.* 2001;**159**:411–15.
- Butrynski JE, D'Adamo DR, Hornick JL, et al. Crizotinib in ALK-rearranged inflammatory myofibroblastic tumor. *N Engl J Med.* 2010;**363**:1727–33.
- Cessna MH, Zhou H, Sanger WG, et al. Expression of ALK1 and p80 in inflammatory myofibroblastic tumor and its mesenchymal mimics: a study of 135 cases. *Mod Pathol.* 2002;**15**:931–8.
- Cheuk W, Chan JK. IgG4-related sclerosing disease: a critical appraisal of an evolving clinicopathologic entity. *Adv Anat Pathol.* 2010;**17**:303–32.
- Coffin CM, Hornick JL, Fletcher CD. Inflammatory myofibroblastic tumor: comparison of clinicopathologic, histologic, and immunohistochemical features including ALK expression in atypical and aggressive cases. *Am J Surg Pathol.* 2007;**31**:509–20.
- Coffin CM, Humphrey PA, Dehner LP. Extrapulmonary inflammatory myofibroblastic tumor: a clinical and pathological survey. *Semin Diagn Pathol.* 1998;**15**:85–101.
- Coffin CM, Patel A, Perkins S, et al. ALK1 and p80 expression and chromosomal rearrangements involving 2p23 in inflammatory myofibroblastic tumor. *Mod Pathol.* 2001;**14**:569–76.

- Coffin CM, Watterson J, Priest JR, Dehner LP. Extrapulmonary inflammatory myofibroblastic tumor (inflammatory pseudotumor). A clinicopathologic and immunohistochemical study of 84 cases. *Am J Surg Pathol*. 1995;**19**:859–72.

- Corradi D, Maestri R, Palmisano A, et al. Idiopathic retroperitoneal fibrosis: clinicopathologic features and differential diagnosis. *Kidney Int*. 2007;**72**:742–53.

- Harik LR, Merino C, Coindre JM, et al. Pseudosarcomatous myofibroblastic proliferations of the bladder: a clinicopathologic study of 42 cases. *Am J Surg Pathol*. 2006;**30**:787–94.

- Hirsch MS, Dal Cin P, Fletcher CD. ALK expression in pseudosarcomatous myofibroblastic proliferations of the genitourinary tract. *Histopathology*. 2006;**48**:569–78.

- Hornick JL, Sholl LM, Dal Cin P, Childress MA, Lovly CM. Expression of ROS1 predicts ROS1 gene rearrangement in inflammatory myofibroblastic tumors. *Mod Pathol*. 2015;**28**:732–9.

- Lee JC, Li CF, Huang HY, et al. ALK oncoproteins in atypical inflammatory myofibroblastic tumours: novel RRBP1-ALK fusions in epithelioid inflammatory myofibroblastic sarcoma. *J Pathol*. 2017;**241**:316–23.

- Mariño-Enríquez A, Wang WL, Roy A, et al. Epithelioid inflammatory myofibroblastic sarcoma: An aggressive intra-abdominal variant of inflammatory myofibroblastic tumor with nuclear membrane or perinuclear ALK. *Am J Surg Pathol*. 2011;**35**:135–44.

- Mossé YP, Voss SD, Lim MS, et al. Targeting ALK with crizotinib in pediatric anaplastic large cell lymphoma and inflammatory myofibroblastic tumor: a Children's Oncology Group study. *J Clin Oncol*. 2017;**35**:3215–21.

- Nascimento AF, Ruiz R, Hornick JL, Fletcher CD. Calcifying fibrous 'pseudotumor': clinicopathologic study of 15 cases and analysis of its relationship to inflammatory myofibroblastic tumor. *Int J Surg Pathol*. 2002;**10**:189–96.

- Parra-Herran C, Quick CM, Howitt BE, et al. Inflammatory myofibroblastic tumor of the uterus: clinical and pathologic review of 10 cases including a subset with aggressive clinical course. *Am J Surg Pathol*. 2015;**39**:157–68.

- Pettinato G, Manivel JC, De Rosa N, Dehner LP. Inflammatory myofibroblastic tumor (plasma cell granuloma). Clinicopathologic study of 20 cases with immunohistochemical and ultrastructural observations. *Am J Clin Pathol*. 1990;**94**:538–46.

- Rossi GM, Rocco R, Accorsi Buttini E, Marvisi C, Vaglio A. Idiopathic retroperitoneal fibrosis and its overlap with IgG4-related disease. *Intern Emerg Med*. 2017;**12**:287–99.

- Sharma P, Yadav S, Needham CM, Feuerstadt P. Sclerosing mesenteritis: a systematic review of 192 cases. *Clin J Gastroenterol*. 2017;**10**:103–11.

- Sirvent N, Hawkins AL, Moeglin D, et al. ALK probe rearrangement in a t(2;11;2)(p23;p15;q31) translocation found in a prenatal myofibroblastic fibrous lesion: toward a molecular definition of an inflammatory myofibroblastic tumor family? *Genes Chromosomes Cancer*. 2001;**31**:85–90.

- Sukov WR, Cheville JC, Carlson AW, et al. Utility of ALK-1 protein expression and ALK rearrangements in distinguishing inflammatory myofibroblastic tumor from malignant spindle cell lesions of the urinary bladder. *Mod Pathol*. 2007;**20**:592–603.

- Weaver J, Goldblum JR, Turner S, et al. Detection of MDM2 gene amplification or protein expression distinguishes sclerosing mesenteritis and retroperitoneal fibrosis from inflammatory well-differentiated liposarcoma. *Mod Pathol*. 2009;**22**:66–70.

- Yamamoto H, Yamaguchi H, Aishima S, et al. Inflammatory myofibroblastic tumor versus IgG4-related sclerosing disease and inflammatory pseudotumor: a comparative clinicopathologic study. *Am J Surg Pathol*. 2009;**33**:1330–40.

# Follicular Dendritic Cell Sarcoma

- Agaimy A, Michal M, Hadravsky L, Michal M. Follicular dendritic cell sarcoma: clinicopathologic study of 15 cases with emphasis on novel expression of MDM2, somatostatin receptor 2A, and PD-L1. *Ann Diagn Pathol*. 2016;**23**:21–8.

- Andersen EF, Paxton CN, O'Malley DP, et al. Genomic analysis of follicular dendritic cell sarcoma by molecular inversion probe array reveals tumor suppressor-driven biology. *Mod Pathol*. 2017;**30**:1321–34.

- Chan AC, Chan KW, Chan JK, et al. Development of follicular dendritic cell sarcoma in hyaline-vascular Castleman's disease of the nasopharynx: tracing its evolution by sequential biopsies. *Histopathology*. 2001;**38**:510–18.

- Chan JK, Fletcher CD, Nayler SJ, Cooper K. Follicular dendritic cell sarcoma. Clinicopathologic analysis of 17 cases suggesting a malignant potential higher than currently recognized. *Cancer*. 1997;**79**:294–313.

- Chen T, Gopal P. Follicular dendritic cell sarcoma. *Arch Pathol Lab Med*. 2017;**141**:596–9.

- Choe JY, Go H, Jeon YK, et al. Inflammatory pseudotumor-like follicular dendritic cell sarcoma of the spleen: a report of six cases with increased IgG4-positive plasma cells. *Pathol Int*. 2013;**63**:245–51.

- Griffin GK, Sholl LM, Lindeman NI, Fletcher CD, Hornick JL. Targeted genomic sequencing of follicular dendritic cell sarcoma reveals recurrent alterations in NF-κB regulatory genes. *Mod Pathol*. 2016;**29**:67–74.

- Jain P, Milgrom SA, Patel KP, et al. Characteristics, management, and outcomes of patients with follicular dendritic cell sarcoma. *Br J Haematol*. 2017;**178**:403–12.

- Lorenzi L, Döring C, Rausch T, et al. Identification of novel follicular dendritic cell sarcoma markers, FDCSP and SRGN, by whole transcriptome sequencing. *Oncotarget*. 2017;**8**:16,463–72.

- Pang J, Mydlarz WK, Gooi Z, et al. Follicular dendritic cell sarcoma of the head and neck: Case report, literature review, and pooled analysis of 97 cases. *Head Neck*. 2016;**38** Suppl 1: E2241–9.

- Pileri SA, Grogan TM, Harris NL, et al. Tumors of histiocytes and accessory dendritic cells. An immunohistochemical approach to classification from the International Lymphoma Study Group based on 61 cases. *Histopathology*. 2002;**41**:1–29.

- Shek TW, Ho FC, Ng IO, et al. Follicular dendritic cell tumor of the liver. Evidence for an Epstein-Barr virus-related clonal proliferation of follicular dendritic cells. *Am J Surg Pathol*. 1996;**20**:313–24.

- Shia J, Chen W, Tang LH, et al. Extranodal follicular dendritic cell sarcoma: clinical, pathologic, and histogenetic characteristics of an underrecognized disease entity. *Virchows Arch*. 2006;**449**:148–58.

- Sun X, Chang KC, Abruzzo LV, et al. Epidermal growth factor receptor expression in follicular dendritic cells: a shared feature of follicular dendritic cell sarcoma and Castleman's disease. *Hum Pathol*. 2003;**34**:835–40.

- Vermi W, Lonardi S, Bosisio D, et al. Identification of CXCL13 as a new marker for follicular dendritic cell sarcoma. *J Pathol*. 2008;**216**:356–64.

## Interdigitating Dendritic Cell Sarcoma

- Gaertner EM, Tsokos M, Derringer GA, et al. Interdigitating dendritic cell sarcoma. A report of four cases and review of the literature. *Am J Clin Pathol.* 2001;**115**:589–97.
- Magro CM, Olson LC, Nuovo G, Solomon GJ. Primary cutaneous interdigitating dendritic cell sarcoma is a morphologic and phenotypic simulator of poorly differentiated metastatic melanoma: A report of 2 cases and review of the literature. *Ann Diagn Pathol.* 2017;**30**:59–65.
- Ohtake H, Yamakawa M. Interdigitating dendritic cell sarcoma and follicular dendritic cell sarcoma: histopathological findings for differential diagnosis. *J Clin Exp Hematop.* 2013;**53**:179–84.
- O'Malley DP, Zuckerberg L, Smith LB, et al. The genetics of interdigitating dendritic cell sarcoma share some changes with Langerhans cell histiocytosis in select cases. *Ann Diagn Pathol.* 2014;**18**:18–20.
- Pillay K, Solomon R, Daubenton JD, Sinclair-Smith CC. Interdigitating dendritic cell sarcoma: a report of four paediatric cases and review of the literature. *Histopathology.* 2004;**44**:283–91.
- Stowman AM, Mills SE, Wick MR. Spindle cell melanoma and interdigitating dendritic cell sarcoma: do they represent the same process? *Am J Surg Pathol.* 2016;**40**:1270–9.

## Fibroblastic Reticular Cell Sarcoma

- Chan AC, Serrano-Olmo J, Erlandson RA, et al. Cytokeratin- positive malignant tumors with reticulum cell morphology: a subtype of fibroblastic reticulum cell neoplasm? *Am J Surg Pathol.* 2000;**24**:107–16.
- Goto N, Tsurumi H, Takami T, et al. Cytokeratin-positive fibroblastic reticular cell tumor with follicular dendritic cell features: a case report and review of the literature. *Am J Surg Pathol.* 2015;**39**:573–80.
- Martel M, Sarli D, Colecchia M, et al. Fibroblastic reticular cell tumor of the spleen: report of a case and review of the entity. *Hum Pathol.* 2003;**34**:954–7.
- Schuerfeld K, Lazzi S, De Santi MM, et al. Cytokeratin-positive interstitial cell neoplasm: a case report and classification issues. *Histopathology.* 2003;**43**:491–4.

## Histiocytic Sarcoma

- Ansari J, Naqash AR, Munker R, et al. Histiocytic sarcoma as a secondary malignancy: pathobiology, diagnosis, and treatment. *Eur J Haematol.* 2016;**97**:9–16.
- Feldman AL, Minniti C, Santi M, et al. Histiocytic sarcoma after acute lymphoblastic leukaemia: a common clonal origin. *Lancet Oncol.* 2004;**5**:248–50.
- Foucar E, Rosai J, Dorfman R. Sinus histiocytosis with massive lymphadenopathy (Rosai-Dorfman disease): review of the entity. *Semin Diagn Pathol.* 1990;**7**:19–73.
- Howard JE, Dwivedi RC, Masterson L, Jani P. Langerhans cell sarcoma: a systematic review. *Cancer Treat Rev.* 2015;**41**:320–31.
- Kordes M, Röring M, Heining C, et al. Cooperation of BRAF(F595L) and mutant HRAS in histiocytic sarcoma provides new insights into oncogenic BRAF signaling. *Leukemia.* 2016;**30**:937–46.
- Lauwers GY, Perez-Atayde A, Dorfman RF, Rosai J. The digestive system manifestations of Rosai-Dorfman disease (sinus histiocytosis with massive lymphadenopathy): review of 11 cases. *Hum Pathol.* 2000;**31**:380–5.
- Liu Q, Tomaszewicz K, Hutchinson L, et al. Somatic mutations in histiocytic sarcoma identified by next generation sequencing. *Virchows Arch.* 2016;**469**:233–41.
- Nakamine H, Yamakawa M, Yoshino T, et al. Langerhans cell histiocytosis and Langerhans cell sarcoma: current understanding and differential diagnosis. *J Clin Exp Hematop.* 2016;**56**:109–18.
- Rosai J, Dorfman RF. Sinus histiocytosis with massive lymphadenopathy. A newly recognized benign clinicopathological entity. *Arch Pathol.* 1969;**87**:63–70.
- Sun W, Nordberg ML, Fowler MR. Histiocytic sarcoma involving the central nervous system: clinical, immunohistochemical, and molecular genetic studies of a case with review of the literature. *Am J Surg Pathol.* 2003;**27**:258–65.
- Thakral B, Khoury JD. Histiocytic sarcoma: secondary neoplasm or "transdifferentiation" in the setting of B-acute lymphoblastic leukemia. *Blood.* 2016;**128**:2475.
- van der Valk P, Meijer CJ, Willemze R, et al. Histiocytic sarcoma (true histiocytic lymphoma): a clinicopathological study of 20 cases. *Histopathology.* 1984;**8**:105–23.
- Vos JA, Abbondanzo SL, Barekman CL, et al. Histiocytic sarcoma: a study of five cases including the histiocyte marker CD163. *Mod Pathol.* 2005;**18**:693–704.

# Chapter 10

# Intermediate Malignant and Malignant Tumors of Soft Tissue Resembling Normal Tissue

Angelo Paolo Dei Tos MD

## Introduction

A diagnostic approach primarily based on recognition of a combination of cell shape, pattern of growth, background, and vascularization is certainly tremendously effective. However, sometimes soft tissue malignancies simply tend to recapitulate the morphologic features of normal tissues. The best example is represented by well-differentiated liposarcoma (atypical lipomatous tumor), wherein tumors are, for the vast majority, represented by a proliferation of mature fat cells.

Other good examples are represented by vascular neoplasms of intermediate malignancy such as retiform hemangioendothelioma and malignant vascular tumors such as angiosarcoma. In both situations, vasoformative features can be prominent, somewhat mimicking a normal vascular architecture and often generating significant diagnostic difficulties. As repeatedly emphasized, the correct diagnosis will be the result of a rational integration of clinical, immunomorphologic, and molecular features.

# Atypical Lipomatous Tumor/Well-Differentiated Liposarcoma

## Definition and Epidemiology

Atypical lipomatous tumor/well-differentiated liposarcoma (ALT/WDLPS) represents by far the largest subgroup of adipocytic malignancies and accounts for approximately 40 to 45% of all liposarcomas. Three subtypes of ALT/WDLPS are currently recognized by the 2013 WHO classification of soft tissue tumors: (1) adipocytic (or lipoma-like), (2) sclerosing, and (3) inflammatory. All of them represent genetically (along with dedifferentiated liposarcoma) *MDM2*-driven lesions. By contrast, spindle cell liposarcoma (atypical spindle cell lipomatous tumor) does not share involvement of the *MDM2* oncogenic pathway and is therefore currently regarded as a distinct entity. Spindle cell sarcoma is discussed in detail in Chapter 4. Well-differentiated liposarcoma occurs predominantly in middle-aged adults, with a peak incidence between the fourth and fifth decade.

As mentioned in the introductory chapter, the alternative term "atypical lipomatous tumor" was introduced for WDLPS arising at surgically amenable soft tissue sites. Although WDLPS has a tendency to recur locally in approximately 30% of cases (the rate depends on the anatomic site), it is incapable of metastasizing unless it undergoes dedifferentiation. Based on this assumption, in 1979 Evans and colleagues suggested adopting the term "atypical lipoma." Aiming to avoid either inadequate or excessive treatment, the use of the label "ALT" should be restricted to lesions arising at anatomic locations for which a complete (even marginal) surgical excision is regarded as adequate. By contrast, the label "WDLPS" is preferred for deep-seated neoplasms (e.g., retroperitoneal), for which multivisceral surgery is currently regarded as the most effective treatment.

## Clinical Presentation and Outcome

For practical reasons (but further stressing that the both ALT and WDLPS identify the same entity, however, arising superficially or at deep sites, respectively), in this chapter we will use the label WDLPS.

Well-differentiated liposarcoma occurs equally commonly in the retroperitoneum and the limbs. The spermatic cord, the mediastinum, the head and neck region, including the oral cavity, the hypopharynx, and the upper respiratory tract represent more rare but well-recognized anatomic locations. Most often, the clinical history is that of a long-standing, slowly growing mass. Tumors occurring at visceral locations generally tend to attain a large size, and in fact

WDLPS of the retroperitoneum ranks among the largest tumors in humans (Fig. 10-1). Distinct morphologic variants of WDLPS tend to exhibit a predilection for specific anatomic sites. Whereas adipocytic WDLPS is observed in both the limbs and retroperitoneum, the sclerosing subtype is most often detected in the retroperitoneum and the spermatic cord. Inflammatory WDLPS is also most commonly observed in the retroperitoneum. Well-differentiated liposarcoma is associated with an extremely variable overall risk of local recurrence that depends entirely on anatomic location (the risk being, of course, highest at deep-seated visceral locations). By contrast, distant metastases are never observed unless dedifferentiation occurs (see Chapter 7). As the anatomic location is by far the most important prognostic factor and the main predictor of relapse, the long-term, overall mortality rate is nearly 0% for lesions arising in surgically amenable soft tissue sites (e.g., the extremities), but rises to 80% for lesions occurring in the retroperitoneum or other visceral sites, wherein the risk for repeated, local (and eventually destructive) recurrences approaches 100%.

Standard treatment for WDLPS is complete surgical removal with negative margins, if possible. Of course, negative surgical margins are almost impossible to achieve when dealing with retroperitoneal tumors. Nonetheless, radical multivisceral

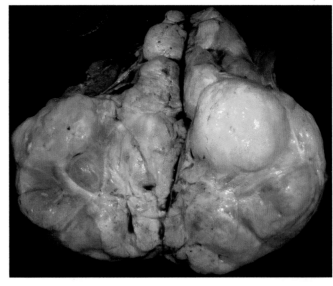

**Fig. 10-1.** Well-differentiated liposarcoma. Retroperitoneal liposarcoma can attain a huge size. Current surgical strategy is based on multivisceral resection.

surgery is currently regarded as the most effective strategy to increase the time to local relapse.

## Morphology and Immunophenotype

The gross appearance of WDLPS depends on the variable combination of fat and fibrous tissue. The lipoma-like variant is most often a well-circumscribed mass exhibiting a uniformly yellow cut surface (Fig. 10-2). When the fibrous component is more abundant, such as in the sclerosing subtype, the presence of firm, white-gray areas can predominate (Fig. 10-3). Extensive sampling is recommended, as key diagnostic features could be represented only focally and therefore easily overlooked.

Microscopically, adipocytic (lipoma-like) WDLPS is composed of a mature adipocytic proliferation superficially resembling normal fat, but upon closer examination exhibiting striking variation in cell size (Fig. 10-4) with at least focal nuclear atypia in fat cells (Fig. 10-5) or in stromal spindle cells (Figs. 10-6A and 10-6B). Fibrous septa are seen relatively commonly, wherein hyperchromatic stromal cells are easier to

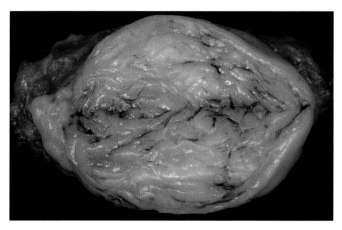

**Fig. 10-2.** Well-differentiated liposarcoma, lipoma-like. Cut surface is uniformly yellow, closely mimicking a benign lipoma.

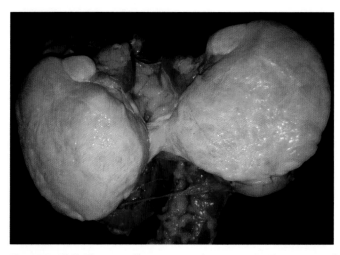

**Fig. 10-3.** Well-differentiated liposarcoma, sclerosing variant. The presence of abundant collagen generates a firm, gray, cut surface.

detect (Fig. 10-7). A key point is represented by the fact that the number of lipoblasts (uni- or multivacuolated fat cells containing a hyperchromatic, scalloped nucleus) (Fig. 10-8) in ALT/WDLPS may be extremely variable (from many to none). Lipoblasts have been traditionally regarded as a main diagnostic clue in favor of a diagnosis of liposarcoma; however, it is currently broadly accepted that the presence of lipoblasts does not make and is not required for a diagnosis of liposarcoma. Moreover, lipoblasts are seen in benign fat-forming neoplasms such as spindle cell/pleomorphic lipoma (see Chapter 4), lipoblastoma (see Chapter 8), and chondroid lipoma (see below). Very rarely, foci of metaplastic bone, scattered rhabdomyoblasts, or areas of smooth muscle differentiation can be observed.

Sclerosing ALT/WDLPS, as mentioned, tends to occur most frequently in the retroperitoneum and in the paratesticular region. Paradoxically, again the main diagnostic clue is not the presence of lipoblasts (which when present tend to be multivacuolated), but instead the identification of scattered bizarre, hyperchromatic stromal cells set in a distinctively fibrillary collagenous matrix (Figs. 10-9 and 10-10). The amount of mature fat is very variable and, not infrequently, the fibrous component can predominate to the extent that lipogenic areas are overlooked, especially in core biopsy specimens (Fig. 10-11).

In rare examples of ALT/WDLPS (most often located in the retroperitoneum), a dense chronic inflammatory infiltrate can be so prominent as to obscure the adipocytic nature of the tumor (Fig. 10-12). As the adipocytic component can be minimal, the detection of scattered atypical stromal cells represents the key morphologic clue to diagnosis (Fig. 10-13). In most cases, the inflammatory component is represented by a lymphoplasmacytic cell population associated with formation of lymphoid follicles (Fig. 10-12), but in some cases T cells are the main inflammatory component. The presence of epithelioid non-necrotizing granulomas can be observed but is exceedingly rare (Fig. 10-14).

Immunohistochemically, most adipocytic tumors express S100 protein; however, this finding plays a minor diagnostic role. MDM2 in particular and CDK4 have become popular confirmatory immunohistochemical markers because they are essentially never overexpressed in benign lipomas (Fig. 10-15). Whereas MDM2/CDK4 immunohistochemistry is relatively straightforward when dealing with sclerosing WDLPS (and, of course, with the far more cellular dedifferentiated liposarcoma), it has to be admitted that in the case of lipoma-like WDLPS immunostains may at times prove unsatisfactory, making fluorescence in situ hybridization (FISH) analysis a more consistent diagnostic tool (Fig. 10-16). MDM2 immunohistochemistry also seems to be very helpful in highlighting neoplastic cells in the context of inflammatory WDLPS (Fig. 10-17). The situations in which MDM2 immunohistochemistry appears to be of diagnostic utility are summarized in Table 10.1.

**Table 10.1** Diagnostic utility of MDM2 immunohistochemistry

- Well-differentiated liposarcoma vs benign lipoma
- Dedifferentiated liposarcoma vs undifferentiated pleomorphic sarcoma or other sarcoma subtypes
- Myxofibrosarcoma-like dedifferentiated liposarcoma vs myxofibrosarcoma
- Well-differentiated/dedifferentiated liposarcoma with myxoid change vs myxoid liposarcoma
- Homologous dedifferentiated liposarcoma vs pleomorphic liposarcoma
- Well-differentiated liposarcoma vs angiomyolipoma

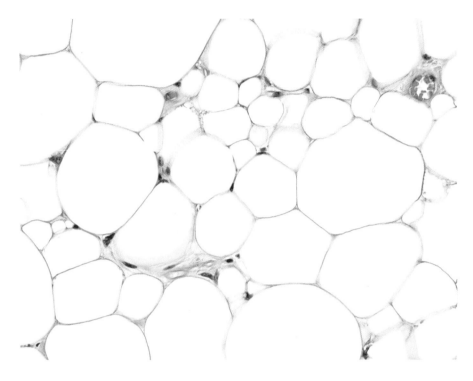

**Fig. 10-4.** Well-differentiated liposarcoma, lipoma-like. Significant variation in cell size is almost always observed.

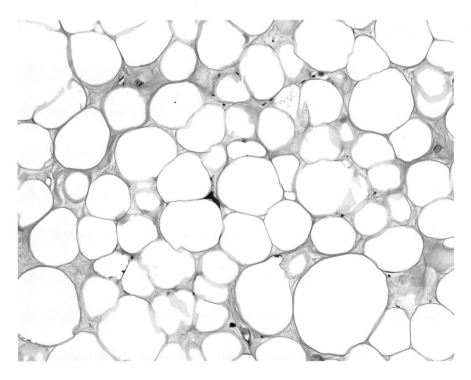

**Fig. 10-5.** Well-differentiated liposarcoma, lipoma-like. Nuclear hyperchromasia is seen within mature fat cells.

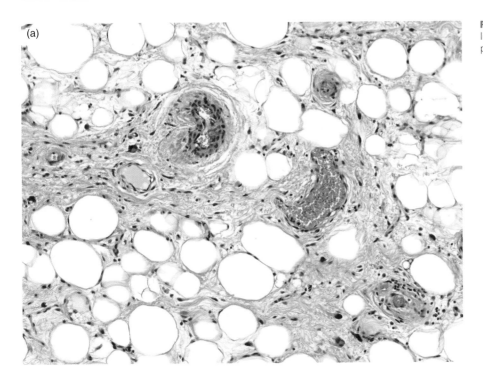

**Fig. 10-6A.** Well-differentiated liposarcoma, lipoma-like. Cell size variation is associated with the presence of atypical stromal cells.

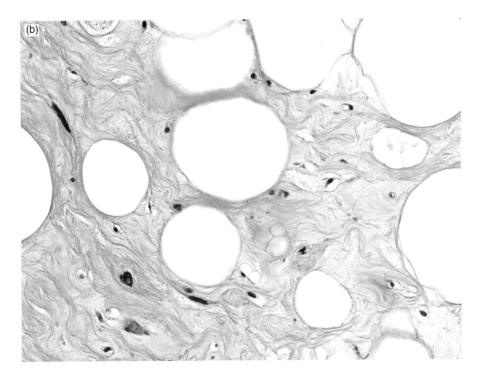

**Fig. 10-6B.** Well-differentiated liposarcoma, lipoma-like. At high power, the presence of nuclear hyperchromasia in stromal cells is easily appreciated.

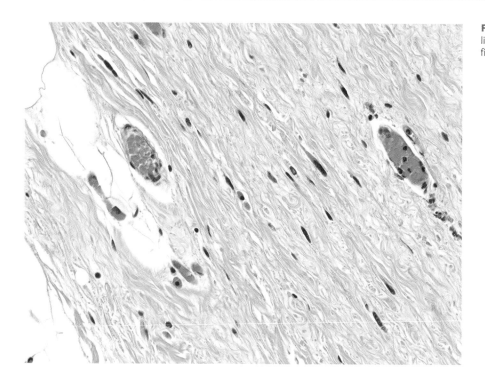

**Fig. 10-7.** Well-differentiated liposarcoma, lipoma-like. Stromal atypia is easier to detect within fibrous septa.

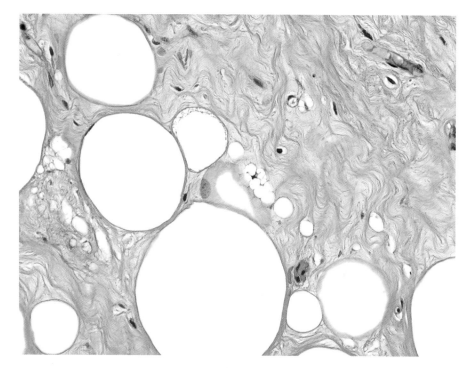

**Fig. 10-8.** Well-differentiated liposarcoma, lipoma-like. Cell size variation is associated with the presence of a multivacuolated lipoblast.

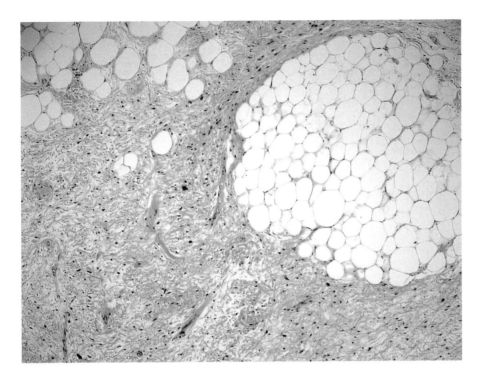

**Fig. 10-9.** Well-differentiated liposarcoma, sclerosing variant. A variable amount of mature adipocytes is associated with the presence of atypical stromal cells set in an abundant fibrillary collagenous background.

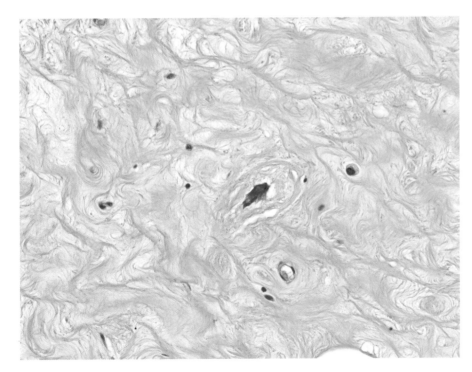

**Fig. 10-10.** Well-differentiated liposarcoma, sclerosing variant. Scattered stromal cells exhibiting marked nuclear hyperchromasia are set in a densely sclerotic stroma.

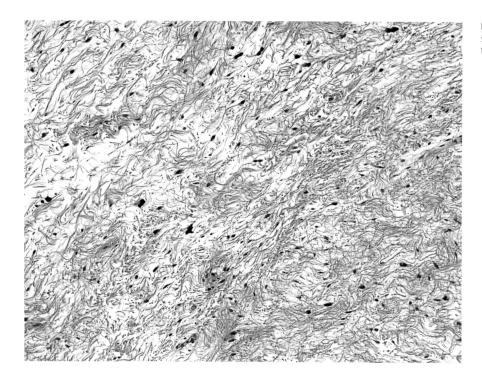

**Fig. 10-11.** Well-differentiated liposarcoma, sclerosing variant. An adipocytic component can be totally lacking.

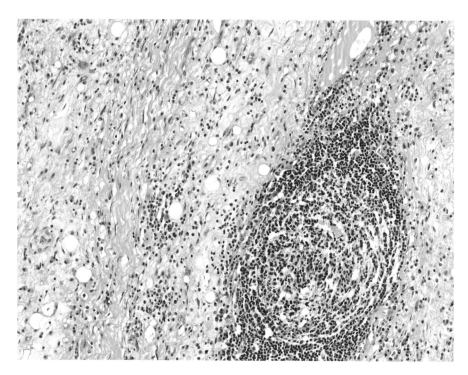

**Fig. 10-12.** Well-differentiated liposarcoma, inflammatory variant. The inflammatory component can obscure the adipocytic nature of the tumor.

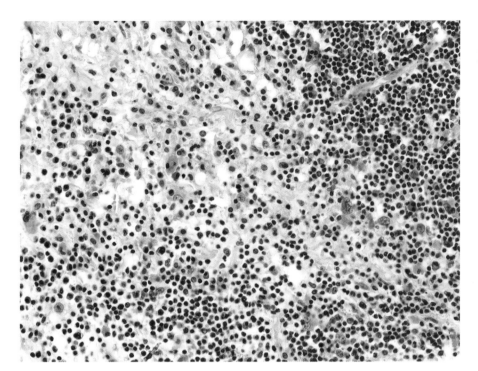

**Fig. 10-13.** Well-differentiated liposarcoma, inflammatory variant. The presence of scattered atypical cells may represent the only diagnostic clue.

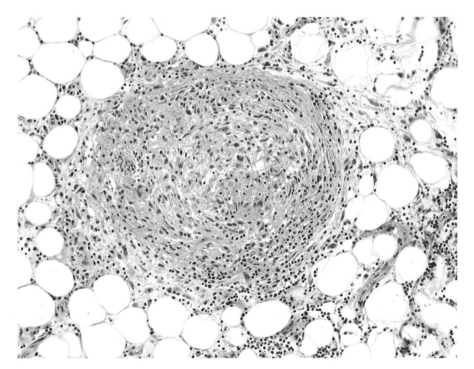

**Fig. 10-14.** Well-differentiated liposarcoma, inflammatory variant. The inflammatory component can be rarely represented by non-necrotizing granulomas.

**Fig. 10-15.** Well-differentiated liposarcoma. Nuclear expression of MDM2 is observed in both fat and stromal cells.

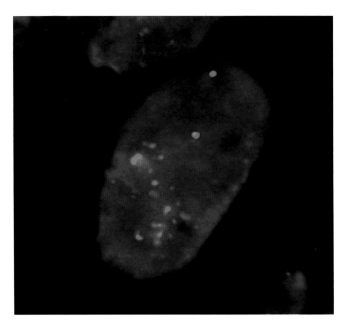

**Fig. 10-16.** Well-differentiated liposarcoma. Fluorescence in situ hybridization shows amplification of the *MDM2* gene (red signal).

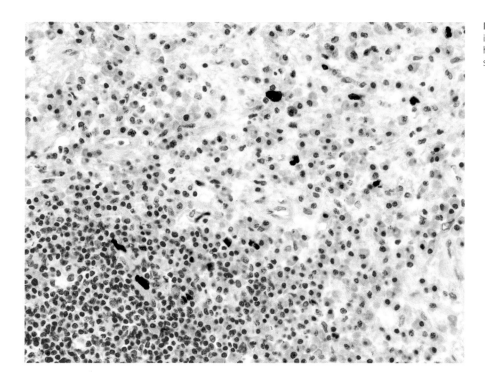

**Fig. 10-17.** Well-differentiated liposarcoma, inflammatory variant. MDM2 immunostains highlight the presence of enlarged neoplastic stromal cells.

## Genetics

Cytogenetically, WDLPS is characterized by the presence of distinctive ring or giant marker chromosomes containing amplified sequences derived from the 12q13-15-chromosome region. Amplification of *HMGA2* and *MDM2*, as well as overexpression of the encoded proteins, appears to be characteristic of WDLPS, and recently it has been shown that the cell cycle regulator *CDK4* is also amplified, but in the context of a distinct amplicon that may also include *DDIT3*. As a consequence, both immunohistochemistry and molecular genetic techniques are rather systematically used as diagnostic confirmatory tools. Recently, it has been shown that the vast majority of WDLPS also harbors amplification of the fibroblast growth factor receptor substrate 2 (FRS2), which also maps 12q13-15. The main genetic aberrations observed in lipomatous tumors are summarized in Table 10.2.

## Differential Diagnosis and Diagnostic Pitfalls

The differential diagnosis of WDLPS is with both non-neoplastic lesions and benign tumors. Among non-neoplastic lesions. the most important mimic of WDLPS is represented by **fat necrosis** and a condition labeled **massive localized lymphedema**.

First reported in 1998 by Sharon Weiss, "massive localized lymphedema" is a pseudosarcomatous condition of unknown etiology, observed invariably in middle-aged, morbidly obese adults. The association with trauma, surgeries, and hypothyroidism has been reported. It presents most often as unilateral, ill-defined masses that histologically consist of lobules of mature fat entrapped by expanded connective tissue septa (Fig. 10-18). A major pitfall is represented by the fact that the widened septa may simulate the fibrous bands of sclerosing

well-differentiated liposarcoma. However, massive localized lymphedema lacks the degree of nuclear atypia seen in the former (Fig. 10-19). The presence of dystrophic calcifications, perivascular chronic inflammation (Fig. 10-20), and metaplastic ossification is also rarely observed. The association of cutaneous angiosarcoma with massive lymphedema has been reported.

A major point is represented by the separation of WDLPS from **benign solitary lipoma**, a benign proliferation of mature white fat representing the most commonly encountered human mesenchymal neoplasm. Interestingly, benign lipomas represent a genetically distinct lesion with approximately half of the cases featuring an aberrant karyotype. Main genetic abnormalities are as follows: (1) rearrangements of the 12q13-15 region primarily with 3q22; (2) deletion of 13q; and (3) rearrangement of 6p21-23. The target gene in 12q13-15 is a member of the high-mobility group (HMG) protein gene family *HMGA2*.

In approximately 5% of cases, benign lipomas can present as multiple lesions, a condition that needs to be kept distinct from lipomatosis, a rare disease in which a diffuse overgrowth of fatty tissue is observed. Benign lipomas most often occur as a subcutaneous, solitary, painless mass of long duration occurring in an adult. Males are more frequently affected than females and the peak incidence is between the fourth and sixth decade. Benign lipomas may locate at any anatomic site and can involve both superficial and deep soft tissues. When they occur within or between skeletal muscles, they are labeled as "intramuscular" and "intermuscular" lipomas, respectively, and they occur most often in the large muscles of the thigh, shoulder, and upper arm. More rarely, benign lipomas can also occur in the head and neck region and at visceral sites such as the small and large bowels and the respiratory tract. Rare

**561**

**Table 10.2** Genetic alterations in lipomatous tumors

| Tumor type | Gene fusion or genetic aberrations | Cytogenetics |
|---|---|---|
| Lipoma | *EBF1-LOC204010* | t(5;12)(q33;q14) |
| | *HMGA2-CXCR7* | t(2;12)(q37;q14) |
| | *HMGA2-EBF1* | t(5;12)(q33;q14) |
| | *HMGA2-LHPF* | t(12;13)(q14;q13) |
| | *HMGA2-LPP* | t(3;12)(q28;q14) |
| | *HMGA2-NFIB* | t(9;12)(p22;q14) |
| | *HMGA2-PPAP2B* | t(1;12)(p32;q14) |
| | *HMGA2-LPP* | t(3;6)(q27;p21) |
| | *LPP-C12orf9* | t(3;12)(q28;14) |
| Lipoblastoma | *COL1A2-PLAG1* | t(7;8)(q21;q12) |
| | *HAS2-PLAG1* | Del(8)(q12;q24) |
| | *PLAG1-RAD51L1* | t(8;14)(q12;q24) |
| | *COL3A1-PLAG1* | t(2;8)(q31;q12.1) |
| Spindle cell lipoma | *RB* loss | 12q loss |
| Chondroid lipoma | *C11orf95-MKL2* | t(11;16)(q13;p13) |
| Hibernoma | Deletions of *MEN1* and *AIP* | 11q13 rearrangement |
| Well-differentiated liposarcoma | *MDM2, CDK4, HGMA2, FRS2* amplification | Ring and giant marker chromosomes |
| Dedifferentiated liposarcoma | *MDM2, CDK4, HGMA2* amplification | Ring and giant marker chromosomes |
| Pleomorphic liposarcoma | *NF1* | Complex karyotypic aberrations |
| Myxoid/round liposarcoma | *FUS-DDIT3* | t(12;16)(q13;p11) |
| | *EWSR1-DDIT3* | t(12;22)(q13;q12) |

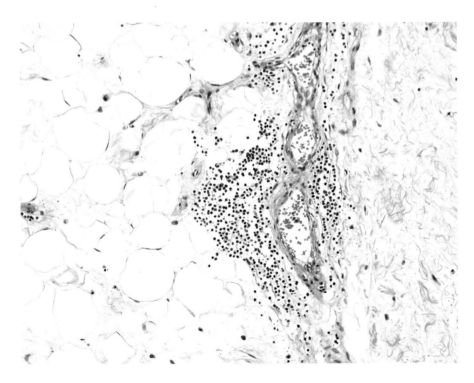

**Fig. 10-18.** Massive localized lymphedema. Fat lobules are entrapped by thick, fibrous septa. A chronic inflammatory infiltrate is seen.

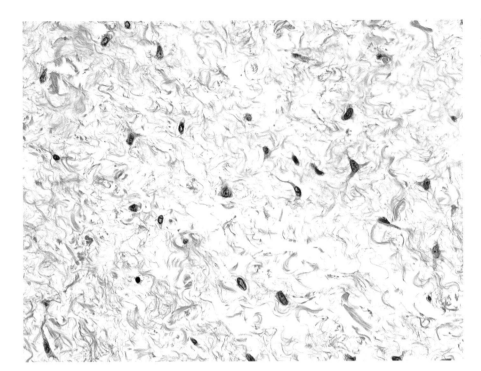

**Fig. 10-19.** Massive localized lymphedema. Stromal fibroblasts never feature nuclear hyperchromasia as typically observed in sclerosing WDLPS.

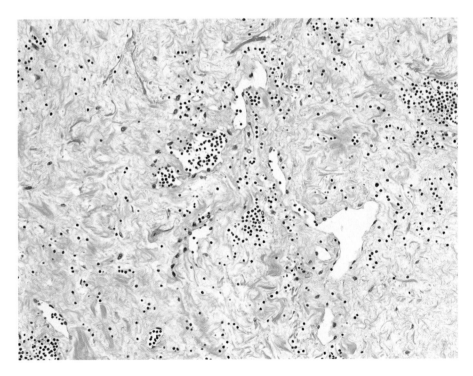

**Fig. 10-20.** Massive localized lymphedema. Patchy chronic inflammation is often seen.

563

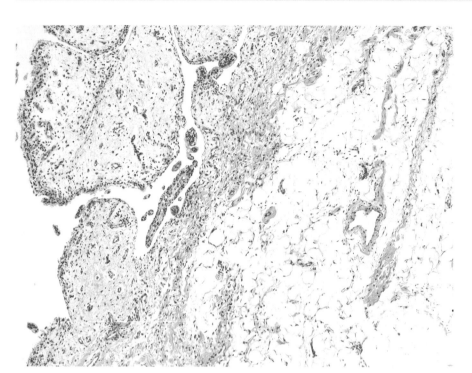

**Fig. 10-21.** Synovial lipoma. A mature adipocytic proliferation underlines a hyperplastic synovia.

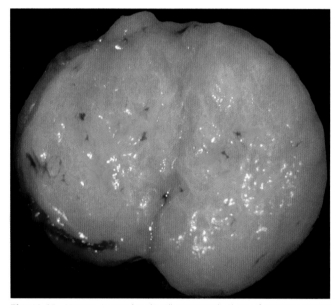

**Fig. 10-22.** Lipoma. A capsulated, well-circumscribed mass featuring a yellow cut surface is most often observed.

variants of lipomas are represented by dermal lipoma and synovial lipoma. Dermal lipomas most often occur as polypoid lesions. The term "nevus lipomatosus superficialis" traditionally describes the occurrence of multiple dermal lipomas usually located around lower limb girdles. Synovial lipoma occurs in the joints of adults and is also labeled as "lipoma arborescens," to reflect its villous, gross appearance. As synovial lipoma is almost always associated with inflammation and synovial hyperplasia, it seems likely that, rather than a true neoplasm, it represents a reactive process secondary to chronic local traumatism (Fig. 10-21).

An extremely rare condition termed "lipomatosis" is represented by the occurrence of diffuse mature adipose tissue. Lipomatosis arises most often in the extremities and the trunk and is further classified clinically as symmetric, asymmetric, pelvic, and mediastino-abdominal. The best-known example of symmetric lipomatosis is represented by Madelung disease. This rare condition occurs predominantly in adult patients of Mediterranean descent, and presents clinically as a massive, ill-defined lipomatous overgrowth localized at the neck and infiltrating into the underlying muscular structures. Asymmetric lipomatosis tends to occur in the extremities, the trunk, and, rarely, the viscera, and may lead to gigantism of the involved anatomic segment. Pelvic lipomatosis is also characterized by diffuse adipose tissue overgrowth, often leading to compression of the urinary tract, sigmoid colon, and rectum.

Macroscopically, benign lipomas are well circumscribed and surrounded by a thin capsule and feature a yellow cut surface (Fig. 10-22). Superficial size tends not to exceed 5 cm, whereas deep-seated lesions may attain larger dimensions. Microscopically, benign lipoma is composed of a uniform proliferation of mature adipocytes with minimal or no variation in size and shape (Fig. 10-23). Ordinary lipomas may rarely contain fibrous tissue (and therefore are named "fibrolipoma") and sometimes may exhibit extensive myxoid change reflected by the use of the term "myxolipoma." Occasionally, the presence of metaplastic bone or cartilage justifies the terms "osteolipoma" and "chondrolipoma" (Fig. 10-24). Intramuscular lipomas are easily recognized by the presence of mature skeletal muscle fibers showing variable degrees of atrophy (Fig. 10-25). Most intramuscular lipomas are infiltrative, whereas a minority (not exceeding 10%) of these tumors appears to be well circumscribed. When dealing with

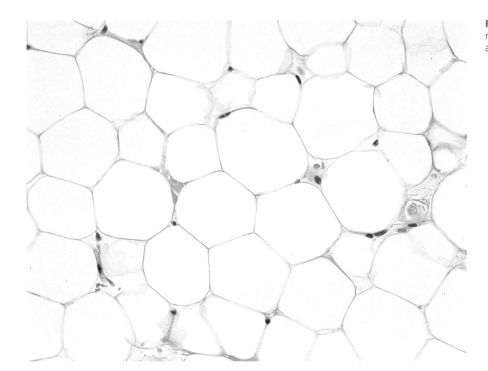

**Fig. 10-23.** Lipoma. The diagnostic hallmark is represented by a uniform proliferation of mature adipocytes lacking nuclear atypia.

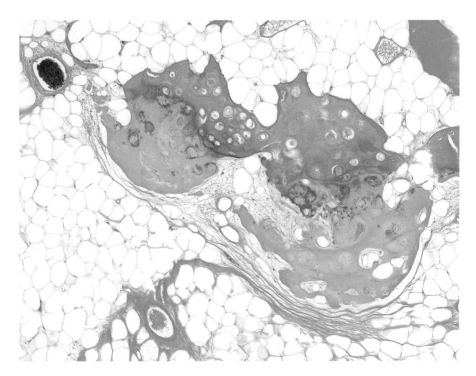

**Fig. 10-24.** Chondro-osseous metaplasia can be rarely observed in benign lipomas.

intramuscular adipocytic proliferation, a major diagnostic pitfall is represented by "intramuscular hemangioma," which may induce extensive fatty atrophy of muscle fibers and therefore mimic intramuscular lipoma (Fig. 10-26).

The key diagnostic clue for separating benign lipoma from lipoma-like WDLPS, in addition to cell size uniformity, is represented by the absence of nuclear atypia in both fat and stromal cells. A major diagnostic pitfall is, in fact, represented by the fact that benign lipoma can exhibit significant variation in cell size as a consequence of fat atrophy secondary to **fat necrosis** (Fig. 10-27). In this context, an additional source of diagnostic confusion is represented by the detection of MDM2 nuclear immunopositivity within the scattered histiocytes (highlighted by CD68 immunostain) that are invariably associated with fat necrosis. Another pseudosarcomatous condition that can be associated with fat necrosis and induce the suspicion of WDLPS is represented by ischemic fasciitis, a reactive process most often (but not necessarily)

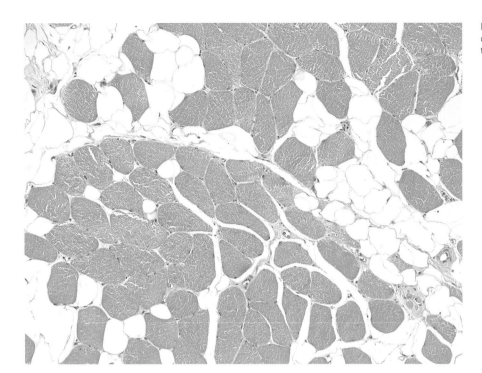

**Fig. 10-25.** Intramuscular lipoma. A combination of mature fat and striated muscle fibers represents the typical microscopic appearance.

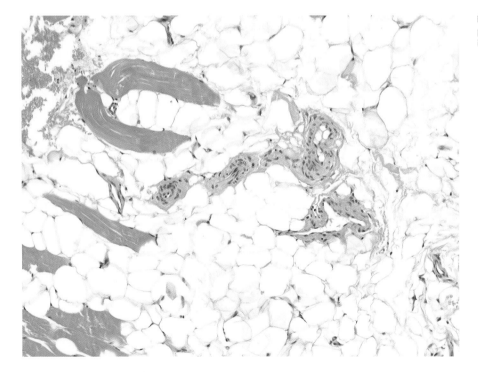

**Fig. 10-26.** Intramuscular hemangioma. The presence of fat atrophy can simulate an intramuscular lipoma.

related to local chronic compression of soft tissue overlying bone prominences (Fig. 10-28). Importantly, it has to be reiterated that WDLPS can also, though rarely, exhibit fat necrosis, the presence of which does not exclude per se a diagnosis of malignancy. Again, the presence of nuclear hyperchromasia represents the most important diagnostic clue (Fig. 10-29).

Again, the absence of lipoblasts in a mature adipocytic tumor cannot be regarded as a morphologic feature that excludes a diagnosis of malignancy. However, as a practical matter, when dealing with superficially located lesions, misdiagnosing a lipoma for a lipoma-like WDLPS actually may not represent a major issue. In fact, in both situations even a marginal resection is currently deemed acceptable, and in the case of a WDLPS, most surgeons will await a local recurrence, which will happen in approximately 10% of cases. By contrast, with deep-seated lesions, a diagnosis of benign lipoma should be made with extreme caution and supported

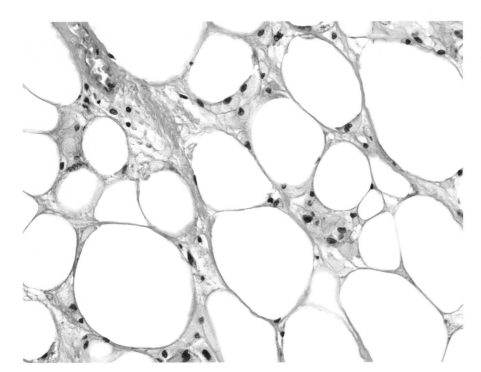

**Fig. 10-27.** Fat necrosis. Secondary atrophy generated by fat necrosis determines variation in cell size and may raise diagnostic confusion with WDLPS.

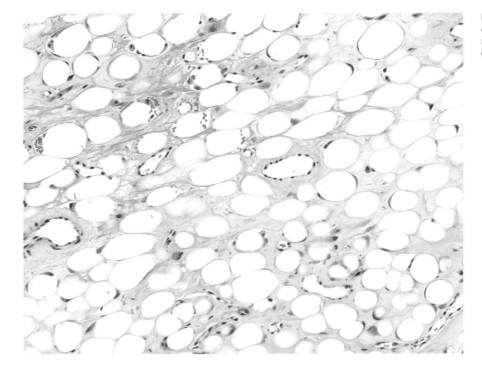

**Fig. 10-28.** Ischemic fasciitis. Fat cells may exhibit cell variation. Because ischemic fasciitis may form a mass, this feature may often represent a source of concern.

by evidence of the absence of MDM2/CDK4 overexpression and/or amplification.

Another lesion that enters the differential diagnosis with lipoma-like WDLPS (which may rarely harbor benign smooth muscle fibers) is represented by **myolipoma**. Myolipoma of soft tissue, first described by Enzinger and Meis in 1991, is a benign adipocytic neoplasm occurring almost exclusively in women, characterized morphologically by the coexistence of mature adipocytic and smooth muscle cell proliferations.

Myolipoma presents as a slow-growing, often large (myolipoma may reach a maximum diameter of 15–20 cm), deep-seated, painless mass, most frequently arising in the pelvis, retroperitoneum, and abdomen of women, with a peak incidence between the fourth and fifth decade. Rare examples have been reported in the groin and extremities.

Macroscopically, myolipoma most often presents as a well-circumscribed, encapsulated or partially encapsulated mass, featuring a glistening, white to yellow cut surface. The presence

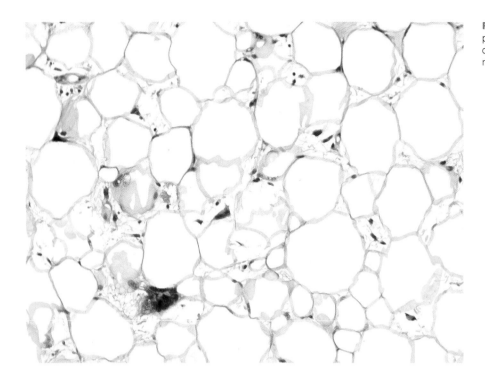

**Fig. 10-29.** Well-differentiated liposarcoma. The presence of fat necrosis does not exclude per se a diagnosis of WDLPS that is based on the presence of nuclear atypia.

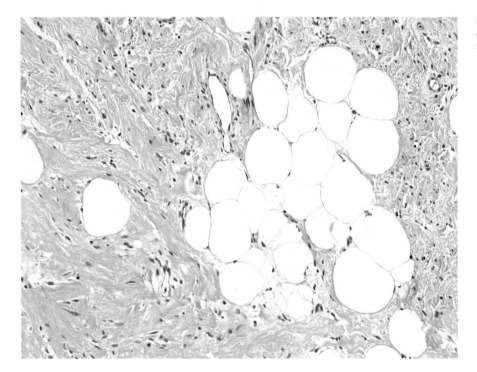

**Fig. 10-30.** Myolipoma of soft tissue. A variable combination of mature, benign adipocytic and smooth muscle components is observed.

of firmer areas correlates with the amount of smooth muscle differentiation. Foci of necrosis are never observed. Microscopically, myolipoma exhibits a distinctive biphasic morphology originated by the coexistence of mature adipose tissue and variable amounts of differentiated smooth muscle fibers organized in short bundles (Fig. 10-30). Notably, both the smooth muscle and adipocytic components lack any cytologic atypia. Immunostains for smooth muscle actin and desmin will help in highlighting the presence of the smooth

muscle component. As myolipoma is entirely benign with no reported recurrences or metastases following complete removal, distinguishing it from WDLPS containing foci of smooth muscle differentiation is crucial. However, myolipoma never shows adipocytic or stromal atypia, and never exhibits overexpression/amplification of MDM2 and/or CDK4. In consideration of the intra-abdominal location, myolipoma also needs to be kept separate from angiomyolipoma (a member of the family of PEComas that often is misclassified as WDLPS

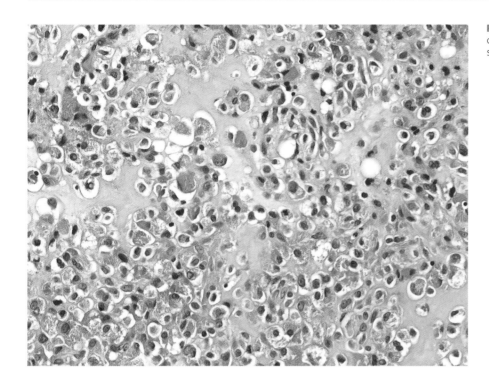

**Fig. 10-31.** Chondroid lipoma. Epithelioid, chondroblast-like cells set in a chondroid matrix are seen.

and is discussed in Chapter 5), which, in addition to the adipocytic component, features a biphenotypic spindle cell population characterized by concomitant expression of melanocytic (HMB45 or Melan-A) and myogenic markers. Angiomyolipoma, of course, also enters the differential diagnosis with WDLPS; however, in addition to the expression of the above-mentioned melanocytic markers, it never exhibits MDM2 and/or CDK4 nuclear expression.

Among benign adipocytic neoplasms that may enter in the differential diagnosis of WDLPS, a particularly challenging as well as rare lesion is represented by **chondroid lipoma**. First formally reported in 1993 by Meis and Enzinger, chondroid lipoma most likely corresponds to an entity previously labeled by John Chan as "extraskeletal chondroma with lipoblast-like cells." The name suggested a chondrogenic differentiation that was subsequently disproved. Clinically, chondroid lipoma presents as a long-standing, most often painless, slow-growing, deep-seated lesion located in the proximal limbs and limb girdles, followed by the trunk, distal extremities, and head and neck region. Approximately 20% of cases arise superficially. The peak incidence is in the third and fourth decades, with female predominance. Chondroid lipoma is a benign adipocytic neoplasm that never recurs or metastasizes, making complete surgical removal curative. The presence in chondroid lipoma of an abundant lipoblastic cell population further underscores the idea that lipoblasts cannot be considered exclusive to adipocytic malignancies.

Grossly, chondroid lipoma is usually well circumscribed and most often (but not always) encapsulated. One-third of cases appear multilobular. The cut surface is white to yellowish, depending on the extent of the mature adipocytic component. Microscopically, chondroid lipoma is composed of a variable admixture of mature adipocytes, eosinophilic chondroblast-like cells often featuring a granular cytoplasm, and

vacuolated cells set in a myxochondroid background, often organized in a lobular growth pattern (Fig. 10-31). One of the most striking features of this lesion is the presence of vacuolated cells that are virtually indistinguishable from ordinary lipoblasts (Fig. 10-32). In the original description, this distinctive cell type was designated as a "pseudolipoblast"; however, these vacuolated elements share all the morphologic and ultrastructural features of lipoblasts and therefore should be regarded as such. Chondroid lipoma is also characterized by a rich vascular network composed of thick-walled blood vessels alternating with large, gaping, thin-walled vascular spaces. Immunohistochemically, S100 protein is positive in most neoplastic cells; however, this finding does not play a major role in the differential diagnosis. Chondroid lipoma is genetically characterized by a t(11;16)(q13;p13) translocation resulting in the fusion of the *MGC3032* and *MKL2* (megakaryoblastic leukemia 2) genes. In addition to WDLPS, the differential diagnosis of chondroid lipoma includes myxoid liposarcoma, extraskeletal myxoid chondrosarcoma (discussed in Chapter 8), and soft tissue myoepithelioma (discussed in Chapter 5). In brief, myxoid liposarcoma is distinguished by its distinctive plexiform, capillary-sized (crow's feet) vascular network, as well as more prominent myxoid stroma. Extraskeletal myxoid chondrosarcoma shows a more pronounced lobular architecture, with abundant myxoid stroma containing a proliferation of uniform, spindled to epithelioid cells, arranged in cords and strands. Soft tissue myoepithelioma also often contains myxoid stroma and shows a reticular architecture, but is distinguished by a distinctive immunophenotype that usually includes variable reactivity for S100 protein, cytokeratins, epithelial membrane antigen, and glial fibrillary acidic protein in approximately 50% of cases.

569

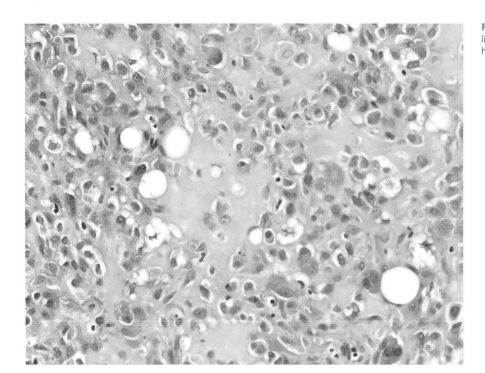

**Fig. 10-32.** Chondroid lipoma. The presence of lipoblasts represents one of the diagnostic hallmarks.

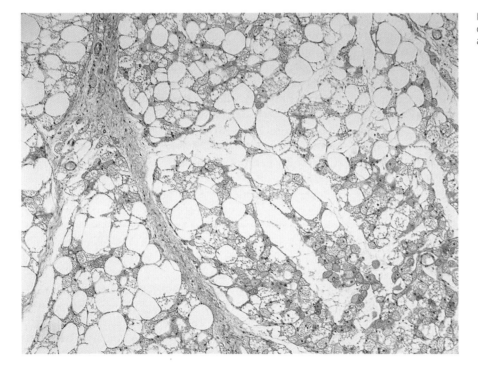

**Fig. 10-33.** Hibernoma. At low power, its distinctive lobular pattern of growth is better appreciated.

Another adipocytic lesion deserving mention is **hibernoma**. Hibernoma represents a benign neoplasm composed of a predominant brown (fetal) fat cell proliferation, variably admixed with mature white adipose tissue. It most often presents as a long-standing, slow-growing mass located in the subcutis in young adults, with a peak incidence between the third and fourth decade and with a slight male predominance. Approximately 10% may arise within somatic muscles. The most frequently affected anatomic site is the thigh, followed by the trunk, upper limbs, and head and neck. Rarely, hibernomas arise at visceral locations, such as the retroperitoneum and mediastinum. Hibernomas are associated with specific genetic changes represented by structural rearrangements of the 11q13-21 chromosome region and, less often, 10q22. At the molecular level, deletion of the multiple endocrine neoplasia-1 (*MEN1*) gene has been reported.

Grossly, hibernomas are well circumscribed, ranging in size from 2 to 20 cm. The cut surface shows an easily recognizable lobulation, with color varying from yellow to red-brown, depending on the relative amounts of brown and white

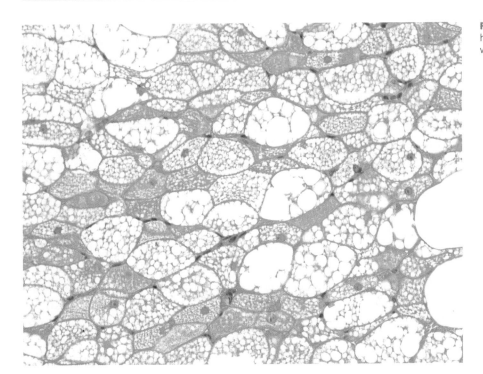

**Fig. 10-34.** Hibernoma. Microscopically, hibernoma is composed of a variable proportion of white and brown fat cells.

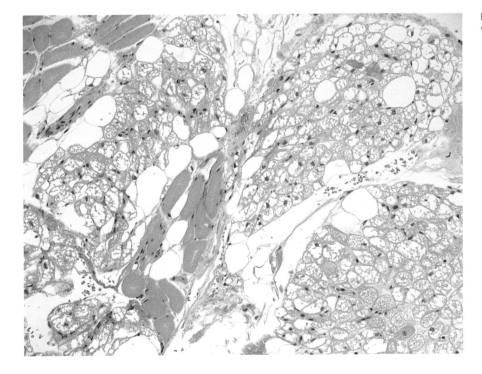

**Fig. 10-35.** Hibernoma. The deep-seated location within muscles can be observed.

adipocytic components. Microscopically, hibernomas are composed of multivacuolated adipocytes containing coarsely granular cytoplasm and centrally located nuclei, organized in a distinctive lobular growth pattern (Fig. 10-33). The cytoplasm of brown fat cells may vary from pale to intensely eosinophilic (Fig. 10-34). In fewer than 10% of cases, the white fat cell component is predominant and scattered or small clusters of brown fat cells are seen. When hibernoma occurs within muscles, it characteristically grows in between striated muscle fibers (Fig. 10-35). Mitotic activity is usually absent, as is cytologic atypia. Absence of nuclear atypia is the main morphologic feature (along with absence of MDM2 expression/amplification) that allows distinction from WDLPS, exhibiting hibernoma-like features (Fig. 10-36).

571

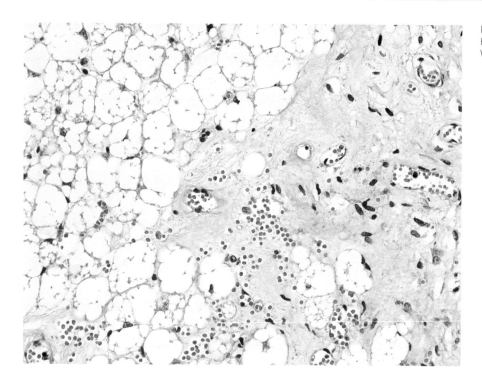

**Fig. 10-36.** Well-differentiated liposarcoma. Hibernoma-like features can be rarely observed in WDLPS.

### Key Points in Well-Differentiated Liposarcoma Tumor Diagnosis

- Adult patients
- Most frequent in the limbs and retroperitoneum
- Mature fat cell proliferation featuring variation in size and presence of nuclear atypia in fat cells or stromal cells
- Lipoblasts vary from many to none; however, not required for diagnosis
- *MDM2/CDK4* gene amplification and MDM2/CDK4 protein overexpression
- Clinical behavior dependent on anatomic location
- No metastatic potential unless dedifferentiation occurs

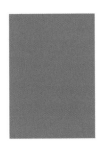

# Retiform Hemangioendothelioma

## Definition and Epidemiology

Retiform hemangioendothelioma (RH) is a locally aggressive vascular tumor originally described by Calonje et al. in 1994 as a low-grade angiosarcoma. Its name reflects the histomorphology, somewhat simulating the appearance of the rete testis. Retiform hemangioendothelioma occurs over a wide age range; however, most cases are observed in young adults, with no sex predilection.

## Clinical Presentation and Outcome

Retiform hemangioendothelioma presents as a poorly circumscribed lesion involving the skin and the subcutaneous soft tissues of the extremities, primarily the lower limb, and the trunk. It is associated with a high local recurrence rate (approximately 60% of cases), but so far metastases to regional lymph nodes have been described only exceptionally. Neither distant metastases nor tumor-related deaths have been reported. Surgical excision is the treatment of choice, but free margins are difficult to obtain because of the highly infiltrative growth pattern.

## Morphology and Immunophenotype

Grossly, RH most often appears as a poorly circumscribed, multinodular lesion involving the dermis or the subcutis and measuring up to 6 cm (most lesions are smaller than 3 cm). Microscopic examination shows a poorly circumscribed vascular proliferation composed of elongated, arborizing, thin-walled vessels infiltrating the dermis and extending into the subcutis (Fig. 10-37). Vessels are lined by a single layer of endothelial cells with a prominent, atypical hyperchromatic nucleus bulging into the lumen, producing a so-called hobnail or matchstick appearance, often associated with the presence of a patchy lymphocytic infiltrate (Fig. 10-38). Mitoses are usually not identified. Intraluminal papillary projections can be detected. Immunohistochemically, neoplastic endothelial cells diffusely express most common vascular markers such as CD31 and ERG.

## Genetics

No major genetic aberrations have been reported thus far.

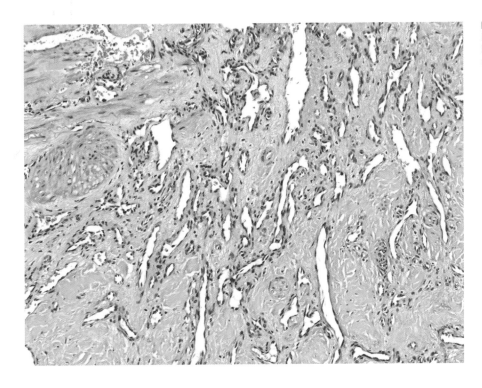

**Fig. 10-37.** Retiform hemangioendothelioma. At low power, RH is composed of gaping, thin-walled blood vessels somewhat resembling the normal rete testis.

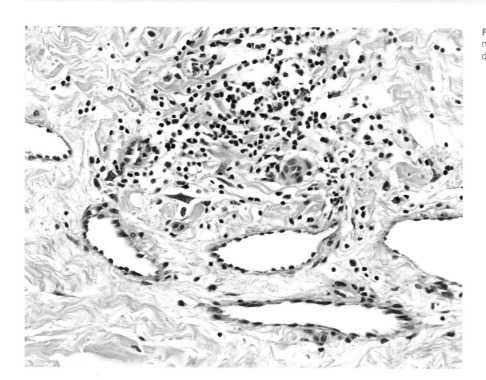

**Fig. 10-38.** Retiform hemangioendothelioma. The nuclei of neoplastic endothelial cells feature distinctive "hobnail" morphology.

## Differential Diagnosis and Diagnostic Pitfalls

Retiform hemangioendothelioma exhibits several histologic features in common with **papillary intralymphatic angioendothelioma** (PILA). PILA was formerly known eponymically as **Dabska tumor**. In 1969, Maria Dabska first reported six cases of a vascular neoplasm arising in children and adolescents, suggesting it be labeled "malignant intravascular hemangioendothelioma." Morphologic overlap includes an infiltrative growth pattern (Fig. 10-39), the presence of a hobnail cytomorphology (Fig. 10-40), and the variable association with a lymphocytic infiltrate. However, papillary tufts with hyaline cores represent the hallmark of PILA and are only rarely observed in RH (Fig. 10-41). It has been suggested that RH may be the adult counterpart of PILA; however; as there exist morphologic as well as immunohistochemical (D2-40 is strongly expressed in PILA but not in RH) differences, the two entities are still kept distinct.

**Hobnail hemangioma** represents the benign end of the spectrum of lesions exhibiting hobnail endothelial cells, and occurs most commonly in the limbs and the trunk of young adults as a small, superficial papule, sometimes exhibiting a targetoid appearance. This is caused by hemosiderin depositions that, in some cases, may form an ecchymotic rim (therefore justifying the alternative term "targetoid hemosiderotic hemangioma"). Despite a partial histologic resemblance to RH,

the lesion is more superficial, the hobnail endothelial cells are seen in only the most superficial vessels, and an inflammatory infiltrate, although present, is not usually prominent (Fig. 10-42). Focal luminal papillary projections may be encountered, but endothelial multilayering is consistently absent.

The most important differential diagnosis of RH is **cutaneous angiosarcoma**, which has a dismal prognosis with very high incidence of recurrence and metastasis and a high mortality rate. Histologically, although angiosarcoma and RH have an infiltrative pattern in common, conventional angiosarcoma is characterized by a more disorganized growth pattern, and the vascular spaces formed tend to be more irregular and jagged than those in RH. In addition, cutaneous angiosarcoma always shows cytologic atypia, multilayering, and mitotic activity.

Retiform hemangioendothelioma can be extremely rarely associated with other distinctive neoplastic vascular components (most often epithelioid hemangioendothelioma and morphologically low-grade angiosarcoma) (Fig. 10-43A and B). This variable combination has been labeled as **composite hemangioendothelioma**. Composite hemangioendothelioma appears to favor the limbs of young adults. Multiple local recurrences seem to be frequent, and progression to full-blown angiosarcoma has been observed. Synaptophysin expression has been recently reported, which would correlate with more aggressive behavior.

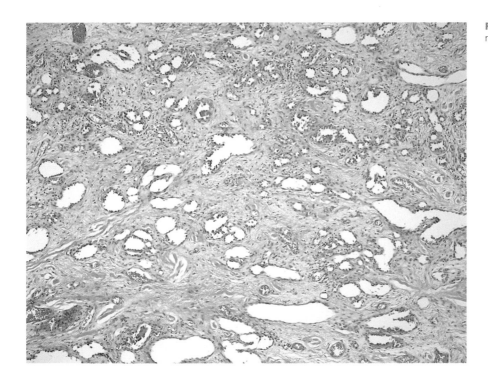

**Fig. 10-39.** PILA. At low power, a superficial resemblance to RH is observed.

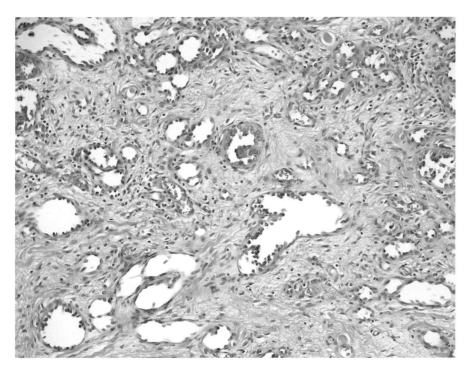

**Fig. 10-40.** PILA. The nuclei of neoplastic endothelial cells feature a "hobnail," matchstick-like morphology. Intraluminal papillae are seen.

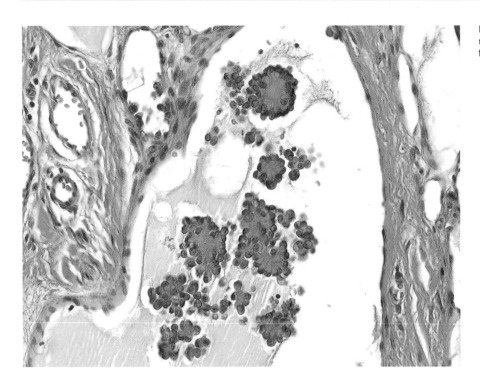

**Fig. 10-41.** PILA. The diagnostic hallmark is represented by the presence of intraluminal papillae featuring a hyaline core.

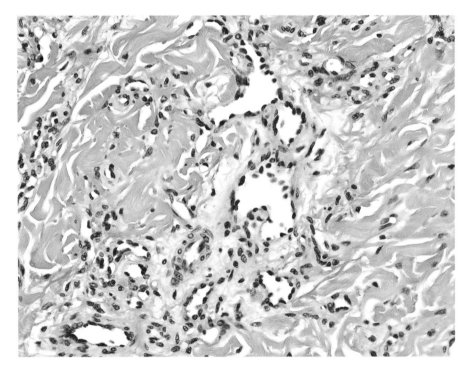

**Fig. 10-42.** Hobnail hemangioma. The benign end of the spectrum of hobnail vascular neoplasia. Hobnailing is predominantly observed in only the most superficial vessels.

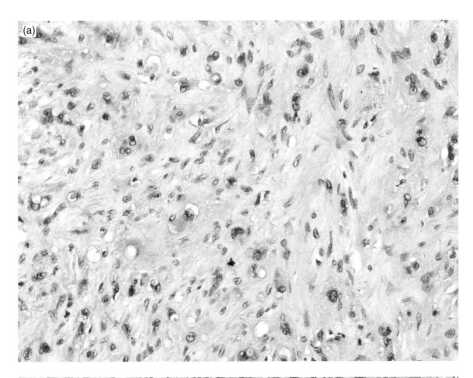

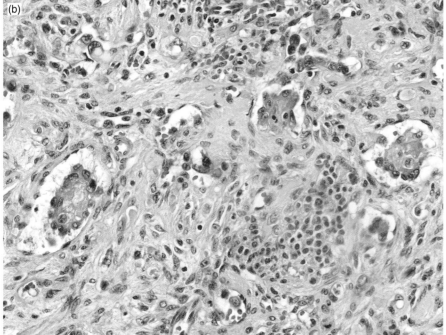

**Fig. 10-43.** Composite hemangioendothelioma. (A) An epithelioid hemangioendothelioma-like morphology is associated with PILA-like (B) features.

**Key Points in Retiform Hemangioendothelioma Diagnosis**

- Locally aggressive vascular tumor
- Most frequent in skin and subcutis of young adults
- Arborizing thin-walled vessels lined by a single layer of endothelial cells with a hobnail appearance
- Rarely associated with other low-grade vascular malignancies to form composite hemangioendothelioma

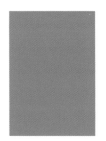

# Angiosarcoma

## Definition and Epidemiology

Angiosarcoma of soft tissue most often exhibits an epithelioid morphology and therefore is discussed in detail in Chapter 5. However, cutaneous angiosarcoma may exhibit distinctive vasoformative features that may somewhat mimic normal tissue. Angiosarcoma is very rare and accounts for approximately 2% of all mesenchymal malignancies. Overall, angiosarcoma tends to occur more frequently in males, with a peak incidence in the sixth decade. However, a broad age range is observed, and great variation is observed based on clinical presentation.

## Clinical Presentation and Outcome

A practical approach to angiosarcoma classification takes into account its clinical presentation. Excluding angiosarcoma of bone, in addition to the already mentioned angiosarcoma of deep soft tissue (including visceral sites), which accounts for approximately 30% of cases, the following occur: cutaneous angiosarcoma (40% of cases), radiation- and lymphedema-associated angiosarcomas (12%), vascular angiosarcoma (10%), and breast parenchymal angiosarcoma (8%).

Several clinicopathologic groups can be distinguished:

1. **Angiosarcoma of the skin.** Primary cutaneous angiosarcoma occurs most often in the scalp or face of elderly males. More rare locations are represented by the extremities, wherein a male predominance is not observed. Peak incidence is between the seventh and eighth decade. Clinically, it presents as enlarging erythematous plaques and nodules with a tendency to ulcerate at late stage. Prognosis is dismal, with 50% mortality within 1 year after diagnosis.

2. **Secondary angiosarcoma.** Angiosarcoma can arise as a consequence of previous radiation therapy or following chronic lymphedema. In both situations, the most common anatomic locations are the thoracic wall and the breast as a consequence of surgery and post-surgical irradiation of breast cancer. Post-radiation angiosarcoma appears approximately 5 to 8 years after treatment and may be preceded by potential precursor lesions labeled as "atypical vascular proliferations." Independently from morphology, post-radiation angiosarcoma is very aggressive, with an overall survival at 5 years not exceeding 15%. Lymphedema-associated angiosarcoma (also known eponymically as Stewart-Treves syndrome) represents an exceedingly rare complication of radical breast and axillary lymph node surgery. Considering that breast cancer

surgery has significantly evolved toward far less radical surgical procedures, the incidence of lymphedema-associated angiosarcoma is rapidly declining. The interval between surgery and onset of angiosarcoma tends to be lengthy, with a median of 10 years, but there have been cases that occurred decades after local treatment. Overall survival overlaps with that of post-radiation angiosarcoma.

3. **Angiosarcoma of breast parenchyma.** Deep-seated angiosarcoma of the breast occurs in woman between the third and fifth decade. It presents as large, ill-defined breast parenchymal masses. In this clinical context, prognosis is extremely poor, with early onset of lung, liver, bone, and cutaneous systemic spread.

4. **Angiosarcoma of deep soft tissue.** This clinical variant is discussed in detail in Chapter 5. It occurs most often in the deep soft tissue of the extremities, trunk, and retroperitoneum. Overall survival at 1 year is less than 50%.

5. **Angiosarcoma of visceral sites.** Visceral sites include liver, spleen, heart (wherein angiosarcoma is the most common sarcoma and most often occurs in the right atrium), adrenal, thyroid, lungs, pleura, and gastrointestinal tract. Hepatic angiosarcoma represents an occupational malignancy related to exposure to vinyl chloride, thorotrast (a now-abandoned radioactive radiologic contrast medium), and arsenic. Again, visceral angiosarcoma is clinically aggressive with an extremely high rate of early disease-related deaths.

As all clinical variants of angiosarcoma are extremely aggressive and radical surgery is often impossible to achieve, systemic treatment is administered, typically with doxorubicin and taxanes. Significant activity is generally observed but unfortunately tends to be of short duration, with onset of early local and systemic recurrences. Some controversy exists concerning the value of histologic grading; however, most recent data would indicate that angiosarcoma behaves aggressively, independent of morphology.

## Morphology and Immunophenotype

Microscopically, angiosarcoma is extremely heterogeneous, showing a spectrum of morphologies ranging from clearly vasoformative to a solid neoplastic proliferation featuring spindle or epithelioid cell morphology. The whole spectrum can often be encountered within the same lesion. When vasoformative, angiosarcoma is composed of anastomosing channels, dissecting the stroma and featuring nuclear hyperchromasia

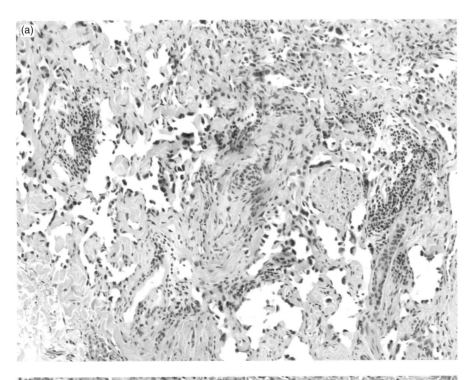

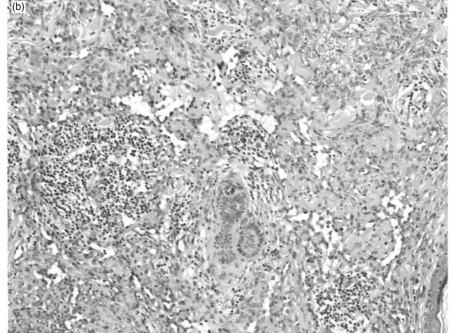

**Fig. 10-44** Angiosarcoma. (A) A dissecting vasoformative proliferation is seen. Neoplastic endothelial cells feature significant nuclear atypia with formation of micropapillae. (B) Anastomosing vascular channels lined by atypical endothelial cells are associated with an infiltrating neoplastic cell population.

(Fig. 10-44A and B), multilayering (Fig. 10-45), and formation of micropapillae (Fig. 10-46). As mentioned, epithelioid morphology is most often observed in deep-seated lesions and may still assume vasoformative features (Figs. 10-47 and 10-48) or exhibit a solid, carcinoma-like appearance (Fig. 10-49). In these non-vasoformative cases, CD31/ERG immunopositivity plays a major diagnostic role (Fig. 10-50). Focal spindle cell morphology can be observed anywhere as part of the histologic spectrum of angiosarcoma; however, it can be predominant in angiosarcomas occurring at visceral sites (Fig. 10-51). Intraparenchymal breast angiosarcoma may appear extremely vasoformative and

well differentiated. A main clue is represented by extensive infiltrative growth of adipose tissue (Fig. 10-52A and B), whereas benign angiomas are always well circumscribed.

Immunohistochemically, both ERG and CD31 represent sensitive differentiation markers. Evaluation of CD31 can be tricky, as intratumoral histiocytes are typically positive. ERG is strongly expressed in the nuclei of normal vessels and of any type of benign and malignant vascular neoplasms. The only caveat is related to the fact that ERG is not entirely specific, as it also decorates prostatic adenocarcinoma, 40% of epithelioid sarcoma, and a small subset of Ewing sarcoma. CD34 is less commonly

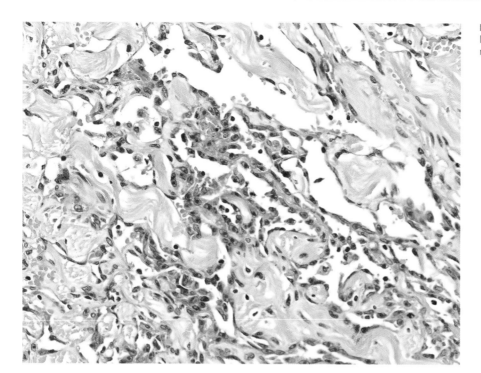

**Fig. 10-45.** Angiosarcoma. Vascular spaces are lined by atypical endothelial cells featuring multilayering.

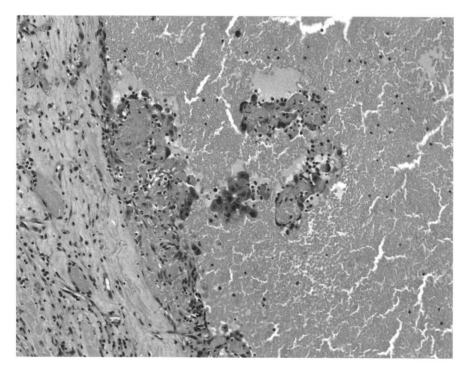

**Fig. 10-46.** Angiosarcoma. Papillary structures lined by markedly atypical neoplastic cells bulge into a hemorrhagic space.

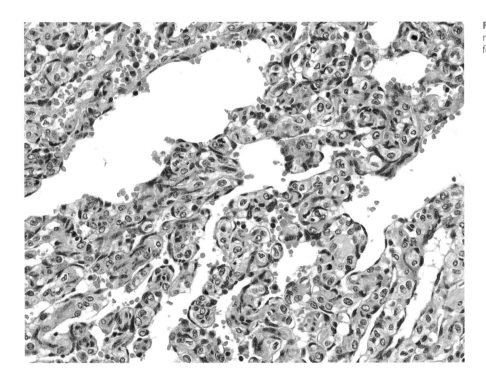

**Fig. 10-47.** Angiosarcoma. Epithelioid morphology can be associated with vasoformative features.

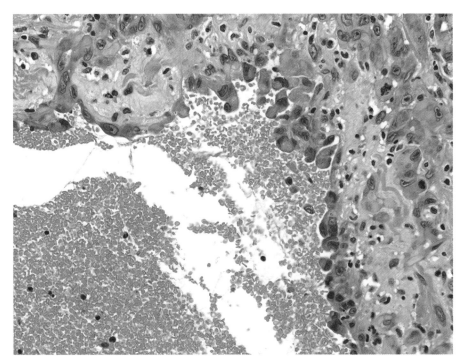

**Fig. 10-48.** Angiosarcoma. Epithelioid morphology can be associated with vasoformative features. Neoplastic cells exhibit extreme nuclear atypia.

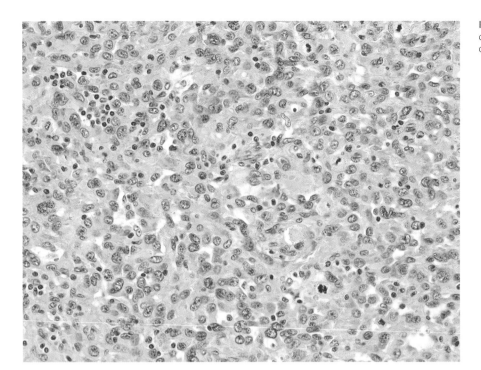

**Fig. 10-49.** Epithelioid angiosarcoma. A solid, carcinoma-like morphology is more commonly observed in deep-seated neoplasms.

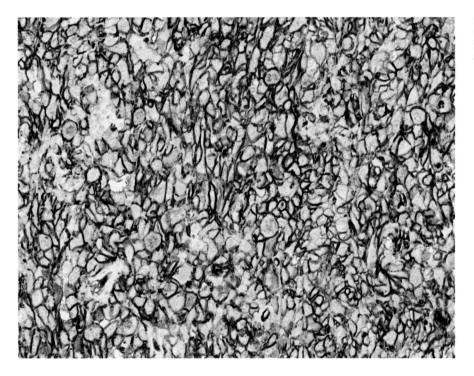

**Fig. 10-50.** Epithelioid angiosarcoma. Strong membrane immunopositivity for CD31 is extremely helpful when dealing with non-vasoformative angiosarcomas.

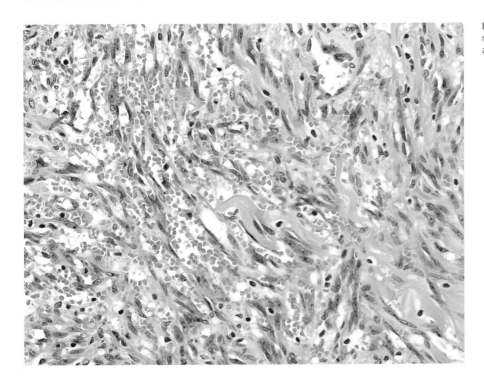

**Fig. 10-51.** Angiosarcoma. A spindle cell morphology is relatively more often observed in angiosarcomas occurring at visceral sites.

**Table 10.3** Immunophenotypic characterization of vascular tumors

| Diagnostic marker | Diagnostic application | Diagnostic pitfalls |
|---|---|---|
| CD31 | All vascular tumors | Expression in histiocytes |
| CD34 | All vascular tumors | Extremely broad pattern of expression |
| ERG | All vascular tumors | Expressed in prostatic carcinoma, epithelioid sarcoma, and a subset of Ewing sarcoma |
| FLI1 | All vascular tumors | Expressed in Ewing sarcoma |
| FVIII-RA | All vascular tumors | Low sensitivity if tumor poorly differentiated |
| Smooth muscle actin | Visualization of pericytic network | Pericytic network can be rarely partly retained in well-differentiated angiosarcoma |
| c-myc | Secondary angiosarcoma | Rarely observed in non-secondary angiosarcoma |
| Human herpesvirus 8 (HHV-8) | Kaposi sarcoma | None |

used because of its extremely broad pattern of expression. By contrast, factor VIII–related antigen (FVIII-RA) is very specific for both normal and neoplastic endothelia, but unfortunately not at all sensitive unless the angiosarcoma is very well differentiated and vasoformative. As mentioned in Chapter 5, epithelioid angiosarcoma may express EMA and cytokeratin in up to half of the cases. KIT immunopositivity is reported in approximately half of all angiosarcomas, but this is unrelated to *KIT* gene mutations and obviously does not predict a response to any of the available tyrosine kinase inhibitors. Splenic angiosarcomas may co-express histiocytic and endothelial markers, suggesting that some tumors may originate from splenic lining cells (so-called littoral cell angiosarcomas). Importantly, post-radiation angiosarcoma (however, not exclusively) exhibits *MYC* gene amplification that translates into MYC overexpression. The clinical utility of immunohistochemical characterization of vascular tumors is summarized in Table 10.3.

## Genetics

Gain-of-function mutation of *KDR* (*VEGFR2*) has been reported in a subset of breast angiosarcomas. Other, rarely observed molecular aberrations include activating mutation of *PLCG1* and loss-of-function mutation of the down-regulator of angiogenesis *PTPRB*. *MYC* gene amplification is observed in radiation-induced angiosarcomas that translates into immunophenotypic nuclear expression of the protein thereof. A small subset of angiosarcomas featuring *CIC* gene rearrangement has been recently reported.

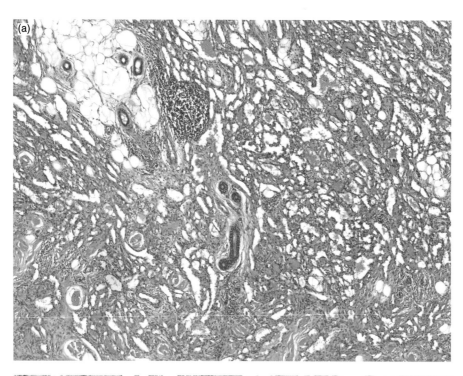

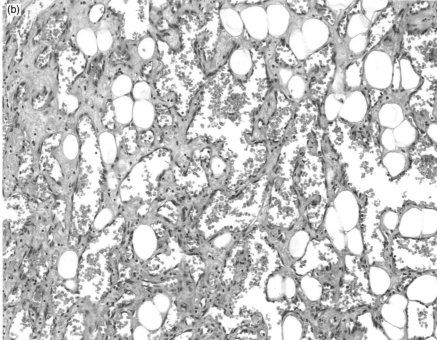

**Fig. 10-52.** Angiosarcoma. Intraparenchymal breast angiosarcoma may exhibit an extremely well-differentiated appearance (A). Diffuse infiltration of the fat represents a major diagnostic clue for diagnosis (B).

## Differential Diagnosis and Diagnostic Pitfalls

When dealing with a well-differentiated form of angiosarcoma, the main problem is the differential diagnosis with **benign hemangiomas**. In consideration of the focus on mesenchymal malignancies, the broad variety of benign vascular neoplasms will not be addressed here. However, with respect to the differential diagnosis with angiosarcoma, it has to be underlined that most often benign hemangiomas exhibit a lobular architecture that is almost never seen in vascular malignancies and typically

lack nuclear atypia as well as multilayering (Fig. 10-53). The presence of a smooth muscle actin–positive pericytic reticulum is also extremely helpful, as it tends to be well formed in hemangiomas, whereas it is almost always absent in angiosarcoma (Fig. 10-54). It has to be underlined that the preservation of the pericytic reticulum is not to be regarded as an absolute rule because, very rarely, well-differentiated angiosarcoma may partly retain it. Importantly, mitotic activity cannot be used in the differential diagnosis (capillary lobular hemangiomas can exhibit amazingly high mitotic counts); however, the

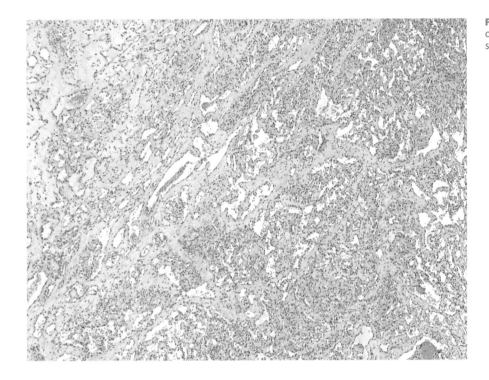

**Fig. 10-53.** Hemangioma. Benign hemangiomas often feature a lobular architecture that is never seen in angiosarcomas.

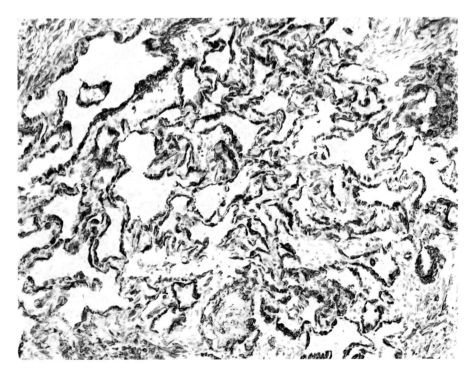

**Fig. 10-54.** Hemangioma. The presence of a well-formed smooth muscle actin-positive pericytic network is most often associated with a benign vascular neoplasm.

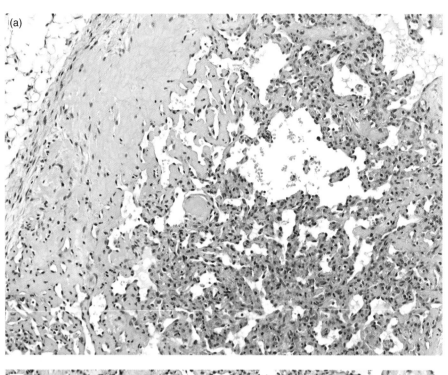

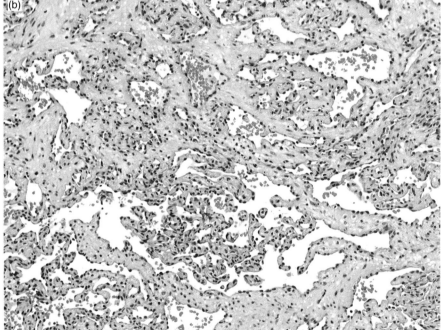

**Fig. 10-55.** Papillary endothelial hyperplasia. In this intravascular form, an exuberant benign papillary endothelial proliferation is seen (A). Note the absence of nuclear atypia and multilayering (B).

presence of atypical mitotic figures is most often associated with angiosarcoma. Another benign lesion that may superficially mimic well-differentiated angiosarcoma is represented by benign lymphangioendothelioma. In fact, as the lesion grows within deeper dermis, the vascular spaces tend to collapse and dissect the collagen in an angiosarcoma-like pattern. However, no monolayering is observed, and cytologic atypia is absent.

An entity that may often raise diagnostic confusion with angiosarcoma is represented by **papillary endothelial hyperplasia** (PEH), also known eponymically as Masson tumor.

Papillary endothelial hyperplasia is currently regarded as an exuberant reactive lesion associated with thrombosis. This may occur with a blood vessel (primary lesion), within a pre-existing benign vascular lesion (secondary), and in the context of organizing hematoma (extravascular). Primary PEH tends to occur most often in the hands and in the head and neck region. Microscopically, PEH is composed of pseudopapillary structures (Fig. 10-55A and B) that at late stage tend to form hyalinized cores lined by flattened endothelial cells (Fig. 10-56). The form of PEH most often suspected of malignancy is the extravascular. In fact, the pathologist can be misled by

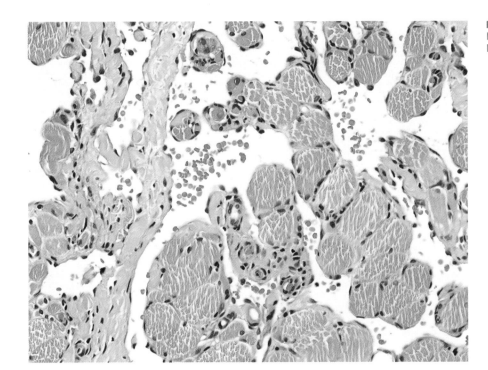

**Fig. 10-56.** Papillary endothelial hyperplasia. At late stage, pseudopapillae feature a hyalinized core lined by flattened endothelial cells.

both the large size and deep location, as well as by the occasional presence of nuclear hyperchromasia. The absence of endothelial multilayering, atypical mitotic figures, necrosis, and infiltration of surrounding soft tissue all represent key diagnostic features against a diagnosis of malignancy.

Secondary well-differentiated angiosarcoma of the breast needs to be differentiated from so-called **atypical vascular lesion** (AVL). Clinical presentation plays a major role in the differential diagnosis. Atypical vascular lesions appear as small papules organized as single lesions or in clusters and differ from angiosarcoma that most often appears as a violaceous plaque. Microscopically, nuclear atypia is at best mild and no atypical mitoses or multilayering is observed (Fig. 10-57A and B). Importantly, *MYC* amplification/overexpression is never observed. As both local recurrence and progression to angiosarcoma is possible, complete surgical removal of the lesion(s) is strongly advised.

When dealing with predominantly spindle cell angiosarcoma, the main differential diagnosis is with Kaposi sarcoma (KS). Four different clinical forms of KS are recognized:

1) **Classic endemic**, occurring in elderly men (>60 years), with a higher incidence in people of Mediterranean and Ashkenazi Jewish descent;

2) **Endemic African form**, occurring in children and having an aggressive clinical course, and in middle-aged adults of sub-Saharan Central African descent, with indolent clinical course;

3) **Iatrogenic**, recognized in patients receiving immunosuppressive treatments, including renal transplant recipients, and which can regress on discontinuation of treatment; and

4) **AIDS-related**, which is characterized by rapid evolution and mucosal and visceral involvement.

Kaposi sarcoma involves the skin, mucosal membranes, lymph nodes, and viscera (mainly the gastrointestinal tract and lungs), according to the clinical form. In the classic type, lesions are usually limited to the skin of distal extremities, while in the endemic African form the disease may be localized to the skin and have an indolent course or may involve lymph nodes in pediatric patients and be rapidly progressive. Iatrogenic forms are characterized by skin involvement and late visceral lesions, and in AIDS-related KS there is skin involvement of the head and neck area, the external genitals, and lower extremities, as well as of oral mucosa, gastrointestinal tract, lungs, and lymph nodes.

Cutaneous lesions of KS are usually multiple and present as slowly growing patches, plaques, or nodules of bluish to purple color ranging in size from a few millimeters to several centimeters; in mucosal or visceral involvement, lesions appear as hemorrhagic nodules. Microscopically, in early stages KS features dilated vascular spaces accompanied by a proliferation of spindle-shaped cells (Figs. 10-58A and 10-58B) infiltrating between collagen bundles, and by extravasated erythrocytes and a variable number of inflammatory cells, including lymphocytes and plasma cells (Fig. 10-59). In plaque and nodular stages there are cellular aggregates of spindle cells within the dermis, showing moderate atypia, frequent mitotic figures, and delimiting, slit-like spaces containing erythrocytes (Fig. 10-60). Immunohistochemically, KS expresses the endothelial markers CD34 and CD31, but only focally to FVIII-RA, as well as to the lymphatic marker D2-40. Nuclear positivity to HHV-8 is observed in virtually all cases. Immunohistochemistry plays an even greater role when dealing with the so-called lymphangioma-like variant of KS (Figs. 10-61 and 10-62) that closely mimics both benign lymphangioendothelioma and well-differentiated cutaneous angiosarcoma.

**587**

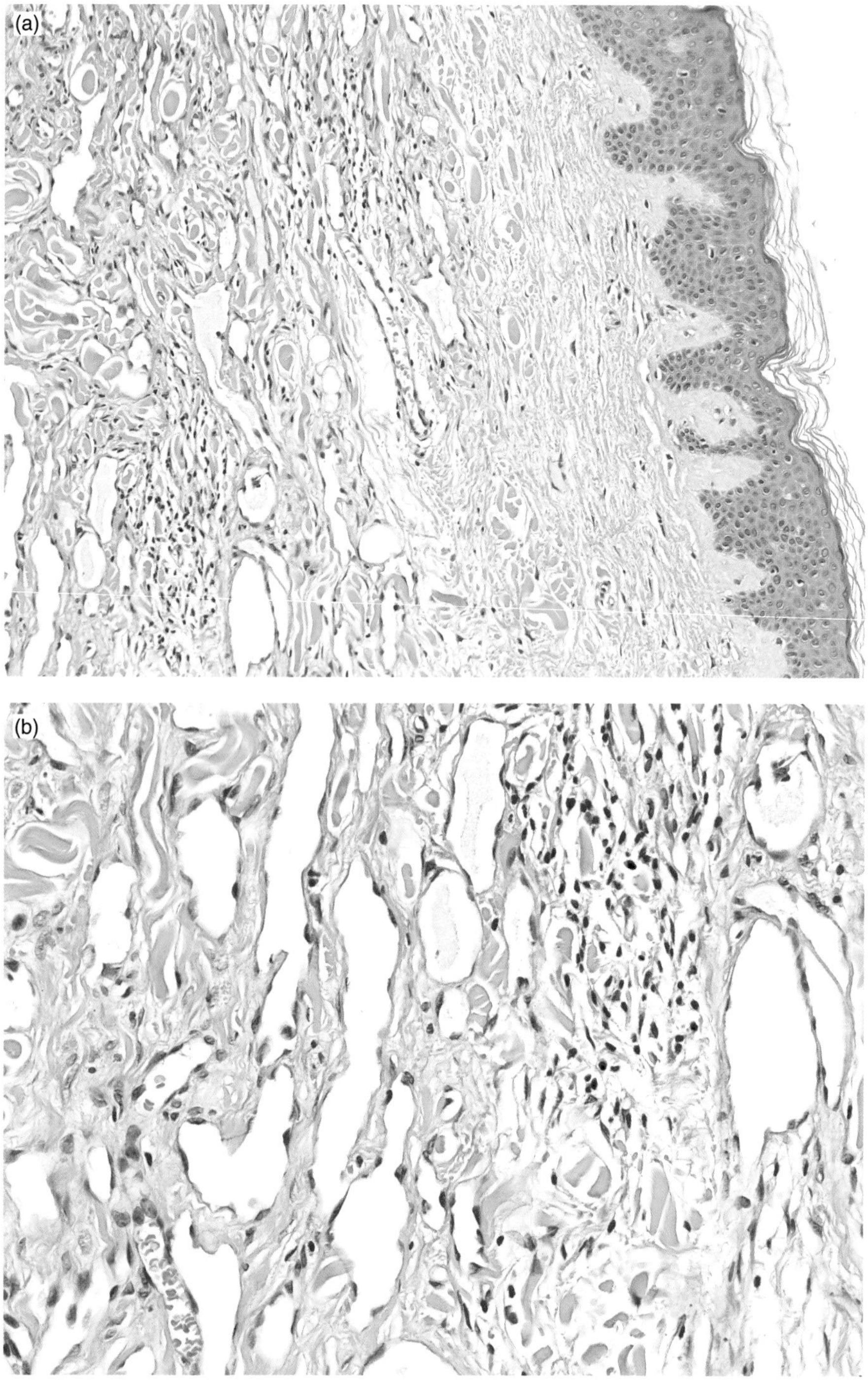

**Fig. 10-57.** Atypical vascular lesion. Superficial location (A) and absence of both severe atypia and multilayering (B) represents important diagnostic features.

As mentioned and discussed in more detail in Chapter 5, angiosarcomas may assume a predominantly epithelioid morphology to the extent that the differential diagnosis includes poorly differentiated carcinoma. Most epithelioid angiosarcomas actually arise in the deep soft tissue, whereas they are comparatively much rarer in the skin. Keeping in mind that both can be keratin positive and that prostatic adenocarcinoma expresses ERG, CD31 immunopositivity represents a very helpful diagnostic tool. Epithelioid sarcoma may also exhibit significant morphologic and immunophenotypic overlap with epithelioid angiosarcoma (both may express ERG, keratins, and CD34), but loss of nuclear expression of INI1 is not reported in epithelioid angiosarcoma.

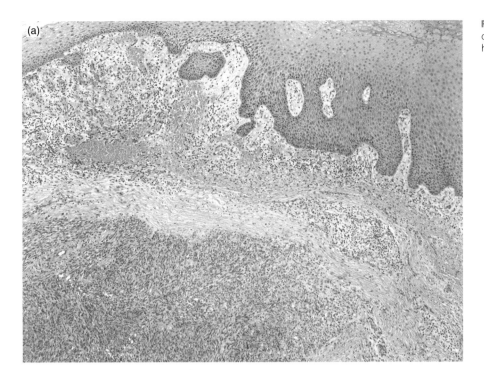

**Fig. 10-58A.** Kaposi sarcoma. A hypocellular dermal spindle cell proliferation merges into a hypercellular, ill-defined nodule.

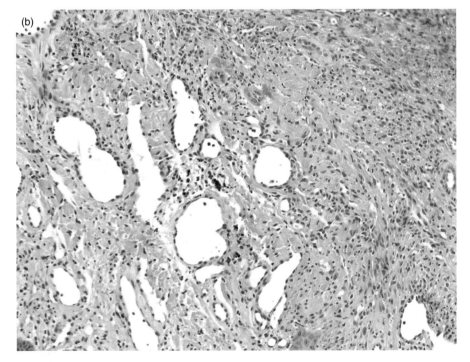

**Fig. 10-58B.** Kaposi sarcoma. Dilated lymphatic vessels are associated with a spindle cell proliferation organized in fascicles.

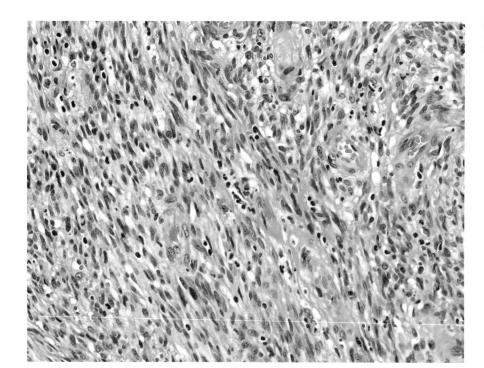

**Fig. 10-59.** Kaposi sarcoma. The spindle cell proliferation is often associated with an inflammatory component.

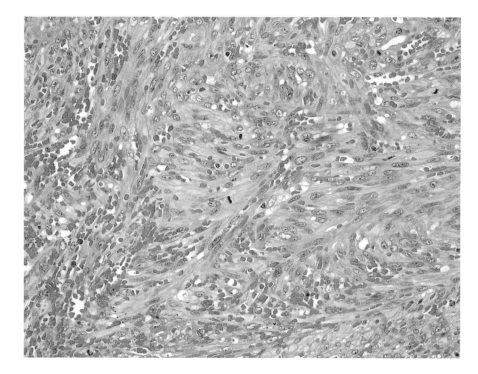

**Fig. 10-60.** Kaposi sarcoma. In the nodular stage, KS is very cellular and features the presence of easily detectable mitotic figures.

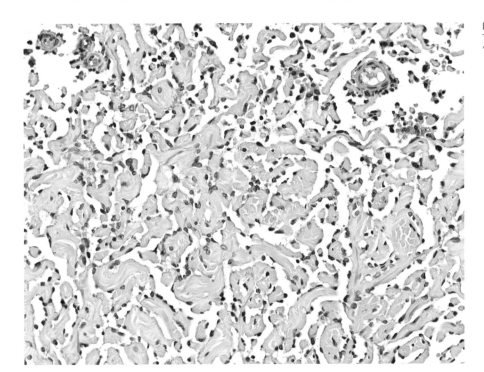

**Fig. 10-61.** Lymphangioma-like Kaposi sarcoma. This variant of KS is characterized by a distinctively "dissecting" pattern of growth.

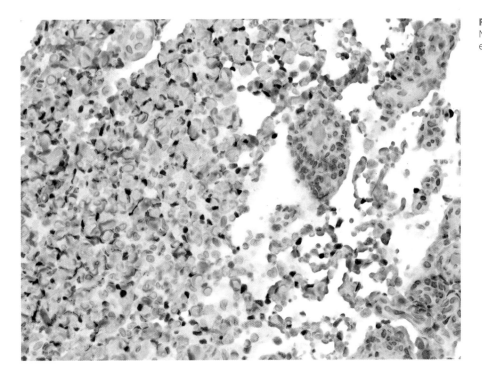

**Fig. 10-62.** Lymphangioma-like Kaposi sarcoma. Nuclear expression of HHV-8 represents an extremely useful diagnostic finding.

### Key Points in Angiosarcoma Diagnosis

- Heterogeneous clinical presentation
- Occurrence in the skin, breast parenchyma, deep soft tissue, and visceral sites
- Broad morphologic spectrum from vasoformative to solid spindle/epithelioid cell proliferation
- Main diagnostic features are nuclear atypia and multilayering
- Consistently positive for CD31 and ERG
- Extremely aggressive clinical behavior irrespective of histologic grade

# Chapter 10 Selected Key References

## Atypical Lipomatous Tumor/ Well-Differentiated Liposarcoma and Its Differential Diagnosis

- Adair FE, Pack GT, Farrior JH. Lipoma. *Am J Cancer.* 1932;**16**:1104–20.
- Argani P, Facchetti F, Inghirami G, Rosai J. Lymphocyte-rich well-differentiated liposarcoma: report of nine cases. *Am J Surg Pathol.* 1997;**21**:884–95.
- Azumi N, Curtis J, Kempson RL, Hendrickson MR. Atypical and malignant neoplasms showing lipomatous differentiation. A study of 111 cases. *Am J Surg Pathol.* 1987;**11**:161–83.
- Ballaux F, Debiec-Rychter M, De Wever I, Sciot R. Chondroid lipoma is characterized by t(11;16)(q13;p12–13). *Virchows Arch.* 2004;**444**:208–10.
- Binh MB, Sastre-Garau X, Guillou L, et al. MDM2 and CDK4 immunostainings are useful adjuncts in diagnosing well-differentiated and dedifferentiated liposarcoma subtypes: a comparative analysis of 559 soft tissue neoplasms with genetic data. *Am J Surg Pathol.* 2005;**29**:1340–7.
- Bonvalot S, Rivoire M, Castaing M, et al. Primary retroperitoneal sarcomas: a multivariate analysis of surgical factors associated with local control. *J Clin Oncol.* 2009;**27**:31–7.
- Cai YC, McMenamin ME, Rose G, et al. Primary liposarcoma of the orbit: a clinicopathologic study of seven cases. *Ann Diagn Pathol.* 2001;**5**:255–66.
- Chan JKC, Lee KC, Saw D. Extraskeletal chondroma with lipoblast-like cells. *Hum Pathol.* 1986;**17**:1285–7.
- Clay MR, Martinez AP, Weiss SW, et al. MDM2 and CDK4 immunohistochemistry: should it be used in problematic differentiated lipomatous tumors? a new perspective. *Am J Surg Pathol.* 2016;**40**:1647–52.
- Dei Tos AP, Doglioni C, Piccinin S, et al. Coordinated expression and amplification of the MDM2, CDK4 and HMGI-C genes in atypical lipomatous tumours. *J Pathol.* 2000;**190**:531–6.
- Enzi G, Busetto L, Ceschin E, et al. Multiple symmetric lipomatosis: clinical aspects and outcome in a long-term longitudinal study. *Int J Obes Relat Metab Disord.* 2002;**26**: 253–61.
- Enzi G, Digito M, Marin R, et al. Mediastino-abdominal lipomatosis: deep accumulation of fat mimicking a respiratory disease and ascites. Clinical aspects and metabolic studies in vitro. *Q J Med.* 1984;**53**:453–63.
- Enzi G, Inelmen EM, Baritussio A, et al. Multiple symmetric lipomatosis: a defect in adrenergic-stimulated lipolysis. *J Clin Invest.* 1977;**60**:1221–9.
- Enzinger FM, Winslow DJ. Liposarcoma. A study of 103 cases. *Virchows Arch Path Anat.* 1962;**335**: 367–88.
- Evans HL. Liposarcoma and atypical lipomatous tumors: a study of 66 cases followed for a minimum of 10 years. *Surg Pathol.* 1988;**1**:41–54.
- Evans HL, Soule EH, Winkelmann RK. Atypical lipoma, atypical intramuscular lipoma, and well differentiated retroperitoneal liposarcoma. A reappraisal of 30 cases formerly classified as well-differentiated liposarcoma. *Cancer.* 1979;**43**:574–84.
- Farshid G, Weiss SW. Massive localized lymphedema in the morbidly obese: a histologically distinct reactive lesion simulating liposarcoma. *Am J Surg Pathol.* 1998;**22**:1277–83.
- Fletcher CD, Martin-Bates E. Intramuscular and intermuscular lipoma: neglected diagnoses. *Histopathology.* 1988;**12**:275–87.
- Fukushima M, Schaefer IM, Fletcher CD. Myolipoma of soft tissue: clinicopathologic analysis of 34 cases. *Am J Surg Pathol.* 2017;**41**:153–60.
- Furlong MA, Fanburg-Smith JC, Childers EL. Lipoma of the oral and maxillofacial region: site and subclassification of 125 cases. *Oral Surg Oral Med Oral Pathol Oral Radiol Endod.* 2004;**98**:441–50.
- Furlong MA, Fanburg-Smith JC, Miettinen M. The morphologic spectrum of hibernoma: a clinicopathologic study of 170 cases. *Am J Surg Pathol.* 2001;**25**:809–14.
- Gaffney EF, Hargreaves HK, Semple E, et al. Hibernoma: distinctive light and electron microscopic features and relationship to brown adipose tissue. *Hum Pathol.* 1983;**14**:677–87.
- Gisselsson D, Domanski HA, Hoglund M, et al. Unique cytological features and chromosome aberrations in chondroid lipoma: a case report based on fine-needle aspiration cytology, histopathology, electron microscopy, chromosome banding, and molecular cytogenetics. *Am J Surg Pathol.* 1999;**23**:1300–4.
- Gronchi A, Lo Vullo S, Fiore M, et al. Aggressive surgical policies in a retrospectively reviewed single-institution case series of retroperitoneal soft tissue sarcomas. *J Clin Oncol.* 2009;**27**:24–30.
- Hahn HP, Fletcher CD. Primary mediastinal liposarcoma: clinicopathologic analysis of 24 cases. *Am J Surg Pathol.* 2007;**31**:1868–74.
- Hallel T, Lew S, Bansal M. Villous lipomatous proliferation of the synovial membrane (lipoma arborescens). *J Bone Joint Surg Am.* 1988;**70**(2):264–70.
- Hallin M, Schneider N, Thway K. Well-differentiated liposarcoma with hibernoma-like morphology. *Int J Surg Pathol.* 2016;**24**:620–2.
- Hostein I, Pelmus M, Aurias A, et al. Evaluation of MDM2 and CDK4 amplification by real-time PCR on paraffin wax-embedded material: a potential tool for the diagnosis of atypical lipomatous tumours/well-differentiated liposarcomas. *J Pathol.* 2004;**202**:95–102.
- Huang D, Sumegi J, Dal Cin P, et al. C11orf95-MKL2 is the resulting fusion oncogene of t(11;16)(q13;p13) in chondroid lipoma. *Genes Chromosomes Cancer.* 2010;**22**:810–18.
- Italiano A, Bianchini L, Keslair F, et al. HMGA2 is the partner of MDM2 in well-differentiated and dedifferentiated liposarcomas whereas CDK4 belongs to a distinct inconsistent amplicon. *Int J Cancer.* 2008;**122**(10):2233–41.
- Jing W, Lan T, Chen H, et al. Amplification of FRS2 in atypical lipomatous tumour/well-differentiated liposarcoma and dedifferentiated liposarcoma: a clinicopathological and genetic study of 146 cases. *Histopathology.* 2018 Jan 25. [Epub ahead of print]
- Jones EW, Marks R, Pongsehirun D. Naevus superficialis lipomatosus. A clinicopathological report of twenty cases. *Br J Dermatol.* 1975;**93**:121–33.
- Kindblom LG, Angervall L, Fassina AS. Atypical lipoma. *Acta Pathol Microbiol Scand.* 1982;**90**:27–36.
- Kindblom LG, Angervall L, Stener B, Wickbom I. Intermuscular and intramuscular lipomas and hibernomas. A clinical, roentgenologic, histologic, and prognostic study of 46 cases. *Cancer.* 1974;**33**: 754–62.
- Kindblom LG, Meis-Kindblom JM. Chondroid lipoma: an ultrastructural and immunohistochemical analysis with further observations regarding its differentiation. *Hum Pathol.* 1995;**26**:706–15.
- Kraus MD, Guillou L, Fletcher CDM. Well-differentiated inflammatory

liposarcoma: an uncommon and easily overlooked variant of a common sarcoma. *Am J Surg Pathol.* 1997;**21**: 518–27.

- Laurino L, Furlanetto A, Orvieto E, Dei Tos AP. Well-differentiated liposarcoma (atypical lipomatous tumors). *Semin Diagn Pathol.* 2001;**18**:258–62.

- Lucas DR, Nascimento AG, Sanjay BKS, Rock MG. Well differentiated liposarcoma. The Mayo Clinic experience with 58 cases. *Am J Clin Pathol.* 1994;**102**:677–83.

- Macarenco RS, Erickson-Johnson M, Wang X, et al. Retroperitoneal lipomatous tumors without cytologic atypia: are they lipomas? A clinicopathologic and molecular study of 19 cases. *Am J Surg Pathol.* 2009;**33**:1470–6.

- Mandahl N, Höglund M, Mertens F, et al. Cytogenetic aberrations in 188 benign and borderline adipose tissue tumors. *Genes Chromosomes Cancer.* 1994;**9**:207–15.

- Meis JM, Enzinger FM. Myolipoma of soft tissue. *Am J Surg Pathol.* 1991;**15**:121–5.

- Meis JM, Enzinger FM. Chondroid lipoma. A unique tumor simulating liposarcoma and myxoid chondrosarcoma. *Am J Surg Pathol.* 1993;**17**:1103–12.

- Michal M. Retroperitoneal myolipoma. A tumour mimicking retroperitoneal angiomyolipoma and liposarcoma with myosarcomatous differentiation. *Histopathology.* 1994;**25**:86–8.

- Montgomery E, Fisher C. Paratesticular liposarcoma: a clinicopathologic study. *Am J Surg Pathol.* 2003;**27**:40–7.

- Muraoka M, Oka T, Akamine S, et al. Endobronchial lipoma: review of 64 cases reported in Japan. *Chest.* 2003;**12**:293–26.

- Nascimento AF, McMenamin ME, Fletcher CD. Liposarcomas/atypical lipomatous tumors of the oral cavity: a clinicopathologic study of 23 cases. *Ann Diagn Pathol.* 2002;**6**:83–93.

- Nielsen GP, O'Connell JX, Dickersin GR, Rosenberg AE. Chondroid lipoma, a tumor of white fat cells. A brief report of two cases with ultrastructural analysis. *Am J Surg Pathol.* 1995;**19**:1272–6.

- Petit MR, Mols R, Schoenmakers EFPM, et al. LPP, the preferred fusion partner gene of HMGIC in lipomas, is a novel member of the LIM protein gene family. *Genomics.* 1996;**86**:118–29.

- Pilotti S, Della Torre G, Mezzelani A, et al. The expression of MDM2/CDK4 gene product in the differential diagnosis of

well differentiated liposarcoma and large deep-seated lipoma. *Br J Cancer.* 2000;**82**:1271–5.

- Rosai J, Akerman M, Dal Cin P, et al. Combined morphologic and karyotypic study of 59 atypical lipomatous tumours: evaluation of their relationship and differential diagnosis with other adipose tissue tumours. *Am J Surg Pathol.* 1996;**20**:1182–9.

- Rydholm A, Berg NO. Size, site and clinical incidence of lipoma. Factors in the differential diagnosis of lipoma and sarcoma. *Acta Orthop Scand.* 1983;**54**:929–34.

- Schoenmakers EFPM, Wanchura S, Mols R, et al. Recurrent rearrangements in the high mobility group protein gene, HMGI-C, in benign mesenchymal tumours. *Nature Genet.* 1995;**10**:436–44.

- Sciot R, Akerman M, Dal Cin P, et al. Cytogenetic analysis of subcutaneous angiolipoma: further evidence supporting its difference from ordinary pure lipomas: a report of the CHAMP Study Group. *Am J Surg Pathol.* 1997;**21**:441–4.

- Shimada S, Ishizawa T, Ishizawa K, et al. The value of MDM2 and CDK4 amplification levels using real-time polymerase chain reaction for the differential diagnosis of liposarcomas and their histologic mimickers. *Hum Pathol.* 2006;**37**:1123–9.

- Shon W, Ida CM, Boland-Froemming JM, Rose PS, Folpe A. Cutaneous angiosarcoma arising in massive localized lymphedema of the morbidly obese: a report of five cases and review of the literature. *J Cutan Pathol.* 2011;**38**:560–4.

- Sirvent N, Coindre JM, Maire G, et al. Detection of MDM2-CDK4 amplification by fluorescence in situ hybridization in 200 paraffin-embedded tumor samples: utility in diagnosing adipocytic lesions and comparison with immunohistochemistry and real-time PCR. *Am J Surg Pathol.* 2007;**31**:1476–89.

- Stoll G, Alembik Y, Truttmann M. Multiple familial lipomatosis with polyneuropathy, an inherited autosomal condition. *Ann Genet.* 1996;**39**:193–7.

- Stout AP. Liposarcoma: the malignant tumour of lipoblasts. *Ann Surg.* 1944;**119**:86–107.

- Weaver J, Downs-Kelly E, Goldblum JR, et al. Fluorescence in situ hybridization for MDM2 gene amplification as a diagnostic tool in lipomatous neoplasms. *Mod Pathol.* 2008;**21**:943–9.

- Willen H, Akerman M, Dal Cin P, et al. Comparison of chromosomal patterns with clinical features in 165 lipomas: a

report of the CHAMP study group. *Cancer Genet Cytogenet.* 1998;**102**:46–9.

## Retiform Hemangioendothelioma and Its Differential Diagnosis

- Calonje E, Fletcher CD, Wilson-Jones E, Rosai J. Retiform hemangioendothelioma. A distinctive form of low grade angiosarcoma delineated in a series of 15 cases. *Am J Surg Pathol.* 1994;**18**: 115–25.

- Dabska M. Malignant endovascular papillary angioendothelioma of the skin in childhood. Clinicopathologic study of 6 cases. *Cancer.* 1969;**24**:503–10.

- Duke D, Dvorak A, Harris TJ, Cohen LM. Multiple retiform hemangioendotheliomas. A low-grade angiosarcoma. *Am J Dermatopathol.* 1996;**18**:606–10.

- El Darouti M, Marzouk SA, Sobhi RM, Bassiouni DA. Retiform hemangioendothelioma. *Int J Dermatol.* 2000;**39**:365–8.

- Fanburg-Smith JC, Michal M, Partanen TA, Alitalo K, Miettinen M. Papillary intralymphatic angioendothelioma (PILA): a report of twelve cases of a distinctive vascular tumor with phenotypic features of lymphatic vessels. *Am J Surg Pathol.* 1999;**23**:1004–10.

- Fukunaga M, Endo Y, Masui F, et al. Retiform haemangioendothelioma. *Virchows Arch.* 1996;**428**:301–4.

- Guillou L, Calonje E, Speight P, Rosai J, Fletcher CD. Hobnail hemangioma: a pseudomalignant vascular lesion with a reappraisal of targetoid hemosiderotic hemangioma. *Am J Surg Pathol.* 1999;**23**:97–105.

- Leduc C, Jenkins SM, Sukov WR, Rustin JG, Maleszewski JJ. Cardiac angiosarcoma: histopathologic, immunohistochemical, and cytogenetic analysis of 10 cases. *Hum Pathol.* 2017;**60**:199–207.

- Mentzel T, Partanen TA, Kutzner H. Hobnail hemangioma ("targetoid hemosiderotic hemangioma"): clinicopathologic and immunohistochemical analysis of 62 cases. *J Cutan Pathol.* 1999;**26**:279–86.

- Nayler SJ, Rubin BP, Calonje E, Chan JK, Fletcher CD. Composite hemangioendothelioma: a complex, low-grade vascular lesion mimicking angiosarcoma. *Am J Surg Pathol.* 2000;**24**:352–61.

- Perry KD, Al-Lbraheemi A, Rubin BP, et al. Composite hemangioendothelioma with neuroendocrine marker expression:

an aggressive variant. *Mod Pathol.* 2017;**30**:1589–1602.

- Santa Cruz DJ, Aronberg J. Targetoid hemosiderotic hemangioma. *J Am Acad Dermatol.* 1988;**19**:550–8.
- Sanz-Trelles A, Rodrigo-Fernandez I, Ayala-Carbonero A, Contreras-Rubio F. Retiform hemangioendothelioma. A new case in a child with diffuse endovascular papillary endothelial proliferation. *J Cutan Pathol.* 1997;**24**:440–4.
- Schommer M, Herbst RA, Brodersen JP, et al. Retiform hemangioendothelioma: another tumor associated with human herpesvirus type 8? *J Am Acad Dermatol.* 2000;**42**:290–2.
- Tan D, Kraybill W, Cheney RT, Khoury T. Retiform hemangioendothelioma: a case report and review of the literature. *J Cutan Pathol.* 2005;**32**:634–7.

# Angiosarcoma

- Billings SD, McKenney JK, Folpe AL, Hardacre MC, Weiss SW. Cutaneous angiosarcoma following breast-conserving surgery and radiation: an analysis of 27 cases. *Am J Surg Pathol.* 2004;**28**:781–8.
- Brenn T, Fletcher CD. Radiation-associated cutaneous atypical vascular lesions and angiosarcoma: clinicopathologic analysis of 42 cases. *Am J Surg Pathol.* 2005;**29**:983–96.
- Cossu S, Satta R, Cottoni F, Massarelli G. Lymphangioma-like variant of Kaposi's sarcoma: clinicopathologic study of seven cases with review of the literature. *Am J Dermatopathol.* 1997;**19**:16–22.
- Deyrup AT, McKenney JK, Tighiouart M, Folpe AL, Weiss SW. Sporadic cutaneous angiosarcomas: a proposal for risk stratification based on 69 cases. *Am J Surg Pathol.* 2008;**32**:72–7.
- Duprez R, Lacoste V, Brière J, et al. Evidence for a multiclonal origin of multicentric advanced lesions of Kaposi sarcoma. *J Natl Cancer Inst.* 2007;**99**:1086–94.
- Fletcher CD. Vascular tumors: an update with emphasis on the diagnosis of angiosarcoma and borderline vascular neoplasms. *Monogr Pathol.* 1996;**38**:181–206.
- Fletcher CD, Beham A, Bekir S, Clarke AM, Marley NJ. Epithelioid angiosarcoma of deep soft tissue: a distinctive tumor readily mistaken for an epithelial neoplasm. *Am J Surg Pathol.* 1991;**15**:915–24.
- Gange RW, Jones EW. Lymphangioma-like Kaposi's sarcoma. A report of three cases. *Br J Dermatol.* 1979;**100**:327–34.
- Guillou L, Fletcher CD. Benign lymphangioendothelioma (acquired progressive lymphangioma): a lesion not to be confused with well-differentiated angiosarcoma and patch stage Kaposi's sarcoma: clinicopathologic analysis of a series. *Am J Surg Pathol.* 2000;**24**:1047–57.
- Hiatt KM, Nelson AM, Lichy JH, Fanburg-Smith JC. Classic Kaposi sarcoma in the United States over the last two decades: a clinicopathologic and molecular study of 438 non-HIV-related Kaposi sarcoma patients with comparison to HIV-related Kaposi sarcoma. *Mod Pathol.* 2008;**21**:572–82.
- Kuo T, Sayers CP, Rosai J. Masson's "vegetant intravascular hemangioendothelioma:" a lesion often mistaken for angiosarcoma: study of seventeen cases located in the skin and soft tissues. *Cancer.* 1976;**38**:1227–36.
- McKay KM, Doyle LA, Lazar AJ, Hornick JL. Expression of ERG, an Ets family transcription factor, distinguishes cutaneous angiosarcoma from histological mimics. *Histopathology.* 2012;**61**:989–91.
- Meis-Kindblom JM, Kindblom LG. Angiosarcoma of soft tissue: a study of 80 cases. *Am J Surg Pathol.* 1998;**22**:683–97.
- Mentzel T, Schildhaus HU, Palmedo G, Büttner R, Kutzner H. Postradiation cutaneous angiosarcoma after treatment of breast carcinoma is characterized by MYC amplification in contrast to atypical vascular lesions after radiotherapy and control cases: clinicopathological, immunohistochemical and molecular analysis of 66 cases. *Mod Pathol.* 2012;**25**:75–85.
- Miettinen M, Lehto VP, Virtanen I. Postmastectomy angiosarcoma (Stewart-Treves syndrome). Light-microscopic, immunohistological, and ultrastructural characteristics of two cases. *Am J Surg Pathol.* 1983;**7**:329–39.
- Nascimento AF, Raut CP, Fletcher CD. Primary angiosarcoma of the breast: clinicopathologic analysis of 49 cases, suggesting that grade is not prognostic. *Am J Surg Pathol.* 2008;**32**:1896–904.
- Neuhauser TS, Derringer GA, Thompson LD, et al. Splenic angiosarcoma: a clinicopathologic and immunophenotypic study of 28 cases. *Mod Pathol.* 2000;**13**:978–87.
- Patton KT, Deyrup AT, Weiss SW. Atypical vascular lesions after surgery and radiation of the breast: a clinicopathologic study of 32 cases analyzing histologic heterogeneity and association with angiosarcoma. *Am J Surg Pathol.* 2008;**32**:943–50.
- Penel N, Bui BN, Bay JO, et al. Phase II trial of weekly paclitaxel for unresectable angiosarcoma: the ANGIOTAX Study. *J Clin Oncol.* 2008;**26**:5269–74.
- Ramirez JA, Laskin WB, Guitart J. Lymphangioma-like Kaposi sarcoma. *J Cutan Pathol.* 2005;**32**:286–92.
- Ray-Coquard IL, Domont J, Tresch-Bruneel E, et al. Paclitaxel given once per week with or without bevacizumab in patients with advanced angiosarcoma: a randomized phase II trial. *J Clin Oncol.* 2015;**33**:2797–802.
- Robin YM, Guillou L, Michels JJ, Coindre JM. Human herpesvirus 8 immunostaining: a sensitive and specific method for diagnosing Kaposi sarcoma in paraffin-embedded sections. *Am J Clin Pathol.* 2004;**121**:330–4.
- Rosai J, Sumner HW, Kostianovsky M, Perez-Mesa C. Angiosarcoma of the skin. A clinicopathological and fine structural study. *Hum Pathol.* 1976;**7**:83–109.
- Russell Jones R, Orchard G, Zelger B, Wilson Jones E. Immunostaining for CD31 and CD34 in Kaposi sarcoma. *J Clin Pathol.* 1995;**48**:1011–16.
- Schneider JW, Dittmer DP. Diagnosis and treatment of Kaposi sarcoma. *Am J Clin Dermatol.* 2017;**18**:529–39.
- Suchak R, Thway K, Zelger B, Fisher C, Calonje E. Primary cutaneous epithelioid angiosarcoma: a clinicopathologic study of 13 cases of a rare neoplasm occurring outside the setting of conventional angiosarcomas and with predilection for the limbs. *Am J Surg Pathol.* 2011;**35**:60–9.
- Wynn GR, Bentley PG, Liebmann R, Fletcher CD. Mammary parenchymal angiosarcoma after breast-conserving treatment for invasive high-grade ductal carcinoma. *Breast J.* 2004;**10**:558–9.

# Index

Locators in **bold** refer to tables; those in *italic* to figures